Second Edition

Goldberg's Genetic and Metabolic Eye Disease

Edited by
William Andrew Renie, M.D.
Wyman Park Health System
and Johns Hopkins University
School of Medicine
Baltimore, Maryland

Foreword by
Morton F. Goldberg, M.D.
Professor and Head,
Department of Ophthalmology,
Illinois Eye and Ear Infirmary,
Lions of Illinois
Eye Research Institute,
University of Illinois
College of Medicine,
Chicago, Illinois

Little, Brown and Company
Boston / Toronto

Contents

Foreword

A decade has elapsed since the appearance of the first edition of *Genetic and Metabolic Eye Disease*. At the time of its publication, it was apparent, as we stated in the Preface to that edition, "that sufficiently new information [had] accrued in the field of ophthalmic genetics to justify dissemination of the factual material and interpretive analyses that constitute[d] this book." The past ten years have seen an exponential outpouring of innovative research and clinical discoveries, making mandatory the compilation of a new edition.

Much of the exciting new work relates to the technology of recombinant DNA. The use of gene probes promises enhanced understanding, and eventually prevention or therapy, for many disabling diseases, including retinitis pigmentosa, retinoblastoma, choroideremia, gyrate atrophy, and others. Development of new biochemical assays proceeds uninterruptedly. These advances make ophthalmic genetics one of the most exciting fields in modern medicine.

The current edition is the combined work of gifted investigators, dedicated clinicians, and a perceptive, enlightened editor. Readers will appreciate their efforts, and affected families will be grateful for their continued commitment.

Morton F. Goldberg

Preface

The changes in genetics that have taken place in the last few years have been so explosive as to make a second edition of this book mandatory for ophthalmologists interested in genetic eye disease. The development of recombinant DNA has opened up a whole new field in molecular biology. Therefore a whole chapter in the new edition is devoted to DNA technologies. Furthermore, some of the old chapters, such as those on biochemical techniques and cytogenetics, now draw substantially on the new DNA methodology for their continued vitality.

This new edition retains the outstanding features of the clinical information found in the old edition; there has been new and additional information included—for example, there are new descriptions of techniques in the treatment of craniosynostoses and ectopia lentis.

It must be noted, sadly, that two contributing authors—Samuel Pruzansky and Charles D. Phelps—died while this edition was being prepared. Marilyn T. Miller, who coauthored Chapter 9 with Dr. Pruzansky, and Robert B. Nixon, who coauthored Chapter 11 with Dr. Phelps, completed the revision and updating of the material in their chapters.

Throughout the second edition we have tried to present a vision of the future—a future that will be heavily shaped by the emerging recombinant DNA technology. This future includes more sophisticated and frequent detection of prenatal disease and carrier status. Ultimately it is hoped that these techniques will eventually lead to gene therapy and treatment of existing genetic diseases.

W. A. R.

Contributing Authors

Gustavo Aguirre, V.M.D.
Associate Professor of Clinical Studies, School of Veterinary Medicine, The University of Pennsylvania; Associate Professor of Ophthalmology, The University of Pennsylvania School of Medicine, Philadelphia
Chapter 6

David J. Apple, M.D.
Professor of Ophthalmology and Pathology, University of Utah School of Medicine; Professor of Ophthalmology and Pathology, University of Utah Medical Center, Salt Lake City
Chapter 8

Michelle Ann Bené Bain, M.D.
Clinical Assistant Professor of Dermatology, University of Illinois at Chicago College of Medicine, Chicago
Chapter 19

John C. Carey, M.D.
Assistant Professor of Pediatrics, University of Utah School of Medicine; Assistant Professor of Pediatrics, University of Utah Medical Center, Salt Lake City
Chapter 8

Edward Cotlier, M.D.
Professor of Ophthalmology, and Director, Genetic Section, Cornell University Medical College, New York
Chapter 20

Eugene R. Folk, M.D.
Professor, University of Illinois at Chicago School of Medicine; Co-Director, Pediatric Ophthalmology, Eye and Ear Infirmary, Chicago
Chapter 10

Brenda L. Gallie, M.D.
Associate Professor of Ophthalmology, University of Toronto Faculty of Medicine; Active Staff, Department of Ophthalmology, The Hospital for Sick Children, Toronto
Chapter 16

Ira Garoon, M.D.
Attending Surgeon, Department of Ophthalmology, Michael Reese Hospital, Chicago
Chapter 15

Stephen C. Gieser, M.D.
Fellow in Ophthalmic Pathology, Department of Ophthalmology, University of Utah School of Medicine, Salt Lake City; James Scholar Program for Independent Study, University of Illinois at Chicago School of Medicine, Chicago
Chapter 8

Joel S. Glaser, M.D.
Professor of Ophthalmology and Neurological Surgery, University of Miami School of Medicine; Bascom Palmer Eye Institute, Miami
Chapter 18

Mark Haskins, V.M.D., Ph.D.
Associate Professor of Pathobiology and Clinical Studies, The University of Pennsylvania School of Veterinary Medicine, Philadelphia
Chapter 6

William H. Havener, M.D.
Professor and Chairman, Department of Ophthalmology, Ohio State University College of Medicine; Chairman, Department of Ophthalmology, The Ohio State University Hospitals, Columbus
Chapter 7

P. C. Huang, Ph.D.
Professor of Biochemistry, The Johns Hopkins University, Baltimore
Chapter 2

Suber S. Huang, M.D.
Intern, Department of Medicine, Bronx Municipal Hospital Center, Albert Einstein College of Medicine, Bronx, New York
Chapter 2

Peter Jezyk, V.M.D., Ph.D.
Associate Professor of Clinical Studies, The University of Pennsylvania School of Veterinary Medicine, Philadelphia
Chapter 6

Joel A. Kaplan, M.D.
Assistant Professor of Ophthalmology, The University of Illinois–Abraham Lincoln School of Medicine; Director, Ocular Disease Center, Resurrection Hospital, Chicago
Chapter 15

Kenneth R. Kenyon, M.D.
Associate Professor of Ophthalmology, Harvard Medical School; Associate Chief of Ophthalmology and Director, Cornea Service, Massachusetts Eye and Ear Infirmary; Senior Scientist, Eye Research Institute of Retina Foundation, Boston
Chapter 5

Jay H. Krachmer, M.D.
Professor of Ophthalmology, University of Iowa College of Medicine; Professor, University of Iowa Hospitals, Iowa City
Chapter 12

Frank P. La Franco, M.D.
Assistant Professor of Ophthalmology, Northwestern University Medical School, Chicago; Chief, Division of Ophthalmology, Evanston Hospital, Evanston, Illinois
Chapter 19

Jacques Libert, M.D.
Assistant, Université Libre de Bruxelles; Chef de Clinique Adjoint, Service d'Ophtalmologie, Hôpital Universitaire Saint-Pierre, Brussels, Belgium
Chapter 5

Irene H. Maumenee, M.D.
Associate Professor of Ophthalmology, The Johns Hopkins University School of Medicine, Baltimore
Chapter 14

Saul Merin, M.D.
Professor of Ophthalmology, Hebrew University; Head, Unit of Ophthalmology, Hadassa Mt. Scopus Hospital, Jerusalem
Chapter 13

Marilyn Baird Mets, M.D.
Assistant Professor, Department of Ophthalmology and Pediatrics, The University of Chicago-Pritzker School of Medicine; Director, Pediatric Ophthalmology, University of Chicago Hospitals, Chicago
Chapter 3

Corey A. Miller, M.D.
Clinical Assistant Professor, University of Utah School of Medicine; Attending Physician, Department of Surgery, Latter-Day Saints Hospital, Salt Lake City
Chapter 12

Marilyn T. Miller, M.D.
Associate Professor, University of Illinois at Chicago School of Medicine; Director, Pediatric Ophthalmology Service, Eye and Ear Infirmary, Chicago
Chapters 9 and 10

Maria Musarella, M.D.
Staff, Ophthalmology, and Research Associate, Department of Ophthalmology, The Hospital for Sick Children, Toronto
Chapter 16

Leonard B. Nelson, M.D.
Associate Professor of Ophthalmology and Pediatrics, Jefferson Medical College of Thomas Jefferson University, Philadelphia
Chapter 14

Robert B. Nixon, M.D.
Fellow, Pediatric Ophthalmology, Indiana University School of Medicine, Indianapolis
Chapter 11

Kenneth G. Noble, M.D.
Clinical Associate Professor, Department of Ophthalmology, New York University Medical Center; Assistant Attending Physician, University Hospital, New York
Chapter 17

Charles D. Phelps, M.D.†
Former Professor and Head, Department of Ophthalmology, University of Iowa College of Medicine; Professor, Department of Ophthalmology, University of Iowa Hospitals and Clinics, Iowa City
Chapter 11

Samuel Pruzansky, D.D.S.†
Former Director, Center for Craniofacial Anomalies, The Abraham Lincoln School of Medicine, University of Illinois College of Medicine; Professor of Orthodontics, University of Illinois, Chicago
Chapter 9

William Andrew Renie, M.D.
Wyman Park Health System and Johns Hopkins University School of Medicine, Baltimore
Chapter 1

George H. Sack, Jr., M.D.
Associate Professor of Medicine, Pediatrics, and Biological Chemistry, The Johns Hopkins University School of Medicine; Physician, Department of Medical Genetics, The Johns Hopkins Hospital, Baltimore
Chapter 4

Lawrence Stramm, Ph.D.
Research Assistant Professor of Ophthalmology, The University of Pennsylvania School of Medicine, Philadelphia
Chapter 6

Sophie Marie Worobec-Victor, M.D.
Assistant Professor of Dermatology, University of Illinois at Chicago School of Medicine; Chief, Dermatology Section, Department of Medicine, West Side Veterans Administrations Hospital; Attending Physician, University of Illinois Hospital, Chicago
Chapter 19

†Deceased

I

Methods of Study in Genetic Eye Disease

1

Fundamentals of Genetics

William Andrew Renie

HISTORY

Concepts of clinical genetics have been with humanity since the Chaldeans 6,000 years ago [87]. Among the first observations that the ancients made regarding genetics were those that dealt with agriculture and the breeding of domestic animals. Human genetics was practiced by the Greeks; they engaged in infanticide by leaving deformed infants out in the countryside to die from exposure [77]. The Talmud of Jewish society recognized the sex-linked nature of hemophilia by permitting circumcision to be omitted in newborn boys who had had two preceding brothers who had bled to death from the procedure [88].

The scientific era of the 1700s stressed the importance of making observations in various fields of study. Maupertius in 1752 was the first to record the transmission of a human genetic trait, polydactyly, in four generations of the Rube family [31]. At the same time, Dalton made observations regarding the transmission of color blindness [16].

At this time the fields of probability and statistics were not well developed. Two mathematical geniuses, Francis Galton and his successor Karl Pearson, laid the foundations in these two fields that made it possible to analyze the different outcomes of matings. Their techniques and methods are still used to analyze genetic data and also have broad applications in many diverse fields ouside genetics [87].

The father of modern-day genetics is usually recognized to be Gregor Mendel. Until his time, because of the complex nature of the interaction between genetic traits and the environment, it was believed that the components from two parents "mixed" or "blended" in their offspring and that the offspring therefore passed on traits that were different from those received from their parents [88]. Mendel's great contribution came from observations on breeding of peas and the inference that genetic traits were determined by factors from both parents that were preserved (i.e., they did not mix) and passed on (without blending) from generation to generation. Mendel realized that these traits were passed on by a statistical process—one that eventually was shown to be describable by the statistical methods developed by Galton and Pearson [87].

Shortly after Mendel's work was rediscovered in 1900, after having lain dormant for 35 years, W. Johannsen in 1911 proposed calling Mendel's nonmixing traits *genes* and introduced the idea of differentiating between an individual's genotype or genetic makeup and his or her phenotype or external appearance [88].

The father of modern day biochemical genetics is A. E. Garrod, who presented his work—the first description of an inborn error of metabolism, alkaptonuria—in 1902. He even guessed correctly that this disease was a mendelian recessive trait, and he speculated that it might some day be shown to be secondary to a missing enzyme. He also clearly delineated the potentially adverse effects of consanguinity on the expression of recessive traits [30].

By the early 1900s genes were known to be unmixable entities that were passed from generation to generation by a statistical process of independent segregation. These concepts can be demonstrated by observing the transmission of physical

3

traits from generation to generation, as Mendel had done. However, the physical and chemical structural basis of the gene was totally unknown. This century has seen the elucidation of the physical and chemical structure of the gene.

By the late 1800s cytologists had made extensive and detailed observations regarding the process of cell division. They observed that during cell division the nucleus was always divided and that the chromosomes were divided and segregated without mixing in a manner similar to that proposed for genes. In 1903 Sutton and Boveri proposed that chromosomes were the physical structures on which genes were localized. This has subsequently been confirmed by myriad other observations and experiments. [87].

Many genetic diseases have been shown to be associated with demonstrable chromosomal aberrations. In 1956 it was firmly established that humans have 46 chromosomes [89], and in 1959 Lejeune and colleagues demonstrated that Down's syndrome is the result of chromosome 21 trisomy [51]. Many other diseases (Patau's syndrome [66], Edwards' syndrome [22], some forms of aniridia [37], and some retinoblastomas [97]) have been shown to be associated with chromosomal abnormalities.

In 1944 Avery, MacCleod, and McCarty demonstrated that DNA, not protein, was the hereditary material [2]. Watson and Crick proposed their famous double-helix model of DNA (Fig. 1-1), which explained both DNA's ability to direct protein synthesis and its ability to self-replicate, in 1953 [95, 96]. In 1961 Nirenberg broke the genetic code and was able to show that each triplet consisting of three DNA bases codes for a specific amino acid in a protein (Table 1-1) [59]. In the 1970s Nathans and Smith discovered restriction enzyme DNA endonucleases that allow pieces of DNA to be removed from one cell (e.g., a human cell) and inserted into another cell (e.g., a bacterium) to make so-called recombinant DNA [83].

These restriction enzyme endonucleases and recombinant DNA hold great potential for the future. They have already been used to harness bacteria to make commercial human insulin [29] and to map genes [81]. Recombinant DNA techniques (see Chap. 4) have also been used in the prenatal diagnosis of sickle cell anemia and thalassemia [7]. With the recent insertion of rat growth hormone genes into mouse embryos, which subsequently developed into supermice [64], this technology brings us one step closer to the goal

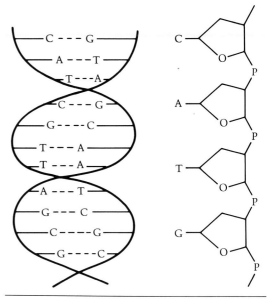

Fig. 1-1. *Model of DNA. The double helix consists of two strands of DNA hydrogen-bonded to each other. Each purine (adenine [A] or guanine [G]) or pyrimidine (thymidine [T] or cytosine [C]) on a DNA strand hydrogen-bonds to its complementary pyrimidine or purine on the other strand (C with G and A with T). On the right is shown the backbone of a DNA strand, composed of alternating sugar and phosphate moieties. Each sugar has a base bound to it that points toward the inner part of the helix.*

of replacing missing or defective DNA in persons with genetic diseases.

GENE STRUCTURE

Genes are chemically represented by DNA (deoxyribonucleic acid) physically located on chromosomes. It has been amply demonstrated that DNA directs the synthesis of proteins through the intermediary of RNA (ribonucleic acid) [94].

DNA and RNA are chemically similar in that both are made up of a base, a pentose sugar (deoxyribose in DNA and ribose in RNA), and phosphoric acid. The bases are either purines (adenine or guanine) or pyrimidines (cytosine or thymine in DNA, cytosine or uracil in RNA) [94].

The pentose sugar has both a base and phosphoric acid bound to it. The phosphoric acid binds to the pentose sugar of the next nucleoside in the chain. Therefore the primary or covalently bound structure or chain of DNA or RNA consists of

Table 1-1. *The Genetic Code*

Amino acid	DNA triplet		Amino acid	DNA triplet
Alanine	CGA		Serine	AGA
	CGG			AGG
	CGT			AGT
	CGC			AGC
Arginine	TCT			TCA
	TCC			TCG
	GCA		Threonine	TGA
	GCG			TGG
	GCT			TGT
	GCC			TGC
Asparagine	TTA		Tryptophan	ACC
	TTG		Tyrosine	ATA
Aspartic acid	CTA			ATG
	CTG		Valine	CAA
Chain end	ATT			CAG
	ATC			CAT
	ACT			CAC
Cysteine	ACA			
	ACG			
Glutamic acid	CTT			
	CTC			
Glutamine	CTT			
	GTC			
Glycine	CCA			
	CCG			
	CCT			
	CCC			
Histidine	GTA			
	GTG			
Isoleucine	TAA			
	TAG			
	TAT			
Leucine	AAT			
	AAC			
	GAA			
	GAG			
	GAT			
	GAC			
Lysine	TTT			
	TTC			
Methionine	TAC			
Phenylalanine	AAA			
	AAG			
Proline	GGA			
	GGG			
	GGT			
	GGC			

A = adenine; G = gaunine; T = thymine; C = cytosine.

alternating phosphoric acid and ribose sugar moieties [94].

Since each ribose sugar has a base attached to it, the result is a structure with a linear sequence of bases. Each purine and pyrimidine then binds by hydrogen bonding to a purine or pyrimidine from another chain (adenine with thymine and cytosine with guanine) to form a double helix. This forms the structure of DNA that was first elucidated by Watson and Crick (Fig. 1-1) [94].

While any sequence of bases along a single strand of DNA is possible, it must be accompanied by a complementary sequence of bases along the other strand of DNA. For example, if on one strand the base sequence is CGA, then the complementary sequence must be GCT. This arrangement can give rise to many different possible sequences. Since there are four possible bases at any given site, there can be 4^n possible DNAs in a piece of DNA consisting of n bases [94].

The arrangement of the DNA on the chromosomes is not entirely clear. It is clear that the DNA must be extensively folded since the DNA on a chromosome may have a molecular weight of 2×10^6. The DNA is believed to be continuous, with no non-DNA components interspersed between DNA. The DNA in the smallest chromosome, if stretched out, would have a total length of about 1 cm. Chromosomes are about 1 to 10 μm long, usually 1 to 2 μm, and therefore it is clear the DNA must be coiled or folded. The DNA is known to be closely associated with histones (very basic proteins), nonhistone proteins, and small amounts of RNA. Obviously each chromosome contains thousands of genes [24].

Chromosomes can be stained with various dyes. The staining material is called chromatin, and chromosomes have been found to have two regions based on their staining properties. Areas of a chromosome that stain well are said to be made up of heterochromatin; those that stain poorly are called euchromatin [24].

The DNA in a chromosome may be either repetitive (5–15%) or nonrepetitive. The repetitive DNA stains as heterochromatin and the nonrepetitive sequences as euchromatin [24].

DNA not only directs the synthesis of protein, but it also self-replicates. This self-replication takes place by a separation of the two strands of a DNA helix and synthesis of a complementary new strand onto each single strand. Replication occurs simultaneously at several points along the DNA. Complete replication of the DNA takes place well before the chromosomes actually physically divide [94].

Protein synthesis is directed by DNA through the synthesis of RNA. RNA differs from DNA in several respects. Instead of thymine, RNA has a base called uracil. RNA is single stranded instead of double stranded. RNA contains the pentose sugar ribose, and DNA has the pentose sugar deoxyribose. There are different types of RNA—messenger RNA (mRNA), ribosomal RNA, and transfer RNA; they all have molecular weights that are much less than that of DNA [94].

For protein synthesis to occur, DNA, as in replication, must first unravel to form single-stranded DNA in the region of the gene being transcribed. The transcription begins on an area of the DNA known as a promoter or initiator region [94].

The DNA is used to make a complementary strand of mRNA. This process is called transcription. Surprisingly, the whole sequence of DNA may be transcribed, but not every part of the DNA eventually is translated into amino acids in a protein [14]. Apparently there is post-transcriptional processing of the messenger RNA that excises the segments of RNA that are not to be translated. The terms *exon* and *intron* have been coined to designate translated DNA and untranslated DNA, respectively [14, 17].

The mRNA then tranverses the nuclear membrane and goes to the cytoplasm where it attaches to structures called ribosomes. Ribosomes consist of proteins and ribosomal RNA. On the ribosomes, mRNA is "read," and a specific amino acid is brought onto the ribosome by a transfer RNA. The specific amino acid is then linked to the growing polypeptide chain by formation of a peptide bond. The whole process is called translation [94].

The code of the DNA has been established (Table 1-1). An amino acid is coded for by a triplet of DNA bases called a codon. Since there are four DNA bases, there are 4^3 or 64 different possible codons. Because there are only 20 amino acids, there is some degree of redudancy in the code. Furthermore, three different sequences, ATT, ATC, and ACT code for no amino acid [59]. That is, they are protein synthesis terminators [59].

Changes in the sequence of DNA are called mutations and can be caused by many different mechanisms. These mutations may be of different types and have many diverse effects, as will be discussed later.

Genes are either structural genes (which code for structural proteins such as enzymes, hormones, or hemoglobins) or control genes, which either accelerate or decelerate translational processes of other structural genes (turn a gene on or off).

CHROMOSOMES

Chromosomes are the structural components on which the genes or DNA are located. Besides DNA, proteins such as histones and protamines help to make up the chromosome [24]. Human chromosomes are not visible or stainable unless one is observing dividing cells at metaphase. Since only a few tissues have a high percentage of cells that are dividing, chromosome or karyotype analysis has been relatively difficult.

Chromosomes are intimately involved in the two different types of cell division that take place in humans—mitosis and meiosis (Figs. 1-2 and 1-3). Normally a cell is said to be in the diploid state, which means that each cell has two homologous copies of each chromosome. In humans, there are 23 pairs of chromosomes. Each pair is homologous; that is, each member of the pair contains the same gene loci although the actual genes may be different on each chromosome. The two genes at the same site on the paired chromosomes are said to be alleles [86]. For example, chromosome 11 contains the gene locus for the

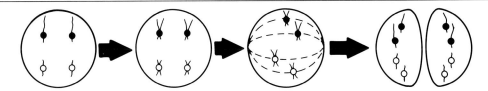

Fig. 1-2. *Mitosis, cell division in which the mother cell divides into two daughter cells, each of which has a diploid number of chromosomes. In this diagram, two homologous pairs of chromosomes are shown. The nucleus and many of the intermediate steps have been eliminated.*

β chain of hemoglobin, although one member of the pair may contain the gene for hemoglobin A and the other chromosome may carry the gene for hemoglobin S.

Mitosis is a cell division that takes place in somatic cells (Fig. 1-2). During mitosis each chromosome duplicates, and then duplicates are pulled to opposite ends of the cell. The cell then divides into two daughter cells, each of which has the full complement of genetic material, that is, each daughter cell has 23 pairs of chromosomes [86].

Meiosis is a much more complicated form of

Fig. 1-3. *Meiosis, cell division in which the mother cell divides into four daughter cells, each of which has a haploid number of chromosomes. This process results in the formation of gametes. In this diagram two homologous pairs of chromosomes are shown. The nucleus and many of the intermediate steps have been eliminated.*

cell division that takes place in the formation of gametes (Fig. 1-3). It results in four daughter cells, each of which has only one-half the full complement, or a haploid complement, of genetic material. Thus a sperm or oocyte formed from meiosis has only 23 chromosomes or only one member of each pair of chromosomes [86].

In meiosis the chromosomes thicken, and highly precise pairing of homologous chromosomes takes place. The chromosomes duplicate, and each arm of a chromosome is then called a chromatid (the arms of a chromosome are joined at the centromere). The pair of chromosomes thus consists of four chromatids or a tetrad consisting of homologous chromosomes held together by chiasmata or bridges. It is in these chiasmata between non-sister chromatids that exchange of homologous chromosomal material or crossing over may take place. Crossing over allows the constant reshuffling of genes since there are thousands of genes on each chromosome [86].

In the next stage of meiosis, the two members (each of which is in duplicate form) of a pair of chromosomes are pulled to opposite ends of the cell, which then divides. This results in two cells,

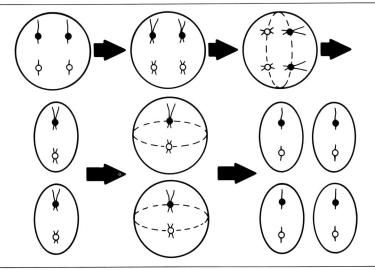

each with 23 duplicate chromosomes. These duplicates are then divided into two cells. The final result is four cells, each of which has the genetic material of 23 chromosomes, not 23 pairs of chromosomes. These cells go on to become the gametes of the organism—either spermatozoa or oocytes. The diploid state or 23 pairs of chromosomes is restored during fertilization when the two gametes come together or fuse to form a zygote, which develops into a new organism [86].

The study of chromosomes by cytologic techniques requires that cells be undergoing mitosis at the time they are fixed or else they will not have chromatin sufficiently condensed to be visible. It is very difficult to take a sample of tissue and find an adequate number of cells in metaphase to allow one to do a karyotypic analysis.

However, several technical advances now allow for routine karyotypic analysis. First, cell culture techniques have developed to the point of allowing for routine culture of dividing cells such as leukocytes, fibroblasts, or bone marrow cells [65]. Second, colchicine has been found to arrest the cells in metaphase, when all the chromosomes are visible, by interfering with spindle contraction [28]. Third, brief exposure of cells to hypotonic saline causes them to swell slightly and makes the chromosomes less clumped and more easily separable on viewing [40, 41]. Finally, phytohemagglutinin is a mitogen for lymphocytes and greatly increases the number of lymphocytes going into mitosis [60].

All of these techniques made it easy to harvest cells showing all of their chromosomes in a nonoverlapping display. However, these techniques only allowed the chromosomes seen to be classified into seven autosomal groups and the sex chromosomes on the basis of their relative length and centromere position (the centromere is the place where the two chromosome arms are joined; it is metacentric if located near the middle and acrocentric if located near the end of the chromosome). These techniques did not allow for individual identification of chromosomes or help elucidate their internal morphology.

Subsequently, various high-resolution banding or staining techniques have been developed to help identify the individual chromosomes and to delineate better their gross morphology (see Chaps. 3 and 8). If quinacrine hydrochloride is introduced early in the cell cycle, when the cell goes into metaphase the quinacrine hydrochloride will appear as fluorescent bands transverse to the long axis of the chromosome [13]. The chromosomes

may also be gently denatured with heat or chemical agents and then stained with Giemsa stain. This will produce the same banding pattern, which is unique and constant to any one chromosome (Fig. 1-4) [67].

Each band is thought to contain at least 1,000 kilobases (kb) of DNA so that several genes may be contained in each band. The bands are thought to be areas rich in AT or CG pairs, depending on whether the particular banding technique stains these regions positively or negatively [63]. A chromosome position is designated by the chromosomal number, by p for the short arm and q for the long arm relative to the centromere, and by the band position. For example, a deletion on band 14 of chromosome 13q has been associated with retinoblastoma [97]. Aniridia, in association with Wilms' tumor, genitourinary anomalies, and mental retardation, has been associated with a chromosome 11p, band 13 deletion [37]. Undoubtedly, more examples will be described in the coming years.

This high-resolution banding, when combined with data from other techniques, is being used to construct a map of the human genome (see Chap. 3). Clearly, pedigree analysis can be used to map

Fig. 1-4. *Normal karyotype. The chromosomes have been stained during metaphase using a Giemsa stain, which results in high-resolution banding. Photographs of the chromosomes have been cut out and rearranged in numerical order. (Courtesy of K. Au. Published in J. H. Priest [Ed.],* Medical Cytogenetics and Cell Culture *[2nd ed.], Philadelphia: Lea & Febiger, 1977.)*

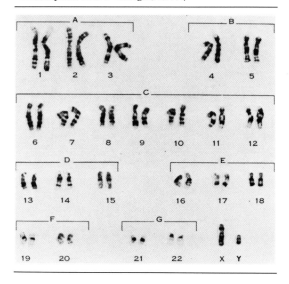

genes to the X chromosome. Linkage analysis can help map genes to specific chromosomes if they are linked to genes with known positions on a chromosome [21, 69]. Linkage analysis was used to assign the Coppock cataract to chromsome 1. Renwick and Lawler found a strong linkage of the cataract to the Duffy blood group locus [69], which has been shown to be on chromosome 1 by linkage to a cytogenetic marker [21]. Deletion mapping has also been used to assign genes to chromosomes [97]. Somatic cell hybridization is a very powerful technique of assigning specific genes to specific chromosomal regions. It involves hybridizing a human cell that has a detectable trait necessary for growth with a mouse cell that does not have the trait. As the cells grow and divide, eventually the human chromosomes will be lost—but they are lost randomly and not all at once. Since cells will grow only if they have the trait in question, one can make a direct correlation between the presence of a specific chromosome and the

ability of the cell to grow, thereby assigning the trait to a specific chromosome [74, 84].

Recombinant DNA is being used to map the relative positions of genes located closely together on a chromosome [80]. A summary and current record of the human genome is kept up-to-date by McKusick [55].

In various genetic disorders there are gross changes in chromosome numbers. Addition of a whole set or one of a pair of chromosomes (to make three or more of a given chromosome) is called *polyploidy*. For example, Down's syndrome is an example of trisomy 21 (Fig. 1-5). Loss of one member of a pair of chromosomes is called *aneuploidy* and is actually more common. Loss of parts of chromosomes (deletions) and exchange of chromosomal material between chromosomes (translocations) can also be detected much more easily now with the development of high-resolution chromosome banding.

It is useful here to recall the terms and draw the distinction between genotype and phenotype. *Genotype* refers to the genes that an individual has for certain traits, whether or not they are actually expressed. The gene sites are called loci, and each member of the pair of genes at a given locus is called an allele. These alleles are often represented by *A* for the dominant allele and *a* for the recessive allele. An individual who has the same two alleles for a trait, such as *AA* or *aa*, is

Fig. 1-5. *Karyotype of a patient with Down's syndrome. This high-resolution banding has been accomplished by staining the chromosomes with a Giemsa stain during metaphase. Notice the chromosome 21 trisomy characteristic of this syndrome. (Courtesy of K. Au. Published in J. H. Priest [Ed.],* Medical Cytogenetics and Cell Culture *[2nd ed.], Philadelphia: Lea & Febiger, 1977.)*

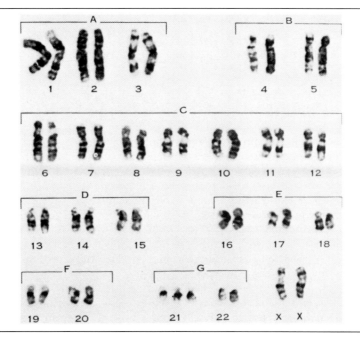

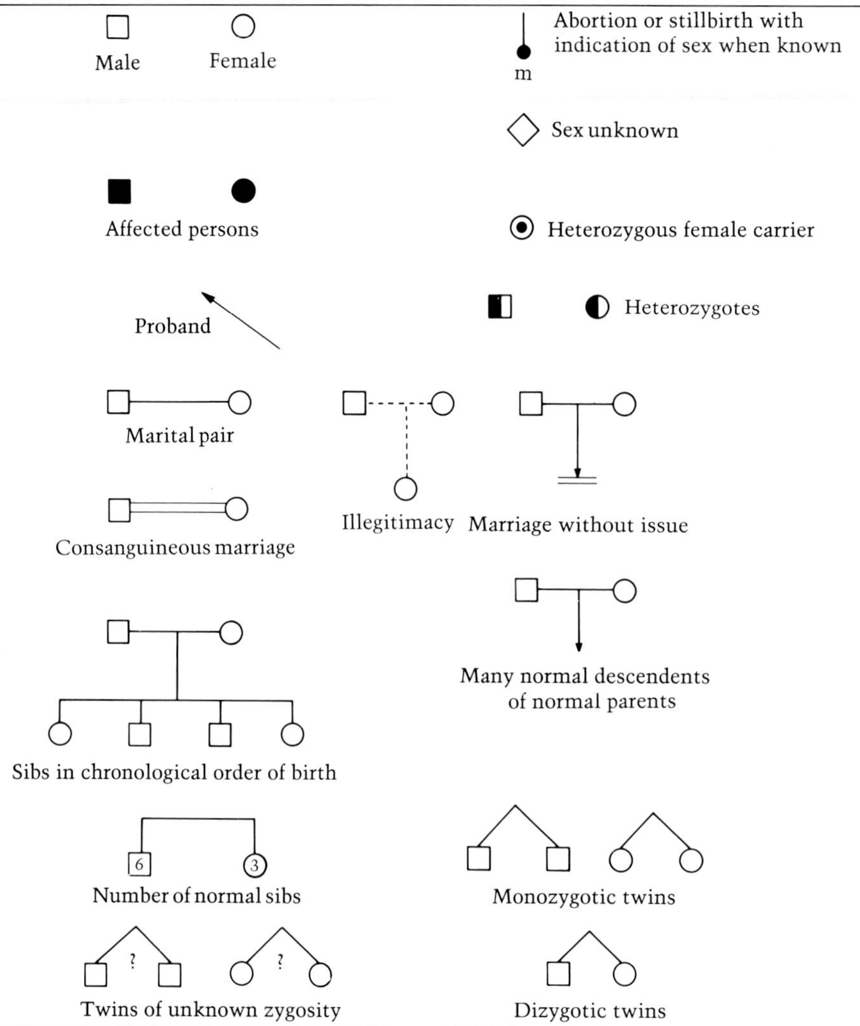

Fig. 1-6. *Symbols frequently used in constructing pedigrees. (Courtesy M. H. Abbott.)*

called a homozygote for that allele. The phenotype is the clinically or laboratory observable expression of the genotype. It may directly correlate with the genotype; however, often the phenotype is the result of an interaction between the genotype and either the internal or the external environment. It is often possible to make inferences by looking at phenotypes of individuals or of pedigrees. This has been the major way of inferring genotypes in the past. Now with recombinant DNA methods, it is possible to use probes to examine the alleles and hence the genotypes directly [88].

The terms *hereditary, familial,* and *congenital* are not synonymous. *Hereditary* refers to a trait that is determined by the presence or absence of

specific genes for that trait. The trait may or may not be expressed, depending on whether it is dominant or recessive and depending on modifying effects of the environment [77].

A condition is *familial* if it occurs in families or family members. Familial occurrence may be secondary to genetic or hereditary factors. However, other causes, such as infectious diseases or toxins, which are environmental and not genetic, may produce the clustering of traits in families [77].

Congenital conditions are those present at birth. While many congenital conditions are genetic, many birth defects can occur from teratogens in utero that are clearly environmental and not ge-

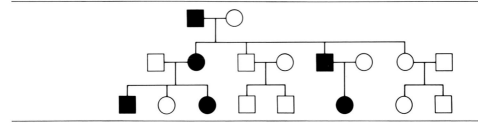

Fig. 1-7. *Pedigree of an autosomal dominant trait. Notice that transmission of the trait is vertical, both sexes are affected, and the trait is passed from either sex to both sexes.*

netic. Finally, not all genetic diseases are congenital; for example, Huntington's chorea may not be clinically expressed until the fourth decade of life [77].

Genetic diseases cannot be adequately studied by an examination of individuals. Family histories and family examinations must be done to delineate adequately a genetic disease. To examine a genetic disease, one must take a history from and examine the first patient, called the proband. This person's disease is the index case. One then takes a history from and, if possible, examines other members of the family. One can then construct a pedigree, which is a symbolic or schematic representation of a family history such that it may be seen at a glance [42]. Pedigree symbols and sample pedigrees are shown in Fig. 1-6.

One should inquire as to whether there is any consanguineous marriage in the family, as this increases the possibility of an autosomal recessive disease being present. Determining the ethnic background of the family may be important since some diseases are more common in certain ethnic groups. For example, Gaucher's disease is more frequent in Jewish families, as is Tay-Sachs disease. One should inquire as to whether any relatives have or have had a genetic condition or any diseases considered to be rare. One should also determine if anyone else in the proband's family is known to have or have had the trait or disease in question or any of its features [42].

AUTOSOMAL DOMINANT TRAITS

Simple mendelian traits are said to be inherited either as X-linked traits, autosomal dominant traits, or autosomal recessive traits. Autosomal dominant traits are those in which the definable abnormality is present in the heterozygote. In classical mendelian thinking, this implies that homozygotes and heterozygotes are identical in appearance. Clearly this is not always the case. For example, sickle cell trait can be detected by Sickledex testing, but clinically it is not nearly as severe as the homozygous sickle cell disease or state [42, 77, 88].

A trait can be said to be autosomal dominant if it satisfies certain criteria on analysis of a pedigree [42, 77, 88]:

1. The trait must appear in every generation; that is, there is vertical transmission.
2. The trait must be expressed in some way in the heterozygote.
3. The affected person transmits the trait to the offspring on the average of 50 percent of the time. This is because, for a relatively rare dominant trait like Marfan's syndrome or some forms of retinoblastoma, most matings will be of the *Aa* × *aa* type. Clearly, a homozygous patient (*AA*) would have virtually a 100 percent chance of passing the trait to each of his or her children.
4. Unaffected persons do not transmit the trait to their children.
5. Affected children have affected parents except in isolated cases caused by mutations.
6. Usually there is equal sex incidence of affected persons.
7. The trait is transmitted to either sex from either sex.

A representative autosomal dominant pedigree is shown in Fig. 1-7.

Autosomal dominant traits usually involve structural proteins (e.g., Marfan's syndrome or neurofibromatosis), while autosomal recessive traits usually involve enzyme deficiencies. Autosomal dominant traits are often of late onset, as in Huntington's chorea. Other properties or concepts that relate to autosomal dominant conditions include penetrance, expressivity, pleiotropy, and anticipation [42, 77, 88].

Penetrance and expressivity are considered only

when the clinician has to rely on external phenotype to make a diagnosis, that is, when biochemical testing cannot be used to determine the presence or absence of a trait. Penetrance is an all-or-none concept. It refers to the ability to detect a gene in a person who is known by pedigree analysis to have a genotype containing the gene. If a gene is penetrant and therefore is dectectable clinically, it may have gradings of severity of manifestations. This is known as variability of expression or degree of expressivity. For example, bilateral retinoblastoma and multiple retinoblastomas are dominantly inherited, whereas single unilateral cases are thought to be somatic mutations. However, offspring of affected individuals with a dominant gene have retinoblastomas in only 45 percent instead of the expected 50 percent of cases. Clearly, in some individuals, the gene is nonpenetrant. In some of these "nonpenetrant" cases, scleral depression and indirect ophthalmoscopy will reveal involuted retinoblastomas, which clearly indicate the presence of the gene with a low degree of expressivity [48]. Another example of expressivity is found in the manifestation of cataracts in myotonic dystrophy. The cataracts may develop, even in the same family, any time from the second to the seventh decade of life [42].

Pleiotropy refers to multiple, apparently unrelated, clinical expressions or manifestations of a single gene. It does not refer to secondary changes, such as thrombosis seen in sickle cell disease. For example, in Marfan's syndrome, there may be involvement of the skeletal system (pectus excavatum or carinatum, arachnodactyly, dolichostenomelia, kyphoscoliosis), cardiovascular system (mitral valve prolapse, aortic root dilatation), and ocular system (ectopia lentis, myopia); there may also be spontaneous pneumothorax, poor muscular development, and an increased incidence of hernias. While these manifestations are found in different organs, they are all primary manifestations of a single gene. These pleiotropic expressions of a single gene comprise a syndrome—in this example, Marfan's syndrome [42, 77, 88].

Because of the presence of vertical transmission in autosomal dominant traits, the concept of anticipation developed. *Anticipation* refers to an apparent earlier onset of a genetic condition in successive generations. It is an artifact of ascertainment since, once a condition is known to be present in a family, family members are more aware of its possible presence in succeeding generations and it is often diagnosed earlier as a result [42, 77, 88].

Not every affected person has an affected parent. In every autosomal dominant disease, a certain proportion of cases represent a new mutation. The estimated gene mutation frequency is 1×10^{-5} per gene per offspring. Therefore, the presence of a new mutation is about 1 in 100,000 births [92].

The percentage of cases of dominant disorders that represent new mutations is inversely proportional to the effect of the disease on the ability of the affected individual to reproduce. For example, new mutations account for 80 percent of cases of tuberous sclerosis, 40 percent of cases of neurofibromatosis, 30 percent of cases of Marfan's syndrome, and 25 percent of cases of myotonic dystrophy [42].

New mutations appear in germ cells of fathers of a relatively advanced age. The age of an unaffected father of a child with Marfan's syndrome is on the average 37 years; the mean age of fathers as a whole and fathers affected with Marfan's syndrome who have Marfan offspring is 30 years [42].

However, before one concludes that an individual case represents a new mutation, one must exclude the presence of low expressivity or extramarital paternity (at least 5% of children randomly sampled) [42].

AUTOSOMAL RECESSIVE TRAITS

Autosomal recessive genetic conditions are those that are fully clinically expressed only when two alleles for the trait are present. A representative autosomal recessive pedigree is shown in Fig. 1-8.

The criteria for an autosomal recessive trait are as follows [42, 77, 88]:

1. The trait does not cause clinical disease in the heterozygote.
2. Individuals with both genes (homozygotes) express the disorder.
3. The trait appears only in siblings, not in parents, offspring, or other relatives (a horizontal distribution of cases in a pedigree).
4. Parents of affected patients may be related (this is increasingly likely the rarer the defect).
5. There is equal sex incidence among affected persons.
6. One-fourth of siblings of the proband are affected on the average. This may be difficult to prove because of small family size in the United States today. For example, in 40 percent of cases

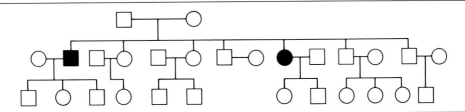

Fig. 1-8. *Pedigree of an autosomal recessive trait. Notice that the trait appears horizontally in the pedigree, it does not appear in successive generations, and either sex is affected.*

of retinitis pigmentosa there is no other family history of the disease.

Autosomal recessive conditions are almost always penetrant. They usually have an early onset in life—usually being diagnosed during childhood and often lethal at an early age. Within a given family, they are often uniformly expressed, although expressivity may vary between different families [42, 77, 88].

Unlike autosomal dominant traits, autosomal recessive traits often represent defects in specific enzymes. If the enzyme is known, often the heterozygote will have 50 percent of the normal level of enzyme; however, because of the functioning of normal regulatory mechanisms, this is usually enough to prevent clinical consequences. However, the drop in enzyme levels to near 0 percent in the homozygous state does have adverse clinical effects [42, 77, 88].

Since homozygotes usually have reduced biologic fitness, most of the deleterious genes reside in the heterozygotes. This can be easily demonstrated with the Hardy-Weinberg equilibrium law. If p = the frequency of the normal gene and q = the frequency of the mutant gene, then q^2 = the frequency of affected autosomal recessive individuals. In metachromatic leukodystrophy, for example, the frequency of affected persons is 1 in 40,000, so $q^2 = (\frac{1}{4}) \times 10^{-4}$ or $q = \frac{1}{200}$. Therefore, $p = 1 - (\frac{1}{200}) = \frac{199}{200}$, and the number of heterozygotes is $2pq = 2(\frac{199}{200})(\frac{1}{200}) = \frac{1}{100}$ or 400 times more than the number of homozygotes [42, 77].

However, because the homozygote often has a reduced fitness, these autosomal recessive genes have, over a long period of time, been reduced to a relatively low frequency. Occasionally, the heterozygote may have a selective advantage over the normal homozygote and this may keep the gene at a relatively high frequency (e.g., in sickle cell

disease, those with sickle cell trait have a resistance to malaria that people with normal β hemoglobin chains do not have [42, 77, 88]).

Consanguineous marriage may also play a role in modifying the clinical presence of a genetic trait. While consanguineous marriage does not increase the frequency of a gene, it does increase the chances of homozygotes being produced. In the United States, there is a relatively low frequency or level of consanguineous marriage (incest must be considered a form of consanguineous sexual relations), so this is often a factor only in the rarer of the autosomal recessive diseases. However, one should always keep the possibility in mind in analyzing patients with autosomal recessive diseases [42, 77, 88].

Since most of the abnormal genes are in carriers, the matings of interest are usually of the form $Aa \times AA$ or $Aa \times Aa$. In the first case 50 percent of the offspring will be carriers and 50 percent will not be. There will be no affected offspring. In the second mating, 25 percent of the offspring will be normal, 50 percent will be carriers, and 25 percent will be affected. An affected individual can be involved in the following matings: $aa \times AA$, $aa \times Aa$, or $aa \times aa$. In the first case, all the offspring will be carriers. In the second mating, 50 percent of the offspring will be carriers, and 50 percent will be affected. This may superficially mimic autosomal dominant inheritance, but matings in subsequent generations will reveal the true character of the trait. In the third case, all the offspring will be affected [42, 77, 88].

Since most of the genes are located in the heterozygote and since most matings that produce children with clinical disease are of the form $Aa \times Aa$, much effort and interest has gone into identifying the carrier state. Often this can be detected biochemically. For example, one can detect decreased levels of ornithine ketoacid transferase in fibroblasts cultured from skin in carriers of hyperornithinemia gyrate atrophy of the choroid and retina [49], decreased levels of enzymes in the serum of carriers of Tay-Sachs [61], abnor-

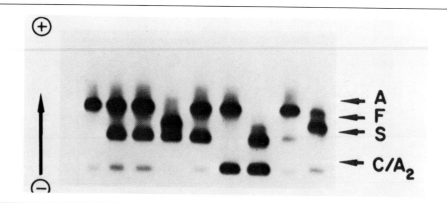

Fig. 1-9. *Hemoglobin electrophoresis demonstrating different gene products (hemoglobins). Shown from left to right are hemoglobins AA, AS, S-HPFH (hereditary persistence of fetal hemoglobin), AS, AC, SC, A-Lepore, and AC in newborn. (From T. H. J. Huisman,* The Hemoglobinopathies. *New York: Marcel Dekker, 1977, by courtesy of Marcel Dekker, Inc.)*

mal proteins in carriers of galactokinase deficiency [53], and hemoglobin S (Fig. 1-9) in sickle cell trait [73]. While great strides are being made in our scientific ability to detect carriers, there remains great ethical consternation as to how best use this information [70].

Finally, a slightly different type of recessive disorder should be mentioned here. It occurs when, at each homologous locus, there is a mutant or abnormal gene, but they are not identical. This is seen when, for example, an individual has hemoglobin SC disease [10]. In this case one gene codes for hemoglobin S and the other for hemoglobin C. The Hurler-Scheie syndrome is thought to result from the presence of an abnormal gene for Hurler's syndrome at one gene locus and an abnormal gene for Scheie's syndrome at the homologous locus [54]. Such recessives are called genetic compounds.

X-LINKED TRAITS

X-linked traits are those in which the trait is located on the X chromosome. Since men have only one X chromosome, if they have a gene for a trait, they will express it. Since they do not pass on the X chromosome to their sons, they will not pass the trait on to their sons (although a son could receive the trait from his mother) [42, 77, 88].

Since women have two X chromosomes, they may or may not clinically express the trait in the heterozygous state. If the trait is usually expressed in the heterozygous state, it is said to be an X-linked dominant. Examples are vitamin D–resistant rickets [11] and pseudohypoparathyroidism [55]. If the trait is not expressed in the heterozygous state, it is said to be an X-linked recessive trait. Examples include red-green color blindness [55], choroidermia [35, 79], and ocular albinism [44, 93]. A representative X-linked pedigree is shown in Fig. 1-10.

The criteria for an X-linked recessive trait are as follows [42, 77, 88]:

1. The carrier female ordinarily does not manifest clinical disease.
2. The trait is much more common in males.
3. The trait is passed from males through all the daughters (obligate carriers) and to one-half of those daughters' sons.
4. The trait never is transmitted from an affected father to his children of either sex.
5. The affected males in a family are either brothers or related to one another through carrier females, for example, maternal uncles (oblique pedigree).
6. Unaffected males transmit the trait to no one.

As one can easily infer, the great majority of individuals affected with an X-linked recessive trait are males, since these genes are relatively rare and therefore most of the women are heterozygotes.

The criteria for an X-linked dominant condition are as follows [42, 77, 88]:

1. The trait is always expressed in a heterozygous individual.

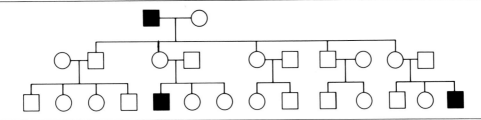

Fig. 1-10. *Pedigree of an X-linked trait. Notice that only males are affected, and there is no male-to-male transmission of the trait.*

2. Heterozygous females transmit the trait to both sexes with equal frequency.
3. Affected males transmit the trait to all their daughters but none of their sons.
4. There are about twice as many affected women as men (because women have two-thirds of all X chromosomes).

X-linked traits in general are less severe than autosomal recessive ones but more severe than autosomal dominant traits. In general women with X-linked conditions with manifestations (even as heterozygotes) are more mildly affected than men. In fact, there are some X-linked traits that are so severe in men that they are never able to reproduce. Examples include Duchenne's muscular dystrophy [55] and incontinentia pigmenti, a disease in which all affected males die in utero and there are normal girls, normal boys, and affected girls, in the ratio 1 : 1 : 1 [12].

These concepts of X-linked inheritance must be further modified by the phenomenon of lyonization, a process whereby one of the two X chromosomes in each somatic cell of a woman is normally randomly inactivated [52]. A heterozygote woman for an X-linked trait may have a disproportionately high percentage of cells in which the normal X chromosome is inactivated. As a consequence, she may have mild manifestations of the trait [52]. An example of this is the mottled mosaic fundus seen in women heterozygous for X-linked ocular albinism [44, 93] or choroideremia [35, 79]. Another example is the lenticular opacities seen in women heterozygous for Lowe's syndrome [20].

There are other explanations for the clinical expression of an X-linked recessive trait in a woman besides lyonization. If the woman's father was affected and her mother was a carrier, the woman could be homozygous for the trait in question. Similarly, a woman could receive one gene for the trait from either a carrier mother or an affected father and a new mutant gene from the other parent. If the woman had Turner's syndrome or some form of monosomy X (either complete or partial—with deletion of that part of the X chromosome carrying the trait in question), she would appear clinically to be affected. Finally, an autosomal genocopy (a copy of the gene located on an autosome) could be present, which would produce a clinically affected woman [62].

While consanguineous marriage is not a factor in influencing X-linked disease, new mutations are. As in autosomal dominant diseases, the proportion of cases resulting from new mutations is inversely proportional to the biologic fitness of the affected individual [42, 77, 88].

SPORADIC CASES

Sporadic cases are isolated cases of a disease. Such cases add no new information regarding the genetic nature of a disease. In fact, as in the case of congenital cataracts secondary to intrauterine infection, they may be the result of environmental influences, not genetic factors. An isolated case may be secondary to a new dominant mutation, a rare autosomal recessive, or an X-linked disease carried by the mother. It may be a phenocopy, that is, an environmentally induced replica of a genetic disease (e.g., methemoglobinemia may be inherited or produced by exposure to nitrites). Even if the disease is inherited, the particular mode of inheritance may be obscure. For example, retinitis pigmentosa has autosomal recessive [3], autosomal dominant [4], and X-linked [6] forms. As was noted earlier, autosomal dominant forms are usually less severe than X-linked forms, which in turn are usually less severe than autosomal recessive forms [42, 77, 88].

MULTIFACTORIAL TRAITS

Many complex traits are genetically inherited or influenced, but not as simple mendelian genetics would predict. They are the result of additive effects of many genes, instead of being determined by just one gene. Traits can also be the result of interaction of polygenic inheritance and environment, in which case they are called multifactorial. It has been speculated that the sum of all the effects of genes must reach a certain threshold to become clinically apparent. The environment may change the threshold. Such traits may often have a continuous variation, such as iris color, refractive error, intelligence, or height. Other polygenic traits may be even more complex to describe. Some of the more common polygenic conditions include congenital heart disease, cleft palate, diabetes, some forms of open-angle glaucoma, some forms of strabismus, club foot, coloboma, myopia, and buphthalmos [42, 77, 88].

Recurrence risks are usually empirically determined. However, some general rules can be stated [77, 88]:

1. There is an increased risk for recurrence among first-, second-, and third-degree relatives of the proband.
2. The empirical risk is often about 3 to 5 percent for first-degree relatives, and often one-half that for second-degree relatives, assuming only the proband is affected.
3. The recurrence risk increases as the number of affected relatives increases.
4. If there is a sex difference in the population as a whole for the trait (e.g., buphthalmos is more common in males) and the proband is of the less-affected sex, then the recurrence risk is greater than if the proband were of the more-affected sex. This is said to be because the occurrence of the condition in the less likely sex is more unlikely from the genetic point of view and therefore the parents have a higher prior probability of producing children with a deleterious number of genes.
5. As the severity of the disorder increases, so does the recurrence risk.

GENETIC HETEROGENEITY

Genetic heterogeneity refers to the production of similar or identical phenotypes by different gene changes. Often this is secondary to different changes in the same gene. For example, hemoglobin$_{Harlem}$, hemoglobin$_{Georgetown}$, and hemoglobin S all are manifested by sickling of red blood cells but are the result of different alterations in the β chain of the hemoglobin molecule. With the newer techniques of DNA analysis, we are finding many different gene level changes in the same gene giving rise to the same clinical effects. Genetic heterogeneity may also be caused by changes in different genes. Pseudoachondroplasia and pseudoxanthoma elasticum are examples of this, with some forms of clinically identical disease being autosomal recessive and some forms being autosomal dominant [42, 77, 88]. Another example is retinitis pigmentosa, which, as mentioned, has autosomal recessive, autosomal dominant, and X-linked forms.

MUTATIONS

Heritable changes in the DNA of genes are called mutations. These changes can be secondary to random changes in base pairing during DNA replication, viruses [42], chemicals [94], or radiation [5, 62]. Among chemicals, alkylating agents are among the most mutagenic [94]. These agents interact with DNA in such a way as to alter it and cause mispairing during replication. For example, 5-bromouracil may pair with either guanine or cytosine. This may result in a base substitution [94]. Other agents may insert themselves into a DNA sequence and then pair with a base, which leads to an addition of a base pair [94]. Other agents may interact with DNA to cause a deletion in a base pair [94]. Ultraviolet radiation causes adjacent thymine residues to form covalent bonds, rendering them unable to pair with other bases in replication [94]. Ionizing radiation causes formation of free radicals, which can interact with DNA to cause changes in base pairing [42]. High doses of ionizing radiation and some chemicals can actually break the covalent structure of DNA, which leads to chromosome breakage [25].

Any mutation in a single base pair of DNA is called a point mutation. If the change in the DNA causes the codon to code for a different amino acid, it is called a missense mutation. For example, in the sixth position of the β hemoglobin chain is the DNA sequence CTT or CTC, which codes for glutamic acid. In hemoglobin C, the first C in the codon is changed to T. Subsequently, TTT or TTC codes for lysine, which gives rise to hemoglobin C. If the normal CTT or CTC sequence is changed to CAT or CAC, the DNA codes for valine at the sixth amino acid; this produces hemoglobin S [94].

Missense mutations may have no, mild, or profound clinical consequences. A change in a DNA base may result in a new codon that codes for the same amino acid or another amino acid. The mutation may result in a codon that codes for an amino acid far removed from the functional part of the protein (and thus have no apparent effect) or a codon that produces a protein that is almost totally nonfunctional [94].

The change in a base pair may result in a termination codon. This is called a nonsense mutation, and at this point the protein chain will be terminated. Hence, the protein will be shorter and often nonfunctional compared with normal protein [93]. A termination codon may be changed to an amino acid codon, in which case the normal protein will be initially synthesized, but protein synthesis will continue and a much longer than normal protein will be produced, as is seen with hemoglobin$_{Constant\ Spring}$ [10].

Deletions or additions of bases may have drastic effects. If the deletion or addition of bases involves a multiple of three adjacent bases, there may be only a loss or addition of amino acids. However, if there is a loss or addition of only one or two bases, this will cause a so-called frameshift mutation, in which all subsequent codons, and therefore amino acids, will be altered. Clearly, this almost always results in a nonfunctional protein [94].

Repair mechanisms exist for excising abnormal DNA and replacing it with properly paired bases. This reduces the frequency of mutations but clearly does not eliminate them [94]. Most mutations, but not all, are harmful—so there is often environmental selection and subsequent elimination of mutant genes from the gene pool, especially for autosomal dominants [34].

Structural abnormalities of chromosomes, as opposed to numerical abnormalities, are thought to be comparable to mutations of genes. These include inversions, deletions, duplications, ring chromosomes, and translocations. Their effects depend on the genetic information carried in the involved segments of the chromosome [88].

It is difficult to estimate or determine the mutation rate in humans, although several methods have been attempted. All of them have limitations. Clearly, autosomal dominant mutations will be seen in the succeeding generation. Mutation rates of dominant genes are known with better accuracy than are those of others because dominant traits are readily observed in the heterozygous state. However, for such an analysis to be accurate, the gene must not be lethal in early age,

a high proportion of cases must be from mutations, and confusion from phenocopies must be minimal [88]. Aniridia is an example [80], but often in other diseases these seemingly simple requirements cannot be met. However, analysis of various diseases has established a mutation rate between 10^{-6} and 10^{-5} per locus per gamete for autosomal dominant genes [92].

Autosomal recessive genes are difficult to study because, unless an extensive pedigree analysis is available, it is often difficult to determine if a clinically apparent recessive disease or trait in an individual is the result of a new mutation. Under the assumptions that the genetic fitness of a recessive homozygote is zero and that the reproductive fitness of the heterozygote and normal homozygote are equal, it can be shown, in a population at equilibrium that μ = the mutation rate = q^2 where q is the frequency of the recessive gene. However, the specific requirements are rarely met and deviation from them seriously alters this relationship [57].

A similar analysis, subject to the same qualifications, shows that for X-linked recessives μ = $q/3$. Again, the requirements are rarely met, and this method fails when they are not satisfied. For X-linked recessives, the trait will not become apparent until it is passed on to a male [34].

Chromosomal structural abnormalities have also been studied, and new abnormalities appear to be present in about 2 in 1,000 newborns. Obviously this does not take into account the number of spontaneous abortions secondary to chromosomal abnormalities in concepti [88].

There is clear evidence that the mutation rate may be altered by various factors. Clearly, exposure to radiation or various chemicals can lead to mutations—although the blood-sperm barrier seems to be relatively effective [88].

Paternal age has clearly been shown to be a factor that increases the rate of mutation. This is because oocytes do not undergo mitosis, while spermatozoa are always dividing. This observation has been amply confirmed in autosomal dominant traits such as achondroplasia or Marfan's syndrome [68].

For some conditions, such as hemophilia, there is strong evidence that the mutation rate is higher in men than in women [15].

Certain genetic conditions predispose to high rates of mutation—both in gametes and somatic cells. These conditions include Bloom's syndrome [76], ataxia telangiectasia [32], and xeroderma pigmentosum [19, 71].

TWIN STUDIES

One way of studying traits on the phenotypic level, especially complex traits, is to take advantage of the fact that nature produces twins. Twin studies help determine whether or not a trait is genetic but say nothing about the nature of genetic control (e.g., single gene vs. polygenic). Twin studies have many limitations and are being supplanted in importance by more powerful methods of analysis such as the growing ability to analyze genes directly by recombinant DNA methods [9].

Twins have classically been described as being of two different types—monozygotic and dizygotic. Monozygotic twins result when one sperm fertilizes one ovum to form a zygote that subsequently divides to form two genetically identical, but separate, organisms. Dizygotic twins are the result of separate fertilization by different sperm of two different ova. Dizygotic twins are related to each other genetically as any two siblings are; on average, they have about one-half their genes in common [9].

Because monozygotic twins have identical genotypes at every gene, any differences in any trait can be secondary only to environmental influences. Dizygotic twins represent a good comparison group because, in many ways, the variation in a trait owing to environment is similar for both monozygotic and dizygotic twins. Any difference in the degree of variation for a trait can be ascribed to the genetic difference of the dizygotic twins. Therefore, dizygotic twins can be compared with monozygotic twins to analyze the variation resulting from either genetic or environmental influences [9].

Unfortunately, there are many difficulties in these studies, and the underlying assumptions are not always fulfilled. Often the environmental influences are not the same for monozygotic and dizygotic twins. Monozygotic twins show an increased number of congenital abnormalities, which may bias the results [9]. There may be unusual types of twins—such as when a polar body of the fertilized egg is also fertilized or when two separate eggs are fertilized by different sperm from different fathers [9]. In the latter case the twins are related as half-sibs, not sibs. Twins may have different types of fetal circulations; monozygotic twins have a mutual circulation that can result in intrapair environmentally induced differences that may not be present for dizygotic twins [9].

Other environmental differences in monozygotic twins may be introduced with different frequency than for dizygotic twins because of perinatal and postnatal factors. Perinatal mortality is higher for monozygotic twins than for dizygotic twins. In the postnatal environment, there is evidence that dizygotic twins, even like-sex dizygotic twins, have a different environmental interaction than do monozygotic twins. All of these factors tend to detract from the assumption that environmental influences are the same for monozygotic and dizygotic twins [9]. However, with these qualifications, it is possible to make some inferences from the use of twin data.

The first step in doing a twin study is to determine the zygosity of each twin pair. If the twins are of different sex, they are clearly dizygotic [9]. Other traits that can be used include blood groups [9], salivary secretion of antigens [82], and major histocompatibility antigen (HLA) typing [9]. More complex traits such as dermatoglyphics [9], hair [82], eye color [82], or gross morphology [82] may also be considered by experienced observers.

Fetal membranes have often been used in the past to help determine zygosity, but either type of twin may have separate placentas with separate amnions and chorions, or a single fused placenta. While dizygotic twins always have two chorions, this may sometimes be appreciated only by special examination. This method has led to many errors in the past [9].

Skin grafting is currently accepted as the definitive test but is done only when it is absolutely necessary to establish zygosity, as in the case of organ transplantation [9, 88].

Both discontinuous traits (e.g., diabetes or schizophrenia) and continuous traits (e.g., height or intelligence) can be studied in twins. For discontinuous traits, one studies concordance (similarity between twins of all-or-none traits) rates and determines if they are the same in monozygotic and dizygotic twins. Any difference, especially if the concordance rate is higher for the monozygotic twins, is strongly suggestive of a genetic influence [9, 88].

Continuous traits are studied by analyzing variance, if the traits can be quantified. The investigator determines the amount of variance for dizygotic twins and compares it to the variance for monozygotic twins. Under the assumption that variance secondary to environment is the same, any increase in variance in dizygotic twins over monozygotic twins is said to be caused by genetic variation and influences [9, 88].

Various statistical techniques are used to analyze variances. The most satisfactory uses the F

test to determine the significance of a ratio of variances V_{dz}/V_{mz} [9, 88]. While it may be easy to demonstrate a genetic component, a quantitative estimation of the magnitude of the genetic component is usually more difficult, if not impossible [9].

CARRIER DETECTION

We are in a unique position with genetic diseases and conditions in that not only can we often identify people who are affected by abnormal genes (e.g., Marfan's syndrome), but we can also identify individuals whose future offspring will be at definite risk ($>10^{-6}$) of having a given disease. This is possible because we can often identify the carriers of abnormal genes. Patients with autosomal dominant genes are usually obvious, although occasionally a gene may be nonpenetrant or have a low expressivity. Patients with a single autosomal recessive gene are often not completely normal clinically, and it is these people, or heterozygotes for autosomal recessive genes, who are the subject of much investigation to determine if they harbor an abnormal gene for a specific condition [42, 77, 88].

The ethics of this type of information and screening are not entirely clear. Does someone who has the autosomal dominant gene for Huntington's chorea really want to know, and is it in his or her best interests to know? There have been adverse social effects of screening for the carriers of sickle cell and Tay-Sachs disease [39]. In one study it was found that patients who were carriers for sickle cell were actually avoided by noncarriers so that they more often ended up marrying carriers than before the screening began [85].

There are two major ways of detecting carriers. The patient can be examined thoroughly for the telltale signs that suggest he or she is a carrier, or DNA or protein product of DNA can be directly examined on the molecular level. Phenotypic examination may reveal the same quality, but much less severe, of changes seen in the homozygote. For example, in ocular albinism, a female heterozygote may have abnormal iris transillumination or pigment clusters in the ocular fundus [44]. In oculocutaneous albinism, there may be freckling, nystagmus, or both [62]. Recessive genes often code for enzymes, and the quantity of enzyme activity may be reduced in the heterozygote without clinical effect. For example, normally there

are 1,000 units of galactose 1-phosphate uridyl transferase activity (a deficiency of this enzyme results in galactosemia) per red blood cell, but in heterozygotes there are only 500 units of activity. This can be demonstrated even if the patient is clinically completely normal [43]. Similarly, the recessive gene may take an abnormal protein, even though the patient is clinically normal. An example is seen in the hemoglobinopathies such as hemoglobin S [73] or hemoglobin C [10], in which the abnormal hemoglobin is easily detected by hemoglobin electrophoresis (see Fig. 1-9). Some genes can now be examined directly. For example, the hemoglobin genes can be studied directly to determine if an individual is a carrier for a hemoglobinopathy such as hemoglobin S [47]. The gene regions for Huntington's chorea [33] and diabetes [72] have also recently been directly investigated.

Often the same biochemical techniques that can be used to determine if an individual is a carrier can also be used to determine if a fetus is affected. This forms the basis of one mode of prenatal detection and again raises many ethical questions. The biochemical techniques, especially the DNA methods, are certainly very powerful, and undoubtedly our ability to detect carriers on the molecular level will continue to grow dramatically in the years ahead.

BAYESIAN ANALYSIS

Sometimes it is not possible to detect the carrier state by either clinical or molecular means. If one is able to construct a pedigree, one may be able to determine the probability of being a carrier and the probability of having an affected offspring. The method of using all the information in a pedigree to compare alternate genotypes is called bayesian analysis, after T. Bayes [77]. It is best explained by the example that follows (see Fig. 1-11), but the principle can be explained here. One first determines whose offspring are at risk, that is, the individual whose genotype is in question. This individual is called the consultand. The pedigree is then divided into the ancestors and the descendants of the consultand [57].

For example, say we are dealing with a woman who has in her family someone with X-linked Duchenne's muscular dystrophy and there is a possibility that she may be a carrier. That is, on the basis of phenotype she may have one of two alternate genotypes. One uses the information on her ancestors to calculate the probability that she is or is not a carrier based on simple mendelian methods. These are called prior probabilities and should sum up to one [57].

One then takes each genotype separately and calculates the probability of obtaining the pedigree represented by her descendants using simple mendelian methods. This is known as the conditional probability, because it is conditional on the assumption of that particular genotype [57]. The product of the prior probability and the conditional probability is known as the joint probability.

Usually the joint probabilities will not add to 1. The reason for this is as follows. A probability of one encompasses all possible outcomes. If the mother in this example had two sons, under the assumption that she was a carrier, all the possibilities are represented by no affected sons, one affected son, or two affected sons. However, if she has already had two sons, they cannot simultaneously represent all possibilities. They can represent only one possible outcome (having already occurred) and, therefore, the other possibilities should no longer be included in the total probability space [57].

The new total probability space is represented by the sum of the joint probabilities. The probabilities of having obtained the entire pedigree, given different consultand genotypes, is normalized or corrected to the new total probability space by taking each joint probability and dividing it by the sum of the joint probabilities (the new total probability space). This gives so-called posterior probabilities for the alternate genotypes, which sum to 1. These posterior probabilities can then be used to calculate the risk of having affected offspring [57].

In Fig. 1-11 the consultand has one affected brother, so her mother must have been a carrier. Given the fact that her mother must have been a carrier, the consultand had a prior probability of ½ of being a carrier and ½ of not being a carrier [57].

Under the assumption that the consultand is not a carrier, there is a conditional probability of 1 that her two sons will be normal. Therefore the joint probability that her two sons will be normal is or was 1 × ½. Under the assumption that the consultand is a carrier, there is a conditional probability of ½ × ½, or ¼, that both sons will be normal. This gives a joint probability of ½ × ¼, or ⅛. Notice that the joint probabilities sum to ⅝. The missing ⅜ would be represented by her having had affected sons and, since this did not

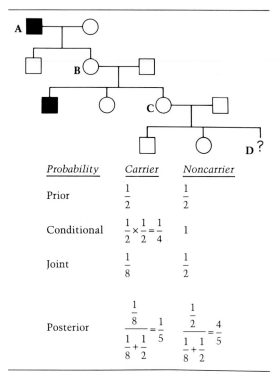

Probability	Carrier	Noncarrier
Prior	$\dfrac{1}{2}$	$\dfrac{1}{2}$
Conditional	$\dfrac{1}{2} \times \dfrac{1}{2} = \dfrac{1}{4}$	1
Joint	$\dfrac{1}{8}$	$\dfrac{1}{2}$
Posterior	$\dfrac{\frac{1}{8}}{\frac{1}{8}+\frac{1}{2}} = \dfrac{1}{5}$	$\dfrac{\frac{1}{2}}{\frac{1}{8}+\frac{1}{2}} = \dfrac{4}{5}$

Fig. 1-11. *Bayesian analysis for an X-linked trait. The question is whether the consultand (C) is a carrier of the trait. Notice that the joint probabilities do not sum to 1. In this example, the consultand has a ⅕ instead of ½ probability of being a carrier when all the information in the pedigree is considered.*

occur, must be eliminated from the total probability space [57].

Therefore the posterior probability for being a carrier is ⅛ ÷ (⅛ + ½) = ⅕; for not being a carrier, ½ ÷ (⅛ + ½) = ⅘. Therefore, using all the information in this pedigree, one can say that the probability of the consultand being a carrier is ⅕. The probability of her next son being affected with X-linked Duchenne's muscular dystrophy is then ⅕ × ½ = ⅒. Such a bayesian analysis often provides the consultand with a more realistic and often reduced risk of affected offspring than could be quoted to him or her using simple mendelian methods [57].

Bayesian analysis can be used to calculate genetic risks in the following situations [57]:

1. Determining the carrier status of a female for an X-linked condition in which there are affected males in the pedigree.
2. With laboratory test values, for X-linked or au-

tosomal recessive conditions. For example, in Duchenne's muscular dystrophy, the carrier female may have an elevated serum creatinine phosphokinase (CPK) level. The higher the CPK value, the greater the probability of her being a carrier. The exact probabilities have been determined empirically and can be used in performing a bayesian analysis to assign prior probabilities in women at risk of being carriers.

3. In calculating risk in a dominant condition which is nonpenetrant or in which there is age dependence in its expression. For example, Huntington's chorea can come on anytime from the second to the seventh decade. If one is at risk of having the disease, the older one bcomes without having been afflicted the less likely one is to have inherited the gene. The age-probability curve has been empirically determined and can be used to modify probabilities in a bayesian analysis.

Bayesian analysis is discussed in much greater detail by Murphy and Chase [57].

LINKAGE

While Mendel asserted that different genes assort independently, he was unaware of the existence of chromosomes. Since chromosomes do not lose their integrity during meiosis, clearly not all genes undergo independent assortment. Instead, many genes or gene loci are located on the same chromosome. Such gene loci are said to be linked or syntenic [42, 77, 88].

The linkage of the genes is not inviolable. When homologous chromosomes pair during meiosis, there may be physical exchange of homologous parts of DNA. This is known as crossing over and is cytologically seen in the formation of chiasmata [42, 77, 88].

While crossing over can occur anywhere, it becomes more likely to occur between two loci the farther apart they are on the chromosome. Genes on different chromosomes would show a crossover or recombination frequency of 50 percent. This is the largest cross-over frequency that can be detected. The distance between gene loci on a chromosome is given by the percentage of crossovers and is measured in centimorgans; that is, 5 percent crossing over indicates the gene loci are 5 centimorgans apart. The gene maps constructed by crossing over can be compared to the gene map made by cytologic studies. Certainly the genes map in the same sequence by both methods; how-

ever, units of recombination are not equal along the length of the chromosome [42, 77, 88]. Furthermore, there is evidence that recombination rates on a given chromosome may be higher in women than in men [26]. Genes on the same chromosome are said to be in the *cis* configuration, while genes on different homologous chromosomes are said to be in the *trans* position [42, 77, 88].

If the two gene loci are far enough apart, there may be a double cross-over, which would not be detected using two loci. Hence, measuring gene map distances between two loci may result in underestimating the degree of crossing over. This underestimation can be demonstrated by using three gene loci. If the gene loci are *ABC*, then the distance between *A* and *B* plus the distance between *B* and *C* by recombinant analysis will be greater than the distance between *A* and *C* measured by recombinants between *A* and *C*. The difference is the number of double cross-overs. Therefore, the most accurate maps between two genes are obtained when there is a short distance between them. Sometimes at very short distances there is interference in crossing over, possibly because of physical factors. If one wants to know the distance between two loci far apart, it is best to divide the distance into short segments and add up the gene map distances of the short segments. This distance may easily be more than 100 centimorgans [42, 77, 88].

Clearly, if the gene map distance between two loci on a chromosome is greater than 50 centimorgans, they behave as if they are not linked. Therefore, failure to demonstrate linkage cannot be taken as evidence that gene loci are on different chromosomes.

It is difficult to perform linkage studies in humans because (1) until recently it was not known which genes were on which chromosomes since this requires having a double heterozygote in known coupling phase, and (2) humans produce relatively few offspring. These two considerations have made linkage studies applicable primarily to X-linked traits. A man's genotype can be established since he has only one X chromosome. If his daughter (because of her offspring) is therefore known to be a double heterozygote, her coupling phase is known since her father's X chromosome could not cross over with his Y chromosome. Her sons can then be listed as recombinant by simple examination. Examination of a few such pedigrees can give good estimates of gene map distances based on recombination frequencies [42, 77, 88].

A more powerful method, known as the lod score method, which requires the presence of a double heterozygote but does not require knowledge of coupling phase, has been devised to investigate linkage of autosomal traits. In this method equal probability is assigned to each coupling phase. One then assumes a recombinant frequency of theta and calculates the probability of obtaining the pedigree represented by the double heterozygote's offspring or F1. This is written as $P(F1/\theta)$ and is expressed in terms of θ. One makes the calculations for various values of θ from 0 to 0.5 and then expresses them as a ratio of $P(F1/\theta$ when $\theta = 0.5)$. One then takes the logarithm of this ratio, which is called the lod score (z).

$$z = \log \{P(F1/\theta)/[P(F1/\theta = 0.5)]\}$$

Clearly, if $P(F1$ for a given $\theta \neq 0.5)$ is greater than $P(F1/\theta = 0.5)$, z will be greater than zero. For all other cases, that is, $P(F1$ for a given $\theta)$ is less than or equal to $P(F1/\theta = 0.5)$, z will be zero or negative. Values of z greater than zero favor linkage, while those zero or negative are against linkage. Calculations of lod scores can also be done when the pedigree is more extensive, in which case they are more informative [88].

An advantage of the z score is that it allows one to overcome the fact that human pedigrees tend to be small. The total probability of a series of pedigrees occurring simultaneously is simply the product of the probabilities. Since lod scores are logarithms, the lod scores of a series of pedigrees can be simply added together to form a cumulative lod score. Thus, lod scores can be added together until z is clearly a maximum at $\theta = 0.5$ or until z reaches a significant value, usually greater than 3.0, for some specific value of θ less than 0.5 [56].

Lod scores were used by Fialkow and colleagues to show measurable linkage between ocular albinism and Xg blood group [28]. In their analysis z was a maximum for $\theta = 0.175$. Renwick and Lawler used lod scores to show that the locus for congenital zonular cataract and the locus for the Duffy blood group are linked [69]. The value of z was at a maximum for $\theta = 0$, indicating that the two loci are closely linked.

PRENATAL DIAGNOSIS

We can now identify many individuals who are carriers for various diseases or who are at risk for having children with genetic diseases. For most conditions it is impossible to determine a priori if a child will be affected before it is conceived. However, one can often perform prenatal diagnosis on the developing fetus to determine if it is affected. The family can then receive genetic counseling, and the option of abortion can be discussed.

Techniques for prenatal diagnosis include both noninvasive and invasive techniques. The principal noninvasive technique is ultrasound visualization, which can help detect gross physical malformations such as skeletal dysplasias, cystic kidneys, myelomeningoceles, and hydrocephalus [45, 75]. Other more sophisticated and powerful techniques, such as focused laser images, are being developed to provide for three-dimensional views [77].

Invasive methods include fetoscopy, amniocentesis, placental blood sampling, and chorionic villi biopsy. Fetoscopy can detect many of the same morphologic abnormalities as ultrasound [77]. It can also be used to sample blood from placental vessels. This latter technique has been employed to screen prenatally for hemoglobinopathies and thalassemias since the fetal cells obtained by amniocentesis do not produce hemoglobin [90].

Amniocentesis is the technique of inserting a needle through the abdomen into the amniotic sac under ultrasonic guidance and withdrawing amniotic fluid for analysis. It is done after the sixteenth week to allow enough fluid to have accumulated to make the procedure technically possible and before the twentieth week to make abortion an option [58, 91].

Amniotic fluid that is withdrawn can be directly analyzed. Fetuses with a neural tube defect or a ventral wall defect will have elevated levels of α-fetoprotein [8]. Cells derived from the fetus will be present in the amniotic fluid. These are usually too few to be analyzed so they are grown in tissue culture for 2 to 4 weeks before being analyzed [91].

After the cells have been cultured, they may be either analyzed directly for their karyotype [91], various enzyme assays may be done [36], or the DNA of the cells may be analyzed using complementary DNA hybridization (this last technique can actually be done without having to culture the cells first) [46]. Analysis of DNA has now been used for prenatal diagnosis of hemoglobinopathies [7], thalassemias [7], and α_1-antitrypsin deficiency [50].

Karyotypic analysis allows for the detection of chromosomal aberrations—abnormalities of both structure and number. Amniocentesis is currently used most frequently for this purpose, usually to screen for Down's syndrome [77].

Many metabolic errors can also now be detected prenatally. These include Tay-Sachs disease [36], Hunter's syndrome [18], and Hurler's syndrome [18]. The fetal cells are assayed for the activity level of the enzyme in question, and consequently the absence of enzymatic activity can be detected. There are too many to enumerate them all here. However, the metabolic diseases that can be detected prenatally fall into several categories: (1) mucopolysaccharidoses, (2) mucolipidoses, (3) sphingolipidoses, (4) lysosomal storage forms of carbohydrate disorders, (5) aminoacidopathies from known ezymatic defects, and (6) miscellaneous disorders [77]. A listing of genetic and metabolic eye diseases that can be detected prenatally is shown in Table 1-2.

Few X-linked recessive conditions can be detected prenatally. One option in this situation is to do prenatal screening of the karyotype for sex determination. The parents can then have only female offspring if they wish since females are known not to be affected. This issue arises in such conditions as Duchenne's muscular dystrophy [1].

Another approach to prenatal diagnosis uses linkage analysis. For example, the specific defect in myotonic dystrophy is unknown. However, the gene for myotonic dystrophy is closely linked to the secretor gene (responsible for the secretion of ABH blood group into blood and amniotic fluid). Hence, if the family is informative for linkage (pedigree can be analyzed and linkage of two genes established; only 10–20% of the cases), prenatal diagnosis or prediction can be done by analyzing ABH type in the amniotic fluid [78].

Chorionic villi biopsy is a recently introduced technique. The biopsy is done at 6 to 10 weeks (earlier than amniocentesis), and the specimen obtained can be used primarily for karyotypic analysis. It has been used more extensively in Europe than in the United States. DNA analysis could also be conceivably done on these samples [23].

While some have advocated doing prenatal amniocentesis in all pregnancies, currently there are neither the facilities nor the funds to make this feasible. Amniocentesis is done primarily when certain indications are present: (1) a previous child with spina bifida or anencephaly—the risk of having a second affected child is 5 percent, (2) a previous child with a chromosomal aberration—2 percent, (3) a balanced translocation for Down's

Table 1-2. *Conditions Affecting the Eye That Can Be Diagnosed Prenatally*

Acephalia

Acute intermittent porphyria

Bermann's disease

Cystinosis

Down's syndrome (trisomy 21)

Epidermolytic hyperkeratosis (congenital bullous ichthyosiform erythroderma)

Fabry's disease (angiokeratoma corporis diffusum)

Familial hypercholesterolemia

Familial lipogranulomatosis

GM_1 gangliosidosis type I (infantile)

GM_1 gangliosidosis type II (juvenile)

GM_2 gangliosidosis type I (Tay-Sach's disease)

GM_2 gangliosidosis type II (Sandhoff's disease)

Gaucher's disease

Globoid cell leukodystrophy (Krabbe's disease)

Glycogenosis type II (Pompe's disease)

Hemangioma

Homocystinuria

Hypophosphatasia, congenital lethal form

Ichthyosis congenita

Mucolipidosis II (I-cell disease)

Mucolipidosis IV

Mucopolysaccharidosis I-H (Hurler's syndrome)

Mucopolysaccharidosis II (Hunter's syndrome)

Mucopolysaccharidosis III (Sanfilippo's syndrome)

Mucopolysaccharidosis VI (Maroteaux-Lamy syndrome)

Myotonic dystrophy (Steinert's disease)

Neuraminidase deficiency

Niemann-Pick disease type A

Osteogenesis imperfecta congenita

Osteogenesis imperfecta tarda

Porphyria

Sialidosis

Sickle cell anemia

α-Thalassemia

β-Thalassemia

Triploidy

Trisomy 13

Trisomy 18

Turner's syndrome

Wolman's disease

syndrome in either parent—5 to 20 percent, (4) high risk for a child with a detectable inborn error of metabolism—25 to 50 percent, or (5) mother 35 years or older—1 to 2 percent [38]. The risk of Down's syndrome increases with the mother's age: Between ages 35 and 39, the risk is 2.2 percent; between 40 and 44 it is 3.4 percent; at age 45, it is 10 percent [38].

As our knowledge continues to expand, our ability successfully to make prenatal diagnoses also expands. Especially exciting are the new molecular biology techniques that allow for direct examination of DNA. These allow us to diagnose or examine diseases and genes whose products are not secreted into amniotic fluid or made by amniotic cells.

REFERENCES

1. Adams, C., et al. Fetal sex determination. *Acta Cytol. (Baltimore)* 17:233, 1973.
2. Avery, O. T., MacLeod, C. M., and McCarty, M. Studies on the chemical nature of the substance inducing transformation of pneumococcal types. *J. Exp. Med.* 79:137, 1944.
3. Baughman, I. A., Conneally, P. M., and Nance, W. E. Population genetic studies of retinitis pigmentosa. *Am. J. Hum. Genet.* 32:223, 1980.
4. Beckershaus, F. Dominante Vererbung der Retinitis pigmentosa. *Klin. Monatsbl. Augenheilkd.* 75:96, 1925.
5. BEIR (Biological Effects of Ionizing Radiation) Report. *The Effects on Populations of Exposure to Low Levels of Ionizing Radiation.* Washington: National Academy of Sciences, National Research Council, 1972. P. 217.
6. Bird, A. C. X-linked retinitis pigmentosa. *Br. J. Ophthalmol.* 59:177, 1975.
7. Boehm, C. P., et al. Prenatal diagnosis using DNA polymorphisms. *N. Engl. J. Med.* 308:1054, 1983.
8. Brock, D. J. H. The prenatal diagnosis of neural tube defects. *Obstet. Gynecol. Surv.* 31:32, 1976.
9. Bulmer, M. G. *The Biology of Twinning in Man.* Oxford, England: Clarendon, 1970.
10. Bunn, H. F., Forget, B. G., and Ranney, H. M. *Human Hemoglobins.* Philadelphia: Saunders, 1977.
11. Burnett, C. H., et al. Vitamin D resistant rickets. *Am. J. Med.* 36:222, 1964.
12. Carney, R. G., and Carney, R. G., Jr. Incontinentia pigmenti. *Arch. Dermatol.* 102:157, 1970.
13. Casperrsson, T., et al. Identification of human chromosomes by DNA-binding fluorescent agents. *Chromosoma* 30:215, 1970.
14. Crick, F. Split genes and RNA splicing. *Science* 204:264, 1979.
15. Crow, J. F. Mutation in man. *Prog. Med. Genet.* 1:1, 1961.
16. Dalton, J. Extraordinary facts relating to the vision of colours: With observations. *Mem. Lit. Philos. Soc. Manchester* 5(1):28, 1798.
17. Darnell, J. E., Jr. Implications of RNA: RNA splicing in evolution of eukaryotic cells. *Science* 202:1257, 1978.
18. Danes, B. S., et al. Antenatal diagnosis of mucopolysaccharidoses (letter). *Lancet* 1:946, 1970.
19. Day, R. S. Xeroderma pigmentosum variants have decreased repair of ultraviolet-damaged DNA. *Nature* 253:748, 1975.
20. Dellman, J.W., Bleeker-Wagemakers, E. M., and van Veelen, A. W. C. Opacities of the lens indicating carrier status in the oculo-cerebro-renal (Lowe's) syndrome. *J. Pediatr. Ophthalmol.* 14:205, 1977.
21. Donahue, R. P., et al. Probable assignment of the Duffy blood group locus to chromosome 1 in man. *Proc. Natl. Acad. Sci. U.S.A.* 61:949, 1968.
22. Edwards, J. H., et al. A new trisomic syndrome. *Lancet* 1:787, 1960.
23. Elles, R. G., et al. Absence of maternal contamination of chorionic villi for fetal gene analysis. *N. Engl. J. Med.* 308:1433, 1983.
24. Evans, H. J. *Advances in Human Genetics: Facts and Fancies Relating to Chromosome Structure in Man.* New York: Plenum, 1977.
25. Evans, H. J., et al. Radiation-induced chromosome aberrations in nuclear-dockyard workers. *Nature* 277:531, 1979.
26. Fenger, K., and Sorenson, S. A. Evaluation of a possible sex difference in recombination for the ABO-AK linkage. *Am. J. Hum. Genet.* 27:784, 1975.
27. Ford, C. E., and Hamerton, J. L. A colchicine, hypotonic citrate, squash sequence for mammalian chromosomes. *Stain Technol.* 31:247, 1956.
28. Fialkow, P. J., Giblett, E. R., and Motulsky, A. G. Measurable linkage between ocular albinism and Xg. *Am. J. Hum. Genet.* 19:247, 1956.
29. Galloway, J. A., and Root, M. A. The use of biosynthetic human insulin in man. In T. Russell et al. (Eds.), *From Gene to Protein: Translation into Biotechnology.* New York, Academic, 1982.
30. Garrod, A. E. *Inborn Errors of Metabolism* (1909; reprinted 1963 with a supplement by H. Harris). London: Oxford University Press, 1963.
31. Glass, B. Maupertius, Pioneer of Genetics and Evolution. In B. Glass, O. Temkin, and W. Straus, Jr. (Eds.), *Forerunners of Darwin: 1745–1859.* Baltimore: Johns Hopkins Press, 1959.
32. Gropp, A., and Flatz, G. Chromosome breakage and blastic transformation of lymphocytes in ataxia telangiectasia. *Humangenetik* 5:77, 1967.
33. Guzella, J. F., et al. A polymorphic DNA marker genetically linked to Huntington's disease. *Nature* 306:234, 1983.
34. Haldane, J. B. S. The rate of spontaneous mutation of a human gene. *J. Genet.* 31:317, 1935.

35. Harris, G. S., and Miller, J. R. Choroideremia: Visual defects in a heterozygote. *Arch. Ophthalmol.* 80:423, 1968.

36. Higami, S., et al. Prenatal diagnosis and fetal pathology of Tay-Sachs disease. *Tohoku J. Exp. Med.* 118:323, 1976.

37. Hitter, H. M., Riccardi, V. M., and Francke, U. Aniridia caused by a heritable chromosome 11 deletion. *Trans. Am. Acad. Ophthalmol. Otolaryngol.* 86:1173, 1979.

38. Horn, E. B. Estimates of maternal age-specific risks of a Down syndrome birth in women aged 34–41. *Lancet* 2:33, 1976.

39. Hsia, Y. E., et al. *Counseling in Genetics.* New York: Liss, 1979.

40. Hsu, T. C. Mammalian chromosomes *in vitro:* I. The karyotype of man. *J. Hered.* 43:167, 1952.

41. Hughes, A. Some effects of abnormal toxicity in dividing cells in chick tissue cultures. *Q. J. Microscopical Sci.* 93:207, 1952.

42. Isselbacher, K. J., et al. *Human Principles of Internal Medicine* (9th ed.). New York: McGraw-Hill, 1980.

43. Isselbacher, K. J., et al. Congenital galactosemia: A single enzymatic block in galactose metabolism. *Science* 123:635, 1956.

44. Jaeger, C., and Jay, B. X-linked ocular albinism: A family containing a manifesting heterozygote, and an affected male married to a female with autosomal recessive ocular albinism. *Hum. Genet.* 56:299, 1981.

45. Kahack, M. M., and Valenti, C. (Eds.). *Intrauterine Fetal Visualization: A Multidisciplinary Approach.* New York: American Elsevier, 1976.

46. Kan, Y. W., and Dozy, A. M. Antenatal diagnosis of sickle cell anemia by DNA analysis of amniotic fluid cells. *Lancet* 2:910, 1978.

47. Kan, Y. W., and Dozy, A. M. Polymorphism of DNA sequence adjacent to human β-globin structural gene: Relationship to sickle mutation. *Proc. Natl. Acad. Sci. U.S.A.* 75:5631, 1978.

48. Keith, G. C. *Genetics and Ophthalmology.* London: Churchill Livingstone, 1978.

49. Kennaway, N. G., Welebur, R. G., and Buist, N. R. M. Gyrate atrophy of choroid and retina: Deficient activity of ornithine ketoacid aminotransferase in cultured skin fibroblasts (letter). *N. Engl. J. Med.* 297:1180, 1977.

50. Kidd, V. J., et al. Prenatal diagnosis of α_1-antitrypsin deficiency by direct analysis of the mutation site in the gene. *N. Engl. J. Med.* 310:639, 1984.

51. Lejeune, J., Gantier, M., and Turpiz, R. Les chromosomes humains en culture de tissus. *C. R. Seances Acad. Sci.* 248:602, 1959.

52. Lyon, M. F. Sex chromatin and gene action in the mammalian X-chromosome. *Am. J. Hum. Genet.* 14:135, 1962.

53. Mayer, J. S., and Guthrio, R. Detection of heterozygotes for galactokinase deficiency in a human population. *Biochem. Genet.* 2:219, 1968.

54. McKusick, V. A. *Heritable Disorders of Connective Tissue.* St. Louis: Mosby, 1972.

55. McKusick, V. A. *Mendelian Inheritance in Man* (6th ed.). Baltimore: Johns Hopkins Press, 1983. Appendix B.

56. Morton, N. E. Sequential tests for the detection of linkage. *Am. J. Hum. Genet.* 7:277, 1955.

57. Murphy, E. A., and Chase, G. *Genetic Counseling.* Chicago: Year Book, 1975.

58. NICHHD Amniocentesis Registry Symposium Report. *JAMA* 236:1471, 1976.

59. Nirenberg, M. W., and Malthaei, J. H. The dependence of cell-free protein synthesis in *E. coli* upon naturally occurring or synthetic polyribonucleotides. *Proc. Natl. Acad. Sci. U.S.A.* 47:1588, 1961.

60. Nowell, P. C. Phytohemagglutinin: An inhibitor of mitosis in cultures of normal human leucocytes. *Cancer Res.* 20:462, 1960.

61. O'Brien, J. S., et al. Tay-Sachs disease: Detection of heterozygotes and homozygotes by serum hexosaminidase assay. *N. Engl. J. Med.* 283:15, 1970.

62. *Ophthalmology Basic and Clinical Science Course,* Section 1. San Francisco: American Academy of Ophthalmology, 1983.

63. Packman, U., and Rigler, R., Quantum yield of acridines interacting with DNA or deferred base sequence. *Exp. Cell Res.* 72:602, 1972.

64. Palmuter, R. D., et al. Dramatic growth of mice that develop from eggs microinjected with metallothionein–growth hormone fusion genes. *Nature* 300:611, 1982.

65. Parker, R. C. *Methods of Tissue Culture* (3rd ed.). New York: Hoeber Med. Div., Harper & Row, 1961.

66. Patau, K., et al. Multiple congenital anomaly caused by an extra autosome. *Lancet* 1:790, 1960.

67. Patil, S. R., Menick, S., and Lubs, H. A. Identification of each human chromosome with a modified Giemsa stain. *Science* 173:821, 1976.

68. Penrose, L. S. Parental age and mutation. *Lancet* 2:312, 1955.

69. Renwick, J. H., and Lawler, S. D. Probable linkage between a congenital cataract locus and the Duffy blood group locus. *Ann. Hum. Genet.* 27:67, 1963.

70. Research Group on Ethical, Social and Legal Issues in Genetic Counseling and Genetic Engineering of the Institute of Society, Ethics and the Life Sciences. Ethical and social issues in screening for genetic disease. *N. Engl. J. Med.* 286:1129, 1972.

71. Robbins, J. H., et al. Xeroderma pigmentosum: An inherited disease with sun sensitivity, multiple cutaneous neoplasms, and abnormal DNA repair. *Ann. Intern. Med.* 80:221, 1974.

72. Rotwein P. S., et al. Polymorphism in the 5′ flanking region of the human insulin gene: A genetic marker for non–insulin dependent diabetes. *N. Engl. J. Med.* 308:65, 1983.

73. Rucknagel, D. L. The Biochemical Genetics of Sickle Cell Anemia and Related Hemoglobinopathies. In

R. D. Levere (Ed.), *Sickle Cell Anemia and Other Hemoglobinopathies.* New York: Academic, 1975.

74. Ruddle, F. H. Linkage analysis using somatic cell hybrids. *Adv. Hum. Genet.* 3:173, 1972.

75. Santo-Ramos, R., and Nuenholten, J. H. Diagnosis of congenital fetal abnormalities by sonography. *Obstet. Gynecol.* 45:279, 1975.

76. Sawitsky, A., Bloom, D., and German, J. Chromosomal breakage and acute leukemia in congential telangiectatic erythema and stunted growth. *Ann. Intern. Med.* 65:487, 1966.

77. Schimke, R. N., and Jackson, L. G. *Clinical Genetics.* New York: Wiley, 1979.

78. Schrott, H. G., and Omenn, S. G. S. Myotonic dystrophy: Opportunities for prenatal diagnosis. *Neurology (NY)* 25:789, 1975.

79. Shapira, T. M., and Sitney, J. A. Choroideremia. *Am. J. Ophthalmol.* 26:182, 1943.

80. Shaw, M. W., Falls, H. F., and Neel, J. V. Congenital aniridia. *Am. J. Hum. Genet.* 12:389, 1960.

81. Shows, T. B., Bernhard, U. Z., and Tricoli, J. V. High Resolution Chromosome Mapping of Cloned Genes and DNA Polymorphisms. In A. Messer and I. Porter (Eds.), *Recombinant DNA and Medical Genetics.* New York: Academic, 1983.

82. Smith, C. A. B., and Penrose, L. S. Monozygotic and dizygotic twin diagnosis. *Ann. Hum. Genet.* 19:273, 1955.

83. Smith, H. O., and Nathans, D. J. A suggested nomenclature for bacterial host modification and restriction systems and their enzymes. *J. Mol. Biol.* 81:419, 1973.

84. Solomon, E., et al. Assignment of the human acid α-glucosidase gene (αGLU) to chromosome 17 using somatic cell hybrids. *Ann. Hum. Genet.* 42:273, 1979.

85. Stamaloyannopoulous, G. Problems of Screening and Counseling in the Hemoglobinopathies. In A. G. Motulsky and F. J. G. Ebling (Eds.), *Birth Defects: Proceedings of the 4th International Conference, Vienna, 1973.* Amsterdam: Excerpta Medica, 1974.

86. Stern, C. *Principles of Human Genetics* (3rd ed.). San Francisco: Freeman, 1973.

87. Stubbe, H. *History of Genetics.* Cambridge, Mass.: MIT Press, 1972.

88. Sutton, H. E. *An Introduction to Human Genetics.* Philadelphia: Saunders, 1980.

89. Tjio, J. H., and Lavan, A. The chromosome number in man. *Hereditas* 42:1, 1956.

90. Valenti, C. Endoamnioscopy and fetal biopsy: A new technique. *Am. J. Obstet. Gynecol.* 114:561, 1972.

91. Valenti, C., and Kehaty, T. Culture of cells obtained by amniocentesis. *J. Lab. Clin. Med.* 73:355, 1969.

92. Vogel, F, and Ruthenberg, R. Spontaneous mutation in man. *Adv. Hum. Genet.* 5:223, 1975.

93. Waardenberg, P. J., and van der Busch, J. X-chromosomal ocular albinism in a Dutch family. *Ann. Hum. Genet.* 21:101, 1956.

94. Watson, J. D. *Molecular Biology of the Gene* (3rd ed.). Menlo Park, Calif.: Benjamin, 1976.

95. Watson, J. D., and Crick, F. H. C. A structure for deoxyribose nucleic acid. *Nature* 171:737, 1953.

96. Watson, J. D., and Crick, F. H. C. Genetical implications of the structure of deoxyribonucleic acid. *Nature* 171:964, 1953.

97. Weischselbaum, R. R., et al. New findings in the chromosome 13 long arm deletion syndrome and retinoblastoma. *Trans. Am. Acad. Ophthalmol. Otolaryngol.* 86:1191, 1979.

2

Biochemical Diagnosis of Genetic and Metabolic Eye Diseases

Suber S. Huang
P. C. Huang

PRIMARY VERSUS SECONDARY EYE DISEASE

Diseases throughout the body often manifest themselves in the eye. Seemingly mild and innocuous ocular or visual change may reflect serious systemic illness. Conversely, a disturbed metabolic process inflicting only a subtle effect on other parts of the body may develop into disabling ophthalmic manifestations. Diabetes mellitus is a well-known example, and similarly a gradual loss in visual field owing to paresis of the cranial nerves may reflect a more serious imbalance in pituitary hormones resulting from tumor formation. Corneal arcus, xanthelasma, and lipemia retinalis are often associated with hyperlipoproteinemia, a disease resulting in premature atherosclerosis.

Indeed, the relationship between various ocular manifestations and diseases not localized in the eye has been well documented; tetanic cataract and hypocalcemia, acute orbital cellulitis and general bacterial infection, marked eyelid and conjunctival edema and acquired syphilis, congenital cataract and rubella syndrome, and ocular toxocariasis and nematode endophthalmitis are further examples. Pallor of the conjunctiva, focal microfarcts of the retina, and hemorrhage are signs of anemia. Episcleritis and uveitis are often diagnostic for inflammatory bowel diseases. More pronounced symptoms of nutritional disease are exemplified by the appearance of Bitot's spots in the bulbar conjunctiva, keratomalacia, and night blindness, all caused by vitamin A deficiency. Anterior lenticonus is an ocular hallmark of Alport's syndrome, a hereditary disorder of progressive nephritis and sensorineural deafness readily detectable by examination of the crystalline lens after dilation of the pupils. In most cases sarcoidosis shows distinct ophthalmic involvements such as sarcoid granuloma of the bulbar conjunctiva and episclera, retinal periphlebitis, and papilledema. Papilledema, a symptom of swollen optic nerve head and elevation of disc tissue, may be due to intracranial, systemic, orbital, or ocular causes and occurs in several neurologic disorders including multiple sclerosis. Another neurologic disorder, myasthenia gravis, is distinguished by blepharoptosis and rapid eye movement.

Several autosomal dominant diseases are characterized by ophthalmic manifestations. Von Recklinghausen's disease is characterized by multiple uveal melanocytes, choroidal nevi, and plexiform fibromas of the eyelids or orbits that lead to a nonexpansile pulsating exophthalmos. Corneal nerves may be enlarged, and colored nodules may be found on the iris. Bourneville's disease (tuberous sclerosis) is typically shown through astrocytic hamartomas of the retina, and sometimes optic nerve glioma, although the former are harmless. Sturge-Weber syndrome (encephalotrigeminal angiomatosis) also produces hemangiomas of episclera and choroid, along with glaucoma. Von Hippel-Lindau disease (retinocerebellar angiomatosis) can be diagnosed in neurologically asymptomatic patients only through ophthalmoscopy. Occasional café au lait spots may be found, and bilateral retinal angioma is seen in 50 percent of patients with von Hippel-Lindau disease, the early sign of which is dilatation of retinal vessels, particularly the retinal veins. An autosomal recessive trait associated with DNA repair deficiency [173], ataxia telangiectasia (Louis-Bar

27

syndrome), is a form of phakomatosis the ophthalmic finding of which is that the conjunctiva is conspicuous. Oculomotor apraxia also is noticeable. Children born with aniridia and deletion in chromosome 11 have been shown to be most likely to develop Wilms' tumor in the kidney.

While the nature of most of these associations is as yet unclear, they illustrate that the eye is a health indicator. Except in those cases in which the eye is the only organ affected, eye disease can extend and reflect disorder elsewhere in the body. Insofar as the eye is a window through which the health of an individual can be viewed, most of the diseases involving the eye can be accurately diagnosed by ophthalmoscopic examinations. Which biochemical procedures are useful or necessary in diagnosis, and how are these procedures applicable to particular genetic eye diseases? These questions are the concerns of this chapter.

BIOCHEMISTRY OF THE EYE

This chapter confines its discussion to the field of metabolic disease with a genetic basis, rather than infectious or inflicted diseases caused by changes in metabolism such as nutritional deficiency, injury, or stress. Genetic diseases often can be defined biochemically. For this reason, a brief review of the biochemistry of the eye and of vision and its possible inborn errors is appropriate.

The eye is an interesting organ in that its structure and function can be reasonably defined in physical and chemical terms. As a well-differentiated photoreceptor equipped with flexible lenses, the eye functions by stereoscopically refracting and focusing light such that the image is focused on the retina. The image, sensed as a matrix of photons of varying intensity and wavelength, is programmed into spatial and temporal signals and transmitted through the connecting optic nerves and sensory organs to the brain, where the signals are decoded. The retinal neurons form a complex matrix with other structures of the eye including the cornea, lens, iris, ciliary body, and pigmented epithelium. The cornea consists of several layers of epithelial cells: epithelium, Bowman's membrane, stroma, Descemet's membrane, and endothelium. The fibrous epithelial cells can regenerate after injury but become anuclear upon aging. The stroma is made up of collagen, glycoproteins, and proteoglycans. Bowman's and Descemet's membranes are made up of collagen fibers also.

They are basal laminae instead of pure phospholipid membranes. Human lenses are encapsulated in these carbohydrate-rich coatings. It is the glycolytic activity of these cells that sustains the transparent property of the lens. Thus inborn errors in carbohydrate metabolism are particularly detrimental to this part of the eye. At least three such disorders have been associated with ocular findings: galactosuria, diabetes mellitus, and the mucopolysaccharidoses (including Hurler's syndrome).

The choroid, ciliary body, and iris constitute the uvea, which contains melanin pigments. The choroid provides nutrients to retinal photoreceptors via the retinal pigmented epithelium, and the ciliary body maintains intraocular pressure. The degree of melanin pigmentation in the iris determines its color. Iris sphincter and dilator muscles contract differentially in response to light. Rhodopsin, a pigment essential in photosensitivity, is also present in the iris.

The retina includes the pigmented epithelium, which is a monolayer of hexagonal cells interconnected by microvilli surrounding the photoreceptor cells. These microvilli serve to maintain the turnover of photoreceptor outer segments and phagocytotic activities. Rod and cone photoreceptors are the visual cells. In their outer segments are visual pigments, the required catabolic enzymes, and surface glycoprotein receptors. The outer segment is continuous with the rhodopsin-containing plasma membranes, which are folded into lobular layers. The inner segments provide the needed components for membrane assembly for the outer segment, which are transported through the connection formed by cilium. The ciliary connection is fragile, because of its chemical composition, and is readily dissociated by mechanical agitation of the retina.

Ail cells are confined by membranes and contain vesicles, both of which require lipid as a component. Disorders of lipid metabolism have been associated with a number of diseases having severe manifestations in the eye. Disorders of lipid storage affect the retina and optic nerve. Macular change has been seen in Tay-Sachs, Niemann-Pick, and Gaucher's diseases. Peripheral retinal changes of retinitis pigmentosa are associated with Refsum's disease. Xanthelasma and arcus lipoides can occur with essential hypercholesterolemia. Fabry's disease (angiokeratoma corporis diffusum universale), which shows irregular conjunctival and retinal veins and tortuous aneurysmal dilatation, is also attributed to a disturbance of the metabolism of a single lipid. Similarly, metachromatic leukodystrophy, a disease characterized by tapetoretinal degeneration, cherry-red macula, and optic atrophy, is the result of sulfatide lipidosis in which the conversion of sulfatides and cerebrosides is disturbed.

The retina also contains the synaptic terminus, which contains the endoplasmic reticulum, mitochondria, and synaptic vesicles. The latter are responsible for the release of neurotransmitters to the bipolar and horizontal cells in the dark. The bipolar cells connect the visual and ganglion cells, transmitting photosignals vertically. The horizontal cells serve as second-order neurons, mediating lateral communication between the vertical connections by connecting cone cells with their dendrites and rod cells with their axons. In addition, lateral interactions are mediated by amacrine cells in which neurotransmitters and neuropeptides have been identified. These molecules are crucial to the transmission of photosignals. Inborn defects in amino acid metabolism, and thus in peptide and protein synthesis, would affect these molecules. Disorders of this nature include cystinosis, homocystinuria, albinism, and alkaptonuria. Since proper synthesis of proteins is essential to the production of enzymes as well as cellular constituents, a deficiency would developmentally retard or affect ocular tissue differentiation and maturation.

Thus a genetic eye disease can be targeted at many ocular tissues or components. A biochemical lesion should be traceable, with the advent of molecular biology, to the alteration of a specific gene, whether in the coding or regulatory sequence. In this sense genetic eye diseases can be expected to be more widely understood as their corresponding molecular biology is understood. Although a genetic defect is classically detected through familial aggregation and pedigree analysis, a definitive diagnosis can now be made at the genomic (the gene), the transcriptional (RNA synthesis), and the translational (protein synthesis) levels.

DIAGNOSTIC ASSAYS

Biochemical Tests—Principles and Limitations

Biochemical procedures are useful in diagnosis as well as therapy, providing that the nature of the defect can be delineated. They are often needed to confirm or establish the diagnosis.

Classically, biochemical diagnostic tests measure the level of either a given enzyme or its substrate. In most cases enzyme deficiency or excess results in disease. Several excellent discussions of various diagnostic procedures can be found in the literature [8, 94, 108, 147, 149, 262, 310].

Molecular Biologic Assays

Assays using molecular biologic techniques have allowed detection of biochemical lesions at the DNA (genomic) or RNA (messenger) level [65, 174]. The rapid advances in human gene mapping have further facilitated these assays. Almost 100 precise chromosomal loci have been mapped. Many other genes have also been assigned to specific regions of various chromosomes, through both linkage or molecular studies. Diagnosis by recombinant DNA probes has been most successfully applied to the hemoglobinopathies and more recently extended to inborn hormonal diseases [8].

At least two forms of childhood tumor that are manifested in the eye can be detected by molecular assays. Translocation involving chromosomes 11 and 12 is detectable cytogenetically in some 55 percent of homozygotes with Wilms' disease. Specific loss of the allele c-Ha-*ras*-1, an oncogene, with concomitant duplication of a nonallelic sequence, has also been demonstrated with DNA probes [101, 201, 259, 270]. Similarly, in primary retinoblastoma, a common intraocular neoplasm of childhood, specific N-*myc* gene amplification has been shown to occur by titration with DNA probes [59, 213]. However, another form of tumor, neuroblastoma, also shows amplified N-*myc* genes [292]. The fact that both retinoblastoma and neuroblastoma originate from neural crest ectodermal cells [207] both suggests a common basis for the action of this oncogene and points out the limits of its applicability as a diagnostic marker. Rearrangements involving chromosome 13 in recessively inherited retinoblastoma [88] can be adequately demonstrated with appropriate gene probes [20, 59].

Gene probes are particularly sensitive when the defective gene product of interest is known biochemically. Thus, insulin and lens crystalline protein deficiency can be directly monitored using DNA probes consisting of their coding sequences. Human DNA sequences capable of restoring DNA repair activity to ultraviolet-damaged genetically deficient cells have recently been cloned [337]. These sequences share a 1.1-kilobase segment that may be the repair gene of interest and are thus potentially useful as probes for monitoring defects in xeroderma pigmentosum. It is not yet clear whether the lesion affects the structural or regulatory sequences of these genes.

Derangement in the regulatory sequence for metallothionein, a metal-binding protein, has been implicated in Wilson's disease and Menkes' syndrome, which also affect the eye. Menkes' syndrome (kinky-hair syndrome) is an X-linked disorder affecting copper metabolism. Increased avidity for copper, zinc, and cadmium in lymphoblasts and fibroblasts has been detected in most adult and fetal extrahepatic tissues [104]. An elevated level of metal in the cell induces a higher than usual level of metallothionein. This protein in turn increases the level of metal accumulation [275], resulting in the formation of the characteristic Kayser-Fleischer ring in the eye [180]. Since human metallothionein genes are located in chromosome 16 and Menkes' is an X-linked disorder, the regulation of metallothionein expression must function by a *trans*-acting mechanism [285].

Maternally inherited eye diseases are being examined for possible defects in the mitochondrial genome. Leber's optic atrophy, for instance, is characterized biochemically as a deficiency in thiosulfate-sulfur transferase, a mitochondrial enzyme. As a result, cyanide reduction metabolism is decreased. If mitochondrial genes code for this enzyme, the exact defect may be detected through molecular hybridization with the now available mitochondrial DNA sequence probes (Zhu, Maumenee, and Huang, in preparation).

In this approach specific DNA fragments are generated by treatment with restriction endonucleases and, upon agarose or polyacrylamide gel electrophoresis, the fragments are transferred to nitrocellulose or other solid support matrices for hybridization analysis [308]. Similarly various species of messenger RNAs (mRNAs) are separated by electrophoresis and likewise transferred to cellulose paper that couples RNA tightly. The RNA so bound is then ready for hybrid monitor and titration using special DNA probes—a procedure known as northern blotting. The matrix material has extended from nitrocellulose to include diazobenzyloxymethyl and aminophenylthio ether–based filters, each of which is useful under different experimental conditions. The limitation of the Southern hydridization procedure is that it can detect possible alterations in gene dosage and position of a given gene but not its location on a particular chromosome or its linkage group.

Mapping of genes on specific chromosomes,

however, has been possible through the availability of panels of Chinese hamster–human cell hybrid lines, each containing a single, specific human chromosome with various terminal deletions [265]. A suspected deletion can therefore be detected by Southern blot analysis with a given gene probe.

Mapping a specific gene by chromosome sorting has been facilitated by the development of a high-resolution dual-laser sorter that separates human chromosomes according to their size and fixes them on a nitrocellulose matrix [211]. The separated chromosomes selectively react to given labeled gene probes, hence locating the desired gene directly. Such a recent approach has been successfully applied to locate the gene for muscle myophosphorylase, which is deficient in McArdle's disease, and assign it to the long arm of chromosome 11 (q13–qter).

Choice of Assay Material

Tissues, blood, and urine are the most commonly available specimens for biochemical assays. It is important to bear in mind that not all genes are expressed in all tissues, so the judicious choice of material for diagnostic tests is crucial.

Blood is useful only for defects in erythrocytes, leukocytes, platelets, granulocytes, and plasma; urine, for detection of substrates, such as amino acids and proteins, that are excreted through the renal system. Tissues differ in their marker proteins. Epithelial cells, for instance, contain keratin, which is absent in fibrolasts. Fibroblasts, on the other hand, show characteristic HLA (major histocompatibility antigen) haplotypes, which are very useful in identification. Normal human fibroblast cells, however, have only a limited life span in culture [329].

The stage of development from which samples are to be taken for analysis depends on the need and availability. For prenatal diagnosis, fetoscopy has been successful in obtaining fetal blood by placental aspiration and skin fibroblasts by biopsy. The procedure involves puncturing a vessel on the chorionic plate to execute direct aspiration from the cord, which usually results in no maternal contamination. A more general and reliable procedure, however, has been the use of amniotic fluid cells, which are obtained by transabdominal amniocentesis and can be used directly for analysis or upon culturing. Chorionic villi of fetal origin may be obtained transvaginally at 6 to 10 weeks of pregnancy. Amniocentesis, however, may be performed only after the 16th week of gestation. Prenatal and adult samples can readily include fibroblasts or lymphocytes, which are analyzed upon culture. The increased use of tears in microassays is also noteworthy.

Newer Assays

A number of novel and more sensitive assays are being developed that may become more generally available as clinical diagnostic tests. These include microassays for enzymes using fluorogenic amplifiers. Batteries of monoclonal antibodies that allow a more precise diagnosis of specific lesions in proteins and enzymes are also being prepared. Immunodetection of proteins and enzymes has been facilitated by a transfer procedure similar to the techniques used for DNA and RNA immobilization, in which proteins (antigens) are immobilized on filters after electrophoretic separation. Specific antibodies identify the protein in question. Hence the procedure is both qualitative and quantitative, something not afforded by other assays such as the enzyme-linked immunosorbent assay (ELISA) and peroxidase-antiperoxidase. This procedure, known as western blotting [36], is nevertheless limited to cell extracts. Conjunctival biopsy specimens or frozen sections of tissues must be used in parallel to ascertain tissue specificity in the accumulation of a given enzyme or protein. This can be done by histochemical [319] or immunochemical [73] methods. The successful use of avidin and biotin represents a newer approach that may eventually replace radioimmunoassays. Subpopulations of damaged ganglion cells in mouse retina can be traced by examining the heavy neurofilaments with antibodies against their specific 200-kilodalton subunits [87]. The observed pathologic changes may be due to ectopic phosphorylation of the neurofilament in response to injury.

Interpretation of Results

Most biologic assay results can be affected by many factors. A useful diagnostic test must be able to demonstrate that the defect is present in the proband or affected relatives. In many assays, including those using DNA probes, one should rule out polymorphism, that is, spontaneous variation in the amino acid sequence of a protein or in the nucleotide sequence of a gene. It would be helpful if the heterozygosity of both parents could be determined for the causal gene. In all assays reference standards from controls should always be included, and for newer procedures it is advisable to share split samples with expert laboratories so that the results can be compared. In general multiple substrates and procedures for a given enzyme should be used if available, within the limits of cost and effectiveness [279].

In designing a diagnostic test and interpreting its results, the problem of expressivity for tissue-specific gene products must also be considered. The cells used must be carefully checked for contamination, particularly by *Mycoplasma*. The absence or partial deficiency of an enzyme may reflect its instability or its concentration in the assay. A number of enzymes, such as β-hexosaminidase and α-galactosidase A, are known to degrade rapidly in cell extracts because of proteases. Further, the addition of exogenous albumin to a diluted enzyme solution helps to stabilize the enzyme's activity. This is often done in restriction and other enzyme assays.

GENETIC DISEASES WITH DEFINABLE BIOCHEMICAL LESIONS

Hereditary eye diseases can be grouped according to their site of manifestation (Table 2-1), their biochemical defects (Table 2-2), or the alteration in known enzyme activity (Table 2-3). In the remainder of this chapter these diseases are presented in alphabetical order. Each disease is numbered according to the classification assigned to it in McKusick's catalog of diseases of mendelian inheritance [234]. The main features of the disease, its chemical pathology, and methods of biochemical detection are discussed.

20010 Abetalipoproteinemia (Bassen-Kornzweig Syndrome)

The hypobetalipoproteinemias consist of two types, both affecting plasma lipoproteins containing apolipoprotein B (apo B), very-low-density lipoprotein (VLDL), and low-density lipoprotein (LDL). Abetalipoproteinemia is characterized by an absence of chylomicrons, VLDL, and LDL. Individuals with hypolipoproteinemia in the homozygous state are indistinguishable from those with abetalipoproteinemia. However, heterozygous individuals have low VLDL and LDL, while heterozygotes with abetalipoproteinemia have normal levels of these lipoproteins [160].

Abetalipoproteinemia has a 2 : 1 male-to-female ratio and presents in infancy with

Table 2-1. *Genetic Disorders and Major Locations of Lesions in the Eyes*

McKusick catalogue number*	Location and disorder
	Eyelids
10480	Amyloidosis (heredofamilial, primary)
17610	Porphyria, hepatic (cutanea tarda hereditaria)
24710	Urbach-Wiethe syndrome (lipid proteinosis)
27870	Xeroderma pigmentosum
	Cornea: Epithelium
22390	Dysautonomia, familial (Riley-Day syndrome)
30150	Fabry's disease (angiokeratoma corporis diffusum)
25887	Hyperornithinemia (chorioretinal gyrate atrophy)
	Cornea: Stroma and Descemet's Membrane
	Cystinosis
21980	Infantile
21990	Juvenile
22000	Adult
14440	Hyperlipoproteinemia type II
24590	Lecithin-cholesterol acyltransferase (LCAT) deficiency
21780	Macular dystrophy (Groenouw's type II)
12220	Lattice dystrophy
	Mucopolysaccharidoses
25280	Type I-H (Hurler; MPS I)
25310	Type I-S (Scheie; formerly MPS V)
25300	Type IV (Morquio; MPS IV)
25320	Type VI (Maroteaux-Lamy; MPS VI)
25270	Mucopolysaccharidoses, unclassified
25260	Pseudo-Hurler polydystrophy (mucolipidosis III)
20540	Tangier disease
27790	Wilson's disease
	Conjunctiva and Sclera
20350	Alkaptonuria
	Porphyria
26370	Congenital erythropoietic (CEP; Günther's disease)
17620	Variegate

Table 2-1 *(continued)*

McKusick catalogue number*	Location and disorder
	Lens: Cataracts
23020	Galactokinase deficiency
23040	Galactosemia (galactose 1-phosphate uridyl transferase deficiency)
30590	Glucose 6-phosphate dehydrogenase (G6PD) deficiency
30900	Lowe's oculocerebrorenal syndrome
30080	Pseudohypoparathyroidism and pseudopseudohypoparathyroidism
27670	Tyrosinemia
	Lens: Dislocation
23620	Homocystinuria
23870	Hyperlysinemia
27230	Sulfite oxidase deficiency
	Retina: Pigment Epithelium
	Albinism
	Oculocutaneous
20310	Tyrosinase negative (type I)
20320	Tyrosinase positive (type II)
30050	Ocular albinism
	Other types of albinism
	Gangliosidoses
23060	GM$_1$ type II (juvenile generalized)
23070	GM$_2$ type III (juvenile form)
23630	Hooft's disease
	Hypobetalipoproteinemias
20010	Bassen-Kornzweig syndrome (abetalipoproteinemia)
—	Hypobetalipoproteinemia, congenital (familial low-density lipoprotein deficiency)
	Mucopolysaccharidoses
30990	Type II (Hunter)
25290	Type III (Sanfilippo)
26650	Refsum's disease
	Retina: Macula
20420	Batten's disease (neuronal ceroidlipofuscinosis; NCL)
22800	Farber's lipogranulomatosis
	Gangliosidoses

Table 2-1 *(continued)*

McKusick catalogue number[*]	Location and disorder
27280	GM$_2$ type I (Tay-Sachs disease)
26880	GM$_2$ type II (Sandhoff's disease)
23050	GM$_1$ type I (generalized gangliosidosis)
23220	Glycogen storage disease type I (von Gierke's disease)
—	Goldberg-Cotlier syndrome [139]
24550	Lactosyl ceramidosis
	Metachromatic leukodystrophy (MLD)
25010	Late infantile form
24990	Variant form (MLD variant)
25720	Niemann-Pick disease, infantile form
27800	Wolman's disease
	Retina: Vasculature
22210	Diabetes mellitus
	Hemoglobinopathies
14170	Sickle cell anemia (Hb S-S)
14170	Sickle cell trait (Hb A-S)
14170	Sickle cell hemoglobin C disease (Hb S-C)
27350	S-thalassemia
	Hyperlipoproteinemias
23860	Type I
14450	Type III
14460	Type IV
23840	Type V
17600	Porphyria, acute intermittent
	Optic Nerve
24520	Globoid cell leukodystrophy (Krabbe's disease)
23900	Hyperphosphatasia (juvenile Paget's disease)
24150	Hypophosphatasia

[*]See McKusick [234].
Source: From E. R. Berman [22].

Table 2-2. *Biochemical Catalog of Genetic Eye Diseases**

Disorders of Amino Acid Metabolism

20350 Alkaptonuria
10480 Amyloidosis (heredofamilial, primary)
21450 Chédiak-Higashi syndrome
Cystinosis
21980 Infantile
21990 Juvenile
22000 Adult
22390 Dysautonomia, familial (Riley-Day syndrome)
23620 Homocystinuria
23870 Hyperlysinemia
25887 Hyperornithemia
12220 Lattice dystrophy
27230 Sulfite oxidase deficiency
20540 Tangier disease
27670 Tyrosinemia

Disorders of Carbohydrate Metabolism

Albinism
  Oculocutaneous
20310 Tyrosinase-negative (type I)
20320 Tyrosinase-positive (type II)
30050 Ocular albinism
  Other types of albinism
22210 Diabetes mellitus
23020 Galactokinase deficiency
23040 Galactosemia (galactose 1-phosphate uridyl
  transferase deficiency)
30590 Glucose 6-phosphate dehydrogenase (G6PD)
  deficiency
23220 Glycogen storage disease type I (von Gierke's
  disease)
24550 Lactosyl ceramidosis—Goldberg-Cotlier
  syndrome

Disorders of Lipid and Lipoprotein Metabolism

Hypobetalipoproteinemias
20010 Bassen-Kornsweig syndrome
  (abetalipoproteinemia)
—Hypobetalipoproteinemia, congenital (familial low-
  density lipoprotein deficiency)
23630 Hooft's disease
Hyperlipoproteinemias
23860 Type I
14440 Type II
14450 Type III
14460 Type IV
23840 Type V
24590 Lecithin-cholesterol acyltransferase (LCAT)
  deficiency
26650 Refsum's disease
20540 Tangier disease
24711 Urbach-Wiethe syndrome (lipid proteinosis)
27800 Wolman's disease

Disorders of Lysosomal Enzymes

20420 Batten's disease (neuronal ceroid lipofuscinosis,
  NCL)

30150 Fabry's disease (angiokeratoma corporis
  diffusum)
22800 Farber's lipogranulomatosis
Gangliosidoses
23050 GM$_1$ type I (generalized gangliosidosis)
23060 GM$_1$ type II (juvenile generalized)
27280 GM$_2$ type I (Tay-Sachs disease)
26880 GM$_2$ type II (Sandhoff's disease)
23070 GM$_2$ type III (juvenile form)
13730 Gaucher's disease
24520 Globoid cell leukodystrophy (Krabbe's disease)
21780 Macular dystrophy (Groenouw's type II)
Metachromatic leukodystrophy (MLD)
25010 Late infantile form
24990 Variant form (MLD variant)
Mucopolysaccharidoses
25280 Type I-H (Hurler; MPS I)
25310 Type I-S (Scheie; formerly MPS V)
30990 Type II (Hunter)
25290 Type III (Sanfilippo)
25300 Type IV (Morquio; MPS IV)
25320 Type VI (Maroteaux-Lamy; MPS VI)
25322 Type VII (Sly)
25270 Mucopolysaccharidoses, unclassified
25720 Niemann-Pick disease, infantile form
25260 Pseudo-Hurler polydystrophy (mucolipidosis III)

*Disorders of Purine or Pyrimidine Metabolism or
DNA Repair Pathway*

27870 Xeroderma pigmentosum

Disorders of Metal Metabolism

27790 Wilson's disease

Disorders of Steroid Metabolism

30080 Pseudohypoparathyroidism and
  pseudopseudohypoparathyroidism

*Disorders of Porphyrin and Heme Metabolism and
Blood Formation*

Porphyria
17600 Porphyria, acute intermittent
17610 Porphyria, hepatic (cutanea tarda hereditaria)
17620 Variegate
Hemoglobinopathies
14170 Sickle cell anemia (Hb S-S)
14170 Sickle cell trait (Hb A-S)
14170 Sickle cell hemoglobin C disease (Hb S-C)
27350 S-thalassemia

Miscellaneous Disorders

26370 Congenital erythropoietic porphyria (CEP;
  Günther's disease)
23900 Hyperphosphatasia (juvenile Paget's disease)
24150 Hypophosphatasia

*Numbering system is from McKusick [234].

Table 2-3. *Enzyme Changes in Genetic Eye Diseases*

Enzyme deficiency	Disease	Site affected
Tyrosinase	Albinism	Eye as a whole
Argininosuccinase	Kinky-hair syndrome (Menkes')	Eyelids
Carbamoyl phosphate synthetase	Hyperammonemia	Ptosis
D-Glyceric dehydrogenase	Oxalosis; hyperoxaluria types I and II	Muscles (myositis)
Ceramide galactosidase	Fabry's disease (angiokeratoma corporis diffusum)	Cornea, iris (epithelial opacities, hyphema)
β-Galactosidase	Gangliosidosis; Landing's disease; pseudo-Hurler polydystrophy	Cornea, retina (epithelial and stromal clouding, cherry-red spot of the macula)
β-Galactosidase	Hunter's disease (MPS II)	Retina (tapetoretinal degeneration)
Homogentisic acid oxidase	Alkaptonuria (ochronosis)	Sclera (pigmentation)
Galactokinase	Juvenile cataract	Lens (cataract)
Galactose 1-phosphate 4-uridyl transferase	Galactosemia	Lens (cataract)
Cystathionine synthetase	Homocystinuria	Lens (subluxation, excessive myopia)
Sulfite oxidase	Lens ectopia	Lens (subluxation)
Sphingomyelinase	Niemann-Pick disease; tyrosinemia	Retina (cherry-red spot)
Uroporphyrinogen decarboxylase	Porphyria	Eyelid
Phytanic acid hydroxylase	Refsum's disease	Retina
Hexosaminidase	Tay-Sachs disease	Retina (cherry-red spot)
β-Glucoronidase, N-acetyl-β-glucosaminidase, α-fucosidase	Sanfilippo's syndrome (MPS III)	Retina (tapetoretinal degeneration)
Acid lipase	Wolman's disease	Retina (periphery)
Glucose 6-phosphate dehydrogenase (G6PD)	G6PD deficiency	Retina, (vascular ischemia, vitreous hemorrhage)
Alkaline phosphatase	Hypophosphatasia	Optic nerve (optic atrophy, exophthalmos)
Alkaline and acid phosphatase	Juvenile Paget's disease	Retina, optic nerve (optic atrophy, angioid streaks)
Pyruvate carboxylase	Leigh's syndrome (infantile subacute necrotizing encephalomyelopathy)	Optic nerve (optic atrophy, ptosis)
Arylsulfatase A	Metachromatic leukodystrophy	Optic nerve, retina (optic atrophy, macular degeneration)
Cerebroside sulfotransferase	Krabbe's disease	Optic nerve (atrophy)
Diphenylnitrohydroazine (DPNH) and ATPase	Canavan's disease, van Bogaert-Bertrand type	Optic nerve (atrophy)
UV endonuclease	Xeroderma pigmentosum	Eyelid and periocular area (sensitivity to UV light)

MPS = mucopolysaccharidosis; UV = ultraviolet.

steatorrhea, hepatomegaly, devastating psychomotor retardation, anemia with acanthocytosis, and numerous ocular findings. A generalized retinal degeneration with night blindness, retinitis pigmentosa, nystagmus, and ophthalmoplegia are common. Ptosis and posterior polar cataracts have occasionally been noted [57, 160]. Massive doses of vitamin A have been shown to partially or completely reverse abnormalities of the electroretinogram and of dark adaptation [146]. Vitamin E deficiency has been likewise linked to photoreceptor changes, retinal pigment epithelium (RPE) changes, and retinitis pigmentosa [245]. Whether vitamin E will prevent the development of retinopathy remains to be seen.

CHEMICAL PATHOLOGY

There is an absence or diminution of nearly all plasma lipids owing to a presumed defect in apo B synthesis or in its intracellular assembly with lipid [160]. Vitamin A, vitamin E, cholesterol, and phospholipid levels are extremely low. Chylomicrons, VLDL, and LDL are virtually absent. Vitamin deficiency and lack of lipid account for nearly all the abnormalities in Bassen-Kornzweig syndrome.

BIOCHEMICAL DETECTION

Serum cholesterol, triglyceride, and lipoprotein levels should be tested sequentially to determine if an individual is afflicted with this disorder. Confirmation of the diagnosis is made immunochemically using antibetalipoprotein to demonstrate the lack of apo B in plasma. Obligate heterozygotes must be tested to differentiate those with normal LDL from heterozygotes with familial hypobetalipoproteinemia, who will demonstrate lower than normal levels of LDL [160].

20350 Alkaptonuria

The main clinical features of alkaptonuria, an inborn error of metabolism that was first described by Garrod in 1902, are the darkening of standing urine, black ochronotic pigmentation of cartilage and connective tissues, and arthritis, characteristically of the spine [122]. Darkening of urine, even in infancy, is diagnostic, while the other signs may take decades before presentation [196].

The most striking ocular abnormality is manifested by a bilateral, dense, brownish black triangular pigmentation of the eyes midway between the limbus and the insertions of the horizontal rectus muscles. Subepithelial pigment globules that may resemble oil drops can be seen at the corneal-scleral limbus, and the episclera may contain pigmented lesions resembling pigmented pingueculas [196]. Vision is unaffected in alkaptonuria. Other important diagnoses in the differential include transcleral extension of a melanoma [304] and long-term exposure to hydroquinones or quinones [6].

CLINICAL PATHOLOGY

A deficiency of homogentisic acid oxidase leads to the accumulation of homogentisic acid, which readily oxidizes to benzoquinoneacetic acid (see Fig. 2-6). Polymers of this melanin-like pigment have a high affinity for connective tissue containing collagen [239]. The resultant breakdown of normal collagen produces potentially crippling degenerative joint disease. The mechanism of the predilection of alkaptonuria for hydroxylysine-rich collagen is unknown, but the inhibition of lysyl hydroxylase activity may play a role [246].

BIOCHEMICAL DETECTION

Since urine is seldom kept standing and alkaptonuria is asymptomatic early in the disease, an individual may live well into adulthood without recognizing that he or she has the disease. Screening for urinary homogentisic acid by thin-layer or paper chromatography is usually diagnostic with up to 8 gm of acid excreted daily [197, 281]. Enzymatic analysis allows precise quantitation in urine and other bodily fluids either by directly assaying [208] or by spectrophotometrically measuring the covalent addition compounds formed as products of homogentisic acid and diethylene triamine [227].

10480 Amyloidosis (Heredofamilial, Primary)

The systemic familial amyloidoses are autosomal dominant diseases that primarily show neurologic, renal, or cardiac involvement. The exception is the familial Mediterranean fever type, which is inherited as an autosomal recessive trait and occurs particularly among Sephardic Jews of Mediterranean origin [237]. In a recent study of 226 patients with systemic generalized amyloidosis the median age at onset of disease was 65 years, with 99 percent over the age of 40. Weakness, fatigue, and occasional profound weight loss were the most common initial findings. Palpable liver and macroglossia were the most common physical findings. Cardiac involvement accounted for 40 percent of the deaths, and the median survival from time of detection was 12 months [206]. The most common ocular involvement is the deposition of amyloid in the eyelids, although purpura and lenticular opacities have also been described [185, 206, 310]. Lattice dystrophy is unrelated to systemic amyloidosis but nonetheless represents an ocular variant in which changes are confined solely to the eyelids and perhaps the vitreous.

CHEMICAL PATHOLOGY AND BIOCHEMICAL DETECTION

Clinical manifestations of amyloidosis result from compression atrophy caused by the extracellular deposition of inert beta-pleated 70- to 100-A protein fibrils [194]. The major component of amyloid in heredofamilial amyloidosis is virtually identical to the variable portion of a monoclonal light-chain protein (the Bence Jones protein). However, an immunoperoxidase technique discloses prealbumin as an amyloid component [219]. Deposition is pericollagenous for amyloidosis I and II but perireticular for the Mediterranean fever type [234]. Lavie and colleagues have suggested that monocytes play an important role in amyloid degradation [210]. Amyloid has an amorphous appearance by light microscopy and exhibits positive staining with Congo red, as well as characteristic red-green birefringence under polarized light [206]. The diagnosis is determined by the clinical picture, optical staining properties of biopsy specimens, and evidence of familial involvement.

30150 Angiokeratoma Corporis Diffusum

See Fabry's Disease.

20010 Bassen-Kornzweig Syndrome

See Abetalipoproteinemia.

20420 Batten's Disease (Neuronal Ceroid Lipofuscinosis)

Neuronal ceroid lipofuscinosis [347] describes a disorder in which ceroid and lipofuscin (two autofluorescent lipopigments) accumulate in the nerve cell perikaryon and in other cells [26]. Of the four

clinical phenotypes now recognized, three present with visual disturbances: (1) The infantile form (Jansky-Bielschowsky) has a rapid onset at 2 years to demise at 5 years. It is the most common form. (2) The juvenile form (Spielmeyer-Vogt) has its onset at 4 to 8 years and a progressive neurologic deterioration leading to death over a span of about 10 years. (3) The adult form is poorly characterized [26].

Seizures and motor, speech, and visual impairment followed by rapid intellectual regression, blindness, and cerebellar dysfunction are nonspecific neurologic findings in the adult form. All patients of the infantile group are blind by the age of 2 years and have optic atrophy, retinal dystrophy, and, in most cases, an extinguished electroretinogram. The juvenile type is notable for the presence of optic atrophy accompanied by macular pigmentary degeneration at an early age [26]. A cherry-red spot is *not* seen in this disorder, although the loss of the foveal red reflex may be an early sign. In general, the picture is one of complete disorganization of the outer segment of the retina [309].

CHEMICAL PATHOLOGY

The biochemical basis for the deposition of autofluorescent ceroid and lipofuscin granules in neuronal tissue is still uncertain. One theory is that this material represents a natural lysosome-derived residual body produced by the nonenzymatic peroxidation of unsaturated fatty acids [102]. Rectal, skeletal muscle, or sural nerve biopsy demonstrates distinct ultrastructural abnormalities in each of the three early forms. The infantile form is characterized by multinucleated phagocyte infiltration with a coarse cytoplasm. In the late infantile form the cytoplasm is filled with densely packed curvilinear bodies. In the juvenile form characteristic "fingerprints" are usually seen [26].

BIOCHEMICAL DETECTION

There are no specific tests for the diagnosis of Batten's disease. Blood cultures of leukocytes may show intense azurophilic staining, and skin fibroblast cultures may show metachromasia [72, 85].

HETEROZYGOTE DETECTION

In a study of 85 individuals in 17 families, 25 with Batten's disease, all parents of affected individuals showed leukocytic granulations [236]. Estimation of the number of azurophilic granules in circulating neutrophils is a crude but useful method of heterozygote detection.

22800 Ceramidase Deficiency

See Farber's Lipogranulomatosis.

25887 Chorioretinal Gyrate Atrophy

An extremely interesting disorder is well described by its main clinical sign, chorioretinal gyrate atrophy, a name given for the curved circular segments of atrophic retina. An autosomal recessive disorder, it is found particularly in Finland and in people of Finnish ancestry [196]. Night blindness presents by age 4 and progresses to total debility by the fourth decade [252].

CHEMICAL PATHOLOGY

The defect that causes the accumulation of ornithine, an amino acid not found in any protein, is a deficiency of ornithine aminotransferase. It is unlikely that ornithine toxicity is primarily responsible for retinal degeneration, since other causes of hyperornithinemia do not cause gyrate atrophy [196].

BIOCHEMICAL PATHOLOGY

Deficiency of ornithine aminotransferase has been shown using fibroblast skin culture [257], and a test for prenatal diagnosis is available [299].

Cystinosis: 21980 Infantile, 21990 Juvenile, 22000 Adult

Cystinosis is a recessively inherited lysosomal storage disorder in which there is a high level of intracellular free cystine but plasma levels are well below saturation. Cystinosis is unique in that, unlike other lysosomal storage diseases, lysosomal acid hydrolase plays no role in the metabolism of cystine [234].

Three types of cystinosis have been described: infantile, juvenile, and adult [234, 286, 291]. The infantile type is the most severe and is marked by failure to thrive and progressive Fanconi-type renal tubular dysfunction starting at about 5 months of age [49]. Affected children have massive systemic intraorgan cystine deposition, but renal deficiency in tubular absorption of water, phosphate, sodium, bicarbonate, glucose, and amino acids leads to severe hypokalemia, acidosis, uremia, and ultimately cardiovascular collapse within the first decade of life [49, 291]. Other signs include rickets and hypopigmentation of skin and hair. Surprisingly, cystinotic patients have shown no increased susceptibility to infection [286, 291].

The cornea, conjunctiva, and retina show characteristic changes and often establish the diagnosis [49, 345, 346]. Severe photophobia develops in most affected children within the first few years of life. Slit-lamp examination shows a carpet of birefringent crystals that reveals preferential localization of cystine throughout the entire peripheral stroma and in the anterior half to two-thirds of the central stroma. This finding suggests that crystal deposition may derive primarily from the limbal blood supply, tears, and aqueous humor. Although the needle-shaped crystals observed in the cornea and sclera have yet to be identified, the rectangular and hexagonal crystals of the conjunctiva and uvea have been determined to be L-cystine by x-ray diffraction [114]. In the conjunctiva the crystals are more prominent in the bulbar conjunctiva and fornix and have a ground-glass appearance. The clinical appearance of the cornea and conjunctiva is consistent and appears in all forms of cystinosis [344].

Peripheral retinopathy is a consistent finding only in the infantile form of cystinosis. A generalized pattern of depigmentation in the RPE occurs peripherally, with superimposed pigment clumps in an irregular distribution. Early in the disease the region behind the equator may thus appear normal [344]. The retinal changes may precede corneal changes by many months and may thus be of special diagnostic importance [345]. The visualization of retinopathy in one case allowed the diagnosis of cystinosis at 5 weeks of age [286, 346].

CHEMICAL PATHOLOGY

Compartmentalization of cystine within the lysosome appears to be the primary manifestation of cystinosis. Experiments with cultured cystinotic fibroblasts, uncultured cystinotic leukocytes, and fibroblasts and leukocytes of healthy heterozygotes have failed to demonstrate crystalline deposits [286, 291]. Numerous electron microscopic studies have also demonstrated cystine crystals or noncrystalline amorphous inclusions within lysosomes of cystinotic conjunctiva, cornea, kidney, lamina propria, and lymphocytes [49, 188, 286, 291]. The fact that the lysosomal membrane is relatively impermeable to unmetabolized amino acids with a molecular weight greater than 200 suggests that a molecular mechanism that normally allows the efflux of cystine or its metabolism may be defective in cystinosis [155].

BIOCHEMICAL DETECTION

Cystinosis is confirmed by demonstrating increased intracellular free cystine in leukocytes, cultured fibroblasts, or biopsy specimens of conjunctiva, spleen, liver, kidney, or lymph node [42]. A comparatively simple technique is the determination of half-cystine content in conjunctival biopsies: cystinosis, 5 to >30 mol/gm wet, compared to only 0.4 mol/gm in heterozygous individuals [291, 346]. A noninvasive diagnostic technique using infrared spectroscopy of hair has recently been applied to diagnose 5 patients with cystinosis [226].

DETECTION OF HETEROZYGOTES

While heterozygotes can be identified using either fibroblasts or leukocytes [288], Schneider and coworkers recommend using leukocytes for the determination of free cystine [287]. Mean intracellular cystine content of heterozygotes is elevated to five to six times normal and is concentrated in the lysosomal fraction of cells, which again suggest a lysosomal membrane defect [286, 291].

PRENATAL DETECTION

Amniocentesis is now a standard procedure for prenatal screening for cystinosis. Cultured amniotic cells are pulse-labeled and grown in media containing (^{35}S)-cystine. Label is incorporated into protein, glutathione, cysteine, and, to a small degree, cystine [286, 291]. Cystinotic cells, however, show greatly increased uptake [289]. The technique is easy and requires less than 48 hours to perform.

JUVENILE CYSTINOSIS

Patients with juvenile cystinosis share the following characteristics with the infantile type: the presence of crystals in the bone marrow, crystalline deposits in the cornea and sclera, and an autosomal mode of inheritance. Onset of the other manifestation is between 18 months and 17 years

and is variable in its severity. Patients generally exhibit near-normal growth patterns and have a more slowly progressing and milder form of glomerular insufficiency rather than the full-blown Fanconi's syndrome. Photophobia, retinopathy, and pigmentary changes of the skin are variably present [142, 286, 291]. As in infantile cystinosis the level of intracellular free cystine is elevated in leukocytes [42, 286, 291].

ADULT CYSTINOSIS

The primary distinction between the adult, benign form of cystinosis and the infantile and juvenile nephropathic forms is the failure of the adult form to express either nephropathic or retinopathic changes. Intracellular crystalline deposits in the cornea, conjunctiva, leukocytes, and bone marrow exist but cause no disability. Intracellular cystine levels appear to be lower than with the nephropathic variants and perhaps reflect the variability of gene expression in this fascinating disorder [288, 291].

22210 Diabetes Mellitus

Only a brief note will be added here to the enormous volume of literature on diabetes. The ocular involvements in this disease are well known to all ophthalmologists and are beyond the scope of this chapter. Although it is obvious that an important genetic component exists, the mode of inheritance is obscure. Recessive, dominant, multifactorial, and "susceptibility" hypotheses may each have validity, as multiple distinct entities probably exist under the heading of diabetes mellitus [278]. Recently three different models of insulin-dependent diabetes mellitus were used to present evidence for the linkage of two different loci: HLA, properdin factor B, and glyoxalase on chromosome 6 and the Kidd blood group on chromosome 2 [164]. A multifactorial inheritance is most likely, but until a specific marker is identified for diabetes susceptibility, the complete story will remain untold [109].

CHEMICAL PATHOLOGY

Diabetes mellitus is characterized by a constellation of effects stemming from the relative or absolute deficiency of insulin and the relative or absolute excess of glucagon. In both type 1 (insulin-dependent) and type 2 (non-insulin-dependent) diabetes, hyperglycemia and hormonal derangements produce chronic metabolic abnormalities especially affecting the eyes, kidneys, nerves, and vasculature.

22390 Dysautonomia, Familial (Riley-Day Syndrome)

Familial dysautonomia (FD) is a rare autosomal recessive disorder characterized clinically by dysfunction of the sensory and autonomic nervous system [50, 130]. The disorder is found mainly, but not exclusively, in Jews of Ashkenazic and eastern European origin, with death usually occurring by the second decade. It is recognized clinically by lack of tearing, emotional lability, paroxysmal hypertension, increased sweating, cold hands and feet, blotching of the skin, and drooling [234, 273]. The tetrad of opththalmologic signs is alacrima, corneal hypoesthesia and exodeviations, with methacholine-induced mitosis [141]. Ulceration may occur secondarily.

CHEMICAL PATHOLOGY

Familial dysautonomia is characterized pathologically by degeneration of sensory and autonomic ganglia and loss of unmyelinated and small myelinated fibers in sensory nerves. Patients with FD have decreased or absent dopamine-β-hydroxyl-

ase (DBH), the enzyme that converts dopamine to norepinephrine [12]. This results in greatly elevated levels of excreted homovanillic acid (HVA) and decreased or absent vanillylmandelic acid (VMA) and 3-methoxy-4-hydroxyphenylethyleneglycol (HMPG). The elevated HVA arises as a breakdown product of alternate dopa and dopamine pathways, while the greatly decreased levels of VMA and HMPG reflect the lack of norepinephrine and epinephrine production (Fig. 2-1). A qualitative (but not quantitative) abnormality of the beta subunit of nerve growth factor has also been reported [301], which suggests a precursor or beta subunit processing defect.

BIOCHEMICAL DETECTION

Both two-dimensional paper chromatography and gas-liquid chromatography can be used for the quantitative assay of urinary VMA, HVA, and HMPG. The use of age-matched controls is mandatory as large differences in the ratio of excreted

Fig. 2-1. *Abbreviated scheme of catecholamine metabolism in adrenal medulla and sympathetic nerve endings. In familial dysautonomia, the deficiency in dopamine-β-hydroxylase activity results in increased urinary excretion of HVA and decreased excretion of HMPG and VMA. (From E. R. Berman [22].)*

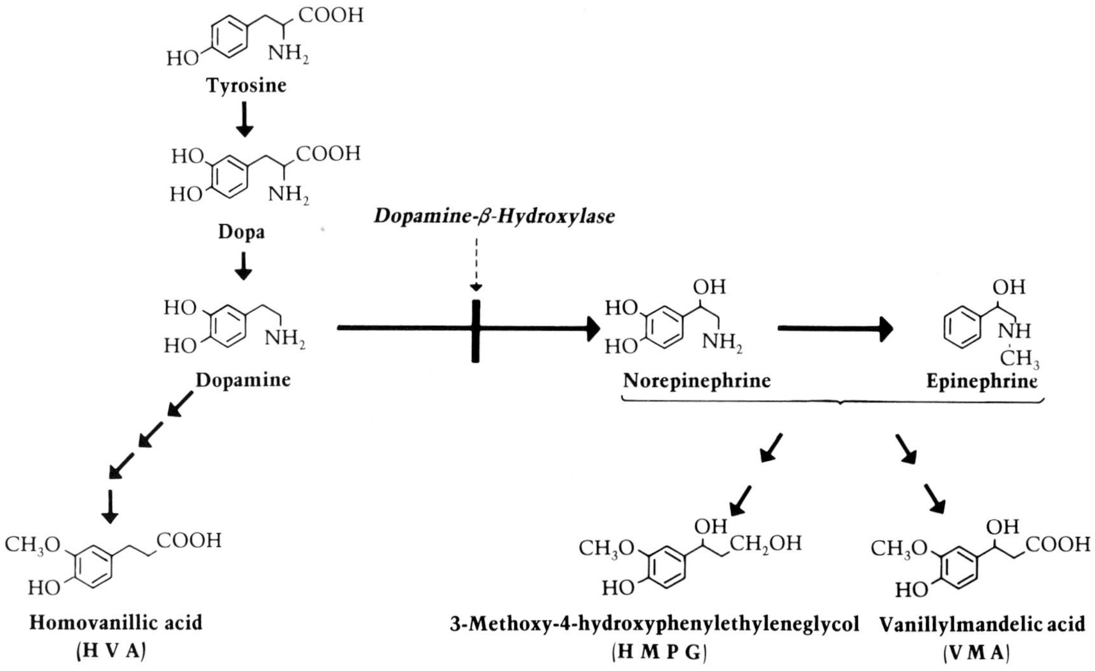

HVA to VMA and HMPG between normal subjects and affected individuals occur only in young children under 2 or 3 years of age [22].

30150 Fabry's Disease (Angiokeratoma Corporis Diffusum)

Fabry's angiokeratoma is an X-linked sphingolipid storage disease caused by a defect in the lysosomal hydrolase α-galactosidase A in the tissues and body fluids of hemizygous males. Progressive deposition of neutral glycosphingolipids usually produces clinical manifestations during early childhood and adolescence. The most debilitating symptom is that of agonizingly painful crises particularly affecting the hands and feet. Angiectases are a common finding. Cardiac, cerebral, and renal symptoms become manifest with age and are the leading causes of mortality [81]. Fabry's disease is unique among the sphingolipid storage diseases in that heterozygous female carriers may manifest some findings of the disease, the most common of which is a whorl-like corneal epithelial dystrophy. Rarely, females may be as severely affected as males [35, 68, 81, 82].

A whorl-like corneal opacity is found in affected males and in virtually all females [110, 296]. Seen only by slit-lamp microscopic examination, the lesions are typically found in the subepithelial layer as a diffuse haziness and progress with time to produce a verticillate pattern of opaque stippling of the epithelium and Bowman's membrane similar to the curved lines of force of a magnetic field. The lines of stippling converge to an inferointernal paracentral point that was first described by Fleischer in 1905 [109]. An identically dystrophic phenocopy is produced in patients undergoing long-term chloroquine and amiodarone therapy.

Two specific lenticular changes have been described. Typically, a propeller-like opacity is seen bilaterally with the apices aligned toward the anterior capsule. A second type, a "Fabry cataract," is located posteriorly and is characterized by linear, spokelike, opaque, granular deposits. Sausagelike tortuous vascular lesions of the conjunctiva and retina are associated systemic involvements. Papilledema, nystagmus, lid edema, and angiokeratoma of the lids have also been reported [110].

CHEMICAL PATHOLOGY

The 10 biochemical defects in Fabry's disease are due to the deficient activity of β-galactosidase A,

which results in the accumulation of ceramide trihexoside and ceramide dihexoside in tissues and plasma. The predilection for vascular endothelial and smooth muscle cells is unique among the glycosphingolipidoses [83]. Circulating β-galactosyl sphingolipids gain access to these cells via a high-affinity receptor-mediated uptake pathway [75]. The major biochemical distinctions between this and other sphingolipid storage diseases are shown in Table 2-4.

BIOCHEMICAL DETECTION

The biochemical detection of Fabry homozygotes may be done by demonstrating the absence of α-galactosidase A activity in plasma, leukocytes, or tears [81, 82, 177, 261]. Analysis of plasma or urinary sediment will show increased levels of ceramide trihexoside. In this X-linked disease, deficient or absent α-galactosidase A activity appears to result from defective activation of this catalytic protein. Studies using radiolabeled globotriosylceramide and chromogenic and fluorogenic substrates have been used to quantitate the level of enzyme activity [40, 81].

HEMIZYGOTE DETECTION

Female hemizygotes can usually be detected by the presence of corneal verticillate opacities and diffuse corneal haziness caused by the accumulation of ceramide trihexoside in the apical portions of basal epithelial cells [22]. Urinary glycosphingolipids may be increased, and residual enzyme activity may only be 10 to 25 percent of that in normal individuals [53]. Immunologic studies have attempted to demonstrate the presence of inactivated α-galactosidase A by detecting cross-reacting immunologic material but so far have had only mixed success [83].

PRENATAL DETECTION

Cultured cells from amniotic fluid have been assayed in at least one case in which marked deficiency of α-galactosidase A was noted in the male fetus. Confirmation of the diagnosis was made after the termination of pregnancy at 21 weeks [40, 81, 82].

22800 Farber's Lipogranulomatosis (Ceramidase Deficiency)

Farber's disease is an autosomal recessive disorder of lipid metabolism associated with intracellular

Table 2-4. *Sphingolipid Storage Diseases*

Disease	Name	Formula	Enzymatic defect
Fabry's	Ceramide trihexoside + ceramide dihexoside	Cer-Glc-Gal-Gal Cer-Gal-Gal	Ceramide-α-trihexosidase
Farber's	Ceramide + GM_3-ganglioside	Cer Cer-Glc-Gal $\mid$ NANA	Unknown
Globoid cell leukodystrophy (Krabbe's)	Galactocerebroside* + sulfatide*	Cer-Gal Cer-Glc-SO_4	Cerebroside-β-galactosidase
Lactosyl ceramidosis	Lactosyl ceramide	Cer-Glc-Gal	Lactosyl ceramide-β-galactosidase
Metachromatic leukodystrophy, late infantile	Sulfatide	Cer-Gal-SO_4	Arylsulfatase A
Metachromatic leukodystrophy, variant	Sulfatide + heparan sulfate	Cer-Gal-SO_4 NAcGlc-$\left\{ \begin{array}{c} GlcUA \\ IdUA \end{array} \right\}$- SO_4	Arylsulfatases A, B, and C
Niemann-Pick	Sphingomyelin + cholesterol	Cer-Phos-choline	Sphingomyelinase

*Decreased, not increased. See text.
Cer = ceramide (sphingosine fatty acid); Glc = glucose; Gal = galactose; NANA = *N*-acetylneuraminic acid (sialic acid); NAcGlc = *N*-acetylglucosamine; IdUA = iduronic acid; GlcUA = glucuronic acid.
Source: From E. R. Berman [22].

ceramide accumulation and a deficiency of lysosomal acid ceramidase. The accumulation of lipid-laden macrophages and granuloma formation involving the joints, larynx, and nervous system in infancy leads to painful joint deformation, hoarseness, neuropathy, and death, usually by 4 years of age [242].

Ocular findings consist of diffuse gray opacifications with pink centers in the parafoveal region but no disturbance of visual function [64]. A granulomatous lesion of the conjunctiva and lenticular opacity have been reported once each in the literature, as well as corneal opacity in 2 patients [242].

CHEMICAL PATHOLOGY

The basic lesion is a granuloma consisting of foamy histiocytes. The material contained stains with periodic acid–Schiff (PAS), but the nature of this substance is still unclear. While the PAS-positive component argues for the classification of this disorder as a mucolipidosis, mucopolysacchariduria is absent, and the massive accumulation of free ceramide, coupled with the known defect in ceramidase, argues for a classification of Farber's syndrome as a sphingolipidosis [26].

BIOCHEMICAL DETECTION

The diagnosis of Farber's syndrome is made clinically. The most useful laboratory test is the demonstration of low or absent ceramidase activity in cultured fibroblasts or peripheral leukocytes [242]. Acid ceramidase activity in heterozygotes is lower than normal, and prenatal detection, using cultured amniotic fluid cells, is also possible with this assay [89, 106].

23020 Galactokinase Deficiency

Galactokinase deficiency and other defects in the utilization of dietary galactose result in bilateral cataract formation within the first year of life. Symptoms of peripheral polyneuropathy have been described in the occasional case, but the only consistent feature appears to be bilateral lens opacification caused by galactitol accumulation [132,

294]. Regression or arrest of cataract formation has resulted from dietary restriction of galactose at an early age [218]. The frequency of the homozygous form is estimated at 1 in 40,000 live births [33].

CHEMICAL PATHOLOGY

The absence of galactokinase leads to galactosemia and galactosuria (Fig. 2-2). In the blood, galactose is reduced by aldose reductase to the alcohol form dulcitol (galactitol), which then accumulates in the lens cortex [132, 193]. The osmotic changes cause the lens to swell, leading to a disruption of the lens structure. While variation in aldose reductase levels in humans has not been established, it is interesting that con-

Fig. 2-2. *Metabolism of galactose in red blood cells, lens, and liver. The absence of galactokinase results in elevated plasma and urinary levels of galactose. The absence of galactose 1-phosphate uridyl transferase in galactosemia results in elevated plasma and urinary levels of galactose and elevated tissue levels of galactose 1-phosphate. (NADPH = reduced form of nicotinamide-adenine dinucleotide; ATP = adenosine triphosphate; ADP = adenosine diphosphate; UDP-glucose = uridine diphosphoglucose; UDP-galactose = uridine diphosphogalactose; PPi = inorganic pyrophosphate; UTP = uridine triphosphate.)*

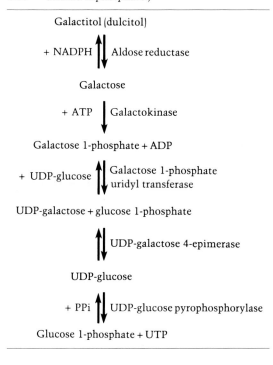

genitally hyperglycemic mice do not develop cataracts, perhaps because mouse lens contains very little aldose reductase [328].

BIOCHEMICAL DETECTION

Major defects in galactose metabolism can be detected by galactosuria or by a spot test such as the Beutler procedure, which assays red blood cell galactose enzyme activity [32, 34]. The ease with which these enzymes can be assayed and the success of early treatment make it imperative that the blood and urine of all children who have cataracts, whether congenital or juvenile, be screened for galactose. The enzyme is both heat and cold labile, so tests are best carried out using fresh red cell lysates.

HETEROZYGOTE DETECTION

The frequency of heterozygotes is approximately 1 percent and is associated with an increased risk of developing bilateral cataracts beginning in the first year of life [33]. Heterozygotes show galactokinase activity reduced to 50 percent of normal, abnormal results on galactose tolerance tests, and increased urinary excretion of galactitol [340]. Siblings should be screened, although wide-scale testing for heterozygotes is as yet unreliable.

23040 Galactosemia (Galactose 1-Phosphate Uridyl Transferase Deficiency)

As opposed to the galactokinase form of galactosemia, galactose 1-phosphate uridyl transferase (G1PUT) deficiency results in widespread tissue damage and mental retardation in addition to bilateral cataracts. The homozygous form of the disease also occurs at a frequency of 1 in 40,000 live births with a carrier frequency of 1 percent [294]. As with galactokinase deficiency, accumulation of galactitol is the presumed mechanism for cataract formation, causing vacuolization, swelling, and eventual rupture of lens fibers, with the subsequent formation of intrafibrillar clefts containing precipitated protein [115]. Early detection is imperative as dietary restriction can prevent the onset and development of the generalized disorder as well as cataracts [294].

Allelic variant forms of this transferase deficiency have been detected by starch gel electrophoresis and immunologic cross-reactivity studies [7, 249]. The most common of these is the Duarte variant in which transferase activity in homozygotes is approximately half that of normals and which is asymptomatic [340]. The Indiana variant, however, has a more classic course and mirrors the severe effects of galactose 1-phosphate uridyl transferase deficiency [172]. At least nine variants have now been described [294]. They are certainly rare, and their frequency and clinical course have yet to be elucidated.

CHEMICAL PATHOLOGY

In addition to the dulcitol (galactitol) that accumulates, a considerable amount of galactose 1-phosphate is also deposited in red cells, brain, liver, lens, and other tissues, which may account for the difference between the relatively benign course of galactokinase deficiency and the rapidly fatal course of the transferase deficiencies. Galactose 1-phosphate in high concentrations is thought to be toxic to the enzymes of the sugar nucleotide pathway [294].

BIOCHEMICAL DETECTION

Several spot tests for the detection of galactosemia are available. Simple screening for glucose and galactose may be done with Clinistix (Ames Co., Elkhart, Ind.). Galactose may then be identified by paper chromatography or specific methods that utilize test strips impregnated with galactose dehydrogenase or galactose oxidase [70]. Positive results on screening tests should be followed by analysis of red cell galactose 1-phosphate levels to distinguish galactosemia from galactokinase deficiency. Several spectrophotometric and fluorometric methods are now available for this purpose [69, 131]. Direct assay of G1PUT in the red cell includes measurements of uridine diphosphoglucose (UDP-glucose) uptake, oxygen consumption, radioactive galactose 1-phosphate incorporation into uridine diphosphogalactose (UDP-galactose) and spectrophotometric measurement of nicotinamide-adenine dinulceotide (NAD) by specific coupling reactions [172, 294].

HETEROZYGOTE DETECTION

Heterozygotes are clinically asymptomatic and without increased risk of cataract. G1PUT activity is decreased, galactitol excretion is not increased, and patients have abnormal galactose tolerance test results [340]. Galactokinase activity

should also be assayed to ruled out deficiency of this enzyme.

The Gangliosidoses

The gangliosidoses are a heterogeneous group of autosomal recessive disorders of ganglioside storage and can be divided into two groups, the GM_1 and GM_2 gangliosidoses. The GM_1 gangliosidoses are due to structural mutations in the acid β-galactosidase gene. The GM_2 gangliosidoses are due to a deficiency of hexosaminidase A or B or both, or a deficiency of an "activating factor" that stimulates hexosaminidase A to cleave the ganglioside GM_2 [253].

27280 GM_2 GANGLIOSIDOSIS TYPE I
(TAY-SACHS DISEASE)

Tay-Sachs disease is by far the most common ganglioside storage disease and has a heterozygote frequency of 1 in 27 among Ashkenazic Jews, 10 times that of the control population. Motor weakness and a startle reflex are the first signs, which usually occur between 3 and 6 months of age. Mental and motor deterioration becomes rapidly progressive, and generalized paralysis, deafness, blindness, convulsions, spasticity, and decerebrate rigidity generally evolve before death at 3 years of age. Ocular signs include a characteristic cherry-red spot of the macular region bilaterally, which is present in over 95 percent of patients, and pale optic discs. The macula may darken to a brownish color as it degenerates [253].

Chemical Pathology. Cerebral ganglioside GM_2 is increased as much as 300 times normal in Tay-Sachs, and the asialoderivative of ganglioside GM_2, GA_2, accumulates up to 20 times normal levels [254]. Enzyme activity of hexosaminidase A (hex A) is nearly absent, but levels of its isozyme, hexosaminidase B (hex B), are three or four times normal. This may be explained by a two-gene hypothesis [31]. Hex A is a paired tetramer consisting of alpha and beta chains, whereas hex B is composed solely of four beta chains [124]. The Tay-Sachs mutation causes a defect in the mechanism of linkage between alpha and beta dimers. The resultant excess in beta chains is thus converted to hex B in abnormal quantities. Genes coding for the alpha and beta subunits as well as an activator gene have been proposed to occupy different loci and are thought to be nonallelic [128].

Detection of Heterozygotes. The method previously described is useful and sensitive for all screening populations except pregnant women, who present with a ratio of hex A to hex B similar to that of obligate heterozygotes and thus have an unacceptably high false-positive rate [253]. The use of lacrimal secretions to assay hexosaminidase activity has proved to be an excellent method of detection, and an automated assay is now in use [56, 135].

26880 GM$_2$ GANGLIOSIDOSIS TYPE II (SANDHOFF'S DISEASE)

The clinical presentation and course of Sandhoff's disease are virtually identical to those of GM$_2$ gangliosidosis type I (Tay-Sachs disease). Sandhoff's disease, however, does not occur in Jewish populations, and visceral involvement of the epithelial cells of the loops of Henle in the kidney may be especially prominent [253]. As with GM$_2$ type I, a macular cherry-red spot is a hallmark in this disorder, and optic atrophy is seen by the second year.

Chemical Pathology. Levels of cerebroganglioside are elevated to levels equivalent to those found in Tay-Sachs disease, but levels of the asialo derivative of GM$_2$ are increased to a far greater degree because of the complete absence of both hex A and hex B. The viscera are highly involved, and intracellular inclusions are seen on ultrastructural examination. These inclusions have also been reported in the ganglion cell layer and the inner nuclear layer of the retina [323].

Biochemical Detection. Because of the deficiency of both hexosaminidase A and B, globoside and *N*-acetylglucosaminyl oligosaccharides (a glycoprotein degradation product) accumulate and are excreted in the urine [253]. These products may be detected in urine by thin-layer chromatography and may be an important clue to Sandhoff's disease. Definitive diagnosis, as well as prenatal and carrier detection, however, rests on the ability to demonstrate the absence of hexosaminidase and is best made using the assays described for Tay-Sachs disease.

23070 GM$_2$ GANGLIOSIDOSIS TYPE III (JUVENILE GM$_2$ GANGLIOSIDOSIS)

The juvenile form of GM$_2$ gangliosidosis has only been described in non-Jewish individuals. Onset

of this disorder is between 2 and 6 years and is characterized by ataxia, loss of speech, and progressive spasticity. The course of neurologic impairment is insidious and results in death by mid-adolescence. The onset of blindness caused by photoreceptor, RPE, macular, and optic nerve degeneration occurs late in the disease, unlike the other ganglioside GM$_2$ disorders [111]. Early retinal involvement also serves to differentiate the juvenile form of GM$_2$ gangliosidosis from the early retinal changes of another disease with a similar phenotype, Batten-Spielmeyer-Vogt disease. Hepatosplenomegaly, skeletal changes, lymphocyte vacuolation, and foam cells of the bone marrow are also seen in juvenile GM$_2$ gangliosidosis [181, 253].

Chemical Pathology. The accumulation and storage of gangliosides in neuronal tissue accounts for the lesions seen in juvenile GM$_2$ gangliosidosis. The enzymatic defect is a partial deficiency of hexosaminidase A [260]. The degree of deficiency and age of onset do not appear to correlate with the clinical severity of this disease [181]. Whether this is a phenomenon of incomplete penetrance or whether this disorder has a multiallelic component is not known.

Biochemical Detection. Cerebral ganglioside levels are markedly elevated in juvenile GM$_2$ gangliosidosis but to levels less than in Tay-Sachs and Sandhoff's diseases. Enzyme activity of hexosaminidase A is variable using synthetic substrates, but if natural GM$_2$ substrate is used, hexosaminidase A activity is almost completely deficient [253]. Thus natural substrate must be used for prenatal and carrier detection. Keys to the differential diagnosis of this disease are the age at onset of clinical symptoms, especially retinal changes, and the level of enzyme activity.

GM$_1$ GANGLIOSIDOSIS: 23050 TYPE I, 23060 TYPE II

The GM$_1$ gangliosidoses are of two main types: type I (infantile form), which manifests itself from birth; and type II (juvenile generalized), which is asymptomatic until about 1 year of age. Type I and type II share many features, including progressive psychomotor retardation, seizures, decerebrate rigidity, and skeletal changes. However, in type I disease visceral involvement is marked and hepatosplenomegaly is common, while this sign is nearly absent in type II. Neurologic changes have an insidious course, and death ensues from bronchopneumonia by age 2 in type I but not until the end of the first decade in the less severe GM_1 type II [253].

The ocular manifestations of type I and type II are varied and inconsistently present. Both, however, have blindness as a late finding. In type I optic atrophy is common, a cherry-red spot is observed in 50 percent of cases, distended conjunctival capillary endothelial cells give rise to microvascular abnormalities, and mild corneal clouding has been noted, as have esotropia and nystagmus. In general, no ocular abnormalities are reported in patients with type II GM_1 gangliosidosis, but ultrastructural examination shows extensive lamellar cytoplasmic bodies in the retinal ganglion cell [25, 96].

Chemical Pathology. At least five phenotypes of GM_1 gangliosidosis have been noted, though all have a deficiency in β-galactosidase A, B, and C, the enzymes needed for the cleavage of β-galactosyl residues. These residues exist as a variety of substrates, most prominently ganglioside GM_1, its asialo derivative, and complex carbohydrates. The genetic defect appears to be a structural mutation of the β-galactosidase A gene. Whether this change is responsible for the occurrence of multiple phenotypes in this disease, is the basis of decreased activity alone, involves a regulatory defect, or is allelic among each GM_1 type is not known [253]. GM_1 gangliosidosis was the first ganglioside storage disease shown to be due to a deficiency in a degradative enzyme.

Biochemical Detection. The biochemical detection of β-galactosidase deficiency can be performed using leukocytes [303], urine [320], and cultured fibroblasts [305]. Carriers demonstrate an intermediate level of enzyme activity [303]. Prenatal detection can be performed by assaying β-galactosidase activity in cultured amniotic cells obtained by amniocentesis in the second trimester of pregnancy [182].

24520 Globoid Cell Leukodystrophy (Krabbe's Disease, Globoid Cell Sclerosis)

Krabbe's disease is a severe neurodegenerative autosomal recessive disorder that progresses from onset in early infancy to death by the second year. Massive infiltration of the white matter by multinucleated macrophages filled with galactocerebroside (globoid cells) and demyelination with astrocytic gliosis provide the morphologic basis for diagnosis [316]. Mental and motor deterioration is rapid, and optic atrophy, cortical blindness, and deafness are common. Histopathologic and ultrastructural studies have shown that the pathogenesis of optic atrophy is similar to that of changes in the brain [95, 154].

CHEMICAL PATHOLOGY

The most characteristic defect in Krabbe's disease is the severe loss of myelin and oligodendrocytes. While normal myelin formation is accompanied by rapid increase in galactocerebroside β-galactosidase activity at $1\frac{1}{2}$ years of age, the lack of this enzyme results in the accumulation of galactocerebroside in globoid cells as well as in galactosyl sphingosine, a cytotoxic substance [327]. Krabbe's disease is unique among the sphingolipidoses in that there is no overt accumulation of galactocerebroside (only in globoid cells) and that galactocerebroside levels in neural tissue are normal. This suggests that the accumulation of galactosyl sphingosine (psychosin), and not galactocerebroside, is responsible for the demise of oligodendroglia [318].

BIOCHEMICAL DETECTION

Specific analyses of lipid composition of white matter are only possible post mortem because of the quantities of brain needed. However, it has been suggested that increased β-galactosidase activity may have value as a diagnostic feature of globoid cell leukodystrophy [316]. Enzymatic assays of β-galactosidase can be performed using leukocytes, cultured fibroblasts, serum, or visceral or nervous tissue [317].

DETECTION OF HETEROZYGOTES

Heterozygotes show enzyme activities intermediate between normal levels and those of affected patients. Demonstration of enzyme activity in leukocytes, fibroblasts, or serum requires the use of natural substrate [317].

PRENATAL DETECTION

Amniocentesis has been performed as a prenatal diagnostic procedure for Krabbe's disease. Amniotic cell cultures incubated with radioactive natural substrate demonstrated a β-galactosidase level only 5 percent of normal, and Krabbe's disease was confirmed after therapeutic abortion [315].

30590 Glucose 6-Phosphate Dehydrogenase Deficiency

Many allelic forms of glucose 6-phosphate dehydrogenase (G6PD) deficiency are now recognized as X-linked inherited traits [234]. Red cell deficiency of this enzyme is the basis of favism, primaquine sensitivity, other drug-related hemolytic anemias, jaundice in the newborn, and chronic nonspherocytic hemolytic anemia [30]. Cataracts have been reported and are particularly prevalent in blacks with type A G6PD deficiency [67].

CHEMICAL PATHOLOGY

G6PD catalyzes the following reaction:

Glucose 6-phosphate + NADPH + H$^+$
$$\longrightarrow 6\text{-phosphogluconate} + NADP^+$$

NADPH functions to maintain glutathione in a reduced state (GSH) in red blood cells according to the following reaction:

GSSG (oxidized glutathione) + NADPH + H$^+$
$$\longrightarrow 2GSH + NADP^+$$

Primaquine phosphate or other drugs deplete the already low levels of erythrocyte glutathione, and the rate of red cell destruction is rapidly increased, leading to the hemolytic anemia that characterizes this disorder [30]. The ratio of NADP$^+$ to NADPH is increased [29], and cataract formation is consistent with the data that aldose reductase inhibitors, which decrease consumption of NADPH and thus increase the level of reduced glutathione, appear to exert a protective effect against the formation of cataract in experimentally induced sugar cataract [192].

BIOCHEMICAL DETECTION

The detection of male hemizygous G6PD-deficient patients is best achieved by the use of a quantitative assay or by one of many screening procedures at a time when the patient is not in crisis. The posthemolytic patient who has few enzyme-deficient cells remaining may show quantitative levels similar to heterozygotes and thus may pose a difficult diagnostic challenge [162, 274].

23220 Glycogen Storage Disease Type I (von Gierke's Disease)

Von Gierke's disease is characterized clinically by massive hepatomegaly, short stature, and en-larged kidneys. Xanthomas frequently present on the extensor surfaces of the extremities, and bleeding may be a major problem, especially after surgery [171]. Vision does not seem to be impaired, though multiple bilateral yellowish paramacular lesions were noted in 3 of 5 patients with glycogen storage disease type I [107].

CHEMICAL PATHOLOGY

Severe hypoglycemia, hyperuricemia, hyperlipemia, and low blood levels of lactic acid result as a consequence of glucose 6-phosphatase deficiency, decreased uric acid secretion, and increased hepatic and extrahepatic production of lactic acid [23, 37].

BIOCHEMICAL DETECTION

Plasma glucose, lactate, ketones, uric acid, and platelets must be carefully monitored in the diagnosed patient, and the prevention of acidosis and seizure is of primary importance [37]. Liver analysis of glycogen, direct enzymatic assays, and erythrocyte and cultured fibroblast cell assays may all be used to detect levels of glucose 6-phosphatase in von Gierke's disease, its carrier state, and for prenatal diagnosis [100, 171].

23325 Goldberg-Cotlier Syndrome (Neuraminidase Deficiency with β-Galactosidase Deficiency)

Goldberg-Cotlier syndrome may be considered a clinical phenotype of mucolipidosis I and shares many of the features of neuraminidase deficiency [321]. As was first described in three siblings, this disease is characterized by dwarfism, gargoyle facies, mental retardation, seizures, corneal clouding, macular cherry-red spot, β-galactosidase deficiency in skin, dysostosis multiplex, and hearing loss, and by the absence of mucopolysacchariduria, vacuolated blood cells, or clinically enlarged viscera [139].

CHEMICAL PATHOLOGY

It has been suggested that in the Goldberg-Cotlier syndrome a post-translational processing mechanism is defective and neuraminidase and β-galactosidase are thus exposed to degradation by other lysosomal enzymes [79]. The addition of a 32,000-dalton glycoprotein "corrective factor" has been shown to restore activity of both enzymes [168]. Although the combined deficiency of this syndrome is clinically indistinguishable from neuraminidase deficiency alone, the apparent lack of a structural defect of β-galactosidase [165] and the evidence supporting a mechanism of intralysosomal degradation indicate that the Goldberg-Cotlier is a unique lysosomal storage disease.

26370 Günther's Disease

See Porphyria, Congenital Erythropoietic.

14170 Hemoglobinopathies

The hemoglobinopathies are a diverse group of hematologic disorders characterized by the production of structurally abnormal hemoglobin. At present more than 300 human hemoglobins have been identified by electrophoretic means or amino acid sequence variation (Fig. 2-3 and Table 2-5), and the number of hemoglobinopathies continues to increase. While many of these are rare and have no ophthalmologic importance, the hemoglobinopathies represent the prototype of genetic disorders that arise from a single gene, and sometimes a single site, mutation. The most important of the hemoglobinopathies are the sickling disorders. The sickle cell diseases result from abnormal hemoglobin structure and usually manifest themselves with the onset of one of four recognized types of sickle cell crisis: vascular occlusive infarctive crisis [341]. Ocular abnormalities arise from vascular occlusive retinal hypoxia. Retinal and vitreous hemorrhage, neovascularization, and rhegmatogenous retinal detachment late in the course are characteristic complications [137, 138].

CHEMICAL PATHOLOGY

Hemoglobin is responsible for the reversible binding and transport of O_2 at the tissue level and is found exclusively in erythrocytes. Hemoglobin is a 46,000-dalton tetramer containing a total of 574 amino acid residues on two pairs of dissimilar globin polypeptide chains. Each chain is covalently linked via a histidine residue to a central heme group (ferroproteoporphyrin IX). Five types of globin chains, designated α, β, γ, δ, and ϵ are made. The α chain contains 141 amino acid residues; the β, γ, and δ chains each contain 146 residues. The hemoglobin (Hb) predominantly

Table 2-5. *Hemoglobinopathies Affecting the Eye*

Type	Chemical pathology
Sickle cell anemia (Hb S-S)	Absence of normal Hb A in red blood cells; 75–95% is Hb S 5–25% is Hb F
Sickle cell trait (Hb A-S)	Carrier of sickle cell anemia; 25–45% is Hb S 55–75% is Hb A
Sickle cell hemoglobin C disease (Hb S-C disease)	Double heterozygote for 2 abnormal hemoglobins; 60–95% is Hb S 5–40% is Hb C
Hemoglobin C trait (Hb A-C)	Carrier of Hb C disease; red blood cells contain both normal (Hb A) and abnormal (Hb C) hemoglobin
Sickle cell thalassemia (S-thalassemia)	Combines β-thalassemia (defective synthesis of β-chain) with sickle cell anemia; 60–95% is Hb S 5–40% is Hb A

Source: E. R. Berman [22].

found in adult erythrocytes is Hb A ($\alpha_2\beta_2$), which accounts for over 90 percent of the total hemoglobin, while Hb A_2 ($\alpha_2\delta_2$) accounts for only 2.5 percent. During fetal development the primary form is Hb F ($\alpha_2\gamma_2$). The ϵ globin chains have been detected only in the first 3 months of fetal life [223, 341].

SICKLE CELL ANEMIA (Hb S-S)

Sickle cell disease by definition affects only those individuals who are homozygotes for the Hb S gene. These individuals retain some fetal hemoglobin (Hb F), but normal Hb A is not found. A simple base change in the globin DNA alters the mRNA triplet coding for glutamic acid (guanine-

Fig. 2-3. *Diagram of human β globin gene. Mutations and polymorphism leading to thalassemia have been located in coding sequences (shaded boxes), intervening sequences (IVS-1 and IVS-2), and regulatory sequences (to the left of the 5' end) by specific molecular probes [8]. Other globin sequences have been similarly analyzed.*

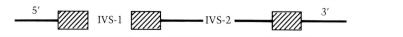

adenine-guanine or GAG) to one coding for valine (guanine-uracil-guanine or GUG) [14]. The solubility of reduced Hb S is decreased at low oxygen tension, and polymerization of Hb S fibers results in the characteristic holly leaf–shaped sickle cell. Condensation of fibers is not an instantaneous event [166], which is an important physiologic consideration as there is wide variability in the transit time through different organ systems.

Deformation of erythrocytes has two major consequences, anemia and ischemic crisis. Abnormal cells are rapidly phagocytized by the reticuloendothelial system, notably in the liver and spleen, which results in a chronic severe anemia. Blockage of vessels by these irregularly shaped cells results in a vicious and painful cycle of ischemia, hypoxia, further deoxygenation, more sickling, and increased blockage, which is aptly named sickle crisis. The site of retinal occlusion is more often in the precapillary arterial branches rather than in the venous circulation where oxygen tension is lowest, which suggests that the retinal lesions may be caused primarily by embolic and occlusive phenomena in the narrow precapillary lumen and not by the sickling process alone [121].

Vascular necrosis from ischemia results in intraretinal hematoma formation, recognized clinically as a "salmon patch." This hemorrhage may extend into the subhyaloid space or subretinal space to cause focal retinoschisis. If accompanied by RPE hyperplasia, a subretinal hemorrhage may produce a so-called black sunburst effect. To some extent, retinal ischemia is diminished because of arteriovenous anastomotic flow. These anastomoses are sites for new capillary formation both on the retinal surface and projecting into the vitreous, causing a "sea fan" pattern of neovascularization. These delicate tufts serve as attachments for the development of crescentic tears and retinal holes. Traction and rhegmatogenous detachment cause significant ocular morbidity [121, 280].

SICKLE CELL TRAIT (Hb A-S)

Heterozygous carriers for sickle cell have 55 to 75 percent normal Hb A in their erythrocytes, with the balance being Hb S (Table 2-5) [121]. Sickling occurs only under extreme conditions of deoxygenation (stasis, high altitudes), and systemic morbidity is rare. Carriers of sickle cell trait are resistant to *Plasmodium falciparum* malaria infection; the postulated mechanism of resistance is a disturbance in K^+ transport in the Hb S red cell membrane [116]. This selective advantage appears to balance the loss of the S gene in homozygotes and may in part account for heterozygote frequencies approaching 50 percent in some African populations [341].

SICKLE CELL HEMOGLOBIN C DISEASE (Hb S-C)

Individuals with Hb S-C disease are double heterozygotes for abnormal proteins, and more than 50 percent of their hemoglobin is Hb S. Although these patients suffer from fewer systemic effects and their longevity is greater than that of patients with sickle cell disease (Hb S-S), the incidence of the retinopathy is greater (32.8% vs. 2.6%) in patients with Hb S-C [66]. One reason for this may be the combination of an anemia more mild and a degree of sickling more pronounced than in Hb S-S and Hb S-A, leading to increased blood viscosity and hence retinal ischemia.

Substitution of lysine for glutamic acid at position 6 of the β chain causes the structural change resulting in Hb S-C.

HEMOGLOBIN C TRAIT (Hb A-C)

Individuals with hemoglobin C trait are the heterozygous carriers of the mutant Hb C gene. Because red cells contain normal hemoglobin A, patients are usually asymptomatic. A few cases of retinopathy similar to those found in Hb S-C disease have been observed [306].

27350 S-THALASSEMIA

The thalassemias are a group of hereditary anemias in which the production of one or more of the four globin components of the hemoglobin tetramer is impaired. The unimpaired chain or chains accumulate and disrupt the normal maturation and function of erythrocytes, causing the premature destruction of the red cell [183].

If there is a structural change in the globin gene in addition to defects in production, as in sickle cell–β-thalassemia, up to 80 percent of the hemoglobin may be Hb S, and symptoms, including retinal lesions, resemble those of sickle cell disease [121].

BIOCHEMICAL DETECTION

Hemoglobin electrophoresis is sensitive and widely used for the detection of sickling disorders, as all known variants show differences in electrophoretic mobility. Samples may be dried on filter paper and later eluted for analysis, which makes electrophoresis an excellent procedure for population screening [91]. Cellulose acetate electrophoresis at pH 8.6 and agar citrate electrophoresis at pH 6.2 are widely used methods. Starch gel electrophoresis is especially useful when sample quantities are small [341].

PRENATAL DIAGNOSIS

Thousands of prenatal testings for thalassemia and sickle cell anemia have been performed [4, 5]. For many years, biochemical analysis has been based on the quantitation of globin synthesis in fetal erythrocytes. Fetal blood is obtained from the placenta by percutaneous transabdominal aspiration or by direct aspiration from blood vessels during fetoscopy. A Coulter Counter Size Distribution Analyzer distinguishes maternal erythrocytes from fetal erythrocytes, which are then incubated with radioactive leucine. Separation and identification of globin chains is performed using an ion-exchange column under denaturing conditions [223]. Fetal loss is a complication approximately 5 percent of the time, and the technique, while quite reliable, is expensive and time-consuming.

Recombinant DNA techniques have allowed the specific determination of changes in DNA structure. Disorders caused by gene mutation, notably the thalassemias and the hemoglobinopathies, have been the prototype for prenatal detection by fetal DNA analysis. Homozygous thalassemias are easily demonstrated by the absence of the α globin gene [86, 258]. The diagnosis of sickle cell anemia can be made by detecting variations in structure caused by the altered structure of the Hb S gene (by restriction enzyme polymorphisms) or by directly detecting the mutation that differentiates Hb A from Hb S [60, 123]. As a general approach DNA analysis has a great advantage in that any nucleated fetal cell can be used, including amniotic cells. The ease and relative safety with which amniocentesis can now be performed suggest that recombinant techniques will assume an even greater role in the prenatal detection of gene disorders.

23630 Hooft's Disease

Hooft's disease has been described only in two sisters who had retarded physical development, erythematosquamous eruption, opague leukonychia, mental retardation, and low serum lipid levels. One had tapetoretinal degeneration [167].

CHEMICAL PATHOLOGY

A generalized hypolipidemia is present. While serum phosphate is high, cholesterol and phospholipids are very low. The nature of this extremely rare defect is not known [234].

25280 Hurler's Syndrome

See Mucopolysaccharidosis I-H.

The Hyperlipoproteinemias

The hyperlipoproteinemias have been classified into five types, I through V, and are characterized by patterns of elevation of specific plasma lipoproteins. Lipoproteins, which serve as the major carrier of cholesterol and triglyceride to the tissues, have variants that occur mainly at three levels: the amino acid level, secondary structure, and macromolecular arrangement of normal peptides. The major lipoproteins are chylomicrons, very-low-density lipoprotein (VLDL), low-density lipoprotein (LDL) (mainly cholesterol), and high-density lipoprotein (HDL) (Table 2-6). Abnormalities in the hyperlipoproteinemias are as follows:

Type I   Elevated chylomicrons
Type II   Increased LDL and cholesterol
Type III   Elevated cholesterol and abnormal VLDL
Type IV   Increased VLDL
Type V   Elevated VLDL and plasma triglycerides

The commonness of lipoprotein disorders and their relation to atherosclerotic and coronary artery disease have stimulated intense interest in the genetic basis of these diseases [293]. While the present classification is useful, it will surely change as the molecular understanding of the enzymatic defects improves.

Hyperchylomicronemia (Type I) and Type IV (increased VLDL) may share clinical features such as impaired glucose tolerance and multiple xanthomas, and the hypercholesterolemias may have corneal arcus and premature atherosclerotic disease as common signs [339]. All of the hyperlipoproteinemias can be detected by (1) chemical analysis of plasma cholesterol and triglyceride, (2) plasma lipoprotein electrophoresis, and (3) analysis of plasma lipoprotein after ultracentrifugation.

Table 2-6. *Properties of Plasma Lipoproteins*

Characteristic	Chylomicrons	VLDL	LDL	HDL
Density (qm/cc)	0.92–0.96	0.95–1.006	1.019–1.063	1.63–1.71
Range or average of molecular weight	5×10^8	$5–100 \times 10^6$	$2–4 \times 10^6$	$2–3 \times 10^5$
Diameter (nm)	75–1000	30–75	17–26	7–10
Composition (% of dry weight)				
Protein	1–2	9–10	25	45–55
Triacylglycerols	80–95	55–65	10	3
Phospholipids	3–8	15–20	22–24	21–30
Cholesterol				
Free	1–3	10	8	3–5
Esters	2–4	5	35–37	15
Type of apoprotein				
Major	B, C	B, C, E	B	A, D
Minor	A	A	—	B, C, E

VLDL = very-low-density lipoproteins; LDL = low-density lipoproteins; HDL = high-density lipoproteins.

23860 HYPERLIPOPROTEINEMIA TYPE I: FAMILIAL
LIPOPROTEIN LIPASE DEFICIENCY

The most severe of the lipoprotein disorders, Type I, is characterized by abdominal pain, pancreatitis, hepatomegaly, and extensive transient xanthomas, which may involve the eyelids. While lipid also may be deposited in the iris, retina, and cornea, lipemia retinalis is a constant feature [339].

Chemical Pathology. Massive postprandial chylomicronemia and triglyceridemia occur as a hereditary defect in lipoprotein lipase deficiency [156, 250]. Pancreatitis is thought to be due to the release of fatty acid emboli; lipemia retinalis, from the deposition of chylomicrons and VLDL in retinal vessels [339].

14440 HYPERLIPOPROTEINEMIA TYPE II: FAMILIAL
HYPERCHOLESTEROLEMIA

Familial hypercholesterolemia is an autosomal dominant disorder. The heterozygous form shows variable penetrance and represents approximately 0.2 percent of live births as recorded in American and British surveys. As a whole, this disorder may be the most common inherited metabolic disorder [144]. It is characterized by hypercholesterolemia, premature coronary artery disease, and cutaneous and tendon xanthomas. Homozygotes typically die before age 30, while heterozygotes survive until ages 40 to 50 [46, 189].

The primary ocular feature, corneal arcus, is present in 10 percent of heterozygotes before the age of 30 and in 50 percent of heterozygotes over age 30. In homozygotes arcus may be observed by age 10 [48]. Xanthelasma and scleral lipid deposits are seen. A possible association between hypercholesterolemia, ocular hypertension, low-tension glaucoma, and deafness remains largely unexplained [339].

Chemical Pathology. The elevation in LDL alone (Type IIa) or with a slight increase in VLDL (Type IIb) occurs as a result of a fractional reduction in catabolism. The rate of LDL synthesis is normal, but there is deficient intracellular suppression of cholesterol synthesis owing to decreased uptake of LDL from the circulation [46–48]. While the regulatory mechanism of this classic example of receptor-mediated endocytosis are still under investigation, dietary therapy and cholesterol diversion remain the major means of preventing premature atherosclerotic disease [19].

14450 HYPERLIPOPROTEINEMIA TYPE III: FAMILIAL
DYSBETALIPOPROTEINEMIA

Clinically, the familial Type III lipoproteinemias are manifest by accelerated atherosclerosis, tuberous xanthomas, and xanthomas of the palms and digits. These manifestations rarely present before age 20 [48]. Several large studies have suggested an autosomal dominant mode of inheritance [158, 240]. Ocular findings are not common but have included xanthelasma, corneal arcus, and in rare instances fundus lipid deposition [339].

This disorder of lipid metabolism is characterized by elevated triglycerides and cholesterol in an approximately even ratio with an abnormal VLDL that migrates with beta mobility (a smaller heavier particle) during electrophoresis. The resulting high ratio of VLDL-cholesterol to plasma triglyceride (70 : 3) is often used as a diagnostic criterion [293]. The defect in the genetic locus coding for the structure of apoprotein E (E^d), a component of remnant lipoproteins made from VLDL and chylomicrons, causes abnormal clearance from plasma and cellular accumulation.

14460 HYPERLIPOPROTEINEMIA TYPE IV: FAMILIAL HYPERTRIGLYCERIDEMIA

Hyperglyceridemia is a common disorder and is most often seen in men. Patients are often obese, have impaired glucose tolerance, and show signs of accelerated atherosclerosis. As with several other hyperlipoproteinemias, atheromatous plaques, xanthelasma, and corneal arcus are often seen. Other features include hyperuricemia, gout, and hepatosplenomegaly [339]. Occasionally, retinal signs including waxy periarterial sheathing that fluctuates in intensity and retinal vascular occlusion secondary to impaired glucose tolerance may be seen [159, 199].

Chemical Pathology. Many cases of hyperlipoproteinemia type IV are nonfamilial and are probably multifactorial or polygenic. The most frequent underlying disorder is diabetes mellitus, although alcoholism and the use of oral contraceptives have also been implicated [339]. No well-defined biochemical or enzymatic features exist at present to explain the onset of this disorder [293].

23840 HYPERLIPOPROTEINEMIA TYPE V: FAMILIAL HYPERTRIGLYCERIDEMIA WITH CHYLOMICRONEMIA

Visible chylomicronemia and elevated VLDL in fasting plasma characterize the type V disorder. Abdominal pain and eruptive xanthomatosis are findings similar to those of type I familial lipoprotein lipase deficiency. Hyperuricemia, diabetes, polyneuropathy, and parotid gland enlargement are other features of type V disease. Important differentiating clues include age of onset (typically in adulthood or middle age in type V) and the association of onset with a predisposing factor, such as pregnancy, the use of estrogenic hormones, diabetes, or alcohol use [250]. More men are affected than women.

Ocular findings include xanthelasma and lipemia retinalis similar to those of type I disease, retinal vascular occlusion, and decreased peripheral retinal circulation secondary to glucose intolerance [204].

Chemical Pathology. There are only speculative reports of the enzymatic defect in the type V disorder. It is thought that an abnormality leading to an increase in VLDL with secondary elevation of chylomicrons is the primary defect. Whether this is due to a defect in lipoprotein lipase (LDL), a kinetic phenomenon, or one of tissue specificity remains unclear [250].

23870 Hyperlysinemia

Only 12 cases of persistent hyperlysinemia have been reported in the literature. This disease appears to be autosomal recessive in inheritance, and several affected individuals have been the product of consanguineous marriages [234]. Hyperlysinemia is characterized by poor growth, muscular and ligamentous asthenia, anemia, convulsions, and mild mental retardation. Ocular findings in four patients included bilateral subluxation of lenses in one and spherophakia in another [307]. The majority of patients have had abnormalities primarily affecting the nervous system; 2 patients had no clinical manifestations of illness. The metabolic changes may be unrelated to the development of clinical symptoms.

The hyperlysinemias comprise three different disorders. Defective activity of lysine-α-ketoglutarate reductase affects two of these, with a concomitant defect in saccharopine dehydrogenase activity in one. In the third disorder lysine-α-ketoglutarate reductase activity is normal [125]. The lack of a lysine degradation pathway results in lysinuria, lysinemia, and an additional increase in saccharopine or pipecolic acid, depending on the site of the defect.

BIOCHEMICAL DETECTION

The diagnosis of hyperlysinemia can usually be made by paper chromatography or high-voltage electrophoresis. Hyperlysinemia, saccharopinuria, or both can be documented by quantitative assay of blood and urine using an amino acid analyzer. Lysine-α-ketoglutarate reductase and saccharopine dehydrogenase should be assayed with cultured fibroblasts and may reveal further clues to this rare disease [71, 105].

25887 Hyperornithinemia

See Chorioretinal Gyrate Atrophy.

23900 Hyperostosis Corticalis Deformans Juvenilis

See Hyperphosphatasia.

23900 Hyperphosphatasia (Juvenile Paget's Disease; Hyperostosis Corticalis Deformans Juvenilis)

Congenital idiopathic hyperphosphatasia is an autosomal recessive disorder characterized in early life by a large head; expanded, bowed, and fragile extremities; premature loss of deciduous teeth; and dwarfism [15, 54, 99]. Some cases show extensive neurologic involvement [230]. Ocular signs include retinal degeneration with optic atrophy, angioid streaks, and blue sclera [15, 334].

CHEMICAL PATHOLOGY

Turnover of bone, both breakdown and production, is markedly elevated in juvenile Paget's disease, and is manifested by increased urinary and serum hydroxyproline. Alkaline phosphatase, acid phosphatase, and elevated leucine aminopeptidase are also seen [54].

BIOCHEMICAL DETECTION

Acid and alkaline phosphatase levels are readily determined by routine laboratory studies. Urinary hydroxyproline is easily detected using thin-layer chromatography.

24150 Hypophosphatasia

Hypophosphatasia is an autosomal recessive disorder characterized by severe skeletal changes that are radiologically indistinguishable from rickets, premature cranial synostosis, and premature loss of deciduous teeth [267]. Blue sclera may be the initial ocular finding. Other signs include band keratopathy, conjunctival calcification, cataracts, pathologic lid retraction, malformation of the or-

bits, proptosis, and papilledema and optic atrophy secondary to the craniostenosis [44, 215]. The severity of the disease varies with the age of onset. Infantile hypophosphatasia often leads to death early in life, whereas the juvenile and adult forms have a significantly longer course.

CHEMICAL PATHOLOGY

Serum alkaline phosphatase is low, and high concentrations of pyrophosphate and phosphorylethanolamine are found in plasma and urine in hypophosphatasia [267]. The incomplete or absent calcification of bone matrix is presumably due to the lack of bone alkaline phosphatase (pyrophosphatase). The role phosphorylethanolamine, pyrophosphates, and inorganic phosphate play in the cascade of bone mineralization is not well understood.

BIOCHEMICAL DETECTION

Low serum alkaline phosphatase, with high urinary pyrophosphate and phosphorylethanolamine, coupled with the histologic and radiographic changes noted, confirm this diagnosis. While heterozygotes present similar laboratory abnormalities, there are no bone changes. Urinary phosphorylethanolamine is elevated in a number of metabolic bone diseases and is thus of limited value as a marker for heterozygosity [220].

23070 Juvenile GM$_2$ Gangliosidosis

See GM$_2$ Gangliosidosis Type III.

23900 Juvenile Paget's Disease

See Hyperphosphatasia.

24520 Krabbe's Disease

See Globoid Cell Leukodystrophy.

24550 Lactosyl Ceramidosis

Lactosyl ceramidosis has been described in only 1 patient, but the partial deficiency in both parents supports recessive inheritance. The disorder is characterized by severe psychomotor retardation, clinically evident by age 25 months, cerebellar ataxia, marked hypotonia, and decreased deep tendon reflexes. Redness of the macula was also noted [76].

Although originally described as a defect of lactosyl ceramide β-galactosidase, it was subsequently found that this was not the case in the original patient, who had normal enzyme activity. However, sphingomyelinase activity was one-sixth of normal activity in this patient, and the possibility that this was an atypical case was proposed [336]. Burton and associates reported that neutral β-galactosidase also cleaved lactosyl ceramide and that fibroblasts from the original patient expressed a very low level of activity of this enzyme, while individuals with Niemann-Pick disease expressed normal levels [52].

CHEMICAL PATHOLOGY

The accumulation of the uncleaved substrate, lactosyl ceramide, in the blood, urine, liver, brain, bone marrow, and fibroblasts severely impairs catabolism of globosides and gangliosides and accounts for the neurosplanchnic pathology found in lactosyl ceramidosis.

BIOCHEMICAL DETECTION

Biochemical detection of neutral β-galactosidase and lactosyl ceramidase activity is best carried out using cultured fibroblasts. The deficiency can be demonstrated only with the use of lactosyl ceramide as an enzyme substrate [21].

24590 Lecithin-Cholesterol Acyltransferase Deficiency

Lecithin-cholesterol acyltransferase (LCAT) deficiency is a rare autosomal recessive lipoprotein abnormality characterized by the failure of LCAT to esterify plasma cholesterol [133]. Unesterified cholesterol and phosphatidylcholine (lecithin) accumulate in the plasma and tissue. While there is a plasma lysolecithin cholesterol ester deficit, tissue deposition is presumably responsible for the development of corneal opacities, anemia, renal failure, and atherosclerosis [133].

Ocular manifestations are characteristic [169]. In addition to a lipoid arcus, a misty-appearing cornea is seen bilaterally. Closer examination reveals minute grayish dots scattered evenly throughout the stroma but without involvement of the corneal epithelium, endothelium, or Descemet's membrane. The increase in dot density at the limbus produces the lipoid arcus. Fundus changes, including ruptures of Bruch's membrane, retinal hemorrhages, disk protrusion, nerv-

ous dilatation, and capillary leakage as observed by fluorescein angiography, have also been observed [169].

CHEMICAL PATHOLOGY

LCAT is a 59,000-dalton protein that circulates in a complex containing HDL and LDL [61]. After its activation by apoprotein AI, LCAT catalyzes the transfer of fatty acid from the C-2 position of lecithin to the hydroxyl group of cholesterol [2, 133]. LCAT deficiency results in the accumulation of unesterified cholesterol and lecithin. Recently a case was reported with cholesterol elevated to 450 mg/dl and triglyceride to over 1600 mg/dl [163].

BIOCHEMICAL DETECTION

LCAT mass can now be measured with ease and sensitivity by a radioimmunoassay, while activity can be quantitated using a synthetic substrate containing egg lecithin [1]. Heterozygotes have been successfully identified using these methods and are found to have one-half the normal activity and mass [61, 117]. Recent reports of genetic heterogeneity in LCAT genes from Sardinian, Canadian, and Norwegian families with varying levels of plasma LCAT activity and mass indicate that much genetic investigation remains [3].

24710 Lipid Proteinosis

See Urbach-Wiethe Syndrome.

24850 Lysosomal α-D-Mannosidase Deficiency

See Mannosidosis.

24850 Mannosidosis (Lysosomal α-D-Mannosidase Deficiency)

Mannosidosis (MAN-B) is characterized by coarse facies, retardation, hepatosplenomegaly, gingival hyperplasia, and dysostosis multiplex. A severe type (I) results in a rapidly progressive course with death in childhood; a mild variant (II) results in survival into adulthood [24, 216]. Spoke-shaped opacities of the posterior cortex are the most common ocular finding.

CHEMICAL PATHOLOGY

A characteristic feature of mannosidosis is visceral storage and urinary excretion of a wide variety of glycoprotein-derived mannose-containing oligosaccharides. Fibrillar granular material is found on ultrastructural examination of conjunctival fibroblasts [24].

BIOCHEMICAL TESTS

The deficiency of the heat-stable lysosomal acidic β form of α-mannosidase isoenzymes can be assayed using leukocytes, cultured fibroblasts, or tears [24]. Analysis of urinary oligosaccharides with high-performance liquid chromatography may also confirm the diagnosis.

25320 Maroteaux-Lamy Syndrome

See Mucopolysaccharidosis VI.

Metachromatic Leukodystrophy: 25010 Late Infantile Form, 24990 Variant Form

Metachromatic leukodystrophy (MLD) is a disorder of myelin metabolism resulting in progressive impairment of mental and motor abilities with peripheral and central nervous system (CNS) demyelination [152, 200]. The disorder is also known by a number of other names: metachromatic leukoencephalopathy, cerebral sclerosis, metachromatic form 4 diffuse, sulfatide lipidosis, arylsulfatase A deficiency, cerebroside sulfatase deficiency. Several MLD variants, including a form caused by a deficiency of cerebroside sulfatase activator and a multiple sulfatase deficiency disorder, have been described in addition to the four established classes of MLD: congenital, late infantile, juvenile, and adult [234]. Only two forms, the late infantile and a variant form, will be described here.

Disturbances of posture and locomotion are the first symptoms to appear, with mental and gross motor deterioration following. Ocular changes are variable and occur late in the course of the disease [200, 224]. These changes consist primarily of optic atrophy with amaurosis, abnormal extraocular movements, and diminished or absent pupillary light reflexes [63, 134, 200, 221]. A graying of the macula with cherry-red spot has been only sporadically reported and, because of its occurrence in other ganglioside storage disorders, should not be definitively associated with MLD [63, 134, 200, 221]. Ultrastructural examination of retinal lesions in late infantile MLD reveals irregularly stained lamellar lipids within a dense granular

matrix distributed in the ganglion cells and several other layers of the retina [134, 221]. Interestingly, cytoplasmic inclusions are found only in the ganglion cell layer in the adult form of MLD [134]. Metachromatic deposits in the optic and ciliary nerves are similarly found throughout the CNS and peripheral nervous system [152, 200].

CHEMICAL PATHOLOGY

MLD is primarily characterized by the accumulation of galactosyl sulfatide in the white matter of the CNS and peripheral nerves. High concentrations of sulfatide in the kidney, gallbladder, and other viscera appear to be clinically insignificant.

The enzymatic basis of MLD is the total lack of arylsulfatase A. The chromogenic substance *p*-nitrocatechol is most frequently used to determine the activity of arylsulfatase A (and under different conditions arylsulfatase B) in a variety of sites [200]. Enzymatic deficiency can be demonstrated in kidney, liver, brain, leukocytes, cultured skin fibroblasts [190, 264], tears [221], and urine [11, 175]. Urinalysis is suggested only as a screening procedure, and low activity levels should be followed up by analysis of cultured fibroblasts or leukocytes.

BIOCHEMICAL DETECTION

Biochemical detection of arylsulfatase A deficiency can be done in a variety of assays as listed above. The most reliable and easiest, however, is the assay of arylsulfatase A activity in leukocyte extracts [152] or in cultured skin fibroblasts [190, 264]. Glycolipid levels are nearly 100 times those of normal subjects [268]. Prenatal diagnosis has been successful [98].

DETECTION OF HETEROZYGOTES

Screening siblings and parents for heterozygosity has important consequences for families of affected individuals. Leukocyte and fibroblast assays can also be used for detection of these individuals, as they express a level of activity approximately 50 percent of normal [200, 348].

25300 Morquio's Syndrome

See Mucopolysaccharidosis IV.

25240 Mucolipidosis I (Lysosomal Enzyme Deficiency, Sialidosis)

Mucolipidosis I is characterized by the presence of dysostosis multiplex, coarse facial features beginning in infancy, and neurologic symptoms that occur by about 6 years of age. Two presentations are noted. In one group adolescents present with decreased visual acuity or myoclonus or both. In the second patients may present in infancy or late childhood with dysmorphic, coarse facies; Hurler-like skeletal abnormalities; and mental retardation. All patients were noted to have macular cherry-red spots [25].

CHEMICAL PATHOLOGY

Sialic acid–containing oligosaccharides have been found in cultured fibroblasts, leukocytes, and urine of patients with mucolipidosis I. A concomitant profound deficiency in *N*-acetylneuraminidase (sialidase) was also noted and has prompted the new classification name of *sialidosis* [238]. In both types of patients there is urinary excretion of sialyloligosaccharides and neuraminidase deficiency. However, in the dysmorphic form, β-galactosidase was found to be low or absent in some patients, while levels were normal in the syndrome with cherry-red spot and myoclonus [25]. Whether these disorders are distinct or reflect variations within the same defect is still not known.

25260 Mucolipidosis III (Pseudo-Hurler Polydystrophy)

Mucolipidosis III (ML III) is an autosomal recessive disorder that is considered to be biochemically related to the lysosomal disorder of mucolipidosis II [27]. The clinical manifestations of ML III, despite its name, are akin to the Maroteaux-Lamy syndrome of intermediate severity (mucopolysaccharidosis VI) and include joint stiffness, growth retardation, carpal tunnel syndrome, and a coarsening of facial features presenting at age 4 to 5 years [247]. Corneal clouding becomes grossly visible by the end of the first decade and is a consistent feature [186]. Conjunctival fibroblasts have been noted to be filled with single-membrane-limited inclusion bodies containing fibrillogranular material, but much less so than in ML II [25]. ML II is known as I-cell disease. It has mental retardation and a MPS (mucopolysaccharidoses) phenotype. It is interesting that the same

type of lysosomal enzyme defect that causes corneal clouding as a reliable feature of ML III should affect the cornea of patients with ML II inconsistently and to an insignificant, mild degree.

CHEMICAL PATHOLOGY

The defect in ML III involves the inappropriate localization of acid hydrolases extracellularly (rather than intralysosomally) as the result of a defect in post-translational phosphorylation. Not all cell types or lysosomal enzymes are affected. Notably, neurons, hepatocytes, acid phosphatase, and β-glucosidase are unaffected with respect to amount, activity, or distribution [247]. The distinguishing feature of this syndrome is the absence of mucopolysaccharides in the urine [186]. Serum levels of β-hexosaminidase, iduronate sulfatase, and arylsulfatase A are elevated as much as 20-fold and are diagnostic of ML II and ML III [186]. Fibroblasts are the cell culture of choice, and the characteristic deficiencies are noted intracellularly. The elevation in culture media activity is approximately equal to the intracellular deficit [186, 214].

BIOCHEMICAL DETECTION

Urine samples from suspected pseudo-Hurler patients give negative results on spot tests with "MPS paper" [28]. Detection of the appropriate serum or fibroblast deficiencies is diagnostic. No biochemical differences between ML II and ML III have yet been noted [247].

PRENATAL DETECTION

Elevated acid hydrolases in amniotic fluid [10], amniotic isoenzyme differences [260], or enzyme deficiency in amniotic cell culture [10] provides ample basis for prenatal detection. Because of a wide overlap between normal individuals and heterozygotes, heterozygote detection is unreliable [247].

25280 Mucopolysaccharidosis I-H (Hurler's Syndrome, Gargoylism)

The clinical features of mucopolysaccharidosis (MPS) I-H (Hurler's syndrome) are the prototype for all the mucopolysaccharide storage diseases. Although normal at birth, affected individuals undergo a severe, rapidly progressive course leading to death, usually before the age of 10 years. Mental and physical deterioration results in moderate to severe hepatomegaly, mental retardation, grotesque facies, hirsutism, cardiovascular disease, dwarfism, and numerous skeletal changes including a widening of the medial end of the clavicle [235]. The latter can be diagnosed radiologically and is characteristic of the mucopolysaccharidoses [150].

Corneal clouding is a prominent feature and develops early, with progression during the first few years of life [136]. Subnormal electroretinographic (ERG) responses, which may eventually become extinct, are present in nearly all cases [217]. Retinal examination reveals features of retinitis pigmentosa including hyperplasia and hypopigmentation of the retinal pigment epithelium, optic atrophy, and arteriolar narrowing [187].

CHEMICAL PATHOLOGY

Absence of α-L-iduronidase, a lysosomal hydrolase required for cleavage of L-iduronic acid residues from mucopolysaccharide polymers, results in deposition and urinary excretion of dermatan sulfate and heparan sulfate (Table 2-7) [231, 235]. Some degradation by glycosidases occurs in the liver, though not in fibroblasts, which also contributes to the detection of mucopolysaccharide fragments in the urine [13, 225]. In vivo correction

of the defect in Hurler fibroblasts has been demonstrated after α-L-iduronidase uptake [13].

BIOCHEMICAL DETECTION

Mucopolysacchariduria is marked in affected individuals and is most easily detected by three common screening procedures: the Berry spot test, the Ames MPS spot test (Ames Co., Elkhart, Ind.), and the gross acid albumin turbidity test (Table 2-8) [225]. As a screening procedure, the Berry spot test is the most sensitive and reliably detects mucopolysacchariduria in all of the mucopolysaccharidoses with as little as 10 ml of urine. However, because of its low specificity, a positive result on the Berry test must be followed up with additional analyses (Table 2-8).

Assays of α-L-iduronidase activity in leukocytes or cultured fibroblasts, using phenyl and 4-methyliumbelliferyl iduronides as well as radioactive iduronic acid disaccharides as substrates, provide specific determination of Hurler's syndrome [13, 235]. Gel filtration followed by colorimetric assessment of sulfoaminohexose and uronate in the macromolecular fraction, electrophoresis, or high-performance liquid chromatography are alternatives that allow assessment of the qualitative as well as quantitative nature of excreted urinary glycosaminoglycans [212].

Table 2-7. *Mucopolysaccharides: Chemical Composition and Distribution**

Name	Disaccharide repeating unit	Tissue
Hyaluronic acid	Glucuronic acid: N-acetylgucosamine	Vitreous; synovial fluid
Chondroitin 4-sulfate	Glucuronic acid: N-acetylgalactosamine-O-SO$_4$	Cartilage; cornea;[†] retina
Chondroitin 6-sulfate	Glucuronic acid: N-acetylgalactosamine-O-SO$_4$	Aorta; umbilical cord
Dermatan sulfate	L-Iduronic acid: N-acetylgalactosamine-O-SO$_4$ (plus some glucuronic acid)	Skin
Heparan sulfate	Glucuronic acid: N-acetylgucosamine -O-SO$_4$ -N-SO$_4$ (plus some L-iduronic acid)	Aorta
Heparin[‡]	Glucuronic acid: N-acetyglucosamine-N-SO$_4$ (plus some L-iduronic acid) plus some -O-SO$_4$	Mast cells
Keratan sulfate	Galactose: N-acetylglucosamine-O-SO$_4$	Cartilage; cornea[†]

*Mucopolysaccharides (glycosaminoglycans) are high molecular weight, negatively charged linear polymers, each having characteristic disaccharide repeating units. All, with the exception of hyaluronic acid, are bound to protein, most of them through the linkage Ser-Xyl-Gal-Gal.
†In cornea both chondroitin sulfate and keratan sulfate are heterogeneous in chemical composition and sulfate content.
‡Heparin has approximately 2.5 mol of sulfate/disaccharide unit. All other sulfated mucopolysaccharides have a statistical average of 1 mol of sulfate/disaccharide.
Source: From E. R. Berman [22].

Table 2-8. *Mucopolysaccharide Screening Tests*

Mucopolysaccharidosis type	Berry spot test	Ames MPS spot test	Gross acid albumin turbidity test
I-H	+	+	+
I-S	+	+	+
II	+	+	+
III	+	+	−
IV	+	−	−
VI	+	−	−

+ = reliable; − = unreliable.

PRENATAL DIAGNOSIS

Midpregnancy microculture of amniotic fluid leukocytes and fibroblasts with specific enzyme testing has shortened the waiting period required between sampling and diagnosis to only 2 weeks [120, 151]. Nonetheless, these techniques require facilities beyond those of many diagnostic laboratories. Recently, it has been reported that two-dimensional electrophoretic analysis of amniotic fluid glycosaminoglycans is a simple, fast, and reliable method of diagnosis [243, 338].

DETECTION OF HETEROZYGOTES

Direct chemical analysis of cultured skin fibroblasts is favored in the detection of heterozygosity in this autosomal recessive disorder [235]. While these cells have a lower level of α-L-iduronidase activity, they exhibit the same degree of ^{35}S-mucopolysaccharide accumulation as do cells of normal individuals [151].

25310 Mucopolysaccharidosis I-S (Scheie's Syndrome)

Scheie's syndrome (formerly known as MPS V) is characterized by severe corneal clouding, deformity of the hands, and involvement of the aortic valve. In contrast to Hurler's syndrome, in Scheie's syndrome stature and intelligence are normal [235]. The cardinal ophthalmologic manifestations of MPS I-S are corneal clouding, glaucoma, and retinal pigmentary degeneration. As in other mucopolysaccharidoses, clouding is due to excessive accumulation of dermatan and heparan sulfate within corneal epithelial cells, subepithelial histiocytes, stromal keratocytes, and endothelial cells and extracellularly throughout the stroma [188]. The accumulation is particularly great in the peripheral and posterior aspect of the stroma [28]. Diminished ERG responses and fundus abnormalities are similar to those described in MPS I-H [187, 217, 235].

CHEMICAL PATHOLOGY

The enzymatic deficiency (of α-L-iduronidase) in Scheie's syndrome is identical to that in Hurler's syndrome and results in deposition and urinary excretion of dermatan sulfate and heparan sulfate. Variability of expression in these two syndromes seems to indicate that there is allelic variance at the iduronidase locus [235]. Interestingly, some investigators have reported iduronidase activity in Scheie fibroblasts when using desulfated heparan but not desulfated dermatan sulfate as a substrate [231].

BIOCHEMICAL DETECTION

Screening tests and chemical analyses available for Hurler's syndrome are applicable to Scheie's syndrome as well. Elucidation of pleiotropic differences in these two syndromes as well as in an intermediate Hurler-Scheie syndrome awaits further molecular genetic investigation.

30990 Mucopolysaccharidosis II (Hunter's Syndrome)

X-linked Hunter's syndrome is similar to MPS I-H (Hurler's syndrome) but is less severe. Mental retardation is not usually a feature of MPS II, and corneal clouding is difficult to appreciate without a slit lamp. A pigmentary retinopathy occurs with loss of photoreceptors, as does vacuolization of ganglion cells and pigment epithelial cells. Retinal pigment epithelial migration to the retina, cornea, sclera, choroidal fibroblasts, and ciliary epithelium has been noted [24]. As with MPS I-

H, large amounts of heparan and dermatan sulfate are excreted in the urine. Severe and mild phenotypes of sulfoiduronate sulfatase deficiency can be explained by two allelic mutations [234].

BIOCHEMICAL TESTS

The same tests used for Hurler's syndrome can be applied to the diagnosis of Hunter's syndrome.

25290 Mucopolysaccharidosis III (Sanfilippo's Syndrome)

In MPS III severe progressive mental retardation, hepatosplenomegaly, and other features of MPS I-H and II are noted. Dermatan sulfate is not excreted, though heparan sulfate is found in the urine. Types A, B, and C nonallelic mutations are recognized and are due to deficiencies in heparan sulfaminidase, *N*-acetyl-α-D-glucosaminidase, and α-glucosaminide *N*-acetyl transferase, respectively. MPS III type C is the only lysosomal storage disease in which acid hydrolase is not defective. Few eyes have been examined in this condition. Pigmentary retinopathy can occur and is associated with photoreceptor and pigment epithelial aberrations.

BIOCHEMICAL TESTS

The diagnostic tests for Hurler's syndrome may be applied to MPS III.

25300 Mucopolysaccharidosis IV (Morquio's Syndrome)

MPS IV is characterized by marked skeletal abnormalities with secondary effects on the nervous system. There is severe growth retardation with deformities of the chest and ribs giving rise to a barrel chest and prominent sternum (pectus carinatum). Joint laxity and hyperplasia of ligaments invariably lead to the development of severe knock knees (genu valgum) and cause atlantoaxial vertebral subluxation to be a major complication. Intelligence is normal [235].

Mild corneal opacities are present in the stroma of nearly all patients but rarely have functional significance [136]. No other ocular involvement has been noted. While the excretion of keratan sulfate constitutes strong evidence of Morquio's syndrome, keratan sulfate is also excreted in patients with fucosidosis, Kniest's syndrome, and

GM$_1$ gangliosidosis, which does not make MPS IV biochemially easy to diagnose.

BIOCHEMICAL DETECTION

Of the screening procedures described for Hurler's syndrome, only the Berry spot test reliably detects the presence of urinary glycosaminoglycans in Morquio's syndrome. The unequivocal diagnosis may be made by assaying *N*-acetylgalactosamine 6-sulfate sulfatase activity in leukocytes, cultured skin fibroblasts, or amniotic cells prenatally, or in leukocytes and cultured skin fibroblasts postnatally using a trisaccharide derivative of chondroitin 6-sulfate: *N*-acetylgalactosamine 6-sulfate $(\beta,1\text{-}4)$-glucuronic acid$(\beta,1\text{-}3)$-1-(^3H)-*N*-galactosaminitol 6-sulfate [202, 232, 330]. The diagnostic use of transmission scanning electron microscopy of conjunctival biopsy specimens and cultured skin fibroblasts has recently been suggested [198].

PRENATAL DIAGNOSIS

Two-dimensional electrophoresis of amniotic fluid glycosaminoglycans may be a rapid and reliable alternative to the cell culture techniques described above [243].

25320 Mucopolysaccharidosis VI (Maroteaux-Lamy Syndrome)

Like Morquio's syndrome, Maroteaux-Lamy syndrome is characterized by marked growth retardation and skeletal dysplasia while intellect remains normal. Genu valgum, lumbar kyphosis, sternal protrusion, cardiac changes, and progressive clawhand deformity become increasingly manifest at age 2 to 3 years. Corneal opacities are of the same character and distribution as in the other mucopolysaccharide storage diseases; the cornea may be grossly opaque [235].

CHEMICAL PATHOLOGY

Deficiency of the enzyme arylsulfatase B (*N*-acetylgalactosamine-4-sulfatase) results in the inability to cleave the *N*-acetylated hexosamine from dermatan sulfate. Interestingly, chondroitin 4-sulfate also has *N*-acetylgalactosamine sulfate as a side group, but chondroitin sulfate is not an excreted urinary mucopolysaccharide.

BIOCHEMICAL DETECTION

While the diagnosis of Maroteaux-Lamy syndrome is often made on the basis of the physical findings, such as the detection of urinary dermatan sulfate and the striking degree of metachromatic inclusion bodies' seen in leukocytes, specific biochemical detection is made by assaying arylsulfatase B activity. This method has also been used successfully in the prenatal diagnosis of this syndrome [326].

23325 Neuraminidase Deficiency

See Goldberg-Cotlier Syndrome.

20420 Neuronal Ceroid Lipofuscinosis

See Batten's Disease.

25720 Niemann-Pick Disease, Infantile Form (Sphingomyelin Lipidosis)

At least five types of Niemann-Pick disease can now be distinguished: the classical infantile form (type A), the visceral form (type B), the subacute or juvenile form (type C), the Nova Scotia variant (type D), and the adult form (type E) [234]. The most commonly occurring type is type A, in which there is severe involvement of the reticuloendothelial, visceral, and nervous systems early in infancy. Emaciation, hypotonia, and failure to achieve developmental milestones ensue, and death usually occurs by the third year. Enlarged foamy histiocytes are present in the bone marrow, liver, splenic pulp, lymph nodes, adrenal medulla, and alveoli of the lungs [39]. Massive hepatosplenomegaly with infiltration by sphingomyelin-laden foam cells is the primary diagnostic characteristic in this disease.

Corneal opacification, brownish discoloration of the anterior lens capsule, retinal opacification, and a macular cherry-red spot are ocular signs that may become manifest in the first year. The macular red spot, although commonly noted, is found in approximately 50 percent of patients [39, 333]. In the juvenile form, two cases of vertical supranuclear ophthalmoplegia have also been reported [41].

Ultrastructural studies reflect the widespread involvement of the disease on the eye. Two types of lamellar inclusion bodies have been described: multilamellar cytoplasmic bodies and a dense pleomorphic type that present as granular, vacuolar, or whorled masses [26, 222, 333]. Conjunctival biopsy in Niemann-Pick disease has been proposed as a method of differential diagnosis for the allelic forms of the disease, types A, B, and C [221]. In type A disease, in addition to the generalized storage of sphingomyelin, cholesterol, or both, lamellar whorls and inclusions are present in Schwann's cells, fibroblasts, epithelial cells, pericytes, and blood endothelial cells. Types B and C demonstrate less disordered ultrastructural morphology.

CHEMICAL PATHOLOGY

Tissue damage is caused by the massive infiltration of histiocytes, swollen by the accumulation of sphingomyelin in secondary lysosomes. The enzymatic deficiency of sphingomyelinase, which is necessary for the conversion of sphingomyelin to ceramide and phosphorylcholine, does not explain the high tissue levels of cholesterol. Sphingomyelinase activity has been shown to be decreased to 4 percent of normal [55], and the enzyme has been found in the visceral organs, fibroblasts, bone marrow, leukocytes, heart, lungs, and in many endocrine and exocrine organs [39].

BIOCHEMICAL DETECTION

Thin-layer chromatography can be used to detect sphingomyelin and cholesterol in a variety of tissue extracts. Coupled with the finding of foamy histiocytes in bone marrow aspirates, this test will establish the diagnosis much of the time. If type A Neimann-Pick disease is suspected, conjunctival biopsy offers another diagnostic procedure [221].

The enzymatic assays of Niemann-Pick disease have been greatly facilitated by the development of a chromogenic analog of sphingomyelin, 2-hexadecanoylamino-4-nitrophenyl phosphorylcholine hydroxine, which is water soluble, has an enzymatic specificity to degradation similar to that of sphingomyelin, and is commericaly available [119]. While the use of fibroblasts has the advantages of higher sphingomyelinase activity and enzyme stability on freezing, control cell cultures show a wide range of activity, and thus two cultures must be grown. Although they have a much lower level of innate activity, leukocytes are the tissue of choice because of the ease of culture and reliable controls [39].

DETECTION OF HETEROZYGOTES

Potential heterozygotes, who may be tested using the sphingomyelinase assays just outlined, have demonstrated activity levels in leukocytes of 54 to 65 percent of control levels. Fibroblast testing is useful in that enzyme activity is preserved in frozen tissue, which allows material to be transported with ease [40, 119]. No information on the detection of type C, D, or E disease is available.

PRENATAL DIAGNOSIS

The chromogenic assay has been successfully used with cultured fetal cells obtained by amniocentesis. While testing appears to be reliable for type A and type B, the prenatal diagnosis of type C disease is not yet possible [290]

30050 Ocular Albinism

Four types of ocular albinism have been described. The Nettleship-Falls type, the Forsius-Eriksson type, and the ocular albinism cum pigmento type are inherited as X-linked traits; punctuate ocular albinism is an autosomal recessive disorder [255, 256]. Melanin pigment is severely reduced in the iris, ciliary body, and retinal epithelium, which makes the choroid circulation especially prominent. The iris is light gray or blue, abnormally translucent, and hypoplastic, although increased pigmentation is often noted with age [196]. Heterozygous females have a characteristic mosaic pattern of retinal pigmentation. Macromelanosomes are present in the skin despite clinically normal pigmentation of the hair and skin [255, 256]. Decreased visual acuity and pendular nystagmus with oscillopsia are common findings [302, 342].

DETECTION OF HETEROZYGOTES

Female heterozygotes in the most common of the X-linked ocular albinisms, the Nettleship-Falls variety (XOAN), are noted for their translucent irises and the tigroid, "splashes of mud" mosaic appearance of their fundi [342]. The phenomenon has been ascribed to the Lyon hypothesis [229], in which a female who is heterozygous for a pair of contrasting genes is a mosaic of two cell types arising as a result of the inactivation of either a paternal (albinotic) or maternal (normal) X chromosome in each cell, resulting in a random pattern of pigmentation.

Oculocutaneous Albinism: 20310 Tyrosinase-negative (Type I), 20320 Tyrosinase-positive (Type II)

At least 10 forms of oculocutaneous albinism (OCA) have been identified. Congenital absence or reduction of skin, hair, and eye melanin are the hallmarks of OCA; associated features include photophobia, decreased visual acuity, nystagmus, and foveal hypoplasia [343]. The major disorders include tyrosinase-negative (ty-neg) OCA; tyrosinase-positive (ty-pos) OCA; Hermansky-Pudlak syndrome; Chédiak-Higashi syndrome; Cross's syndrome; brown OCA; black locks, albinism, and deafness of the sensorineural type (BADS); and yellow mutant (ym) OCA. With the exception of autosomal dominant OCA, all are inherited as autosomal recessive traits. These disorders can be identified by their clinical, biochemical, genetic, and ultrastructural features [342] and by the ability of anagen hair bulbs incubated in L-tyrosine to produce pigment [203]. Contrary to the original belief that deficiency of tyrosinase was the sole defect in OCA, only in tyrosinase-negative OCA does this appear to be true. The literature has recently been reviewed [343; see also Chap. 19]. It is beyond the scope of this chapter to describe the complete range of this burgeoning family of disorders.

CHEMICAL PATHOLOGY

In tyrosinase-negative OCA, there is complete lack of pigment in the skin, hair, and eyes and an absence of tyrosinase activity in tissues incubated with L-tyrosine or L-dopa [203]. Melanocytes are present in a normal distribution but fail to produce mature, stage IV melanosomes, containing only nonpigmented stage I and stage II forms. In contrast, in ty-pos individuals levels of tyrosinase activity are normal or increased as much as fourfold, and melanocytes contain both stage III and stage IV melanosomes, although fewer than normal [343]. The enzymatic defect in ty-pos OCA is unknown but may be a defect in an intracellular inhibitor or the feedback control mechanism of tyrosine utilization (Fig. 2-4).

BIOCHEMICAL DETECTION

The differentiation of ty-neg and ty-pos OCA on biochemical grounds is easily performed by incubating well-developed anagen hair bulbs in a phosphate-buffered solution of tyrosine at 37° C

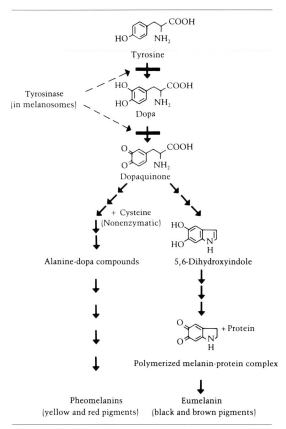

Fig. 2-4. *Production of melanin from tyrosine in melanocytes. The defect in tyrosinase-negative (ty-neg) albinism is a deficiency of tyrosinase, which converts tyrosine to dopa and then to dopaquinone. When this enzyme is absent, no melanin pigments are formed. The enzymatic defects for tyrosinase-positive albinism and ocular (X-linked) albinism are not known. (From E. R. Berman [22].)*

for 12 to 24 hours. Under light microscopy, using reflected light, these bulbs can be compared with formalin-fixed controls for evidence of pigment formation [203]. Normal individuals show a mild to moderate increase in pigment, while ty-pos individuals have a large increase, and ty-neg patients show no increase in pigmented melanosomes.

HETEROZYGOTE DETECTION

Detection of the ty-neg heterozygous state using anagen hair bulbs has been done with some success. As a test for unbound tyrosinase (T_1, T_3), this test measures the amount of ^{3}H-OH produced

when incubated with ^{3}H-tyrosine [191, 192]. Heterozygotes express little or no activity, possibly because T_1 tyrosinase is immediately bound to the melanosome as T_4 in these individuals, and thus have only a small amount of the free, soluble form [343].

26650 Phytanic Acid Storage Disease

See Refsum's Disease.

17600 Porphyria, Acute Intermittent

Acute intermittent porphyria (AIP) is an autosomal dominant disorder caused by the deficiency of porphobilinogen (PBG) deaminase (Fig. 2-5) and is notable as the only disorder of porphyrin metabolism not associated with cutaneous sensitivity. Steroids, drugs, and nutrition may precipitate this disorder by altering liver δ-aminolevulinic acid (ALA) synthetase and porphyrin-heme synthesis.

Attacks of AIP are intermittent and are characterized by acute abdominal pain, often with nausea, vomiting, and ileus; muscle pain; and proximal neuropathy. Mental disturbance and seizure are not uncommon in severe episodes [184]. Retinal edema, retinal hemorrhage, papilledema, and optic atrophy may in the rare case lead to blindness [67, 80, 209].

CHEMICAL PATHOLOGY

Excessive quantities (up to 200 mg/day) of ALA and PBG are excreted in the urine during acute attacks. In individuals who already manifest the disease, ALA, PBG, and uroporphyrin may remain high because of the nonenzymatic formation of uroporphyrin from PBG [184]. For unclear reasons, almost 90 percent of individuals with inherited PBG deaminase deficiency remain clinically and biochemically asymptomatic.

BIOCHEMICAL DETECTION

PBG deaminase activity is readily measured in erythrocytes [282]. Urinary PBG is best measured by the spectrophotometric detection of a reddish purple chromogen after the addition of Ehrlich's aldehyde [233]. A recent procedure for the analysis of whole blood uroporphyrinogen I synthetase from a filter paper dry blood spot has been developed for widespread population screening for AIP [176].

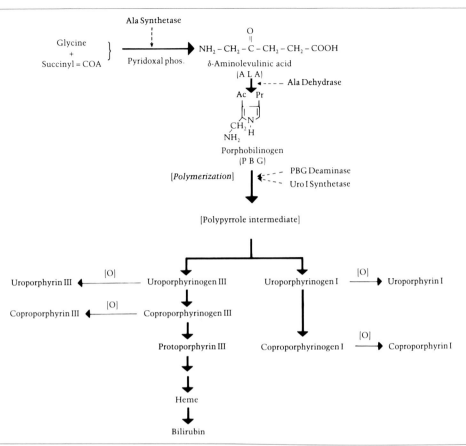

Fig. 2-5. *Abbreviated scheme of porphyrin synthesis in liver and red blood cells. In acute intermittent porphyria, there is elevated urinary excretion of both δ-aminolevulinic acid (ALA) and porphobilinogen (PBG). In congenital erythropoietic porphyria, elevated levels of uroporphyrin I and coproporphyrin I are present in urine, plasma, feces, red blood cells, and spleen. In hepatic porphyria, there is greatly increased urinary excretion of urophorphyrin. In variegate porphyria, both protoporphyrin and coproporphyrin are excreted during acute attacks. (Ac = acetyl; Pr = pyridoxal ; Uro I = urophorphyrinogen I.) (From E. R. Berman [22].)*

26370 Porphyria, Congenital Erythropoietic (Günther's Disease)

A rare but dramatic form of porphyria, congenital erythropoietic porphyria (CEP) is an autosomal recessive disorder often detectable in early infancy. CEP should be considered in any patient with severe photosensitivity beginning in early childhood. The disease may be recognized by the excretion of red urine, hemolytic anemia, splenomegaly, and the formation of serous bullae. The fluid may contain red and white cells as well as various porphyrins that fluoresce under ultraviolet (UV) light. Rupture of bullae, which occurs particularly on the exposed hands, head, and face, leads to cutaneous scarring and depigmentation of the eyelids; corneal scarring and chorioretinitis are the principal ocular signs [67].

CHEMICAL PATHOLOGY

Urine porphyrin excretion results in a red coloration and can be in the range of 50 to 100 mg daily (up to 400 times the normal level). In CEP the excreted porphyrin consists mostly of uroporphyrin I and coproporphyrin I (Fig. 2-5). Uroporphyrin III and coproporphyrin III excretion is elevated, and there is excessive excretion of 5-, 6-, and 7-carboxylated porphyrins [184]. The primary enzymatic defect seems to arise from a homozygous structural gene mutation that decreases uroporphyrinogen III cosynthetase activity [93, 184, 251], leading to an overproduction by erythrocytes of type I porphyrin isomers.

BIOCHEMICAL DETECTION

Diagnosis of CEP must exclude other types of photocutaneous porphyrias (porphyria cutaneous tarda, coproporphyria hereditary, and variegate). CEP is unique in that both urine and erythrocyte porphyrins are increased [184]. Ion-exchange or thin-layer chromatography using purified porphyrin standards may be carried out for qualitative and quantitative assessment.

HETEROZYGOTE DETECTION

Heterozygotes can be detected by studying uroporphyrinogen III cosynthetase activity in cultured fibroblasts [277]. While amniotic fluid analysis and cell culture seem likely directions for prenatal and heterozygote detection, the precise protocols have yet to be established [93, 148].

17610 Porphyria, Hepatic (Porphyria Cutanea Tarda Hereditaria)

An autosomal dominant disorder, hepatic porphyria is characterized by the urinary excretion of large amounts of uroporphyrin coupled with a light-sensitive dermatitis [234]. Porphyria cutanea tarda (PCT) usually has its onset in adult life, but inheritance of this disorder is nonetheless sporadic. Skin lesions consist of small white plaques (milia) that frequently progress to form bullous and fluid-filled vesicles after sun exposure. An almost identical syndrome is found in association with chlorinated cyclic hydrocarbon exposure, liver disease, alcohol abuse, and, rarely, in cases of altered endogenous hormone production such as Klinefelter's syndrome [184].

Scarring of the lids may produce ectropion and conjunctival hyperemia; lacrimation, photophobia, and blepharospasm are frequently found. Recurrent conjunctival vesication may produce erosion and necrosis secondary to the adherence of the conjunctiva to the underlying sclera [171].

CHEMICAL PATHOLOGY

Decreased liver uroporphyrinogen decarboxylase is found in all cases of porphyria and causes a greatly increased urinary excretion of uroporphyrin (Fig. 2-5), resulting in pink or brownish urine [77]. While the pathogenesis of hepatic por-

phyria is unclear, liver cell damage, iron overload, and estrogen appear to be contributing factors [184].

BIOCHEMICAL TESTS

Plasma porphyrin content is invariably increased in PCT as well as the other photocutaneous porphyrias. Plasma porphyrin levels can be determined quantitatively by fluorometry, while qualitative identification of the specific porphyrin defect can be performed using thin-layer or high-performance liquid chromatography to analyze the pattern of porphyrin excretion [92, 184].

17620 Porphyria, Variegate

Variegate porphyria displays an autosomal dominant pattern of inheritance and is especially common in South African whites—approximately 3 in 1,000 have inherited this disorder [184]. The most common symptoms and signs are abdominal pain, tachycardia, vomiting, constipation, hypertension, and neuropathy, all of which occur in more than 60 percent of patients [90]. Photocutaneous sensitivity and neuropsychiatric disturbances that accompany acute attacks are triggered by the administration of barbiturates, sulfonamides, or a variety of hepatotoxic agents [184].

Eye findings include those described under Congenital Erythropoietic Porphyria, with optic neuritis, optic atrophy, and retinal hemorrhage being other rare findings [67].

CHEMICAL PATHOLOGY

The most characteristic finding in variegate porphyria is an increase in stool protoporphyrin content. Stool coproporphyrin is also increased, although to a lesser degree (Fig. 2-5). Urinary ALA and PBG excretion is also greatly increased during acute attacks [184].

The enzymatic defect in the variegate form of porphyria remains unclear. While substantial evidence has shown that there is markedly reduced activity of protoporphyrinogen oxidase [43, 84, 90, 184], decreased ferrochelase activity may also play a role [18].

BIOCHEMICAL DETECTION

Clinical detection of porphyrin in blood plasma may be done using quantitative thin-layer chromatography [78]. Porphobilinogen can be detected using Urobilistic reagent strips (Ames Co., Elkhart, Ind.).

25260 Pseudo-Hurler Polydystrophy

See Mucolipidosis III.

26650 Refsum's Disease (Phytanic Acid Storage Disease)

Refsum's disease was first described in four children aged 4 to 7 years by Sigvald Refsum in 1946 as heredopathia atactica polyneuritiformis [271]. He noted its autosomal family inheritance and the diagnostic triad of retinitis pigmentosa, peripheral polyneuropathy, and cerebellar ataxia. Additional findings of elevated cerebrospinal fluid (CSF) protein levels without pleocytosis; anosmia; nerve deafness; hypertrophic symmetrical polyneuropathy with thickening of ulnar, sural, and auricular nerves; motor weakness; decreased deep tendon reflexes; sensory loss in a glove-and-stocking distribution; ichthyosis of palms and soles; cardiac abnormalities; and epiphyseal dysplasia were also described [271]. One of the earliest signs is failing night vision with progressive visual field constriction. Later, pupillary abnormalities and posterior subcapsular cateracts become manifest [312, 322].

CHEMICAL PATHOLOGY

Characterization of the enzyme defect in cell culture reveals a deficiency of phytanic acid α-hydroxylase [272]. This unique α-hydroxylation constitutes the first step in the phytanic acid degradation cascade. With the enzyme deficiency phytanic acid is deposited in the liver, heart, peripheral nerves, and choroid of the retina and constitutes up to 30 percent of the total plasma fatty acid concentration [161, 312]. The major source is dietary, especially milk, butter, and beef fat and secondarily the phyto group of chlorophyll in leafy vegetables [312]. Treatment by dietary restriction and plasmapheresis appears to limit progression of this disease [127, 241].

BIOCHEMICAL DETECTION

Refsum's disease may be detected by assaying blood phytanic acid levels by gas [312] or thin-layer chromatography, or by measuring CO_2-labeled phytanic acid in cultured fibroblasts [161].

DETECTION OF HETEROZYGOTES

Heterozygotes are asymptomatic and manifest no clinical signs of this disorder on a normal diet [312]. Heterozygote fibroblast cell cultures express about one-half the normal phytanic acid α-hydroxylase activity, whereas affected patients express only about 5 percent of normal activity [161].

PRENATAL DETECTION

While it has long been observed that amniotic cells have the capacity to oxidize phytanic acid [324], there has been a paucity of reports of the successful prenatal detection of homozygotes or heterozygotes of this disease.

22390 Riley-Day Syndrome

See Dysautonomia, Familial.

26880 Sandhoff's Disease

See GM$_2$ Gangliosidosis Type II.

25310 Scheie's Syndrome

See Mucopolysaccharidosis I-S.

25240 Sialidosis

See Mucolipidosis I.

25720 Sphingomyelin Lipidosis

See Niemann-Pick Disease, Infantile Form.

27230 Sulfite Oxidase Deficiency

Sulfite oxidase deficiency has been described only twice in the literature [244, 298]. The disease was manifested in a $2\frac{1}{2}$-year-old boy and a $4\frac{1}{2}$-year-old boy and was characterized by multiple neurologic abnormalities, including mental retardation, seizures, hemiplegia, and bilateral dislocated lenses.

CHEMICAL PATHOLOGY

Patients have increased sulfite in the urine with markedly decreased inorganic sulfate excretion. Metabolites consist of S-sulfocysteine, sulfite, and thiosulfite ions. The enzymatic defect is the absence of sulfite oxidase in liver, kidney, brain [244], and fibroblasts [298], which results in the accumulation of sulfite ion. Oxidation with cysteine to form sulfocysteine removes the toxic sulfite ion and allows for excretion from the body. While a sulfite oxidase deficiency is seen in rats after tungsten adminstration, assays have not been performed in the human condition [178, 179].

BIOCHEMICAL TESTING

It is possible to test for sulfite using a commercially available test paper, and thiosulfate and S-sulfocystathionine can be detected by two-dimensional electrophoresis of urinary amino acids [297]. However, a recent modification of the Sorbo spectrophotometric method, which is based on the cyanolysis of thiosulfate to thiocyanate, provides a reliable screening procedure for urinary thiosulfate [297].

20540 Tangier Disease

Tangier disease, a rare autosomal recessive trait, is characterized clinically by hyperplastic orange tonsils, hepatosplenomegaly, enlarged lymph nodes, and hypocholesterolemia. The thymus is extensively infiltrated by cholesterol esters, and neuropathy and intestinal storage have also been reported [97, 160].

Fine stromal opacities are present in some of the patients [22] but do not impair vision. Other ocular manifestations arise from neurologic changes and may present as ptosis, ocular muscle palsies, or diplopia [160].

CHEMICAL PATHOLOGY

The principal biochemical defect in Tangier disease is the absence of normal plasma HDL (α-lipoprotein). Homozygotes accumulate cholesterol esters, while heterozygotes have plasma HDL levels approximately half the normal level but do not develop neuropathy or excessive storage of cholesterol. Experiments with cell-free translation systems have suggested an enzymatic defect in the proteolytic conversion of proapolipoprotein AI to the apo AI form [145]. Other studies suggest a rapid and altered catabolism [283]. Analphalipoproteinemia results in the formation of abnormal chylomicrons, which are phagocytized by histiocytes and cells of the reticuloendothelial system. Loss of normal histiocyte clearance of cholesterol by HDL accounts, in part, for the observed intracellular accumulation of cholesterol.

BIOCHEMICAL DETECTION

Low plasma cholesterol levels coupled with normal to high triglyceride levels are characteristic of Tangier disease and, with the physical findings previously described, serve to exclude familial LCAT deficiency, obstructive liver disease, acquired HDL deficiency, and other forms of hepatosplenic storage disease [160]. Abnormal HDL can be detected by paper chromatography and analytic ultracentrifugation. In addition, the demonstration of apo AI mRNA in various organs by complementary DNA (cDNA) hybridization is now possible, and the nucleotide sequence of cloned human apolipoprotein AI cDNA is now known.

DETECTION OF HETEROZYGOTES

Serum concentrations of both A apolipoproteins is decreased by 50 percent in heterozygotes. Catabolic activity is normal without evidence of cholesterol ester accumulation. Heterozygotes express no consistent pattern of clinical abnormalities and show no signs or symptoms of premature atherosclerotic disease [160].

27280 Tay-Sachs Disease

See GM$_2$ Gangliosidosis Type I.

27670 Tyrosinemia Type II

The term *tyrosinemia* refers to a group of diseases that have tyrosinemia, tyrosinuria, and phenylaciduria as common findings. The three major diseases are tyrosinemia types I and II and tyrosinosis. Although it is still poorly characterized, the defect in tyrosinemia type II, the most common form, appears to be a deficiency of tyrosine aminotransferase (TAT) (Fig. 2-6) [143]. High levels of plasma tyrosine and urinary p-hydroxyphenylpyruvate and p-hydroxyphenyllactate result, although other amino acid, renal, and hapatic metabolic functions appear to be unimpaired.

Ocular manifestations of tyrosinemia type II begin as early as 2 weeks after birth [51] and consist of bilateral herpetiform keratitis, dendritic ulcer, and, rarely, corneal and conjunctival plaques [17, 51, 129, 142]. Neovascularization may be a prominent finding [17, 51]. The development of cataract may be a long-term sequela in untreated patients.

Other clinical features include painful, nonpruritic, crusty, hyperkeratotic lesions of the tips

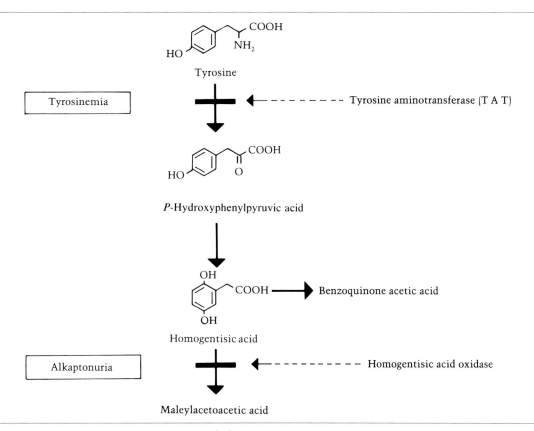

Fig. 2-6. *Abbreviated scheme of tyrosine metabolism in liver and other tissues. In tyrosinemia the deficiency in TAT causes an elevation in plasma tyrosine levels as well as some increase in urinary tyrosine. In alkaptonuria the deficiency in homogentisic acid oxidase results in elevated excretion of homogentisic acid. In the tissues some of this acid is converted to benzoquinoneacetic acid, which is presumed to form ochronotic pigment deposits in connective tissues. (From E. R. Berman [22].)*

of the digits, palms, and soles. Mild to moderate mental retardation with diminished fine motor and verbal abilities are major neurologic features [142].

Type I (hepatorenal) tyrosinemia and tyrosinosis are characterized by chronic nodular cirrhotic liver disease and renal tubular dysfunction [234]. A deficiency of fumarylacetoacetate (FAA) hydrolase is proposed as the metabolic cause of tyrosinosis [143]. Accumulation of succinylacetone malate and fumarylacetoacetate is thought to reduce the level of glutathione and thus impair hepatic detoxification mechanisms.

BIOCHEMICAL DETECTION

The easiest method of evaluating the tyrosinemias is to assay blood tyrosine levels and urine *p*-hydroxyphenylpyruvic acid, *p*-hydroxylphenyllactic acid, or *p*-hydroxyphenylacetic acid [42]. A number of other methods exist for the prenatal diagnosis of hereditary tyrosinemia [153]. The assay for succinylacetone in amniotic fluid has been widely used to date [118, 142], but its sensitivity has been recently challenged [205, 311]. In equivocal cases the additional assay for deficient FAA hydrolase activity in cultured amniotic cells may be indicated. Assays of cord blood at birth indicate that liver toxicity and marked elevation of α-fetoprotein may predate increases in plasma tyrosine and may thus provide another biochemical marker for this disease [170].

24710 Urbach-Wiethe Syndrome (Lipid Proteinosis)

The association of early hoarseness with papular eruptions suggests the diagnosis of Urbach-Wiethe syndrome [234]. While the course of the illness has not been definitively characterized, the disease often starts in early childhood with deposition of plaques on the mucous membranes, eruption on the face and extensor surfaces of the skin, and nodular formation on the margins of the eyelids that, in advanced cases, produces a characteristic picture similar to moniliform blepharitis. Neither madarosis nor trichiasis usually occurs [38, 103]. Drusen and conjunctival granulations have been reported in several early cases [112], as have visceral and CNS involvement.

CHEMICAL PATHOLOGY

The underlying enzymatic defect is unknown. An amorphous infiltrative material is deposited in the skin and throughout the body, which suggests a disease of lysosomal storage. Altered $(SO_4)^{2-}$ incorporation in 70 mucopolysaccharides suggests defects in mucopolysaccharide metabolism [16]. Dermal fibroblasts show striking cytoplasmic vacuolization similar to that in other lysosomal storage diseases such as the mucolipidoses, gangliosidoses, and ceroid lipofuscinosis, as well as membrane-bound cytoplasmic inclusions in cultured skin fibroblasts [16].

BIOCHEMICAL DETECTION

In patients with Urbach-Wiethe syndrome the quantitative levels and qualitative distribution of lipids, protein, and related blood and serum components are normal. Lipid content of the severely affected areas is lower than normal. There is lack of birefringence and amyloid stain uptake on histologic examination [248].

23220 Von Gierke's Disease

See Glycogen Storage Disease Type I.

27790 Wilson's Disease

Wilson's disease is most frequently characterized by progressive liver disease and neurologic impairment presenting in adolescence (between 8 and 16 years of age). Although hemolytic crisis and diffuse bone involvement may also be the initial presentation, symptoms frequently found include jaundice, vomiting, malaise, dysarthria, and incoordination of voluntary movements [74, 284]. The Kayser-Fleischer ring is one of the few pathognomonic signs in clinical medicine. It is a yellowish brown, dull copper–colored granular deposit on Descemet's membrane at the limbus

of the cornea seen earliest and most predominantly at the upper and lower poles [140]. Kayser-Fleischer rings are present in 100 percent of patients with neurologic manifestations of Wilson's disease [284]. Although easily visible in the late stage even to the unaided eye, early definitive diagnosis requires slit-lamp biomicroscopy [74, 335].

Analysis of copper content in various parts of the eye suggests that the Kayser-Fleischer ring is caused by a complex of copper with a sulfur-containing molecule, since there is a relative abundance of sulfur at the corneal limbus but virtually none at the central area [180]. Sunflower cataracts, cause by the deposition of copper on the anterior and posterior lens capsule, have been reported in 15 to 20 percent of cases. Sunflower cataract appears as an axially situated disc-shaped opacity with fine, wispy granular deposits that radiate peripherally in a petal-like distribution [335]. Both the Kayser-Fleischer ring and the sunflower cataract disappear with penicillamine treatment and as falling plasma copper levels reduce the extrahepatic manifestations of this disease. Although pupillary sluggishness is often seen as a clinical sign [284], defects of ocular motility and accommodation are minimal and rare [140, 195]. Other rare signs include blepharoconjunctivitis, retrobulbar neuritis, retinal hemorrhage, and hemeralopia.

CHEMICAL PATHOLOGY

The primary defect in Wilson's disease has not been established. Present evidence indicates that the disease is not caused by a molecular defect in ceruloplasmin. Nonetheless a profound disturbance in copper metabolism causes both a marked reduction in the rate of copper incorporation into ceruloplasmin and a reduction in the excretion of copper by the biliary system [74]. Initially copper is accumulated in the liver. As the plasma nonceruloplasmin copper level rises, extrahepatic deposition in the cornea, brain (especially in the basal ganglia), kidney, muscle, bone, and joints may become evident. In young patients copper tends to accumulate in the cytoplasm after being bound by monomeric metallothionein, whereas in neonates and the elderly copper is bound by polymeric complexes of metallothionein and is stored in the lysosome [74]. Many explanations for cell necrosis and death have been postulated [263, 313]. While theories of membrane lipid oxidation, protein and nucleic acid binding, and free radical generation have been advanced as possible mechanisms, the chemical pathology remains obscure.

BIOCHEMICAL DETECTION

The diagnosis of suspected cases is confirmed by demonstrating a serum ceruloplasmin level less than 20 mg/dl in the presence of Kayser-Fleischer rings, or a concentration of copper in a liver biopsy sample greater than 250 μg/gm dry weight [58]. Most affected patients excrete more than 100 μg copper per day in urine and show changes in hepatocyte histology [332]. Serum and urinary copper, including ceruloplasmin-bound copper, can be measured either by reaction with 2,2'-biquinoline after reduction with ascorbic acid or via a colorimetric assay using dicyclohexanone oxalylhydrazone [325]. Serum ceruloplasmin can be estimated by measurement of its oxidative capacity using phenylenediamine as a substrate, direct measurement of the optical density at 610 nm or by an immunologic assay [22]. Approximately 5 percent of affected individuals have plasma ceruloplasmin levels greater than 20 mg/dl, and Kayser-Fleischer rings and elevated hepatic copper levels are found in other hepatic disorders [74]. The use of radioactive copper as a marker for ceruloplasmin incorporation easily distinguishes Wilson's disease from the other entities [314], since patients with Wilson's disease, despite normal levels of ceruloplasmin, incorporate virtually no isotope into the protein.

HETEROZYGOTE DETECTION

Siblings of affected individuals have a 1 in 4 chance of developing the disease and should be tested using liver biopsy or radioactive copper when initial test results are normal. Heterozygotes are asymptomatic. Because of its relatively low reliability (80–90%), large-scale screening has little value [74]. Since prenatal diagnosis is not possible at this time, early clinical detection remains the most important step in the diagnostic cascade. It is important to remember that early intervention and treatment with penicillamine, if instituted before the onset of hepatic damage, will allow the individual to lead a long and symptom-free life.

27800 Wolman's Disease

Wolman's disease is a rare autosomal recessive disorder characterized by the accumulation of cholesterol esters and triglycerides in most of the tissues of the body, resulting in massive hepatosplenomegaly, abdominal distention, adrenal calcification demonstrable by x-rays, and death by nutritional failure by 2 to 4 months of age [9]. Although case reports note normal-appearing fundi and the lack of a cherry-red spot, histochemical examination reveals swollen retinal ganglion cells with foamy cytoplasm [334]. Sudanophilic droplets, both free and within macrophages, have been observed in the sclera, cornea, and ciliary body [22].

CHEMICAL PATHOLOGY

There is a generalized storage of neutral lipids owing to defective acid lipase activity, especially in the visceral organs and in the adrenal glands. Especially striking is the calcification of the adrenals, an abnormality seen in all but 4 patients [9]. Disseminated foam cell infiltration is seen in many organs including bone marrow and is present as vacuolated lymphocytes in the peripheral blood [234]. The RPE, neuroretina, and urea have all shown high affinity for acid lipase [157].

BIOCHEMICAL DETECTION

The diagnosis of Wolman's disease is made by the clinical picture and by demonstrating acid lipase deficiency in skin fibroblasts, lymphocytes, or affected organs. No specific laboratory tests suggest the diagnosis, although liver function values may be abnormal [9].

27870 Xeroderma Pigmentosum

Xeroderma pigmentosum (XP) is an autosomal recessive disease in which sensitivity to sunlight and the early development of carcinoma is observed. The nature and extent of cutaneous, ocular, and neurologic manifestations vary widely with genetic background and sun exposure [62, 300]. Skin changes include excessive freckling, erythema, keratoses, and the full range of skin cancers (see Chap. 19) [62, 228, 276]. Mild conjunctivitis and photophobia are common ocular findings, and even small amounts of UV radiation may lead to atrophic or malignant changes in the eyelid. Ectropion, entropion, blepharitis, symblepharon, and exposure keratitis may result [276]. Common neurologic findings are microcephaly, mental deficiency, and areflexia [269, 276]. A few cases of XP with severe neurologic symptoms, the

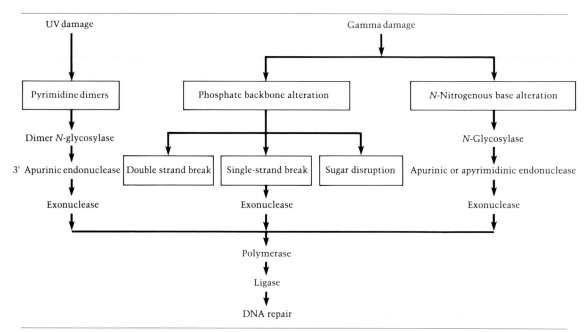

Fig. 2-7. *Major radiation damage to DNA and probable repair pathway. All enzymes listed have been identified in bacteria, and most have been found in humans, although the exact pathway has yet to be established. Repair of chemical damage, including cross-links, probably follows one of these two main paths. (UV = ultraviolet.)*

De Sanctis-Cacchione syndrome, have been reported. In addition to the neurologic lesions just described, these patients exhibit retarded skeletal development, sensorineural deafness, chorioathetosis, ataxia, and gonadal hypoplasia [269].

CHEMICAL PATHOLOGY

The mechanism of the loss of skin resistance to damage by sunlight is a decrease in the capacity of cells to repair or replicate damaged DNA. This type of DNA repair defect should be distinguished from diseases in which there is loss of shielding (albinism), deposition of sensitizing agents (porphyria), and hypersensitivity to DNA-damaging agents [62]. Sunlight in the near-UV spectrum is absorbed by proteins and nucleic acids to form DNA-protein links and the well-characterized cyclobutane pyrimidine dimer [45, 331]. Full understanding of the biochemistry of XP has still not been attained, but the disease is known to involve all three methods of DNA repair: photoreactivation, excision repair, and postreplicative repair [45, 62].

BIOCHEMICAL DETECTION

Fibroblasts, either from patients or from amniotic fluid, can be used for the detection of a DNA repair deficiency (Fig. 2-7) [126, 266]. Cells are cultured in several passages to eliminate nonviable cells, karyotyped for male fetuses to rule out maternal contamination, pulse-chased with tritiated thymidine, exposed to UV radiation, cultured in ^{3}H-TdR medium, and subjected to autoradiographic analysis. Cells undergoing stationary phase (S-phase) replication are heavily labeled, while cells undergoing DNA repair synthesis are only lightly labeled [266]. Despite numerous studies no consistent laboratory abnormality has been demonstrated [62, 300].

REFERENCES

1. Albers, J. J., Adolphson, J. L., and Chen, C. H. Radioimmunoassay of lecithin-cholesterol acyltransferase. *J. Clin. Invest.* 67:141, 1981.
2. Albers, J. J., Chen, C. C., and Adolphson, J. L. Familial lecithin-cholesterol acyltransferase: Identification of heterozygotes with half-normal enzyme activity and mass. *Hum. Genet.* 58:306, 1981.

3. Albers, J. J., and Vtermann, G. Genetic control of lecithin: cholesterol acyltransferase: Measurement of LCAT mass in a large kidney with LCAT deficiency. *Am. J. Hum. Genet.* 33:702, 1981.

4. Alter, B. P. Prenatal diagnosis of hemoglobinopathies and other hematologic disorders. *J. Pediatr.* 95:501, 1979.

5. Alter, B. P. Prenatal diagnosis of haemoglobinopathies: A status report. *Lancet* 2:1152, 1981.

6. Anderson, B. Corneal and conjunctival pigmentation among workers engaged in manufacture of hydroquinone. *Arch. Ophthalmol.* 38:812, 1947.

7. Anderson, M. W., et al. Transferase-deficiency galactosemia: Immunochemical studies of the Duarte and Los Angeles variants. *Hum. Genet.* 65:287, 1984.

8. Antonarakis, S. E., Phillips, J. A., III, and Kazazian, H. H. Genetic diseases: Diagnosis by restriction endonuclease analysis. *J. Pediatr. Genet.* In press, 1986.

9. Assman, G., and Frederickson, D. S. Acid Lipase Deficiency: Wolman's Disease and Cholesterase Ester Storage Disease. In J. B. Stanbury et al. (Eds.), *The Metabolic Basis of Inherited Disease* (5th ed.). New York: McGraw-Hill, 1983.

10. Aula, P., et al. Prenatal diagnosis and fetal pathology of I-cell disease (mucolipidosis II). *J. Pediatr.* 87:221, 1975.

11. Austin, J., McAfee, D., and Shearer, L. Metachromatic form of diffuse cerebral sclerosis: IV. Low sulfatase activity in the urine of a living patient with metachromatic leukodystrophy (MLD). *Arch. Neurol.* 12:447, 1965.

12. Axelrod, F. B., et al. Progressive sensory loss in familial dysautonomia. *Pediatrics* 67:517, 1981.

13. Bach, G., et al. The defect in Hurler and Scheie syndromes: Deficiency of alpha-ʟ-iduronidase. *Proc. Natl. Acad. Sci. U.S.A.* 69:2048, 1972.

14. Baglioni, C. An improved method for the fingerprinting of human haemoglobin. *Biochim. Biophys. Acta* 48:392, 1961.

15. Bakwin, H., Golden, A., and Fox, S. Familial osteoectasia with macrocranium. *Am. J. Roentgenol.* 91:609, 1964.

16. Bauer, E. A., Santa-Cruz, D. J., and Eisen, A. Z. Lipoid proteinosis: *In vivo* and *in vitro* evidence for a lysosomal storage disease. *J. Invest. Dermatol.* 76:119, 1981.

17. Beard, M. E., et al. Histopathology of keratopathy in the tyrosine-fed rat. *Invest. Ophthalmol.* 13:1037, 1974.

18. Becker, D. M., et al. Reduced ferrochelatase activity: A defect common to porphyria variegata and protoporphyria. *Br. J. Haematol.* 36:171, 1977.

19. Beisiegel, V., Schneider, V., and Goldstein, J. L. Monoclonal antibodies for study of receptor-mediated endocytosis and genetics of familial hypercholesterolemia. *J. Biol. Chem.* 256:11923, 1981.

20. Benedict, W. F., et al. Patients with 13 chromosomal deletion: Evidence that the retinoblastoma gene is a recessive cancer gene. *Science* 219:973, 1983.

21. Ben-Yoseph, Y., Burton, B. K., and Nadler, H. L. Sphingolipidosis: The role of neutral beta-galactosidase in the *in vivo* cleavage of lactosyl ceramide (abstract). *J. Pediatr.* 93:317, 1978.

22. Berman, E. R. Biochemical Diagnostic Tests In Genetic and Metabolic Eye Disease. In M. F. Goldberg (Ed.), *Genetic and Metabolic Eye Disease.* Boston: Little, Brown, 1974.

23. Berman, E. R. Glycogen Storage Diseases. In A. Garner and G. K. Klintworth (Eds.), *Pathobiology of Ocular Disease.* New York: Dekker, 1982.

24. Berman, E. R. Glycosaminoglycan and Proteoglycan Disorders. In A. Garner and G. K. Klintworth (Eds.), *Pathobiology of Ocular Disease.* New York: Dekker, 1982.

25. Berman, E. R. Mucolipidoses. In A. Garner and G. K. Klintworth (Eds.), *Pathobiology of Ocular Disease.* New York: Dekker, 1982.

26. Berman, E. R. Sphingolipidoses and Neuronal Ceroid-Lipofuscinosis. In A. Garner and G. K. Klintworth (Eds.), *Pathobiology of Ocular Disease.* New York: Dekker, 1982.

27. Berman, E. R., et al. Acid hydrolase deficiencies and abnormal glycoproteins in mucolipidosis III (pseudo-Hurler polydystrophy). *Clin. Chim. Acta* 52:115, 1974.

28. Berman, E. R., Vered, J., and Bach, G. A reliable spot test for mucopolysaccharidoses. *Clin. Chem.* 17:886, 1971.

29. Beutler, E. Glucose-6-Phosphate Deficiencies. In J. Stanbury et al. (Eds.), *The Metabolic Basis of Inherited Disease* (5th ed.) New York: McGraw-Hill, 1983.

30. Beutler, E. Glucose-6-Phosphate Dehydrogenase Deficiency. In M. M. Wintrobe (Ed.), *Red Cell Metabolism in Hemolytic Anemia.* New York: Plenum, 1978.

31. Beutler, E. The biochemical genetics of the hexosaminidase system in man. *Am. J. Hum. Genet.* 31:95, 1979.

32. Beutler, E., and Baluda, M. C. A simple spot screening test for galactosemia. *J. Clin. Lab. Med.* 68:137, 1966.

33. Beutler, E., and Matsumoto, F. Galactokinase and cataracts. *Lancet* 1:1161, 1978.

34. Beutler, E., Paniker, N. V., and Trinidad, F. The assay of red cell galactokinase. *Biochem. Med.* 5:325, 1971.

35. Bird, T. D., and Lagunoff, D. Neurologic manifestations of Fabry's disease. *Ann. Neurol.* 4:537, 1978.

36. Bittner, M., Kupferer, P., and Morris, C. F. Electrophoretic transfer of proteins and nucleic acids from slab gels to diazobenzyloxymethyl cellulose sheets. *Anal. Biochem.* 102:459, 1980.

37. Blackett, P. R. Secondary metabolic changes in von

Gierke's disease (type I glycogen storage disease). *Ann. Clin. Lab. Sci.* 12:424, 1982.

38. Blodi, F. C., Whinery, R. D., and Hendricks, C. A. Lipid proteinosis (Urbach-Wiethe) involving the lids. *Trans. Am. Ophthalmol. Soc.* 58:155, 1960.

39. Brady, R. O. Sphingomyelin Lipidoses: Niemann-Pick Disease. In J. B. Stanbury et al. (Eds.), *The Metabolic Basis of Inherited Disease* (5th ed.). New York: McGraw-Hill, 1983.

40. Brady, R. O., Johnson, W. G., and Uhlendorf, B. W. Identification of heterozygous carriers of lipid storage diseases. *Am. J. Med.* 51:423, 1971.

41. Breen, L., et al. Juvenile Niemann-Pick disease with vertical supranuclear ophthalmoplegia: Two case reports and a review of the literature. *Arch. Neurol.* 38:388, 1981.

42. Bremer, H. J., et al. *Disturbances of Amino-Acid Metabolism: Clinical Chemistry and Diagnosis.* Baltimore: Urban & Schuarzenberg, 1981. Pp. 250 and 337.

43. Brenner, D. A., and Bloomer, J. R. The enzymatic defect in variegate porphyria. *N. Engl. J. Med.* 302:765, 1980.

44. Brenner, M. S., et al. Eye signs in hypophosphatasia. *Arch. Ophthalmol.* 81:614, 1969.

45. Brown, A. J., et al. Overlapping pathways for repair of damage from UV light and chemical carcinogens in fibroblasts. *Cancer Res.* 39:2522, 1979.

46. Brown, M. S., and Goldstein, J. L. Familial cholesterolemia: Genetic, biochemical, and pathophysiologic considerations. *Adv. Intern. Med.* 20:273, 1975.

47. Brown, M. S., and Goldstein, J. L. Familial hypercholesterolemia: defective binding of lipoproteins to cultured fibroblasts associated with impaired regulation of 3-hydroxy-3-methylglutaryl coenzyme reductase A activity. *Proc. Natl. Acad. Sci. U.S.A.* 71:788, 1974.

48. Brown, M. S., Goldstein, J. L., and Frederickson, D. S. Familial Type 3 Hyperlipoproteinemia (Dysbetalipoproteinemia). In J. B. Stanbury et al. (Eds.), *The Metabolic Basis of Inherited Disease* (5th ed.). New York: McGraw-Hill, 1983.

49. Broyer, M., et al. Infantile cystinosis: A reappraisal of early and late symptoms. *Adv. Nephrol.* 10:137, 1981.

50. Brunt, P. W., and McKusick, V. A. Familial dysautonomia: A report of genetic and clinical studies, with a review of the literature. *Medicine (Baltimore)* 49:343, 1970.

51. Burns, R. P., Gipson, I. K., and Murray, M. J. Keratopathy in tyrosinemia. *Birth Defects* 12(3):169, 1976.

52. Burton, B. K., Ben-Yoseph, Y., and Nadler, H. L. Lactosylceramidosis: A deficiency of neutral beta-galactosidase (abstract). *Am. J. Hum. Genet.* 29:26A, 1977.

53. Cable, W. J. L., et al. Fabry disease: Detection of heterozygotes by examination of glycolipids in urinary sediment. *Neurology (N.Y.)* 32:1139, 1982.

54. Caffey, J. P. Familial Hyperphosphatemia with Ateliosis and Hypermetabolism of Growing Membranous Bone: A Review of the Clinical, Radiographic, and Chemical Features. In H. J. Kaufman (Ed.), *Intrinsic Disease of Bones (Progress in Pediatric Radiology*, Vol. 4). Basel: Karger, 1973.

55. Callahan, J. W., and Khalil, M. Sphingomyelinases in human tissues: III. Expression of Niemann-Pick disease in cultured fibroblasts. *Pediatr. Res.* 9:914, 1975.

56. Carmody, P. J., Rattazi, M. C., and Davidson, R. G. Tay-Sachs disease: The use of tears for the detection of heterozygotes. *N. Engl. J. Med.* 289:1072, 1972.

57. Carr, R. E. Abetalipoproteinemia and the eye. *Birth Defects* 12(3):385, 1976.

58. Cartwright, G. E. The diagnosis of treatable Wilson's disease. *N. Engl. J. Med.* 298:1347, 1978.

59. Cavenee, W. K., et al. Expression of recessive alleles by chromosomal mechanisms in retinoblastoma. *Nature* 305:779, 1983.

60. Change, J. C., and Kan, Y. W. Antenatal diagnosis of sickle cell anemia by direct analysis of the sickle mutation. *Lancet* 2:1127, 1981.

61. Chen, C. H., and Albers, J. J. Distribution of lecithin-cholesterol acyltransferase (LCAT) in human plasma lipoprotein fractions: Evidence for the association of active LCAT low density lipoproteins. *Biochem. Biophys. Res. Commun.* 107:1091, 1982.

62. Cleaver, J. E. Xeroderma Pigmentosum. In J. B. Stanbury et al. (Eds.), *The Metabolic Basis of Inherited Disease* (5th ed.). New York: McGraw-Hill, 1983.

63. Cogan, D. G., Kuwabara, T., and Moser, H. Metachromatic leukodystrophy. *Ophthalmologica* 160:2, 1970.

64. Cogan, D. G., et al. Retinopathy in a case of Farber's lipogranulomatosis. *Arch. Ophthalmol.* 75:752, 1966.

65. Cohen, B. H., Lilienfield, A., and Huang, P. C. (Eds.). *Genetic Issues in Public Health and Medicine.* Springfield, Ill.: Thomas, 1978.

66. Condon, P. I., and Serjeant, G. R. Ocular findings in hemoglobin SC disease in Jamaica. *Am. J. Ophthalmol.* 74:921, 1972.

67. Cotlier, E. Biochemical detection of inborn errors of metabolism affecting the eye. *Trans. Am. Acad. Ophthalmol. Otolaryngol.* 76:1165, 1972.

68. Scully, R. E., Mark, E. J., and McNeely, B. V. (Eds.). CPC of MGH Case 2—1984. *N. Engl. J. Med.* 310:106, 1984.

69. Dahlquist, A. A fluorometric method for the assay of galactose-1-phosphate in red blood cells. *J. Lab. Clin. Med.* 78:931, 1971.

70. Dahlquist, A., and Svenningsen, N. W. Galactose in the urine of newborn infants. *J. Pediatr.* 75:454, 1969.

71. Dancis, J. Abnormalities in the Degradation of Lysin. In W. L. Nyhan (Ed.), *Heritable Disorders of Amino Acid Metabolism.* New York: Wiley, 1974.

72. Danes, B. S., and Bearn, A. G. Metachromasia and skin fibroblast cultures in juvenile familial amaurotic idiocy. *Lancet* 2:855, 1968.

73. Danielson, K. G., Ohi, S., and Huang, P. C. Immunochemical detection of metallothionein in specific epithelial cells. *Proc. Natl. Acad. Sci. U.S.A.* 79:2301, 1982.

74. Danks, D. M. Hereditary Disorders of Copper Metabolism in Wilson's Disease and Menkes' Disease. In J. B. Stanbury et al. (Eds.), *The Metabolic Basis of Inherited Disease* (5th ed.). New York: McGraw-Hill, 1983.

75. Dawson, G. Detection of glycosphingolipid in small samples of human tissue. *Ann. Clin. Lab. Sci.* 2:274, 1972.

76. Dawson, G., and Stein, A. O. Lactosyl ceramidosis: Catabolic enzyme defect of sphingolipid metabolism. *Science* 170:556, 1970.

77. Day, R. S., Blekkenhorst, G., and Eales, L. Hepatic porphyrins in varigate porphyria. *N. Engl. J. Med.* 303:1368, 1980.

78. Day, R. S., Pimstone, N. R., and Eales, L. The diagnostic value of blood plasma porphyrin methyl ester profiles produced by quantitative TLC. *Int. J. Biochem.* 9:897, 1978.

79. d'Azzo, A., et al. Molecular defect in combined beta-galactosidase and neuraminidase deficiency in man. *Proc. Natl. Acad. Sci. U.S.A.* 79:4535, 1982.

80. DeFrancisco, M., Savino, P. J., and Schatz, N. J. Optic atrophy in acute intermittent porphyria. *Am. J. Ophthalmol.* 87:221, 1979.

81. Desnick, R. J., et al. Enzymatic diagnosis of hemizygotes and heterozygotes: Fabry's disease. *J. Lab. Clin. Med.* 81:157, 1973.

82. Desnick, R. J., et al. Prenatal diagnosis of glycosphingoliposes: Sandhoff's and Fabry's disease. *J. Pediatr.* 83:149, 1973.

83. Desnick, R. J., and Sweeley, C. C. Fabry's Disease: Galactosidase-a Deficiency. In J. B. Stanbury et al. (Eds.), *The Metabolic Basis of Inherited Disease* (5th ed.). New York: McGraw-Hill, 1983.

84. Deybach, J. C., de Verneuil, H., and Nordman, Y. The inherited enzymatic defect in prophyria variegata. *Hum. Genet.* 58:425, 1981.

85. Donahue, S., Watanabe, I., and Zeman, W. Morphology of leukocytic hypergranulation in Batten's disease. *Ann. N.Y. Acad. Sci.* 155:847, 1968.

86. Dozy, A. M., et al. Prenatal diagnosis of homozygous alpha-thalassemia. *JAMA* 241:1610, 1979.

87. Drager, U. C., and Hofbauer, A. Antibodies to heavy neurofilament subunit detect a subpopulation of damaged ganglion cells in retina. *Nature* 309:624, 1984.

88. Dryja, T. P., et al. Homozygosity of chromosome 13 in retinoblastoma. *N. Engl. J. Med.* 310:550, 1984.

89. Dulaney, J. T., and Moser, H. W. Farber's Disease (Lipogranulomatosis). In R. H. Glew and S. P. Peters (Eds.), *Practical Enzymology of the Sphingolipidoses.* New York: Liss, 1977.

90. Eales, L., Day, R. S., and Blekkenhorst, G. H. The clinical and biochemical features of variegate porphyria: An analysis of 300 cases studied at Goote Schuur Hospital, Cape Town. *Int. J. Biochem.* 12:837, 1980.

91. Efremor, G. D., and Huisman, T. H. J. The laboratory diagnosis of the haemoglobinopathies. *Clin. Haematol.* 3:527, 1974.

92. Elder, G. H. Porphyrin metabolism in porphyria cutanea tarda. *Semin. Hematol.* 14:227, 1977.

93. Elder, G. H. Recent advances in the identification of enzyme deficiencies in the porphyrias. *Br. J. Dermatol.* 108:729, 1983.

94. Elias, S. Prenatal diagnosis of genetic disorders. *Obstet. Gynecol. Annu.* 12:79, 1983.

95. Emery, J. M., Green, W. R., and Hub, D. S. Krabbe's disease: Histopathology and ultrastructure of the eye. *Am. J. Ophthalmol.* 74:400, 1972.

96. Emery, J. M., et al. GM$_1$-gangliosidosis: Ocular and pathological manifestations. *Arch. Ophthalmol.* 85:177, 1971.

97. Engel, W. K., et al. Neuropathy in Tangier disease: Alpha-lipoprotein deficiency manifesting as a familial recurrent neuropathy and intestinal lipid storage. *Arch. Neurol* 17:1, 1967.

98. Eto, Y., et al. Prenatal diagnosis of metachromatic leukodystrophy: A diagnosis by amniotic fluid and its confirmation. *Arch. Neurol.* 39:29, 1982.

99. Eyring, E. J., and Eisenberg, E. Congenital hyperphosphatasia: A clinical, pathological, and biochemical study of two cases. *J. Bone Joint Surg. [Am]* 50A:1099, 1968.

100. Farmer, P. M. Laboratory diagnosis of the neuromuscular glycogen storage diseases. *Ann. Clin. Lab. Sci.* 12:431, 1982.

101. Fearon, E. R., Vogelstein, B., and Feinberg, A. P. Somatic deletion and duplication of genes on chromosome 11 in Wilms' tumour. *Nature* 309:176, 1984.

102. Feeney, L., and Berman, E. R. Oxygen toxicity: Membrane damage by free radicals. *Invest. Ophthalmol.* 15:789, 1976.

103. Feiler-Ofry, V., et al. Lipoid proteinosis (Urbach-Wiethe sd.). *Br. J. Ophthalmol.* 63:694, 1979.

104. Fell, G. S. Analytical procedures for diagnosis of trace element disorders. *J. Inherited Metab. Dis.* 6(Suppl. 1):5, 1983.

105. Fellows, F. C. I., and Carson, N. A. J. Enzymatic studies in a patient with saccharopinuria: A defect of lysine metabolism. *Pediatr. Res.* 8:42, 1974.

106. Fenson, A. H., et al. Prenatal diagnosis of Farber's disease. *Lancet* 2:990, 1979.

107. Fine, R. N., Wilson, R. A., and Donnell, G. N. Retinal changes in glycogen storage disease type I. *Am. J. Dis. Child.* 115:328, 1968.

108. Forget, B. G. Molecular studies of human beta-glo-

bin gene: A model system for analysis of inborn errors of metabolism. *Recent Prog. Horm. Res.* 38:257, 1982.

109. Foster, D. W. Diabetes Mellitus. In J. B. Stanbury et al. (Eds.), *The Metabolic Basis of Inherited Disease* (5th ed.). New York: McGraw-Hill, 1983.

110. Franceschetti, A. T. Fabry disease: Ocular manifestations. *Birth Defects* 12(3):195, 1976.

111. François, J. Ocular manifestations of inborn errors of carbohydrate and lipid metabolism. *Bibl. Ophthalmol.* 84:1, 1975.

112. Francois, J. The significance of genetic research in ophthalmology. *Birth Defects* 18(6):3, 1982.

113. François, J., Bacskulin, J., and Follmann, P. Manifestation oculaires du syndrome d'Urbach-Wiethe: Hyalinosis cutis et mucosae. *Ophthalmologica* 139:45, 1960.

114. Frazier, P. D., and Wong, V. G. Cystinosis: Histologic and crystallographic examination of crystals in eye tissue. *Arch. Ophthalmol.* 80:87, 1968.

115. Friedenwald, J. S., and Ryfel, D. Contributions to the histopathology of cataract. *Arch. Ophthalmol.* 53:825, 1955.

116. Friedman, M. J., and Trager, W. The biochemistry of resistance to malaria. *Sci. Am.* 3:154, 1980.

117. Frohlich, J., Hon, K., and McLeod, R. Detection of heterozygotes for familial lecithin cholesterol acyltransferase (LCAT) deficiency. *Am. J. Hum. Genet.* 34:65, 1982.

118. Gagne, R., et al. Pre-natal diagnosis of heredity tyrosinemia: Measurement of succinylacetone in amniotic fluid. *Prenatal Diagn.* 2:185, 1982.

119. Gal, A. E. et al. The diagnosis of Type A and Type B Niemann-Pick disease and detection of carrier using leukocyctes and a chromatogenic analogue or sphingomyelin. *Clin. Chim. Acta* 104:129, 1980.

120. Galjaard, H., et al. Microtechniques in Prenatal Diagnosis of Genetic Disease. In S. Armendares and R. Lisker (Eds.), *Proceedings of the 5th International Congress on Human Genetics.* Amsterdam: Excerpta Medica, 1977.

121. Garner, A. Vascular Disorders. In A. Garner and G. K. Klintworth (Eds.), *Pathobiology of Ocular Disease.* New York: Dekker, 1982.

122. Garrod, A. E. The incidence of alkaptonuria: A study in chemical individuality. *Lancet* 2:1616, 1902.

123. Geever, R. F., et al. Direct identification of sickle cell anemia by blot hybridization. *Proc. Natl. Acad. Sci. U.S.A.* 78:5081, 1981.

124. Geiger, B., and Arnon, R. Chemical characterization and subunit structure of human *N*-acetylhexosaminidases A and B. *Biochemistry* 15:3484, 1976.

125. Ghadimi, H. The Hyperlysinemias. In J. B. Stanbury, J. B. Wyngaarden, and D. S. Fredrickson (Eds.), *The Metabolic Basis of Inherited Disease* (5th ed.). New York: McGraw-Hill, 1983.

126. Giannelli, F., Croll, P. M., and Lewin, S. A. DNA repair synthesis in human heterokaryons formed by normal and UV-sensitive fibroblasts. *Exp. Cell. Res.* 78:175, 1973.

127. Gibberd, F. B., et al. Heredopathia atactica polyneuritiformis (Refsum's disease) treated by diet and plasma-exchange. *Lancet* 1:575, 1979.

128. Gilbert, G., et al. Tay-Sachs and Sandhoff's disease: The assignment of genes for hexosaminidase A and B to individual human chromosomes. *Proc. Natl. Acad. Sci. U.S.A.* 72:263, 1975.

129. Gipson, I. K., Burns, R. P., and Wolfe-Lande, J. D. Crystals in corneal epithelial lesions of tyrosine-rats. *Invest. Ophthalmol.* 14:937, 1975.

130. Gitlow, S. E. et al. Excretion of catecholamine metabolites by children with familial dysautonomia. *Pediatrics* 46:513, 1970.

131. Gitzelmann, R. Estimation of galactose-1-phosphate in erythrocytes: A rapid simple enzymatic method. *Clin. Chim. Acta* 26:313, 1969.

132. Gitzelmann, R., Curtius, H. C., and Schneller, I. Galactitol and galactose-1-phosphate in the lens of a galactosaemic infant. *Exp. Eye Res.* 6:1, 1967.

133. Glomset, J. A., Norum, K. R., and Gjone, E. Familial Lecithin: Cholesterol Acyltransferase Deficiency. In J. B. Stanbury et al. (Eds.), *The Metabolic Basis of Inherited Disease* (5th ed.). New York: McGraw-Hill, 1983.

134. Goebel, H. H., et al. The ultrastructure of the retina in adult metachromatic leukodystrophy. *Am. J. Ophthalmol.* 85:841, 1978.

135. Goldberg, J. D., Truex, J. H., and Desnick, R. J. Tay-Sachs disease: An improved fully-automated method of heterozygote identification by tear beta-hexosaminidase assay. *Clin. Chim. Acta* 77:43, 1977.

136. Goldberg, M. F. A review of selected inherited corneal dystrophies associated with systemic diseases. *Birth Defects* 7(3):13, 1971.

137. Goldberg, M. F. Retinal neovascularization in sickle cell retinopathy. *Trans. Am. Acad. Ophthalmol. Otolaryngol.* 83:OP409, 1977.

138. Goldberg, M. F. Retinal Vaso-Occuclusion in Sickling Hemoglobinopathies. In D. Bergsma, A. J. Bron, and E. Cotlier (Eds.), *The Eye and Inborn Errors of Metabolism.* New York: Liss, 1976.

139. Goldberg, M. F., et al. Macular cherry-red spot, corneal clouding, and beta-galactosidase deficiency: Clinical, biochemical, and electron microscopic study of a new autosomal recessive storage disease. *Arch. Intern. Med.* 128:387, 1971.

140. Goldberg, M. F., and von Noorden, G. K. Ophthalmologic findings in Wilson's hepatolenticular degeneration. *Arch. Ophthalmol.* 75:162, 1966.

141. Goldberg, M. F., Payne, J. W., and Brunt, P. W. Ophthalmologic studies of familial dysautonomia: The Riley-Day syndrome. *Arch. Ophthalmol.* 80:732, 1968.

142. Goldman, H., et al. Adolescent cytinosis: Comparison between infantile and adult forms. *Pediatrics* 47:970, 1971.

143. Goldsmith, L. A. Tyrosinemia and Related Disor-

ders. In J. B. Stanbury et al. (Eds.), *The Metabolic Basis of Inherited Disease* (5th ed.). New York: McGraw-Hill, 1983.

144. Goldstein, J. L., and Brown, M. S. Familial Hypercholesterolemia. In J. B. Stanbury et al. (Eds.), *The Metabolic Basis of Inherited Disease* (5th ed.). New York: McGraw-Hill, 1983.

145. Gordon, J. I., et al. Proteolytic processing of human preproapolipoprotein A-I: A proposed defect in the conversion of pro A-I to A-I in Tangier disease. *J. Biol. Chem.* 258:4037, 1983.

146. Gouras, P., Carr, R. E., and Gunkel, R. D. Retinitis pigmentosa in abetalipoproteinemia: Effects of vitamin A. *Invest. Ophthalmol.* 10:784, 1971.

147. Grabowski, G. A. Prenatal diagnosis of inherited metabolic diseases: Principles, pitfalls, and prospects. *Methods Cell Biol.* 26:95, 1982.

148. Grandchamp, B., et al. Studies of porphyrin synthesis in fibroblasts of patients with congenital erythropoietic porphyria and in one patient with homozygous coproporphyria. *Biochim. Biophys. Acta* 629:577, 1980.

149. Grenier, A. Mass screening for hereditary tyrosinemia/detection of succinylacetone. *Clin. Chim. Acta* 123:93, 1982.

150. Grossman, H., and Dorst, J. P. The mucopolysaccharidoses. *Prog. Pediatr. Radiol.* 4:495, 1973.

151. Hall, C. W., et al. Enzymatic diagnosis of the genetic mucopolysaccharide storage disorders. *Metods Enzymol.* 50:539, 1978.

152. Haltia, T., et al. Juvenile metachromatic leukodystrophy: Clinical, biochemical, and neuropathologic studies in nine new cases. *Arch. Neurol.* 37:42, 1980.

153. Halvorsen, S. Screening for Disorders of Tyrosine Metabolism. In H. Bickel, R. Guthrie, and G. Hammersen (Eds.), *Neonatal Screening for Inborn Errors of Metabolism.* New York: Springer, 1980.

154. Harcourt, B., and Ashton, N. Ultrastructure of the optic nerve in Krabbe's leukodystrophy. *Br. J. Ophthalmol.* 57:885, 1973.

155. Harms, E., and Schneider, J. A. The lysosomal localization of free cystine in normal cystinotic cells. *Clin. Res.* 27:457A, 1979.

156. Havel, R. J., and Gordon, R. S., Jr. Idiopathic hyperlipidemia: Metabolic studies in an affected family. *J. Clin. Invest.* 39:1777, 1960.

157. Hayasaka, S. Lysosomal enzymes in ocular tissues and diseases. *Surv. Ophthalmol.* 27:245, 1983.

158. Hazzard, W. R., O'Donnell, T. F., and Lee, Y. L. Broad-beta disease (type III hyperlipoproteinemia) in a large kindred. *Ann. Intern. Med.* 82:141, 1975.

159. Henkes, H. E., et al. Fundus changes in primary hyperlipidemia. *Ophthalmologica* 173:190, 1976.

160. Herbert, P. N., et al. Familial Lipoprotein Deficiency: Abetalipoproteinemia, Hypobetalipoproteinemia, and Tangier Disease. In J. B. Stanbury et al. (Eds.), *The Metabolic Basis of Inherited Disease* (5th ed.). New York: McGraw-Hill, 1983.

161. Herndon, J. H., et al. Refsum's disease: Characterization of the enzyme defect in cell culture. *J. Clin. Invest.* 48:1017, 1969.

162. Herz, F., Kaplan, E., and Scheye, E. S. Diagnosis of erythrocyte glucose-6-phosphate dehydrogenase deficiency in the Negro male despite hemolytic crisis. *Blood* 35:90, 1970.

163. Hesterberg, R. C., Jr., and Tredici, T. J. Corneal opacification and lecithin:cholesterol acyltransferase (LCAT) deficiency: A case report. *Ann. Ophthalmol.* 16:616, 1984.

164. Hodge, S. E., et al. Close linkage between diabetes mellitus and the Kidd blood group. *Lancet* 2:893, 1981.

165. Hoeksema, H. L., DeWit, J., and Westerveld, A. The genetic defect in the various types of beta-galactosidase deficiency. *Hum. Genet.* 53:241, 1980.

166. Hofrichter, J., Rose, P. D., and Eaton, W. A. Kinetics and mechanism of deoxyhemoglobin S gelatin: A new approach to the understanding of sickle cell disease. *Proc. Natl. Acad. Sci. U.S.A.* 70:3604, 1973.

167. Hooft, C., et al. Familial hypolipidaemia and retarded development without steatorrhea: Another inborn error of metabolism? *Helv. Paediatr. Acta* 17:1, 1967.

168. Hoogeveen, A., d'Azzo, A., and Galjaard, H. Correction of combined beta-galactosidase/neuraminidase deficiency in human fibroblasts. *Biochem. Biophys. Res. Commun.* 103:292, 1981. 1981.

169. Horven, I., Gjone, E., and Egge, K. Ocular manifestations in familial LCAT deficiency. *Birth Defects* 12(3):271, 1976.

170. Hostetter, M. K., et al. Evidence of liver disease preceding amino acid abnormalities in hereditary tyrosinemia. *N. Engl. J. Med.* 308:1265, 1983.

171. Howell, R. R., and Williams, J. C. The Glycogen Storage Diseases. In J. B. Stanbury et al. (Eds.), *The Metabolic Basis of Inherited Disease* (5th ed.). New York: McGraw-Hill, 1983.

172. Hsia, D. Y.-Y. (Ed.). *Galactosemia.* Springfield, Ill.: Thomas, 1969.

173. Huang, P. C., and Sheridan, R. B. Genetic and biochemical studies with ataxia telangiectasia: A review. *Hum. Genet.* 59:1, 1981.

174. Huang, P. C., Kuo, T. T., and Wu, R. (Eds.). *Genetic Engineering Techniques: Recent Developments.* New York: Academic, 1982.

175. Hultberg, B. Fluorometric assay of the arylsulfatases in human urine. *J. Clin. Chem. Clin. Biochem.* 17:795, 1979.

176. Johansson, L., Thunell, S., and Wetterberg, L. A filter paper dry blood spot procedure for acute intermittent porphyria population screening by the use of whole blood uroporphyrinogen-I-synthetase assay. *Clin. Chim. Acta* 137:317, 1984.

177. Johnson, D. L., et al. Diagnosis of hemizygotes and heterozygotes by galactosidase A activity in tears. *Clin. Chim. Acta* 63:81, 1975.

178. Johnson, J. L., Cohen, H. J., and Rajagoplan, K. V. Molecular basis of the biological function of molybdenum: Molybdenum-free sulfite oxidase from livers of tungsten-treated rats. *J. Biol. Chem.* 249:5046, 1974.

179. Johnson, J. L., and Rajagopalan, K. V. Human sulfite oxidase deficiency: Characterization of the molecular defect in a multicomponent system. *J. Clin. Invest.* 58:551, 1976.

180. Johnson, R. E., and Campbell, R. J. Wilson's disease: Electron microscopic, X-ray energy spectroscopic, and atomic absorption spectroscopic studies of corneal copper deposition and distribution. *Lab. Invest.* 46:546, 1982.

181. Johnson, W. G., et al. Alpha-locus hexosaminidase genetic compound with juvenile gangliosidosis phenotype: Clinical, genetic and biochemical studies. *Am. J. Hum. Genet.* 32:508, 1980.

182. Kaback, M. M., et al. GM$_1$ gangliosidosis type I: *In utero* detection and fetal manifestations. *J. Pediatr.* 82:1037, 1973.

183. Kan, Y. W. The Thalassemias. In J. B. Stanbury et al. (Eds.), *The Metabolic Basis of Inherited Disease* (5th ed.). New York: McGraw-Hill, 1983.

184. Kappas, A., Sassa, S., and Anderson, K. E. The Porphyrias. In J. B. Stanbury et al. (Eds.), *The Metabolic Basis of Inherited Disease* (5th ed.). New York: McGraw-Hill, 1983.

185. Kaufman, H. E., and Thomas, L. B. Vitreous opacities diagnostic of familial amyloid polyneuropathy. *N. Engl. J. Med.* 261:1267, 1959.

186. Kelly, T. E., et al. Mucolipidosis III (pseudo-Hurler polydystrophy): Clinical and laboratory studies in a series of 12 patients. *Johns Hopkins Med. J.* 137:156, 1975.

187. Kenyon, K. R. Ocular manifestations and pathology of systemic mucopolysaccharidoses. *Birth Defects* 12(3):133, 1976.

188. Kenyon, K. R., and Sensenbrenner, J. A. Electron microscopy of cornea and conjunctiva in childhood cystinosis. *Am. J. Ophthalmol.* 78:68, 1974.

189. Khachadurian, A. K., and Uthman, S. M. Experiences with the homozygous cases of familial hypercholesterolemia: A report of 52 patients. *Nutr. Metab.* 15:132, 1973.

190. Kihara, H., et al. Metachromatic leukodystrophy: Ambiguity of heterozygote identification. *Am. J. Ment. Defic.* 77:389, 1973.

191. King, R. A., and Witkop, R. A., Jr. Detection of heterozygotes for tyrosine-negative oculocutaneous albinism by hair bulb tyrosinase assay. *Am. J. Hum. Genet.* 29:164, 1977.

192. King, R. A., and Witkop, R. A., Jr. Hair bulb tyrosinase activity in oculocutaneous albinism. *Nature* 263:69, 1976.

193. Kinoshita, J. H. Mechanisms initiating cataract formation. *Invest. Ophthalmol.* 13:713, 1974.

194. Kisilevsky, R. Amyloidosis: A familiar problem in the light of current pathogenetic developments. *Lab. Invest.* 49:381, 1983.

195. Klingele, T. G., Newman, S. A., and Burde, R. M. Accommodation defect in Wilson's disease. *Am. J. Ophthalmol.* 90:22, 1980.

196. Klintworth, G. K. Disorders of Amino Acid Metabolism. In A. Garner and G. K. Klintworth (Eds.), *Pathobiology of Ocular Disease.* New York: Dekker, 1982.

197. Knox, W. E., and LeMay-Knox, M. The oxidation in liver of L-tyrosine to acetoacetate through *p*-hydroxyphenylpyruvate and homogentisic acid. *J. Biochem.* 49:686, 1951.

198. Kohn, G., et al. Mucolipidosis IV: Prenatal diagnosis by electron microscopy. *Prenatal Diagn.* 2:301, 1982.

199. Kohner, E. M., et al. Streptokinase in central occlusion: A controlled clinical trial. *Br. Med. J.* 1:550, 1976.

200. Kolodny, E. H., and Moser, H. W. Sulfatide Lipidosis: Metachromatic Leukodystrophy. In J. B. Stanbury et al. (Eds.), *The Metabolic Basis of Inherited Disease* (5th ed.). New York: McGraw-Hill, 1983.

201. Koufos, A., et al. Loss of alleles at loci on human chromosome 11 during genesis of Wilms' tumour. *Nature* 309:170, 1984.

202. Kresse, H., et al. Enzymatic Diagnosis of the Genetic Mucopolysaccharide Storage Disorders: An Extension. In V. Ginsberg (Ed.), *Methods of Enzymology.* New York: Academic, 1981.

203. Kugelman, T. P., and Van Scott, E. J. Tyrosinase activity in melanocytes of human albinos. *J. Invest. Dermatol.* 37:73, 1961.

204. Kurz, G. H., et al. The retina in type V hyperlipoproteinemia. *Am. J. Ophthalmol.* 82:32, 1976.

205. Kvittingen, E. A., Halvorsen, S., and Jellum, E. Deficient fumarylacetoacetate sumarylhydrolase activity in lymphocytes and fibroblasts from patients with hereditary tyrosinemia. *Pediatr. Res.* 14:541, 1983.

206. Kyle, R. A., and Greipp, P. R. Amyloidosis (AL): Clinical and laboratory features in 229 cases. *Mayo Clin. Proc.* 58:665, 1983.

207. Kyritsis, A. P., et al. Retinoblastoma: Origin from a primitive neuroectodermal cell. *Nature* 307:471, 1984.

208. LaDu, B. N. Alkaptonuria. In J. B. Stanbury, J. B. Wyngaarden, and D. S. Fredrickson (Eds.), *The Metabolic Basis of Inherited Disease* (5th ed.). New York: McGraw-Hill, 1978.

209. Lai, C. W., Hung, T., and Lin, W. S. J. Blindness of cerebral origin in acute intermittent porphyria. *Arch. Neurol.* 34:310, 1977.

210. Lavie, G., Zucker-Franklin, D., and Franklin, E. L. Degradation of serum amyloid A protein by surface-associated enzymes of human blood monocytes. *J. Exp. Med.* 148:1020, 1978.

211. Lebo, R. V., et al. High resolution chromosome sorting and DNA spot-blot analysis assign McArdle's syndrome to chromosome 11. *Science* 225:57, 1984.

212. Lee, J.-L. L., et al. Enzymatic studies of urinary isomeric chondroitin sulfates in patients with mucopolysaccharidoses: The appplication of high-performance liquid chromatography. *Clin. Chim. Acta* 104:65, 1980.

213. Lee, W. H., Murphree, A. L., and Benedict, W. F. Expression and amplification of the N-*myc* gene in primary retinoblastoma. *Nature* 309:172, 1984.

214. Leroy, J. G., et al. I-cell disease: Biochemical studies. *Pediatr. Res.* 6:752, 1972.

215. Lessell, S., and Norton, E. W. D. Band keratopathy and conjunctival calcification in hypophosphatasia. *Arch. Ophthalmol.* 71:497, 1964.

216. Letson, R. D., and Desnick, R. J. Punctate lenticular opacities in type II mannosidosis. *Am. J. Ophthalmol.* 85:218, 1978.

217. Leung, L.-S. E., Weinstein, G. W., and Hobson, R. R. Further electroretinographic studies of patients with mucopolysaccharidoses. *Birth Defects* 7(3):32, 1971.

218. Levy, H. L., et al. Galactose-1-phosphate uridyl transferase deficiency due to Duarte/galactosemia combined variation: Clinical and biochemical studies. *J. Pediatr.* 92:390, 1972.

219. Libbey, C. A., et al. Familial amyloid polyneuropathy: Demonstration of prealbumin in a kinship of German/English ancestry with onset in the seventh decade. *Am. J. Med.* 76:18, 1984.

220. Licata, A. A., et al. The urinary excretion of phosphoethanolamine in diseases other than hypophosphatasia. *Am. J. Med.* 64:133, 1978.

221. Liebert, J., and Danis, P. Differential diagnosis of type A, B. and C Niemann-Pick disease by conjunctival biopsy. *J. Submicrosc. Cytol.* 11:143, 1979.

222. Liebert, J., Touissaint, D., and Guisling, R. Ocular findings in Niemann-Pick disease. *Am. J. Ophthalmol.* 80:991, 1975.

223. Liebhaber, S. A., and Manno, C. S. Update on hemoglobinopathies. *DM* 29:1, 1983.

224. Lipert, J., et al. Ocular finding in metachromatic leukodystrophy. *Arch. Ophthalmol.* 97:1495, 1979.

225. Lorincz, A. E., Hurst, R. E., and Kolodny, E. H. The early laboratory diagnosis of mucopolysaccharidoses. *Ann. Clin. Lab. Sci.* 12:258, 1982.

226. Lubec, G., Nauer, G., and Pollak, A. Non-invasive diagnosis of cystinosis by infra-red spectroscopy of hair. *Lancet* 2:623, 1983.

227. Lustberg, T. J., Schulman, J. D., and Seegmillar, J. E. The preparation and identification of various adducts of oxidized homogentisic acid and the development of a new sensitive colorimetric assay for homogentisic acid. *Clin. Chem. Acta* 35:325, 1971.

228. Lynch, H. T., et al. Xeroderma pigmentosum, malignant melanoma, and congenital ichthyosis. *Arch. Dermatol.* 96:625, 1967.

229. Lyon, M. F. Sex chromatin and gene action in the mammalian X-chromosome. *Am. J. Hum. Genet.* 14:135, 1962.

230. Mabry, C. C., et al. Familial hyperphosphatasia with mental retardation, seizures, and neurological deficits. *J. Pediatr.* 77:74, 1970.

231. Matalon, R., and Deauching, M. The enzymatic basis for the phenotypic variations in Hurler and Scheie syndromes. *Pediatr. Res.* 11:519, 1977.

232. Matalon, R., et al. Keratan and heparan sulfanuria: Glucosamine-6-sulfate sulfatase deficiency. *Ann. Clin. Lab. Sci.* 12:234, 1982.

233. Mauzerall, D., and Granick, S. The occurrence and determination of delta-aminolevulinic acid and porphobilinogen in urine. *J. Biol. Chem.* 219:435, 1956.

234. McKusick, V. A. *Mendelian Inheritance in Man* (6th ed.). Baltimore: Johns Hopkins Press, 1983.

235. McKusick, V. A., and Neufeld, E. F. The Mucopolysaccharide Storage Diseases. In J. B. Stanbury et al. (Eds.), *The Metabolic Basis of Inherited Disease* (5th ed.). New York: McGraw-Hill, 1983.

236. Merritt, A. D., et al. Detection of heterozygotes in Batten's disease. *Ann. N. Y. Acad. Sci.* 155:860, 1968.

237. Meyerhoff, J. Familial Mediterranean fever: Report of a large family, review of the literature, and discussion of the frequency of amyloidosis. *Medicine (Baltimore)* 59:66, 1980.

238. Michalski, J. C., et al. Structures of the sialyl-oligosaccharides excreted in the urine of a patient with mucolipidosis I. *FEBS Lett.* 79:101, 1977.

239. Milch, R. A. Biochemical studies on the pathogenesis of collagen tissue changes in alkaptonuria. *Clin. Orthop.* 24:2213, 1962.

240. Morganroth, J., Levy, R. I., and Fredrickson, D. S. The biochemical, clinical and genetic features of type III hyperbetalipoproteinemia. *Ann. Intern. Med.* 82:158, 1975.

241. Moser, H. W., et al. Therapeutic trial of plasmapheresis in Refsum disease and in Fabry disease. *Birth Defects* 16:491, 1980.

242. Moser, H. W., and Chen, W. W. Ceramidase Deficiency: Farber's Lipogranulomatosis. In J. B. Stanbury et al. (Eds.), *The Metabolic Basis of Inherited Disease* (5th ed.) New York: McGraw-Hill, 1983.

243. Mossman, J., and Patrick, A. D. Prenatal diagnosis of mucopolysaccharidosis by two-dimensional electrophoresis of amniotic fluid glycosaminoglycans. *Prenatal Diagn.* 2:169, 1982.

244. Mudd, S. H., Irreverre, F., and Laster, L. Sulfite oxidase deficiency in man: Demonstration of enzymatic defect. *Science* 156:1599, 1967.

245. Muller, D. P. R., Harries, J. T., and Lloyd, J. K. The relative importance of the factors involved in the absorption of vitamin E in children. *Gut* 15:966, 1974.

246. Murray, J. C., Linberg, K. A., and Pinnell, S. R. *In vitro* inhibition of chick embryo lysylhydroxylase by homogentisic acid. *J. Clin. Invest.* 59:1071, 1977.

247. Neufeld, E. F., and McKusick, V. A. Disorders of Lysosomal Enzyme Synthesis and Localization: I-Cell Disease and Pseudo-Hurler polydystrophy. In J. B. Stanbury et al. (Eds.), *The Metabolic Basis of Inherited Disease* (5th ed.). New York: McGraw-Hill, 1983.

248. Newton, F. H., et al. Neurologic involvement in Urbach-Wiethe disease: A clinical, ultrastructural, and chemical study. *Neurology (N.Y.)* 21:1205, 1971.

249. Ng, W. G., Bergren, W. R., and Donnell, G. N. A new variant of galactose-1-phosphate uridyl transferase: Demonstration of multiple activity bands with the Duarte variant. *Biochem. Biophys. Res. Commun.* 37:354, 1969.

250. Nikkila, E. A. Familial Lipoprotein Lipase Deficiency and Related Disorders of Chylomicron Metabolism. In J. B. Stanbury et al. (Eds.), *The Metabolic Basis of Inherited Disease* (5th ed.) New York: McGraw-Hill, 1983.

251. Nordman, Y., and Deybach, J. C. Congenital erythropoietic porphyria. *Semin. Liver Dis.* 2:154, 1982.

252. Nyhan, W. L. *Abnormalities in Amino Acid Metabolism in Clinical Medicine.* East Norwalk, Conn.: Appleton-Century-Crofts, 1984.

253. O'Brien, J. S. The Gangliosidoses. In J. B. Stanbury et al. (Eds.), *The Metabolic Basis of Inherited Disease* (5th ed.). New York: McGraw-Hill, 1983.

254. O'Brien, J. S., et al. Ganglioside storage diseases. *Fed. Proc.* 30:956, 1971.

255. O'Donnell, F. E., Jr., et al. X-linked ocular albinism in blacks: Ocular albinism cum pigmento. *Arch. Ophthalmol.* 96:1189, 1978.

256. O'Donnell, F. E., Jr., et al. X-linked ocular albinism: An oculocutaneous macromelanosomal disorder. *Arch. Ophthalmol.* 94:1883, 1976.

257. O'Donnell, J. J., Sandman, R. P., and Martin, S. R. Gyrate atrophy of the retina: Inborn error of L-ornithine:2-oxoacidaminotransferase. *Science* 200:200, 1978.

258. Orkin, S. H., et al. Application of endonuclease mapping to the analysis of thalassemias caused by globin gene deletion. *N. Engl. J. Med.* 299:166, 1978.

259. Orkin, S. H., Goldman, D. S., and Sallan, S. E. Development of homozygosity for chromosome 11p markers in Wilms' tumour. *Nature* 309:172, 1984.

260. Owada, M., et al. Prenatal diagnosis of I-cell disease by measuring altered alpha-mannosidase activity in amniotic fluid. *J. Inherited Metab. Dis.* 3:117, 1980.

261. Philippart, M., Scarlieve, L., and Manacorda, A. Urinary glycolipid in Fabry's disease: Their examination in the detection of atypical variant and the pre-symptomatic state. *Pediatrics* 43:201 1969.

262. Philips, J. A., 3rd. Clinical applications of restriction endonuclease analysis. *Birth Defects* 19(5):73, 1983.

263. Popper, H., et al. Cytoplasmic copper and its toxic effects: Studies in Indian childhood cirrhosis. *Lancet* 1:1205, 1979.

264. Porter, M. T., et al. A correlation of intracellular cerebroside sulfatase activity in fibroblasts with latency in metachromatic leukodystrophy. *Biochem. Biophys. Res. Commun.* 44:660, 1971.

265. Puck, T. T., and Kao, F. T. Somatic cell genetics and its application to medicine. *Annu. Rev. Genet.* 16:225, 1982.

266. Ramsay, C. A., et al. Pre-natal diagnosis of xeroderma pigmentosum. *Lancet* 2:1109, 1974.

267. Rasmussen, H. Hypophosphaturia. In J. B. Stanbury et al. (Eds.), *The Metabolic Basis of Inherited Disease* (5th ed.). New York: McGraw-Hill, 1983.

268. Reed, C. R. Screening for metachromatic leukodystrophy. *J. Clin. Pathol.* 20:301, 1967.

269. Reed W. B., May, S. B., and Nickel, W. R. Xeroderma pigmentosum with neurologic complications: The de Sanctis-Cacchione syndrome. *Arch. Dermatol.* 91:224, 1965.

270. Reeve, A. E., et al. Loss of a Harvey *ras* allele in sporadic Wilms' tumour. *Nature* 309:174, 1984.

271. Refsum, S. Heredopathia atactica polyneuritiformis. *Acta Psychiatr. Scand. [Suppl.]* 38:39, 1946.

272. Refsum, S. Heredopathia atactica polyneuritiformis, phytanic-acid storage disease, Refsum's disease: A biochemically well-defined disease with a specific dietary source. *Arch. Neurol.* 38:605, 1981.

273. Riley, C. M. Familial dysautonomia: Clinical and pathophysiological aspects. *Ann. N.Y. Acad. Sci.* 228:283, 1974.

274. Ringelhahn, B. A simple laboratory procedure for the recognition of A-(African type) G6PD deficiency in acute haemolytic crisis. *Clin. Chim. Acta* 36:272, 1972.

275. Riordan, J. R., and Jolicoeur, P. L. Metallothionein accumulation may account for intracellular copper retention in Menkes' disease. *J. Biol. Chem.* 257:4639, 1982.

276. Robbins, J. H., et al. Xeroderma pigmentosum: An inherited disease with sun sensitivity, multiple cutaneous neoplasms and abnormal DNA repair. *Ann. Intern. Med.* 80:221, 1974.

277. Romeo, G., Glenn, B. L., and Levin, E. Y. Uroporphyrinogen III cosynthetase in asymptomatic carriers of congenital erythropoietic porphyria. *Biochem. Genet.* 4:719, 1970.

278. Rotter, J. I. The modes of inheritance of insulin-dependent diabetes mellitus, or The genetics of IDDM, no longer a nightmare but still a headache. *Am. J. Hum. Genet.* 33:835, 1981.

279. Rowley, P. T. Genetic screening: Marvel or menace? *Science* 225:1104, 1984.

280. Ryan, S. J. Role of the vitreous in the haemoglobinopathies. *Trans. Ophthalmol. Soc. U.K.* 95:403, 1975.

281. Sankoff, I., and Sourkes, T. L. Determination of thin-layer chromatography of urinary homovanil-

lic acid in normal and disease states. *Can. J. Biochem. Physiol.* 41:1381, 1963.

282. Sassa, S., et al. A microassay for uroporphyrinogen I synthetase, one of three abnormal enzyme activities in acute intermittent porphyrin, and its application to the study of the genetics of this disease. *Proc. Natl. Acad. Sci. U.S.A.* 71:732, 1979.

283. Schaefer, E. J., et al. Metabolism of high-density lipoprotein apolipoproteins in Tangier disease. *N. Engl. J. Med.* 299:905, 1978.

284. Scheinberg, I. H., and Sternlieb, I. Wilson's Disease. In L. H. Smith, Jr. (Ed.), *Major Problems in Internal Medicine*, Vol. 23. Philadelphia: Saunders, 1984.

285. Schmidt, C. J., Hamer, D. H., and McBride, O. W. Chromosomal location of human metallothionein genes: Implications of Menkes' disease. *Science* 224:1104, 1984.

286. Schneider, J. A. Clinical Aspects of Cystinosis. In J. D. Schulman (Ed.), *Cystinosis* (DHEW Publication No. [NIH] 72-249). Washington: U.S. Government Printing Office, 1973.

287. Schneider, J. A., Bradley, K., and Seegmiller, J. E. Increased cystine in leukocytes from individuals homozygous and heterozygous for cystinosis. *Science* 157:1321, 1967.

288. Schneider, J. A., and Schulman, J. D. Cystinosis. In J. B. Stanbury et al. (Eds.), *The Metabolic Basis of Inherited Disease* (5th ed.). New York: McGraw-Hill, 1983.

289. Schneider, J. A., et al. Prenatal disease of cystinosis. *N. Engl. J. Med.* 290:878, 1974.

290. Schoenfeld, A., et al. Chemical and biochemical studies in fetuses affected with Niemann-Pick disease type A. *Prenatal Diagn.* 2:177, 1982.

291. Schulman, J. D., and Bradley, K. H. *In Vitro* Studies on Cystinosis. In J. D. Schulman (Ed.) *Cystinosis* (DHEW Publication No. [NIH] 72-249). Washington: U.S. Government Printing Office, 1973.

292. Schwab, M., et al. Amplified DNA with limited homology to *myc* cellular oncogenes is shared by human neuroblastoma cell lines and a neuroblastoma tumour. *Nature* 305:245, 1983.

293. Segal, P., Rifkind, B. M., and Schull, W. J. Genetic factors in lipoprotein variation. *Epidemiol. Rev.* 4:137, 1982.

294. Segal, S. Disorders of galactose metabolism. In J. B. Stanbury et al. (Eds.), *The Metabolic Basis of Inherited Disease* (5th ed.) New York: McGraw-Hill, 1983.

295. Sevel, D., and Burger, D. Ocular involvement in cutaneous porphyria. *Arch. Ophthalmol.* 85:580, 1971.

296. Sher, N. A., Reiff, W., and Desnick, R. J. The ocular manifestations in Fabry's disease. *Arch. Ophthalmol.* 97:671, 1979.

297. Shih, V. E., Carney, M. M., and Mandell, R. A simple screening test for sulfite oxidase deficiency: De-

tection of urinary thiosulfate by a modification of Sorbo's method. *Clin. Chim. Acta* 95:143, 1979.

298. Shih, V. E., et al. Sulfite oxidase deficiency: Biochemical and clinical investigations of a hereditary metabolic disorder in sulfur metabolism. *N. Engl. J. Med.* 297:1022, 1977.

299. Shih, V. E., and Schulman, J. D. Ornithine-ketoacid transaminase activity in human skin and amniotic fluid cell culture. *Clin. Chim. Acta* 27:73, 1970.

300. Shinohara, K. Lethality and the depression of DNA synthesis in UV-irradiated normal human and xeroderma pigmentosum cells. *Mutat. Res.* 122:385, 1983.

301. Siggers, D. C., et al. Increased nerve-growth-factor beta-chain cross-reacting material in familial dysautonomia. *N. Engl. J. Med.* 295:629, 1976.

302. Simon, J. W., et al. Albinotic characteristics in congenital nystagmus. *Am. J. Ophthalmol.* 97:320, 1984.

303. Singer, H. S., and Schafer, I. A. White cell beta-galactosidase activity. *N. Engl. J. Med.* 282:571, 1970.

304. Skinsnes, O. K. Generalized ochronosis: Report of an instance where it was misdiagnosed as a melanosarcoma, with resultant enucleation of the eye. *Arch. Pathol.* 45:552, 1948.

305. Sloan, H. R., et al. Beta-galactosidase in tissue culture derived from human skin and bone marrow: Enzyme deficiency in GM$_1$ gangliosidosis. *Pediatr. Res.* 3:368, 1969.

306. Smith, E. W., and Krevans, J. R. Clinical manifestations of hemoglobin C disorders. *Bull. Johns Hopkins Hosp.* 104:17, 1959.

307. Smith, T. H., Holland, M. E., and Woody, N. C. Ocular manifestations of familial hyperlysinemia. *Trans. Am. Acad. Ophthalmol. Otolaryngol.* 75:355, 1971.

308. Southern, E. Gel electrophoresis of restriction fragments. *Methods Enzymol.* 68:152, 1979.

309. Spalton, D. J., Taylor, D. S. I., and Sanders, M. D. Juvenile Batten's disease: An ophthalmological assessment of 26 patients. *Br. J. Ophthalmol.* 64:726, 1980.

310. Stanbury, J. B., et al. (Eds.). *The Metabolic Basis of Inherited Disease* (5th ed.). New York: McGraw-Hill, 1983.

311. Steinberg, B., et al. Prenatal diagnosis of hereditary tyrosinemia. *N. Engl. J. Med.* 310:855, 1984.

312. Steinberg, D. Phytanic Acid Storage Disease (Refsum's Disease). In J. B. Stanbury et al. (Eds.), *The Metabolic Basis of Inherited Disease* (5th ed.). New York: McGraw-Hill, 1983.

313. Sternlieb, I. Copper and the liver. *Gastroenterology* 78:1615, 1980.

314. Sternlieb, I., and Scheinberg, I. H. Radiocopper in diagnosing liver disease. *Semin. Nucl. Med.* 2:176, 1972.

315. Suzuki, K., Schneider, E. L., and Epstein, C. J. *In utero* diagnosis of globoid cell leukodystrophy (Krabbe's disease). *Biochem. Biophys. Res. Commun.* 45:1303, 1971.

316. Suzuki, K., and Suzuki, Y. Galactosylceramide Lipidosis: Globoid Cell Leukodystrophy (Krabbe's Disease). In J. B. Stanbury et al. (Eds.), *The Metabolic Basis of Inherited Disease* (5th ed.) New York: McGraw-Hill, 1983.

317. Suzuki, Y., and Suzuki, K. Krabbe's globoid cell leukodystrophy: Deficiency of galactocerebrosidase in serum, leukocytes and fibroblasts. *Science* 171:73, 1971.

318. Svennerholm, L., Vanier, M. T., and Mansson, J.-E. Krabbe disease: A galactosphingosine (psychosine) lipidosis. *J. Lipid Res.* 21:53, 1980.

319. Taylor, D. L., and Wang, Y. L. Fluorescently labeled molecules as probes of the structure and function of living cells. *Nature* 284:405, 1980.

320. Thomas, G. H. Beta-D-galactosidase in human urine: Deficiency in generalized gangliosidosis. *J. Lab. Clin. Med.* 74:725, 1969.

321. Thomas, G. H., et al. Neuraminidase deficiency in the original patient with the Goldberg syndrome. *Clin. Genet.* 16:323, 1979.

322. Toussaint, D., and Danis, P. An ocular pathologic study of Refsum's syndrome. *Am. J. Ophthalmol.* 72:342, 1971.

323. Tripathi, R. C., and Ashton, N. Application of electron microscopy to the study of ocular inborn errors of metabolism. *Birth Defects* 12(3):69, 1976.

324. Uhlendorf, B. W., et al. Cell cultures derived from human amniotic fluids: The possible application in the intrauterine disease of heritable metabolic disease. *In Vitro* 4:158, 1969.

325. Van den Hamer, C. J. A., et al. Physical and chemical studies of ceruloplasmin: IX. The role of galactosyl residues in the clearance of ceruloplasmin from the circulation. *J. Biol. Chem.* 245:4397, 1970.

326. Van Dyke, D. L., et al. Prenatal diagnosis of Maroteaux-Lamy syndrome. *Am. J. Med. Genet.* 8:235, 1981.

327. Vanier, M. T., and Svennerholm, L. Chemical pathology of Krabbe's disease: III. Ceramide hexosides and gangliosides of brain. *Acta Paediatr. Scand.* 64:641, 1974.

328. Varma, S. D., and Kinoshita, J. H. The absence of cataracts in mice with congenital hyperglycemia. *Exp. Eye Res.* 19:582, 1974.

329. Vincent, R. A., and Huang, P. C. The proportion of cells labeled with tritiated thymidine as a function of population doubling level in cultures of fetal, adult, mutant and tumor origin. *Exp. Cell Res.* 102:31, 1976.

330. Von Figura, K., van de Kamp, J. J., and Niermeijer, M. F. Prenatal diagnosis of Moroquio's disease type A (N-acetylgalactosamine 6-sulphate sulphatase deficiency). *Prenatal Diagn.* 2:67, 1982.

331. Walker, I. G. Alkaline sucrose sedimentation analysis as an indication of repair capability of xeroderma pigmentosum fibroblasts for 4-nitro-quinoline-1-oxide damage. *Carcinogenesis* 2:691, 1981.

332. Walshe, J. M. Wilson's Disease (Hepatolenticular Degeneration). In P. J. Vinken (Ed.), *Handbook of Clinical Neurology*, Vol. 27. New York: American Elsevier, 1976.

333. Walton, D. S., Robb, R. M., and Crocker, A. C. Ocular manifestations of group A Niemann-Pick disease. *Am. J. Ophthalmol.* 85:174, 1978.

334. Warburg, M. *Diagnosis of Metabolic Eye Diseases.* Copenhagen: Munksgaard, 1972.

335. Webers, D. O., Hollenhorst, R. W., and Goldstein, N. D. The ophthalmolgic manifestations of Wilson's disease. *Mayo Clin. Proc.* 52:409, 1977.

336. Wenger, D. A., et al. Lactosyl ceramidosis: Normal activity for two lactosyl ceramide-beta-galactosidases. *Science* 188:1310, 1975.

337. Westerveld, A., et al. Molecular cloning of a human DNA repair gene. *Nature* 310:425, 1984.

338. Whiteman, P., and Henderson, H. A method for the determination of amniotic-fluid glycosaminoglycans and its application to the prenatal diagnosis of Hurler and Sanfilippo diseases. *Clin. Chim. Acta* 79:99, 1977.

339. Winder, A. F. Disorders of Lipid and Lipoprotein Metabolism. In A. Garner and G. K. Klintworth (Eds.), *Pathobiology of Ocular Disease*. New York: Dekker, 1982.

340. Winder, A. F. Disorders of monosaccharide metabolism. In G. K. Klintworth (Ed.), *Pathobiology of Ocular Disease: A Dynamic Approach*, Part B. New York: Dekker, 1982.

341. Winslow, R. M., and Anderson, W. F. The Hemoglobinopathies. In J. B. Stanbury et al. (Eds.), *The Metabolic Basis of Inherited Disease* (5th ed.). New York: McGraw-Hill, 1983.

342. Witkop, C. J., et al. Ophthalmologic, biochemical, platelet, and ultra-structural defects in the various types of oculocutaneous albinism. *J. Invest. Dermatol.* 60:443, 1973.

343. Witkop, C. J., Queredo, W. C., Jr., and Fitzpatrick, T. B. Albinism and Other Disorders of Pigment Metabolism. In J. B. Stanbury et al. (Eds.), *The Metabolic Basis of Inherited Disease* (5th ed.). New York: McGraw-Hill, 1983.

344. Wong, V. G. Ocular manifestations in cystinosis. *Birth Defects* 12(3):181, 1976.

345. Wong, V. G., Lietman, P. S., and Seegmiller, J. E. Alterations of pigment epithelium in cystinosis. *Arch. Ophthalmol.* 77:361, 1967.

346. Wong, V. G., Schulman, J. D., and Seegmiller, J. E. Conjunctival biopsy for the biochemical diagnosis of cystinosis. *Am. J. Ophthalmol.* 70:278, 1970.

347. Zeman, W., et al. The neuronal ceroid-lipofuscinoses (Batten-Vogt syndrome). In P. J. Vinken and G. W. Bruyn (Eds.), *Handbook of Clinical Neurology*, Vol. 10. Amsterdam: North-Holland, 1970.

348. Zlotogora, J., et al. Metachromatic leukodystrophy in the Habbanite Jews: High frequency in a genetic isolate and screening for heterozygotes. *Am. J. Hum. Genet.* 32:633, 1980.

3

The Eye and the Chromosome

Marilyn Baird Mets

The eye and its diseases have long been a key to the secrets of the chromosomes. In 1937 Bell and Haldane recognized the first disease linkage on a human chromosome—that between color blindness and hemophilia on the X chromosome [13]. Later, in 1963, Renwick and Lawler assigned the first human disease locus to an autosome, chromosome 1 [121]. This was done by linking the Coppock cataract, studied extensively by Nettleship and Ogilvie [106], to the Duffy blood group locus, which had previously been assigned to chromosome 1. Since then numerous ocular diseases and systemic diseases with ocular involvement have been mapped. The purpose of this chapter is to provide an update on the unfolding of the chromosome map as it relates to the eye.

HUMAN GENETICS

A summary of human genetic terminology will be provided to the reader to assure better comprehension of the text to follow. The word *chromosome* refers to the condensed form the nuclear DNA assumes during cell division. The human species has 46 chromosomes in each somatic cell. These 46 chromosomes, the human *genome*, consist of 22 pairs of *autosomes* and two sex chromosomes. In the woman the sex chromosomes are identical and consist of the two X chromosomes; in the man they are nonidentical and consist of the X and Y chromosomes. The two members of each pair, one from each parent, are called *homologous chromosomes*. Units of genetic information, *genes*, are encoded in the DNA of the chromosome. The relative order of the genes, which are arranged in a linear fashion along the chromosome, is referred to as the *genetic map*. The precise position of a particular gene on the genome is its *locus*. Alternative forms of a particular gene that can occupy the same locus are called *alleles*.

Mendel's law of independent assortment states that genes that are not allelic assort independently of one another. Exceptions to this law occur as the result of linkage. Linked genes have their loci on the same chromosome and are close enough so that they do not assort independently. They are transmitted to the same gamete (haploid reproductive cell) more than 50 percent of the time. The concept of linkage was extended by Renwick to include genes that are too far apart on the same chromosome to show linkage in family studies [120]. Genes on the same chromosome are called *syntenic*.

The human genome may undergo numerical or structural changes in chromosome composition. In addition it may be subject to mutation. According to Crow, a mutation is a change that cannot be shown to be due to a detectable chromosome rearrangement or to a recombination mechanism [39]. Indeed, mutations or so-called point mutations may be due to microscopic changes that are analogous to the numerical or structural changes but are simply too small for us to "view" at present.

Let us now further elaborate on the numerical and structural chromosomal changes.

Numerical Chromosomal Changes

The numerical changes that the human genome may undergo include trisomies and duplications.

Table 3-1. *Ocular Anomalies Found in Trisomy 13 (Patau's Syndrome)*

Microphthalmos
Coloboma (iris, posterior pole, optic nerve)
Retinal dysplasia
Optic nerve hypoplasia
Persistent hyperplastic primary vitreous
Cataract
Anterior cleavage syndrome
Corneal opacity
Cyclopia
Intraocular cartilage

Table 3-3. *Ocular Anomalies Found in Trisomy 21 (Down's Syndrome)*

Oblique palpebral fissures
Prominent epicanthal folds
Blepharitis
Strabismus
Nystagmus
High myopia
Brushfield's spots
Cataract
Keratoconus
Optic atrophy

The more common numerical changes of human autosomes lead to trisomies 13, 18, and 21. The eye findings associated with these entities are outlined in Tables 3-1, 3-2, and 3-3, respectively. The only monosomy commonly compatible with life is Turner's syndrome (45, XO). Monosomy of an autosome is usually lethal. (Exceptions involve G monosomies, of chromosome 21) [78]. Eye findings associated with the Turner's syndrome are listed in Table 3-4. There are similarities in the eye findings in these numerical changes no matter which chromosome is involved. The most common eye findings seen in numerical changes are hypertelorism, epicanthus, slanted palpebral fissures, and strabismus [78]. Less common complications include ptosis, coloboma, nystagmus, and cataract [78]. These abnormalities are also found in patients with large chromosomal deletions.

Structural Chromosomal Changes

Structural changes in the genome occur when there is chromosomal breakage followed by reconstitution in an altered order. These new forms may be stable (capable of passing through cell division

Table 3-2. *Ocular Anomalies Found in Trisomy 18 (Edwards' Syndrome)*

Microphthalmos
Prominent epicanthal folds
Blepharophimosis
Ptosis
Hypertelorism
Optic disc anomalies
Uveal colobomas
Congenital glaucoma
Corneal opacities

unaltered) or unstable. There are several types of stable structural changes: deletions, duplications, inversions, translocations, and isochromosomes. Dicentrics (two centromeres), acentrics (no centromere), and rings are unstable forms. Rings containing a centromere can be stable.

Deletions involve loss of chromosomal material. The loss may involve one break, resulting in a terminal deletion, or two, yielding an interstitial deletion. If the deleted portion has no centromere, it is called an acentric fragment. Acentric fragments are usually lost at the next cell division and are therefore considered unstable, as mentioned above.

Duplications involve addition of chromosomal material. These are usually the result of unequal crossing over or exchange of material between homologous chromosomes during meiosis (Fig. 3-1). The homologous chromosome in such a situation carries a deletion.

Inversions of chromosomal material represent a reversal of the order or sequence of a certain segment; for example, ABCD is inverted to ACBD. Inversions, like interstitial deletions, are the result of two chromosome breaks. Inversions result in gametes that are unbalanced and therefore yield a high incidence of abnormal offspring.

The transfer of a part of one chromosome to a nonhomologous chromosome is called a trans-

Table 3-4. *Ocular Anomalies Found in 45,XO Monosomy (Turner's Syndrome)*

Prominent epicanthal folds
Ptosis
Strabismus
Blue sclera
Cataract
Color blindness (incidence as seen in normal males)

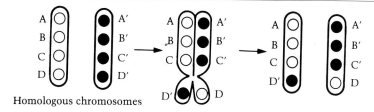

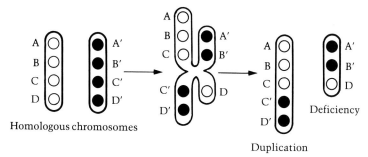

Equal crossing over

Homologous chromosomes

Duplication

Deficiency

Unequal crossing over

Fig. 3-1. *Crossing over at the first meiotic division. A. Equal crossing over between homologous chromosomes. The result is genetic reassortment. B. Unequal crossing over between homologous chromosomes. The result is duplications and deficiencies.*

location (Fig. 3-2). Reciprocal translocations occur when a chromosome segment is exchanged with another chromosome without addition or loss of chromosomal material. Not all translocations are reciprocal. In robertsonian translocations the breaks occur at the centromeres and entire arms are exchanged. Another type of translocation, an insertion, is characterized by the annealing of a chromosome segment in the chain of a nonhomologous chromosome. An insertion requires at least three breaks and occurs rarely. Translocations, like inversions, result in a high incidence of abnormal offspring.

Isochromosomes contain arms of equal length on either side of the centromere. The banding

Fig. 3-2. *Reciprocal translocation. Translocations are exchanges between nonhomologous chromosomes (in this case, chromosomes 1 and 2). In a reciprocal translocation, chromosomal material is exchanged but not lost.*

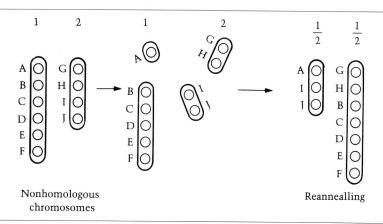

Nonhomologous chromosomes

Reannealling

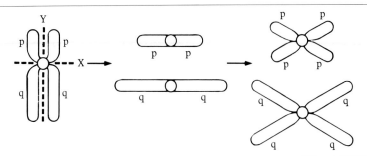

Fig. 3-3. *Isochromosome formation. The y-axis seen here is the plane along which the centromere normally divides. If the division occurs along the x-axis, the resulting chromosomes are defined as isochromosomes. Isochromosomes carry the same information on each arm.*

sequence in these otherwise identical arms is opposite each other. Isochromosomes presumably result from erroneous division of the centromere. That is, the separation occurs between the long and short pairs of arms rather than between homologous chromosomes (Fig. 3-3).

In addition to numerical and structural changes in the chromosomes, which can occur in any of the 22 autosomes or the sex chromosomes, mention should be made of phenomena special to the X chromosome. The Lyon hypothesis or lyonization explains the expression of disease in female carriers of X-linked disease [90]. All females have two X chromosomes, in contrast to the XY constellation in males, which leads to excess genetic material in females since the Y chromosome seems void of genetic information beyond sex determination. This is compensated for by inactivation of one of the two X chromosomes, which becomes pyknotic in early development. The pyknotic chromosome can be identified as the *Barr body*. The inactivation appears to be a random process and may occur to either the paternal or maternal X chromosome. Therefore, all females are mosaics for genetic information coded for by the X chromosome; that is, some of their cells have inactivated paternal X chromosomes, and others have inactivated maternal X chromosomes. Thus, carrier females can be detected in X-linked ocular albinism and X-linked retinitis pigmentosa because of their mosaicism. The female carriers of X-linked albinism often show iris transillumination. The female carriers of X-linked retinitis pigmentosa often show some peripheral bone spicules.

Mapping Techniques

The goal in mapping is first to discover which chromosome a gene is located on and then to find the specific position of the gene on that chromosome. The results thus far for eye-related entities are diagrammed in Fig. 3-4, the human linkage map. Ultimately, this mapping will lead to a knowledge of the specific nucleotide order of the human DNA.

The mapping techniques employed in human genetics include pedigree analysis, gene dosage methods, somatic cell hybridization, and recombinant DNA techniques. Thus far 488 autosomal assignments have been made [118]. Pedigree analysis and deletion mapping are employed mainly in human dominant disease states for which no biochemical marker is available. Somatic cell hybridization is used to assign biochemical markers. The particular gene dosage method I will discuss is deletion mapping, which was used in retinoblastoma. The specific recombinant DNA technique I will discuss employs restriction fragment length polymorphisms. This approach has just recently been developed and may prove to be the most powerful technique for mapping the human genome found thus far. It is a melding of recombinant techniques and classical family linkage studies. These are not all of the mapping techniques being used in human genetics, but they are the ones that have been used for the mapping of eye diseases.

PEDIGREE ANALYSIS

Pedigree analysis, until recently the only source of information on the chromosome map, uses a statistical approach for linkage analysis. The unique genetic pattern of X linkage allows it to be discovered quite readily, though determination

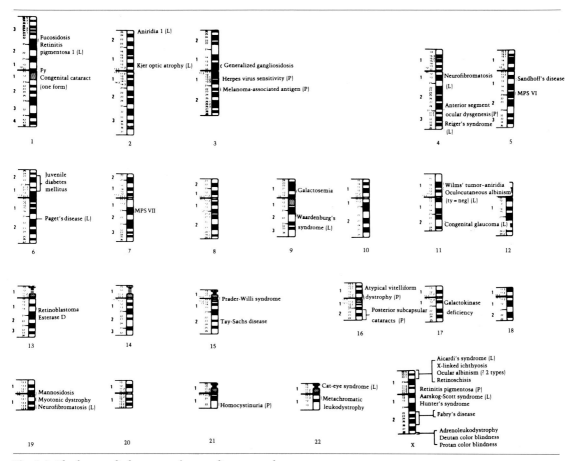

Fig. 3-4. *The human linkage map for eye diseases and systemic diseases with significant eye findings. The number of each chromosome is found beneath it. The bands are numbered sequentially from the centromere out, according to the classification agreed on in the Paris conference of 1971 and updated by McKusick [93]. The centromere is designated by the thick horizontal line to the left. The p or shorter arm is above; the q or longer arm is below. The diseases are written to the right of their normal map position. (L = limbo, P = provisional, MPS = mucopolysaccharidosis.)*

of the gene order on the X chromosome requires sophisticated statistical analysis. Nonetheless, it is not suprising that the first human disease linkage was found on the X chromosome between hemophilia and color blindness. The autosomes are far more difficult to map. However, as more and more genetic markers (traits with more than one allelic gene and often with a known chromosomal assignment) are found, it becomes easier to localize new traits, which fit into the map like pieces into a puzzle.

As previously defined, linkage produces a deviation in Mendel's law of independent assortment. That is, traits physically proximal on a chromosome tend to be inherited together. Chromosomes can undergo recombination or crossing over. Crossing over between traits results in their separation in the offspring. Such offspring are called recombinants. The degree of linkage can be quantified as the recombination frequency, that is, the number of recombinant offspring divided by the total number of offspring observed. When this is expressed as a percentage, it is equivalent, for short distances, to the number of *map units* in *centimorgans* that separate the two traits. That is, by studying recombination frequencies, one can map out the relative distances on the chromosome between traits.

Single (one family) multigeneration pedigrees are preferred for linkage analysis because they are likely to yield more reliable information since one is certain of dealing with a single gene defect. However, in human studies, data are often available for only two generations. Statistical information can be obtained from two-generation family studies and then combined by means of the *lod* (log odds) method [33]. In brief the principle of the lod method is to establish a series of theoretical recombination frequencies. Then one calculates the odds for a given pedigree on the basis of a given recombination frequency compared to the likelihood if the recombination frequency is 50 percent (the frequency for random assortment). If the ratio is expressed as a logarithm, then information from different families may be combined by simple addition. A lod score of 3 (1000 : 1) or greater is considered "proof" of linkage; 2 to 3, "suggestive" of linkage; and 1 to 2, "interesting" [101]. In this manner, one can calculate the probability of linkage and, by using genetic markers, can gradually gather information on new traits [144].

An additional key concept in linkage analysis concerns the polymorph. A polymorphic locus, by definition, is one in which the most common allele has a frequency of no more than 0.99 [144]. Therefore at least 2 percent of the population are heterozygous at that locus [144]. This heterozygosity makes polymorphs especially useful genetic markers. The ABO blood types and the HLA (major histocompatibility) antigens are examples of such polymorphs.

GENE DOSAGE METHODS

Gene dosage methods are another approach for detecting linkage. As mentioned previously, one example of this approach is deletion mapping, which was employed in the chromosomal assignment of retinoblastoma to chromosome 13. Deletion mapping involves the study of the chromosome composition of an individual by means of microscopic examination of a chromosome spread from a human cell in metaphase. Studies of chromosome spreads are referred to as cytogenetics. When this spread is cut from a photomicrograph and arranged according to standard classification, it is called a karyotype. Deletion mapping involves noting an association between a particular phenotype such as retinoblastoma and the loss of a particular region of a chromosome, as demonstrated by study of the individual's karyotype. In the case of retinoblastoma, the deleted portion is part of the long arm of chromosome 13.

The standard of classification that will be employed throughout this chapter is that agreed on the *Paris Conference*, 1971 [116A]. That is, p =

short arm of a chromosome, q = long arm of a chromosome, r = ring, and number = band number and position from the centromere. In the case of retinoblastoma, the deletion is chromosome 13, long arm, region 14, or 13q14.

SOMATIC CELL HYBRIDIZATION

As mentioned before, the two previously described methods, pedigree analysis and deletion analysis, are used primarily in human dominant disease states for which no biochemical marker is available. Somatic cell hybridization, on the other hand, is used to assign biochemical markers. A thorough review of the technique is found in the article by Ruddle and Kucherlapati [125].

The technique of somatic cell hybridization is summarized in Fig. 3-5. It involves the in vitro fusion of cells from different species. For example, mouse cells and human fibroblasts that are adapted to tissue culture are placed in a Petri dish and allowed to remain in contact with each other. The spontaneous fusion that would normally occur only rarely in such a situation is enhanced by inactivated Sendai virus or a similar agent. The Sendai virus enhances fusion by forming intracellular bridges between closely adjacent cells. The situation is further manipulated because the mouse cells used are deficient in enzymes required to metabolize the medium in the Petri dish. The human cells are not deficient. Therefore the mouse cells are selected against and die, leaving the human cells and the fused cells that have now formed a clonal population (a group of cells derived by mitosis from a single cell). Human cells that are in tissue culture grow slowly. Therefore, it is easy to isolate the clonal populations of fused cells. There are two important characteristics of these fused cells. First, for some reason, the human genome is selectively lost. That is, the fused cells

Fig. 3-5. *The technique of somatic cell hybridization.*

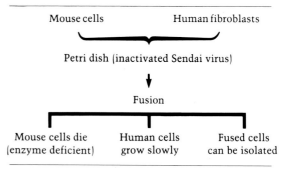

contain essentially intact mouse genome, with small pieces of the human genome. The second characteristic is that all the DNA remains functional. That is, the mouse and human genes are expressed at the same time, each coding for its appropriate proteins. Mouse and human chromosomes can be distinguished from each other by means of amino acid sequence as demonstrated by electrophoresis.

The sequence of events in mapping by means of somatic cell hybridization involves first noting which gene products are consistently formed together. Since the human chromosomes are usually lost from the hybrid cells as discrete units, gene products consistently found together are probably coded for by genes on the same chromosome or syntenic genes. Therefore, by assaying a number of clones, information on synteny may be found. Now one can compare the information on gene expression with the presence or absence of particular chromosomes and thus assign genes to particular chromosomes. Information on the locus of a gene on a chromosome has been obtained by taking advantage of the normally occurring structural changes previously discussed. Specifically, translocations and deletions disturb the normal syntenic relationship of genes. In this way, they provide further information on the chromosomal location of a particular gene. Somatic cell hybridization has greatly expanded our knowledge of the human chromosome map.

RECOMBINANT DNA TECHNIQUES (RESTRICTION FRAGMENT LENGTH POLYMORPHISMS)

A limitation of both pedigree analysis and somatic cell hybridization is the availability of genetic markers. That is, an appropriate polymorph or biochemical marker for detecting linkage to a particular disease may not exist. However, if one goes a step further, to the DNA sequence itself for use as the "marker," then it is certain that appropriate markers can be found. A new method that is rapidly coming into use does this by employing recombinant DNA techniques to detect restriction fragment length polymorphisms (RFLPs). A very good discussion of RFLPs is found in the article by Botstein and colleagues [23]. The technique will be briefly discussed here.

DNA restriction enzymes can "recognize" sequences of DNA and cleave the DNA at specific sites [105]. The result is restriction fragments of defined lengths. When alleles differ in ways that affect the relative location of restriction sites, they may yield fragments of different lengths. These restriction fragments can be separated by electrophoresis according to their molecular size. Then specific polymorphic sequences within these fragments can be identified by hybridization with recombinant radioactive probe sequences after the method of Southern [133]. Thus, one has restriction fragment length polymorphisms that can be tested in human pedigrees for linkage relationships by established methods. Since RFLPs themselves are being used as genetic markers, neither a specific gene isolation nor knowledge of the biochemical nature of the trait is required for mapping.

Recently a close genetic linkage was demonstrated between the X-linked retinitis pigmentosa and an RFLP identified by recombinant DNA probe L1.28 [22]. This suggests that the X-linked retinitis pigmentosa locus is on the proximal part of the short arm of the X chromosome. In the future this RFLP may be used for carrier detection of X-linked retinitis pigmentosa.

AUTOSOMAL ASSIGNMENTS

Table 3-5 summarizes the eye diseases with autosomal assignments. All of these will be discussed except those whose linkage is designated provisional or limbo (Table 3-5). One "limbo" disease, Waardenburg's syndrome, and one "provisional" disease, familial posterior polar cataract, are discussed, because of their significance in ophthalmology.

Chromosome 1

As mentioned previously, the first human disease to be assigned to an autosome was the Coppock cataract, also called Doyne's discoid cataract, central pulverulent cataract, and hereditary nuclear cataract [85]. This autosomal dominant condition involves opacities in the fetal nucleus.

Renwick and Lawler employed pedigree studies for linkage analysis [121]. They analyzed blood and saliva samples from members of the Coppock family for common markers. They found a strong indication of close linkage with the Duffy blood group locus, which was subsequently assigned to chromosome 1 by linkage to a cytogenic marker [42]. Thus the first human disease was mapped on an autosome, chromosome 1.

Fucosidosis is a very rare autosomal recessive disorder first described by Durand and co-workers [44, 45]. There are two types, the first of which

Table 3-5. *Assignment of Genes to Chromosomes*

Chromosome no.	Enzyme or disorder	Chromosome no.	Enzyme or disorder
Chromosome 1	α-L-Fucosidase (fucosidosis)	Chromosome 15	
	Coppock cataract	15q11–15q12	Prader-Willi syndrome
	(L)*Retinitis pigmentosa [71]	15q22–15q25.1	Hexosaminidase A (Tay-Sachs
Chromosome 2			disease)
2p23	(L) Aniridia [52]	Chromosome 16	
2p	(L) Optic atrophy, Kjer type [81]	16p	(P) Macular dystrophy, atypical
Chromosome 3			vitelliform [141]
3p12–3q13**	β-Galactosidase 1 (generalized	16q	(P) Familial posterior polar
	gangliosidosis)		cataract [92]
	(P)*Herpes virus sensitivity [31,	Chromosome 17	
	56]	17q210–17q220	Galactokinase
3q23–3q ter	(P) Melanoma-associated antigen	Chromosome 19	
	[118]	19p ter**–19q13	Lysosomal α-mannosidase B
Chromosome 4	(L) von Recklinghausen		(mannosidosis)
	neurofibromatosis [137]		Myotonic dystrophy
	(P) Anterior segment ocular	19q	(L) Neurofibromatosis [77]
	dysgenesis [73]	Chromosome 22	
4q23–4q27	(L) Rieger's syndrome [89]	22p ter–22q11	(L) Cat-eye syndrome [127]
Chromosome 5		22q13.31–22q	Arylsulfatase A (metachromatic
5q13	Hexosaminidase B (Sandhoff's	ter	leukodystrophy)
	disease)	X chromosome	*Xg Cluster*
	Arylsulfatase B (MPS VI)	Xp	Steroid sulfatase deficiency
Chromosome 6	(L) Juvenile diabetes mellitus [9,		(ichthyosis)
	10]		Ocular albinism (Nettleship-
	(L) Paget's disease of bone [49,		Falls type)
	55]		(P) Ocular albinism (Forsius-
Chromosome 7	Corneal type I procollagen		Eriksson type) [112, 151]
	β-Glucuronidase (MPS VII)		Retinoschisis
Chromosome 9		Xq28	*G6PD Cluster*
9p12–9p13	Galactose 1-phosphate uridyl		Deutan color blindness
	transferase (galactosemia)		Protan color blindness
	(L) Waardenburg's syndrome		Adrenoleukodystrophy
	type I		*Somatic Cell Hybridization*
Chromosome 11		Xp22	(L) Aicardi's syndrome [68]
11p13	Wilms' tumor, aniridia,	Xq26–27	Sulfoiduronate sulfatase (MPS II,
	gonadoblastoma, retardation		Hunter's syndrome)
	(WAGR)	Xq12	(L) Aarskog-Scott syndrome [12]
	(L) Congenital glaucoma [27]	Xq22–Xq24	α-Galactosidase A (Fabry's
	(L) Tyrosinase-negative albinism		disease)
	[93]		*RFLP*
Chromosome 13		Xp	(P) Retinitis pigmentosa
13q14	Retinoblastoma		
	Esterase D		

P = short arm of chromosome; q = long arm of chromosome; L = MPS = mucopolysaccharidosis; G6PD = galactose 6-phosphate dehydrogenase; RFLP = restriction fragment length polymorphisms.

is consistent with the original description and is characterized by progressive cerebral degeneration after the first year of life. The second type presents as delayed psychomotor development. Patients of this latter group develop angiokeratoma similar to that of Fabry's disease around the age of 5 years [17]. These different clinical pictures are probably due to allelism. The ocular findings in fucosidosis with angiokeratoma appear to combine some of the ocular characteristics of Fabry's disease (conjunctival and retinal vessel tortuosity) and an ocular characteristic of the mucopolysaccharidoses (diffuse corneal opacities) [132]. The enzyme defect has been found to be an absence of α-L-fucosidase [147]. The disease was mapped by means of somatic cell hybridization [66].

Chromosome 3

GM$_1$ gangliosidosis type 1, or generalized gangliosidosis, is characterized by (1) severe progressive cerebral degeneration leading to death in the first 2 years of life, (2) accumulation of specific ganglioside in neurons and viscera, and (3) bony deformities like those seen in Hurler's syndrome [108]. The enzyme defect was found to be a deficiency of β-galactosidase [113]. The eye findings consist of a macular cherry-red spot, seen in half the patients. One case of corneal clouding has been reported [108]. Somatic cell hybridization was employed to assign this enzyme deficiency to chromosome 3 [130].

Chromosome 5

Sandhoff's disease, like Tay-Sachs disease and juvenile GM$_2$ gangliosidosis, results in the accumulation of massive amounts of ganglioside GM$_2$ in the central nervous system. In all three diseases, there is an abnormality of the lysosomal enzyme β-D-N-acetylhexosaminidase. This enzyme has at least two isoenzymes, hex A and hex B. Patients with Sandhoff's disease exhibit a deficiency in both of these forms [126]. This disease is also autosomal recessive and presents clinically as Tay-Sachs disease plus visceromegaly. The psychomotor retardation is usually evident by 6 months of age. The disease is progressive and results in death by age 2 to 3 years because of bulbar incompetence and secondary pneumonitis. The eye manifestations are blindness and a cherry-red spot on fundus examination [20]. Somatic cell hybridization has been employed to map the gene for hex B on chromosome 5 [58].

Mucopolysaccharidosis (MPS) VI, or the Maroteaux-Lamy syndrome, is characterized by a Hurler-like appearance (MPS I), including dwarfism, and corneal clouding, but without the intellectual impairment. This autosomal recessive disorder is due to an arylsulfatase deficiency [11, 91]. The corneal clouding seen in this entity, like that in MPS I, begins in the periphery and progresses centrally. It involves the full thickness of the stroma. The mapping of this disease to chromosome 5 was carried out by means of somatic cell hybridization [72].

Chromosome 7

Recently, corneal type I procollagen has been assigned to chromosome 7. Though this is not a disease, it is included here for heuristic reasons. Type I collagen forms the bulk of sclera, conjunctiva, and cornea and is responsible for their tensile strength. Somatic cell hybridization was used to map the structural gene for corneal type I procollagen to chromosome 7 [36].

Mucopolysaccharidosis VII (Sly's disease) has the following clinical features: short stature, hepatosplenomegaly, progressive skeletal deformities of thorax and spine, granular inclusions in the leukocytes, and frequent pulmonary infections. The disease and the enzyme defect, deficiency of lysomal β-D-glucuronidase, were described by Sly and co-workers [131]. Since their first report, there have been several reported cases with corneal clouding [18]. This disease was mapped by means of somatic cell hybridization [82].

Chromosome 9

Waardenburg's syndrome, as originally discribed, has the following eye findings: lateral displacement of the inner canthi and inferior lacrimal puncta (estimated trait penetrance 99%), prominent medial brows (45%), and heterochromia iridis (25%). Key findings in other systems are congenital sensorineural deafness, white forelock, and prominent root of the nose [149, 150]. The syndrome is transmitted in an autosomal dominant manner with almost complete penetrance. Arias has divided this syndrome into three types [4]. Type I, by far the most common, includes the lateral displacement of the inner canthi. The other two do not. Type I has been assigned to chromosome 9. Pedigree analysis was employed to demonstrate loose linkage (recombination frequency 0.175–0.255) between the ABO locus and Waardenburg's syndrome type I [5, 6].

The cardinal features of galactosemia are hepatomegaly, cataracts, and mental retardation. The basic defect is a marked decrease or total absence of galactose 1-phosphate uridyl transferase [80]. The most common presentation is failure to thrive in the newborn period. Cataracts have been seen as early as the first few days of life. They consist of punctate lesions in the fetal nucleus and may be very subtle, seen only on slit-lamp examination. The cataract is caused by galactitol accumulation in the lens [19]. Somatic cell hybridization has been used to assign this autosomal recessive disease to human chromosome 9 [15, 28, 99, 154].

Chromosome 11

The association between sporadic aniridia and Wilms' tumor was first reported in 1964 by Miller and colleagues in an epidemiologic study of Wilms' tumor [97]. Later it was brought to the ophthalmic literature when an additional 4 cases were found [41]. These patients also had genital abnormalities, and the authors noted a high incidence of mental retardation. Deletion analysis was employed by Riccardi and associates to assign the complex of aniridia, ambiguous genitalia, and mental retardation (AGR) to chromosome 11p [124]. They described 3 unrelated patients with 11p interstitial deletions. These deletions were all overlapping band 13. One of the three also had Wilms' tumor. They concluded that a partial deletion of 11p13 causes the characteristic syndrome of AGR and a nephroblastic diathesis, with the tumor developing in only a portion of cases.

Chromosome 13

Work on retinoblastoma, the most common intraocular tumor of childhood, has resulted not only in the mapping of the retinoblastoma gene, but also in an advancement in the understanding of human oncogenesis. There are three recognized patterns of inheritance of retinoblastoma: sporadic (in 55–65% of cases), autosomal dominant (35–40%), and that associated with the chromosomal deletion (3–5%). The third of these types is the most amenable to study; therefore much work has been done on it.

Deletion analysis was employed by various groups over a period of time to assign retinoblastoma to 13q14. Before staining techniques were

well developed, three case reports associated retinoblastoma with chromosome 13, 14, or 15 [86, 142, 148]. Several workers then identified the chromosome in question as chromosome 13 [59, 67, 116, 140, 155]. Taylor suggested that the retinoblastoma locus is situated on the long arm, near the centromere [140]. This suggestion was deduced from the absence of retinoblastoma in the Dr (ring D chromosome) patients and its presence in the Dq-patients (deletion of the long arm of the D chromosome). (The Dr patients had long rings, with presumably small deletions of the distal long arm.) Yunis and Ramsey [157] observed that the 9 known cases [152] of retinoblastoma with 13q deletion, as well as their 2 cases, had a deletion that included band 14. Subsequently, a patient with retinoblastoma and translocation of the 13q14 region to the short arm of the X chromosome was described [38, 107]. Therefore, it seemed that it was not the deletion that resulted in retinoblastoma but the monosomy.

Hence, in the chromosomal deletion form of retinoblastoma, monosomy of 13q14 was associated with manifest retinoblastoma. But what about the familial, autosomal dominant form of retinoblastoma? Esterase D, a polymorphic genetic marker, was assigned to band 13q14 by deletion mapping [135, 146]. Subsequently, Sparkes and colleagues evaluated three families with hereditary retinoblastoma and demonstrated close linkage of the gene for this tumor with the genetic locus for esterase D [136]. Therefore, the gene for retinoblastoma in the autosomal dominant form was mapped on chromosome 13q14 by linkage analysis.

What of oncogenesis? As mentioned previously, it appeared that monosomy for the 13q14 region was necessary for the development of retinoblastoma. Further studies have continued to support this idea: Esterase D levels in tumor cells appear to be about 50 percent of those found in somatic cells of the same patient [14, 64]. It now appears that the retinoblastoma gene is a recessive cancer gene that manifests itself when the normal allele is deleted [34, 43, 104] This is a fundamentally different mechanism of oncogenesis than has been previously described for human cancer oncogenes.

Chromosome 15

The clinical manifestations of Prader-Willi syndrome may be divided into two phases. The first phase, which begins at birth, includes severe muscular atony, hyporeflexia to areflexia, feeding difficulties, and, in males, hypoplastic penis and scrotum and cryptorchidism. Female children may show small labia majora and absent labia minora. As affected children get older, the second phase, which includes polyphagia, obesity, delayed psychomotor development, mental subnormality, muscular hypotonia, short stature, and hypogonadism, begins [21]. The patients also manifest albinoidism—light hair and skin and transillumination of the irides [74]. The latter is the only reported eye manifestation. Prader-Willi syndrome has been assigned to chromosome 15 by deletion mapping [84].

The manifestations of Tay-Sachs disease (GM$_2$ gangliosidosis type I) include developmental retardation in infancy followed by paralysis, dementia, and blindness. The patients die by the second or third year of life. Characteristically, a cherry-red spot is seen on fundus examination. The disease is autosomal recessive and is seen primarily in Ashkenazic Jews. There is an absence of hexosaminidase A with a resultant failure to degrade ganglioside GM$_2$. This results in its accumulation in neurons throughout the body [114]. Somatic cell hybridization was employed to assign hexosaminidase A to chromosome 15 [51].

Chromosome 16

Pedigree analysis was employed to assign one form of familial posterior polar cataract to a locus on chromosome 16 [92]. Linkage to haptoglobin, a chromosome 16 marker, was demonstrated. A lod score of 1.8, which is equivalent to a linkage probability of 64 : 1, was obtained. Therefore this familial posterior polar cataract was provisionally assigned to chromosome 16.

Chromosome 17

Like galactose uridyl transferase deficiency (galactosemia), galactokinase deficiency also has the manifestation of cataracts and galactosuria [62, 63]. However, it shows none of the other systemic manifestations. Apparently, the mechanism of the cataract formation is the same in the two diseases—an accumulation of galactitol, a breakdown produce of galactose, in the lens [88]. The appearance of the cataract in galactokinase deficiency is quite variable and has been described as zonular, Y sutural, nuclear, posterior cortical, and embryonal nuclear opacities [88].

The urine may be negative for galactose if the patient's diet does not include milk. The definitive test is an assay for galactokinase in the red blood cells. Galactokinase deficiency has been assigned to chromosome 17, specifically 17q210–222, by means of somatic cell hybridization [47, 115].

Chromosome 19

Mannosidosis is a rare, autosomal recessive, lysosomal enzyme disorder. Two distinct clinical forms are known. Type I patients exhibit a Hurler-like appearance, hepatosplenomegaly, severe recurrent infections, and death in early childhood, like the patient originally described by Ockerman [109]. Type II patients have a milder disease characterized by hearing loss, mental retardation, mild dysostosis multiplex, and survival into adulthood [40]. Both types show posterior, spokelike cataracts [92]. Two brothers have been described showing the clinical characteristics of types I and II [98]. Therefore it is postulated that the two types may be due to environmental effects rather than genetic ones. The enzyme defect is a deficiency of α-mannosidase, of which there are two types [32]. A deficiency of the lysosomal α-mannosidase B appears to be responsible for mannosidosis. This enzyme has been assigned to chromosome 19 by somatic cell hybridization [35].

Myotonic dystrophy is an autosomal dominant disorder characterized by myotonia, muscle wasting, hypogonadism, frontal balding, electrocardiographic changes, and cataracts. Other eye findings include ptosis, which is usually present, external ophthalmoplegia, sluggish pupils [143], and macular and peripheral retinal pigment epithelial (RPE) dystrophy [30].

As early as 1954 Mohr suspected linkage between the Secretor and the Lutheran (Se : Lu) linkage groups [100]. This was confirmed in 1971, when the genome for myotonic dystrophy was placed on chromosome 19 by linkage analysis [70, 122, 123].

Chromosome 22

The late infantile form of metachromatic leukodystrophy usually has its onset in the second year of life, followed by progression to death before 5 years of age. It was first described by Greenfield and is characterized by normal development in the first year, followed by motor regression [68]. This progresses to involve speech, and at this stage mentation may also deteriorate. The eye findings include maintenance of visual function until terminal stages despite a grayish macular halo seen on fundus examination from early on. Cogan and co-workers describe this finding as a subtle graying of the area surrounding the fovea, with the central area standing out darkly in the manner of a red spot [37]. The enzyme defect in this disease is the deficiency of arylsulfatase A with resultant accumulation of cerebroside sulfate [7, 139]. This disease was assigned to chromosome 22 by means of somatic cell hybridization [29].

X CHROMOSOME ASSIGNMENTS

The characteristic pattern of X-linked inheritance permits direct assignment of a given gene to the X chromosome. To date more than 115 X-linked genetic diseases are known. Of these at least 51 involve the eye (Table 3-6). I will discuss only those diseases that have some regional assignment on the X chromosome. These are summarized in Table 3-5. They can be organized into two groups: those mapped by family linkage studies and those mapped by somatic cell hybridization. The Xg cluster and the glucose 6-phosphate dehydrogenase (G6PD) cluster of assignments have both been charted using pedigree analysis.

Diseases Mapped by Family Linkage Studies

GLUCOSE 6-PHOSPHATE DEHYDROGENASE CLUSTER

The G6PD cluster includes protan and deutan color blindness and adrenoleukodystrophy. As mentioned previously, Bell and Haldane were first to recognize a linkage on human chromosomes in 1937; this was the linkage between color blindness (protanopia and deuteranopia) and hemophilia A on the X chromosome [13]. They tested color vision in hemophilic and nonhemophilic brothers and by means of pedigree analysis deduced linkage between the two. Subsequently, pedigree analysis has been employed with known markers, and linkage has been established between both color blindness and hemophilia A and the polymorphic G6PD locus [24, 25, 119].

Adrenoleukodystrophy is a lipid storage disease that presents in childhood as progressive mental and neurologic deterioration, often associated with bronzing of the skin. The central nervous system signs are due to progressive demyelination; the skin manifestation, to adrenal insufficiency [102]. The eye abnormalities are visual loss owing to optic atrophy. Retinal function as measured by electroretinogram remains normal. Both visual loss and retinal function are probably caused by central demyelination [156]. Regional localization on the X chromosome was ascertained by pedigree analysis and linkage to Xg blood groups [138].

Xg CLUSTER

The Xg cluster includes ichthyosis, ocular albinism, and retinoschisis. X-linked ichthyosis is one of the four forms of this hereditary skin disease, which is characterized by excessive surface scaling [128]. X-linked ichthyosis is thought to be due to steroid sulfatase deficiency [129]. It can be distinguished from the other forms on the basis of eye findings. The X-linked form has discrete opacities in the deep corneal stroma [128]. Regional assignment on the X chromosome has been deduced from linkage to the Xg blood group locus [153].

Males with X-linked ocular albinism demonstrate nystagmus, impaired vision, foveal hypoplasia, iris transillumination, and variable pigmentary dilution in the fundus [110]. They also have some cutaneous involvement in the form of macromelanosomes, as demonstrated by O'Donnell and associates [111]. The female carriers show iris transillumination and patchy fundus pigmentation [50]. These findings are consistent with the Lyon hypothesis, as previously described [90]. Also consistent with the Lyon hypothesis is the fact that one female carrier has been reported with nystagmus [117]. The inactivation of the X chromosome, though random, statistically should lead to individuals at either end of the spectrum with regard to degree of eye involvement.

Juvenile hereditary retinoschisis was first described by Thomson in 1932 [145]. Its major manifestations include a cystic maculopathy with peripheral retinal schisis. Histologically, these correspond to splitting of the nerve fiber layer. Vitreous veils are seen in more severely involved cases. Thomson noted that the disease was seen only in male members of the family he studied [145]. Its X-linked form of inheritance was further clarified by Levy [87]. Since then, its position on the X chromosome has been defined by pedigree analysis, using Xg and the deutan locus as markers [54, 77]. Gieser and Falls saw a macular cyst in a female carrier, which they suggested might be a manifestation of the carrier state [60]. Again, the variability in expressivity in female carriers is consistent with lyonization.

Table 3-6. *Eye Disease Assigned to Chromosome X*

Disease	McKusick catalogue number[*]	Additional feature	Disease	McKusick catalogue number[*]	Additional feature
Adrenoleukodystrophy	30010		Microphthalmos	30980	Or anophthalmia with associated anomalies
Ocular albinism	30050	Nettleship Falls	Mucopolysaccharidosis II	30990	(Hunter's syndrome)
Albinism deafness	30070		Night blindness	31050	Congenital stationary, with myopia
Albright's hereditary osteodystrophy	30080		Norrie's disease	31060	
Alport's syndrome	30105		Nystagmus	31070	(X-linked)
Fabry's disease	30150		Nystagmus, myoclonic	31080	
Cataract	30220	Congenital total	Ophthalmoplegia	31100	
Cataract	30230	Congenital with microcornea	Optic atrophy	31105	
Choroideremia	30310		Optic atrophy	31107	Polyneuropathy and deafness
Choroideremia	30311	With deafness and obesity	Optic atrophy	31110	Spastic paraplegia syndrome
Chorioretinal degeneration	30320		Opticoacoustic nerve atrophy with dementia	31115	(Jensen's syndrome)
Chorioretinal dystrophy	30330		Orofacial-digital syndrome	31120	
Blue cone monochromatism	30370		Pterygium syndrome	31215	(X-linked)
Deutan color blindness	30380		Retinal dysplasia	31255	
Aicardi's syndrome	30405		Retinitis pigmentosa	31260	(X-linked)
Dermoid of the cornea	30473		Retinitis pigmentosa	31265	Plus congenital deafness
Dyskeratosis congenita	30500		Retinoschisis	31270	
Aarskog-Scott syndrome	30540		Spondyloepiphyseal dysplasia	31340	Late
Focal dermal hypoplasia	30560	(Goltz's syndrome)	Spondylometaphyseal dysplasia	31342	X-linked (Richmond type)
Hypertelorism	30710		Telecanthus	31360	With associated abnormalities
Ichthyosis	30810		Van den Bosch's syndrome	31450	
Incontinentia pigmenti	30830		Wildervanck's syndrome	31460	Cervico-oculoacoustic syndrome
Iris hypoplasia	30850	With glaucoma	Zonular cataract and nystagmus	31500	
Leber's optic atrophy	30890				
Lowe's oculocerebrorenal syndrome	30900				
Macular dystrophy	30910				
Megalocornea	30930				
Microphthalmos	30970				

[*]See McKusick [94].

HUNTER'S SYNDROME

Hunter's syndrome or mucopolysaccharidosis II was first described by Hunter in 1917 [75]. Its clinical manifestations include dysostosis with dwarfism; coarse (gargoylelike) facial features; mucopolysaccharide deposits in the intima of the heart (cardiovascular disorder), liver, and spleen (hepatosplenomegaly); urine excretion of chondroitin sulfate B and heparan sulfate; mental retardation; and deafness [96]. There are two types. MPS IIA, the severe form, is associated with profound mental retardation by late childhood. In MPS IIB, the milder form, mentation may be normal [96]. The eye manifestations consist of retinitis pigmentosa–like changes in the fundus. Unlike MPS I (Hurler's syndrome), patients with MPS II have clear corneas [65]. The enzyme defect in Hunter's syndrome is a deficiency of sulfoiduronate sulfatase [8]. Linkage analysis was employed to map MPS II close to the Xm serum system on the X chromosome [16]. Also, a girl with Hunter's syndrome has been described with a translocation whose breakpoint is between Xq26 and Xq27. The severe symptoms in this girl may be explained by nonrandom X inactivation secondary to the translocation [103].

SOMATIC CELL HYBRIDIZATION ASSIGNMENT

Fabry's disease is characterized by acroparesthesias, angiokeratoma, and corneal opacities. The enzyme defect is deficiency of α-galactosidase A (ceramide trihexosidase) [26]. The eye findings include dilated aneurysmal conjunctival vessels, whorled corneal opacities, cataracts, retinal vascular tortuosity [134], and periorbital edema as described by Fabry in his first case [48]. The regional localization of this disease on the X chromosome was deduced by means of somatic cell hybridization [79].

THE MITOCHONDRIAL CHROMOSOME

McKusick states, "Man has 25 chromosomes (not 24)—one in addition to the 22 autosomes and the two sex chromosomes. The 25th is the single circular chromosome resembling that of a bacterium, situated in the mitochondrion" [95]. Indeed, much attention has now been directed toward the circular DNA of the mitochondrion. The entire human mitochondrial genome has been sequenced, all 16,569 base pairs [2]. It has been shown that the human mitochondrial DNA is mater-

nally inherited [61]. That is, the mitochondrial DNA of the offspring is like that of the mother, with very little contribution from the father. This information has been used to provide preliminary information on the inheritance of chronic progressive external ophthalmoplegia (CPEO, Kearns-Sayer, mitochondrial cytopathy) [46]. Egger and Wilson observed that many families with CPEO demonstrate maternal inheritance. They suggest that CPEO is inherited on the mitochondrial genome [46]. If further studies prove this to be the case, then CPEO will be the first human disease to be mapped on the human mitochondrial genome.

CONCLUSIONS

In 1937 the first human chromosomal linkage was described for color blindness and hemophilia. Now that retinoblastoma has been assigned to chromosome 13, the concepts and clinical applications of linkage analysis have again become important to ophthalmologists. There is interest in understanding human genetic mechanisms from a theoretical point of view. In addition, given the rapid advances in gene manipulation, gene assignments may in the future be of major clinical importance. As mentioned previously, recombinant DNA techniques may make it possible for an enzyme-deficient host to produce the deficient enzyme. Eighty-four human ocular diseases have so far been chromosomally mapped, and 488 human systemic diseases or markers have been assigned to specific loci. The total number of well-established human genetic diseases is over 1,700, and an equal number of presumptive genetic diseases have been described. As more and more genetic markers become assigned, further mapping becomes easier, and further progress in the assignment of ophthalmic diseases is likely to occur—with possible benefits in clinical care. The possible use of esterase D for detecting the carrier state in retinoblastoma and recombinant DNA probe L1.28 for detecting the carrier state in X-linked retinitis pigmentosa are examples of mapping information extending clinical care.

REFERENCES

1. Adam, A., et al. Linkage relations of X-borne ichthyosis to the Xg blood groups and to other markers of the X in Israelis. *Ann. Hum. Genet.* 32:323, 1969.
2. Anderson, S., et al. Sequence and organization of

the human mitochondrial genome. *Nature* 290:457, 1981.

3. Arbisser, A. I., et al. Ocular findings in mannosidosis. *Am. J. Ophthalmol.* 82:465, 1976.

4. Arias, S. Genetic heterogeneity of the Waardenburg syndrome. *Birth Defects* 7(4):87, 1971.

5. Arias, S., and Mota, M. Current status of the ABO-Waardenburg syndrome type I linkage. *Cytogenet. Cell Genet.* 22:291, 1978.

6. Arias, S., et al. Probable loose linkage between the ABO locus and Waardenburg syndrome type I. *Humangenetik* 27:145, 1975.

7. Austin, J., et al. Abnormal sulfatase activities in two human diseases (metachromatic leukodystrophy and gargoylism). *Biochem. J.* 93:447, 1964.

8. Bach, G., et al. The defect in the Hunter's syndrome: Deficiency of sulfoiduronate sulfatase. *Proc. Natl. Acad. Sci. U.S.A.* 70:2134, 1973.

9. Barbosa, J., et al. Analysis of linkage between the major histocompatibility system and juvenile insulin-dependent diabetes in multiplex families. *J. Clin. Invest.* 62:492, 1978.

10. Barbosa, J., et al. Genetics of juvenile diabetes. *N. Engl. J. Med.* 298:462, 1978.

11. Barton, R. W., and Neufeld, E. F. A distinct biochemical deficit in the Maroteaux-Lamy syndrome (MPS VI). *J. Pediatr.* 80:114, 1972.

12. Bawle, E., et al. Aarskog syndrome: In full male and female expression associated with an X-autosome translocation. *Am. J. Med. Genet.* 17:595, 1984.

13. Bell, J., and Haldane, J. B. S. The linkage between the genes for colour blindness and haemophilia in man. *Proc R. Soc. Lond. [Biol.]* 123:119, 1937.

14. Benedict, W. F., et al. Patient with 13 chromosome deletion: Evidence that the retinoblastoma gene is a recessive cancer gene. *Science* 219:973, 1983.

15. Benn, P. A., et al. Confirmation of the assignment of the gene for galactose-1-phosphate uridyltransferase (E.C.2.7.7.12) to human chromosome 9. *Cytogenet. Cell Genet.* 24:37, 1979.

16. Berg, K., Danes, B. X., and Bearn, A. G. The linkage relation of the loci for the Sm serum system and the X-linked form of Hurler's syndrome (Hunter's syndrome). *Am. J. Hum. Genet.* 20:398, 1968.

17. Bergsma, D. *Birth Defects Compendium* (2nd ed.). New York: A. R. Liss: 1979. Pp. 450–451.

18. Ibid, pp. 734–735.

19. Ibid, pp. 455–456.

20. Ibid, p. 486.

21. Ibid, pp. 883–885.

22. Bhattacharya, S. S., et al. Close genetic linkage between X-linked retinitis pigmentosa and a restriction fragment length polymorphism identified by recombinant DNA probe L1.28. *Nature* 309:253, 1984.

23. Botstein, D., et al. Construction of a genetic linkage map in man using restriction fragment length polymorphisms. *Am. J. Hum. Genet.* 32:314, 1980.

24. Boyer, S. H., and Graham, J. B. Linkage between the X chromosome loci for glucose 6-phosphate dehydrogenase electrophoretic variation and hemophilia A. *Am. J. Hum. Genet.* 17:320, 1965.

25. Boyer, S. H., Porter, I. H., and Weilbaecher, R. G. Electrophoretic heterogeneity of glucose-6-phosphate dehydrogenase and its relationship to enzyme deficiency in man. *Proc. Natl. Acad. Sci. U.S.A.* 48:1868, 1962.

26. Brady, R. O., et al. Enzymatic defect in Fabry's disease. *N. Engl. J. Med.* 276:1163, 1967.

27. Broughton, W. L., Rosenbaum, K. N., and Beauchamp, G. R. Congenital glaucoma and other ocular abnormalities associated with pericentric inversion of chromosome 11. *Arch. Ophthalmol.* 101:594, 1983.

28. Bruns, G. A. P., et al. Expression of ACONS and GALT in man-rodent somatic cell hybrids. *Birth Defects* 14(4):172, 1978.

29. Bruns, G. A. P., et al. Expression of human arylsulfatase-A in man-hamster somatic cell hybrids. *Hum. Gene Mapping* 4:182, 1977.

30. Burian, H. M., and Burns, C. A. Ocular changes in myotonic dystrophy. *Am. J. Ophthalmol.* 63:22, 1967.

31. Carritt, B., and Goldfarb, P. A human chromosomal determinant for susceptibility to herpes simplex virus. *Nature* 264:556, 1976.

32. Carroll, M., et al. Human mannosidosis: The enzyme defect. *Biochem. Biophys. Res. Commun.* 49:579, 1972.

33. Cavalli-Sforza, L. L., and Bodmer, W. F. *The Genetics of Human Populations.* San Francisco: Freeman, 1971. Pp. 873–878.

34. Cavenee, W. K., et al. Expression of recessive alleles by chromosomal mechanisms in retinoblastoma. *Nature* 305:799, 1983.

35. Champion, M. J., and Shows, T. B. Mannosidosis: Assignment of the lysosomal alpha-mannosidase B gene to chromosome 19 in man. *Proc. Natl. Acad. Sci. U.S.A.* 74:2968, 1977.

36. Church, R. L., Nirmala, S., and Rohrbach, D. H. Gene mapping of human ocular connective tissue proteins. *Invest. Ophthalmol. Vis. Sci.* 21:73, 1981.

37. Cogan, D. G., Kuwabara, T., and Moser, H. Metachromatic leucodystrophy. *Ophthalmologica* 160:2, 1970.

38. Cross, H. E., et al. Retinoblastoma in patient with a 13qXp translocation. *Am. J. Ophthalmol.* 84:548, 1977.

39. Crow, J. F. Mutation in man. *Prog. Med. Genet.* 1:1, 1961.

40. Desnick, R. J., et al. Mannosidosis: Clinical, morphologic, immunologic and biochemical studies. *Pediatr. Res.* 10:985, 1976.

41. Digeorge, A. M., and Harley, R. D. The association of aniridia, Wilms' tumor, and genital abnormalities. *Arch. Ophthalmol.* 75:796, 1966.

42. Donahue, R. P., et al. Probable assignment of the

Duffy blood group locus to chromosome 1 in man. *Proc. Natl. Acad. Sci. U.S.A.* 61:949, 1968.

43. Dryja, T. P., et al. Homozygosity of chromosome 13 in retinoblastoma. *N. Engl. J. Med.* 310:550, 1984.

44. Durand, P., Borrone, C., and Della Cella, G. Fucosidosis. *J. Pediatr.* 75:665, 1969.

45. Durand, P., et al. A new glycolipid storage disease. *Pediatr. Res.* 1:416, 1967.

46. Egger, J., and Wilson, J. Mitochondrial inheritance in a mitochondrially mediated disease. *N. Engl. J. Med.* 309:142, 1983.

47. Elsevier, S. M., et al. Assignment of the gene for galactokinase to human chromosome 17 and its regional localization to band q21–22. *Nature* 251:633, 1974.

48. Fabry, J. Ein Beitrag zur Kenntniss der Purpura haemorrhagica nodularis. *Arch. Dermatol. Syph.* 43:187, 1898.

49. Falk, C. T., Fotino, M., and Haymovits, A. Likely linkage of Paget's disease of bone and HLA. *Hum. Gene Mapping* 5:152, 1979.

50. Falls, H. F. Sex-linked ocular albinism displaying typical fundus changes in the female heterozygote. *Am. J. Ophthalmol.* 34(Suppl. 2):41, 1951.

51. Ferguson-Smith, M. A., and Westerveld, A. Report of the committee on the genetic constitution of chromosomes 13, 14, 15, 16, 17, 18, 19, 20, 21, and 22. *Cytogenet. Cell Genet.* 25:59, 1979.

52. Ferrell, R. E., et al. Autosomal dominant aniridia: Probable linkage to acid phosphatase-1 locus on chromosome 2. *Proc. Natl. Acad. Sci. U.S.A.* 77:1580, 1980.

53. Ferrell, R. E., et al. Anterior segment mesodermal dysgenesis: Probable linkage to the MNS blood group on chromosome 4. *Am. J. Hum. Genet.* 34:245, 1982.

54. Forsius, H., et al. A genetic study of three rare retinal disorders: Dystrophia retinal dysacusis syndrome, X-chromosomal retinoschisis, and grouped pigments of the retina. *Birth Defects* 7(3):83, 1971.

55. Fotino, M., Haymovits, A., and Falk, C. T. Evidence for linkage between HLA and Paget's disease. *Transplant. Proc.* 9:1867, 1977.

56. Francke, U., and Francke, B. R. Assignment of genes required for herpes simplex virus type I (HSVI) replication to the long arm of human chromosome 11. *Hum. Gene Mapping* 5:155, 1979.

57. Gallie, B. L. Gene carrier detection in retinoblastoma. *Ophthalmology (Rochester)* 87:591, 1980.

58. George, D. L., and Francke, U. Regional mapping of human genes for hexosaminidase B and diphtheria toxin sensitivity on chromosome 5 using mouse × human hybrid cells. *Somatic Cell Genet.* 3:629, 1977.

59. Gey, W. Dq−, multiple missbildungen and retinoblastoma. *Humangenetik* 10:362, 1970.

60. Gieser, E. P., and Falls, H. F. Hereditary retinoschisis. *Am. J. Ophthalmol.* 51:1193, 1961.

61. Giles, R. E., et al. Maternal inheritance of human mitochondrial DNA. *Proc. Natl. Acad. Sci. U.S.A.* 77:6715, 1980.

62. Gitzelmann, R. Deficiency of erythrocyte galactokinase in a patient with galactose diabetes. *Lancet* 2:670, 1965.

63. Gitzelmann, R. Hereditary galactokinase deficiency, a newly recognized cause of juvenile cataracts. *Pediatr. Res.* 1:14, 1967.

64. Godbout, R., et al. Somatic inactivation of genes on chromosome 13 is a common event in retinoblastoma. *Nature* 304:451, 1983.

65. Goldberg, M. F., and Duke, J. R. Ocular histopathology in Hunter's syndrome. *Arch. Ophthalmol.* 77:503, 1967.

66. Goss, S. J., and Harris, H. Gene transfer by means of cell infusion: II. The mapping of 8 loci on human chromosome 1 by statistical analysis of gene assortment in somatic cell hybrids. *J. Cell Sci.* 25:39, 1977.

67. Grace, E., et al. The 13q− deletion syndrome. *J. Med. Genet.* 8:351, 1971.

68. Greenfield, J. G. A form of progressive cerebral sclerosis in infants associated with primary degeneration of the interfascicular glia. *Proc. R. Soc. Med.* 26:690, 1933.

69. Grobstein, C. The recombination DNA debate. In *Sci Am Genet: 20th ed*, 122–130, 1981.

70. Harper, P. S., et al. Genetic linkage confirmed between the locus for myotonic dystrophy and the ABH secretion and Lutheran blood group loci. *Am. J. Hum. Genet.* 24:310, 1972.

71. Heckenlively, J., et al. Possible assignment of a dominant retinitis pigmentosa with (R.P.) gene to chromosome 1. *Ophthalmol. Res.* 14:46, 1982.

72. Hellkhul, B., and Grzeschik, K. H. Assignment of a gene for arylsulfatase-B to human chromosome 5 using human mouse somatic cell hybrids. *Hum. Gene Mapping* 4:203, 1977.

73. Hittner, H. M., et al. Autosomal dominant anterior segment dysgenesis with variable expressivity: Probable linkage to MNS blood group on chromosome 4. *Pediatr. Res.* 15:56, 1981.

74. Hittner, et al. Oculocutaneous albinoidism as a manifestation of reduced neural crest derivatives in the Prader-Willi syndrome. *Am. J. Ophthalmol.* 94:328, 1982.

75. Hunter, C. A rare disease in two brothers. *Proc. R. Soc. Med.* 10:104, 1917.

76. Ichikawa, K., et al. Coincidence of neurofibromatosis and myotonic dystrophy in a kindred. *J. Med. Genet.* 18:134, 1981.

77. Ives, E. J., Ewing, C. C., and Innes, R. X-linked juvenile retinoschisis and Xg linkage in five families. *Am. J. Hum. Genet.* 22:17A, 1970.

78. Jay, M. *The Eye in Chromosome Duplications and Deficiencies.* New York: Dekker, 1977. Pp. 139, 213.

79. Johnston, A. W., et al. Linkage relationships of the

angiokeratoma (Fabry) locus. *Am. J. Hum. Genet.* 32:369, 1969.

80. Kalckar, H. M., Anderson, E. P., and Isselbacher, K. J. Galactosemia, a congenital defect in nucleotide transferase. *Biochim. Biophys. Acta* 20:262, 1956.

81. Kivlin, J. D., et al. Linkage analysis in dominant optic atrophy. *Am. J. Hum. Genet.* 35:1190, 1983.

82. Knowles, B. B., et al. Complement-mediated antiserum cytotoxic reactions to human chromosome 7 coded antigens: Immunoselection of rearranged human chromosome 7 in human-mouse somatic cell hybrids. *J. Exp. Med.* 145:314, 1977.

83. Lally, P. A., Rattazzi, M. C., and Shows, T. B. Human β-D-N-acetylhexosaminidases A and B: Expression and linkage relationships in somatic cell hybrids. *Proc. Natl. Acad. Sci. U.S.A.* 71:1569, 1974.

84. Ledbetter, D. H., et al. Chromosome 15 abnormalities and the Prader-Willi syndrome: A follow-up report of 40 cases. *Am. J. Hum. Genet.* 34:278, 1982.

85. Lee, J. B., and Benedict, W. L. Hereditary nuclear cataract. *Arch. Ophthalmol.* 44:643, 1950.

86. Lele, K. P., Penrose, L. S., and Stallard, H. B. Chromosome deletion in a case of retinoblastoma. *Ann. Hum. Genet.* 27:171, 1963.

87. Levy, J. Inherited retinal detachment. *Br. J. Ophthalmol.* 36:626, 1952.

88. Levy, N. S., Krill, A. E., and Beutler, E. Galactokinase deficiency and cataracts. *Am. J. Ophthalmol.* 74:41, 1972.

89. Ligutič, I., et al. Interstitial deletion of 4 q and Reiger syndrome. *Clin. Genet.* 20:323, 1981.

90. Lyon, M. R. Sex chromatin and gene action in the mammalian X chromosome. *Am. J. Hum. Genet.* 14:135, 1962.

91. Maroteaux, P., and Lamy, M. Hurler's disease, Morquio's disease and related mucopolysaccharidoses. *J. Pediatr.* 67:312, 1965.

92. Maumenee, I. H. Classification of hereditary cataracts in children by linkage analysis. *Ophthalmology (Rochester)* 86:1554, 1979.

93. McKusick, V. A. The human gene map. Personal communication, 7/15/81. P. 19.

94. McKusick, V. A. *Mendelian Inheritance in Man* (6th ed.). Baltimore: Johns Hopkins Press, 1983.

95. McKusick, V. A. The human genome through the eyes of a clinical geneticist. *Cytogenet. Cell Genet.* 32:7, 1982.

96. McKusick, V. A. *Heritable Disorders of Connective Tissue* (4th ed.). St. Louis: Mosby, 1972.

97. Miller, R. W., Fraumeni, J. F., Jr., and Manning, M. D. Association of Wilms' tumor with aniridia, hemihypertrophy, and other congenital malformations. *N. Engl. J. Med.* 270:922, 1964.

98. Mitchell, M. M., et al. Mannosidosis: Two brothers with different degrees of disease severity. *Clin. Genet.* 20:191, 1981.

99. Mohandas, T., et al. Assignment of GALT to chromosome 9 and regional localization of GALT, AK_1, AK_3, and ACONS on chromosome 9. *Birth Defects* 14(4):456, 1978.

100. Mohr, J. *A study of linkage in man (Opera ex Domo Biologie Hereditariae Humanae Universitatis Hafniensis 33).* Copenhagen: Munksgaard, 1954.

101. Morton, N. E. Segregation and Linkage. In W. J. Burdette (Ed.), *Methodology in Human Genetics.* San Francisco: Holden Day, 1962. Pp. 17–52.

102. Moser, H. W., et al. Adrenoleukodystrophy: Studies of the phenotype, genetics and biochemistry. *Genet. Clin. Johns Hopkins Hosp.* 147:217, 1980.

103. Mossman, J., et al. Hunter's disease in a girl: Association with X : 5 chromosomal translocation disrupting the Hunter gene. *Arch. Dis. Child.* 58:911, 1983.

104. Murphree, A. L., and Benedict, W. F. Retinoblastoma: Clues to human oncogenesis. *Science* 223:1028, 1984.

105. Nathans, D., and Smith, H. Restriction endonucleases in the analysis and restructuring of DNA molecules. *Annu. Rev. Biochem.* 44:273, 1975.

106. Nettleship, E., and Ogilvie, F. M. A peculiar form of hereditary congenital cataract. *Trans. Ophthalmol. Soc. U.K.* 26:191, 1906.

107. Nichols, W. W., et al. Further observations on a 13q Xp translocation associated with retinoblastoma. *Am. J. Ophthalmol.* 89:621, 1980.

108. O'Brien, J. S. GM$_1$ Gangliosidoses. In J. B. Stanbury, J. B. Wijngaarden, and D. S. Fredrickson (Eds.), *The Metabolic Basis of Inherited Disease.* New York: McGraw-Hill, 1972. Pp. 639–662.

109. Ockerman, P. A. A generalized storage disease resembling Hurler syndrome. *Lancet* 2:239, 1967.

110. O'Donnell, F. E., Jr., and Green, W. R. The Eye in Albinism. In T. E. Duane (Ed.), *Clinical Ophthalmology 4.* Hagerstown, Md.: Harper & Row, 1979. Chap. 38.

111. O'Donnell, F. E., Jr., et al. X-linked ocular albinism: An oculocutaneous macromelanosomal disorder. *Arch. Ophthalmol.* 94:1883, 1976.

112. O'Donnell, F. E., Jr., et al. Forsius-Eriksson syndrome: Its relation to the Nettleship-Falls X-linked ocular albinism. *Clin. Genet.* 17:403, 1980.

113. Okada, S., and O'Brien, J. S. Generalized gangliosidosis: Beta-galactosidase deficiency. *Science* 160:1002, 1968.

114. Okada, S., and O'Brien, J. S. Tay-Sachs disease: Generalized absence of a beta-D-N-acetylhexosaminidase component. *Science* 165:698, 1969.

115. Orkwiszewski, K. G., Tedesco, T. A., and Croce, C. M. Assignment of the human gene for galactokinase to chromosome 17. *Nature* 252:60, 1974.

116. Orye, E., Delbeke, M. J., and Vendenabeele, B. Retinoblastoma and D-chromosome deletions. *Lancet* 2:1376, 1971.

116A. Paris Conference, 1971. *Birth Defects* 3(7), 1972.

117. Pearce, W. G., Johnson, G. J., and Gillian, J. G.

Nystagmus in a female carrier of ocular albinism. *J. Med. Genet.* 9:126, 1972.

118. Plowman, G. D., et al. Assignment of the gene for human melanoma-associated antigen p 97 to chromosome 3. *Nature* 303:70, 1983.

119. Porter, I. H., Schultze, J., and McKusick, V. A. Genetical linkage between the loci for glucose-6-phosphate dehydrogenase deficiency and colour blindness in American Negroes. *Ann. Hum. Genet.* 26:107, 1967.

120. Renwick, J. H. Progress in mapping human chromosomes. *Br. Med. Bull.* 25:65, 1969.

121. Renwick, J. H., and Lawler, S. D. Probable linkage between a congenital cataract locus and the Duffy blood group locus. *Ann. Hum. Genet.* 27:67, 1963.

122. Renwick, J. H., and Bolling, D. R. An analysis procedure: Illustrated in a triple linkage of use for prenatal diagnosis of myotonic dystrophy. *J. Med. Genet.* 8:399, 1971.

123. Renwick, J. H., et al. Confirmation of linkage of the loci for myotonic dystrophy and ABH-secretion. *J. Med. Genet.* 8:407, 1971.

124. Riccardi, V. M., et al. Chromosomal imbalance in the aniridia–Wilm's tumor association: 11p interstitial deletion. *Pediatrics* 61:604, 1978.

125. Ruddle, F. H., and Kucherlapati, R. S. Hybrid cells and human genes. *Sci. Am. Genet.* (20th ed). Pp. 122–130, 1981.

126. Sandhoff, K., et al. Enzyme alterations and lipid storage in three variants of Tay-Sachs disease. *J. Neurochem.* 18:2469, 1971.

127. Schinzel, A., et al. The "cat-eye syndrome": Dicentric small marker chromosome probably derived from a no. 22 tetrasomy (22 pter q11) associated with a characteristic phenotype. *Hum. Genet.* 57:148, 1981.

128. Sever, R. J., Frost, P., and Weinstein, G. Eye changes in ichthyosis. *JAMA* 206:2283, 1968.

129. Shapiro, L. J., et al. X-linked ichthyosis due to steroid-sulphatase deficiency. *Lancet* 1:70, 1978.

130. Shows, T. B., et al. GM$_1$ gangliosidosis: Chromosome 3 assignment of the beta-galactosidase-A gene (beta GALA). *Somatic Cell Genet.* 5:147, 1979.

131. Sly, W. S., et al. Beta-glucuronidase deficiency: Report of clinical, radiologic, and biochemical features of a new mucopolysaccharidosis. *J. Pediatr.* 82:249, 1973.

132. Snyder, R. D., et al. Ocular findings in fucosidosis. *Birth Defects* 12(3):241, 1976.

133. Southern, E. M. Detection of specific sequences among DNA fragments separated by gel electrophoresis. *J. Mol. Biol.* 98:503, 1975.

134. Spaeth, G. L., and Frost, P. Fabry's disease: Its ocular manifestations. *Arch. Ophthalmol.* 74:760, 1965.

135. Sparkes, R. S., et al. Regional assignment of genes for human esterase D and retinoblastoma to chromosome band 13q 14. *Science* 208:1042, 1980.

136. Sparkes, R. S., et al. Gene for hereditary retinoblastoma assigned to human chromosome 13 by linkage to esterase D. *Science* 219:971, 1983.

137. Spence, M. A., et al. Linkage analysis of neurofibromatosis (von Recklinghausen disease). *J. Med. Genet.* 20:334, 1983.

138. Spira, T. J., Adam, A., and Goodman, R. M. Recombination between cerebral sclerosis–Addison's disease and the Xg blood groups. *Lancet* 2:820, 1971.

139. Stumpf, D., and Austin, J. Metachromatic leukodystrophy (MLD): IX. Qualitative and quantitative differences in urinary arylsulfatase A in different forms of MLD. *Arch. Neurol.* 24:117, 1971.

140. Taylor, A. I. Dq−, Dr and retinoblastoma. *Humangenetik* 10:209, 1970.

141. Terrell, R. E., Hittner, H. M., and Antoszyk, J. H. Linkage of atypical vitelliform macular dystrophy (VMD-1) to the soluble glutamate pyruvate transaminase (GPT1) locus. *Am. J. Genet.* 35:78, 1983.

142. Thompson, H., and Lyons, R. B. Retinoblastoma and multiple congenital anomalies, associated with complex mosaicism with deletion of D-chromosome and probable DC translocation. *Hum. Chromosome Newsletter* 15:21, 1965.

143. Thompson, H. S., van Allen, M. W., and von Noorden, G. K. The pupil in myotonic dystrophy. *Invest. Ophthalmol.* 3:325, 1964.

144. Thompson, J. S., and Thompson, M. W. *Genetics in Medicine* (3rd ed.). Philadelphia: Saunders, 1980.

145. Thomson, E. Memorandum regarding family in which neuroretinal disease of unusual kind occurred only in the males. *Br. J. Ophthalmol.* 16:681, 1932.

146. Van Heyningen, V., et al. Chromosome assignment of some human enzyme loci: Mitochondrial malate dehydrogenase to 7, mannosiphosphate isomerase and pyruvate kinase to 15 and probably, esterase D to 13. *Ann. Hum. Genet.* 38:295, 1975.

147. Van Hoof, F., and Hers, H. G. Mucopolysaccharidosis by absence of alpha-fucosidase. *Lancet* 1:1198, 1968.

148. Van Kempen, C. A case of retinoblastoma, combined with severe mental retardation and a few other congenital anomalies, associated with complex aberrations of the karyotype. *Maandschr. Kindergeneesk* 34:92,1966.

149. Waardenburg, P. J. A new syndrome combining developmental anomalies of the eyelids, eyebrows, and nose root, with pigmentary defects of the iris and head hair and with congenital deafness. *Am. J. Hum. Genet.* 3:195, 1951.

150. Waardenburg, P. J., Franceschetti, A., and Klein, D. *Genetics and Ophthalmology.* Assen, Netherlands: Royal Van Gorcum, 1963, Vol. 1. P. 361.

151. Waardenburg, P. J. Some notes on publications of Professor Arnold Sorsby and on Aland eye disease (Forsius-Eriksson syndrome). *J. Med. Genet.* 7:194, 1970.

152. Walbaum, R., et al. Un cas de retinoblastome bilateral avec monosomie 13 partielle (q12 q14). *Hum. Genet.* 44:219, 1978. (Engl. abstract.).

153. Went, L. N., et al. X-linked ichthyosis: Linkage relationship with the Xg blood groups and other studies in a large Dutch kindred. *Ann. Hum. Genet.* 32:333, 1969.

154. Westerveld, A., Beyersbergen van Henegouwen, H. M. A., and van Someren H. Evidence for synteny between human loci for galactose-1-phosphate uridyl transferase and aconitase in man–Chinese hamster somatic cell hybrids. *Birth Defects* 11(3):283, 1975.

155. Wilson, M. G., Towner, J. W., and Fujimoto, A. Retinoblastoma and D-chromosome deletions. *Am. J. Hum. Genet.* 25:57, 1973.

156. Wray, S. H., et al. Adrenoleukodystrophy with disease of the eye and optic nerve. *Am. J. Ophthalmol.* 82:480, 1976.

157. Yunis, J. J., and Ramsay, N. Retinoblastoma and subband deletion of chromosome 13. *Am. J. Dis. Child.* 132:161, 1978.

4

Recombinant DNA Technology: Applications to Ophthalmology

George H. Sack, Jr.

Many biologic systems can now be studied in molecular detail, which yields unprecedented information regarding structure, control, genetics, development, and pathophysiology. The rapidly emerging techniques will ultimately be applicable to a wide range of basic and clinical questions in ophthalmology. The purpose of this chapter is to provide an introduction to molecular genetics, to provide references to established applications in eye physiology, and to indicate areas for future thought and experimentation. Basic references are also included.

EUKARYOTIC GENE STRUCTURE

Determination of the organization of human (and other eukaryotic) genes has provided a broad view of their chromosomal organization. Fig. 4-1 shows a hypothetical human chromosomal gene and its relation to the messenger RNA (mRNA) molecule that will serve to direct protein synthesis. There are several conspicuous features. First, the chromosomal region encompassing the transcription unit is much larger than the length of coding information in the mRNA used for protein synthesis. Moreover, the mRNA is not the first transcription product. The initial product of RNA transcription (the *primary transcript*, which is made in the cell nucleus), is an RNA homolog of the bases in the entire length of DNA in the gene region.

As shown, the primary transcript is a faithful copy of the gene region but is much longer than

The author wishes to acknowledge the support of the Kroc, Garrett, and Kennedy Foundations during preparation of this work.

the mRNA. This primary transcript undergoes a series of reactions that remove entire regions of the RNA; this is the process of *splicing.* Nucleotides removed from the RNA will, obviously, not become part of the coding information used to make the protein product. As the figure indicates, delineation of coding and noncoding regions of genes permits division of the original length of nuclear DNA into *exons*—regions of coding and control information—and *introns*—regions separating exons (also called *intervening sequences*). The mRNA will thus have lost many (perhaps thousands) of the bases in the homologous nuclear DNA region.

Splicing is only one of the events that occur in the cell nucleus before RNA maturation. A second conspicuous feature is the set of reactions (which may occur concurrent with splicing) that modify ends of the RNA. As shown in Fig. 4-1, these reactions add modified nucleotide(s) to form a "cap" structure at the 5' end of the strand. This cap aids recognition of the 5' end of the mRNA and also may prolong its survival. The 3' end also is modified by the addition of a stretch of adenylates to form the *3' poly A tail*. This may lengthen the RNA by several hundred nucleotides and often proves useful in gene isolation strategies, as will be discussed below. After splicing and terminal modifications, the mature mRNA is ready to enter the cytoplasm and direct the synthesis of proteins by aligning the appropriate amino acid transfer RNAs on the ribosome for polymerization. Ultimately, the mRNA will be degraded in the cytoplasm and must be resynthesized in the nucleus if synthesis of the specific protein is to continue. Control of mRNA production and degradation permits regulation of protein synthesis.

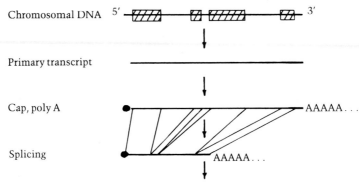

Fig. 4-1. *Outline of relationship between chromosomal DNA (top) and cytoplasmic messenger RNA (mRNA) (bottom). Exons (hatched boxes) are destined to be part of the mRNA sequence. Introns (regions between exons) are ultimately removed by splicing as shown. Addition of the "cap" of modified nucleotides at the 5' end and polyadenylate (poly A) to the 3' end helps define the mRNA precursor. Note that the mRNA (exclusive of the 3' poly A) is considerably shorter than the corresponding nuclear gene.*

The third conspicuous feature of chromosomes, implied by the steps in mRNA production previously outlined, is that each is a complex set of specific regions. Even genes themselves are now envisaged as a mosaic of coding (exon) and noncoding (intron) sequences as well as signals for control of specific protein synthesis under changing developmental or physiologic requirements. In addition, various groups of genes are sometimes organized in so-called *gene families*. Best studied for the globin genes [7], a family may span many thousands of bases (the term *kilobase*, which means 1000 bases and is abbreviated *kb*, thus becomes convenient). Members of a family generally share structural and functional features but also may show divergence for specific applications (for example, the crystallin family of proteins in the lens); presumably they are evolutionarily related.

Not all chromosomal DNA encodes proteins. In addition to introns, there are nucleotide sequences that probably contribute to chromosomal structure. Frequently these are regions of repetition of short sequences called *reiterated DNA*. While some are concentrated in physically distinct regions such as the centromere, others can be found throughout the chromosomes. Details of chromosomal structure including the precise form of DNA packing and interaction with nuclear proteins are not fully established.

BASIC TECHNIQUES

Most genetic manipulations are based on several features of bacterial physiology. Bacteria grow rapidly (dividing as frequently as every 20 minutes), and large numbers can be obtained with relative ease. Foreign DNA can be introduced into

bacteria in several forms. As shown in Fig. 4-2, when bacterial viruses (or bacteriophages) infect cells they introduce their genetic material. Such phages as lambda are well studied, and appropriate alterations (particularly deletion mutants) accomodate foreign DNA (see page 105 and 106). Plasmids (also known as episomes or resistance transfer factors) are independently replicating circular DNA molecules of varying length that originally were selected as carriers of antibiotic resistance genes. It is now possible to exploit the

Fig. 4-2. *Basic features of bacteriophage and plasmid growth. Both processes amplify (increase the number of copies of) the original genome, but the new copies of the phage DNA ae released as progeny phage, while those of a plasmid are transferred to the cell's descendants. Appropriate insertions of additional DNA do not change the basic features of these processes.*

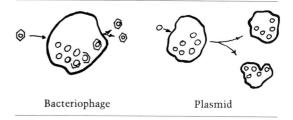

Bacteriophage   Plasmid

independent replication ability of plasmids together with their antibiotic resistance markers to
produce selectable recombinant molecules that
can multiply to very high numbers (thousands) in
a single bacterial cell. Such plasmids can then
amplify DNA molecules of interest that, under
appropriate circumstances, can direct the cell to
synthesize a desired protein or that can themselves be objects of further study—for example,
sequence analysis (see below).

Recombinant DNA techniques involve several
basic enzymatic tools. The first group are the *restriction enzymes*, bacterial proteins whose name
was derived from their physiologic function—
protecting their host organism from exogenous
DNA. These proteins have the common feature
of producing a double-stranded DNA break at a
specific base sequence (or, occasionally, sequences). As shown in Fig. 4-3, this cleavage leads
to a collection of DNA fragments with specific
ends. Much recombinant DNA technology is based
on isolating specific DNA fragments, and many
restriction enzymes are commercially available,
permitting cleavage of DNA at hundreds of specific sites. An important characteristic of a given
DNA molecule is the location of restriction enzyme cleavage sites along it—this is known as a
restriction map [6]. Disclosed by separation techniques such as gel electrophoresis, the size of fragments from DNA cleavage can serve as a rough
basis for comparison of various DNAs.

Other bacterial enzymes also are useful in DNA
studies. DNA ligase forms the phosphodiester
bonds between adjacent DNA bases and can thus
regenerate an intact DNA strand from individual
fragments (Fig. 4-4). Also, a variety of DNA
polymerases can be used to synthesize new DNA.
Generally, these work by using the complementary strand as a *template*, as shown.

The ultimate level of genetic reduction is the
actual sequence of DNA bases. Several methods
now exist for *DNA sequencing*, and these can
yield the sequence of several hundred contiguous
bases at a time. When such data are combined
with computer analysis, one obtains long lengths
of sequence information. Such data permit detection of important structural, coding, splicing, and
control information; sequences also serve as the
ideal basis for comparison of different genes and
for in vitro construction of special recombinants.

Structures of control regions of some eukaryotic genes are known, and gene expression can
be detected in vitro. These methods permit delineation of precise transcription regions, termi-

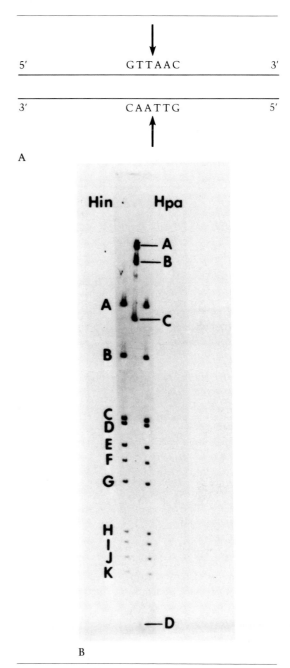

Fig. 4-3. *A. The hexanucleotide DNA recognition
sequence of restriction endonuclease Hpa I. Note the
symmetry of the base sequence on opposite DNA
strands. Cleavage occurs at arrows, leaving "blunt-
ended" fragments [15]. B. Autoradiogram of ^{32}P-
labeled simian virus 40 (SV40) viral DNA after
cleavage by restriction endonucleases Hin dII/dIII or
Hpa I/II and separation by slab gel electrophoresis.
Large fragments are at the top of the figure; smaller
fragments migrate toward the bottom [6].*

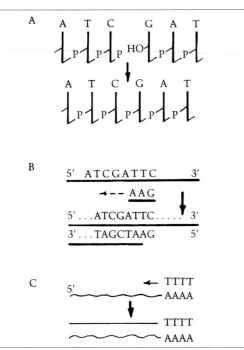

Fig. 4-4. *Important enzyme reactions in recombinant DNA technology. A. DNA ligase creates a phosphodiester bond and connects two DNA strands. B. DNA polymerase synthesizes a DNA strand complementary to a template strand beginning at a short complementary primer. C.* Reverse transcriptase *(RNA-directed DNA polymerase) synthesizes a single DNA strand complementary to an RNA template. Here the template is mRNA and an oligo thymidine primer is used to hybridize with the 3' poly A; the product is cDNA (complementary DNA).*

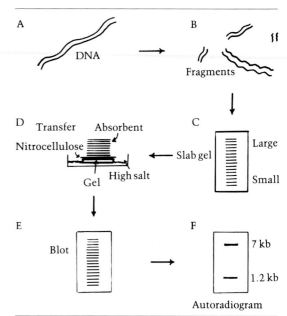

Fig. 4-5. *Basic features of DNA fragment "blotting" [17] and hybridization. High molecular weight DNA (A) is cleaved into fragments by restriction endonuclease digestion (B). The fragments are separated by slab gel electrophoresis (C) on the basis of length. The transfer (D) mobilizes the DNA of the separated fragments (which is separated into single strands by denaturation within the gel slab) by eluting it from the gel in a high-salt solution and into a sheet of nitrocellulose. After the transfer, the nitrocellulose sheet is baked to attach the DNA strands tightly (E). The blot represents a direct transfer of the fragments as originally separated by electrophoresis. Radioactive probe DNA fragments can then attach to homologous DNA sequences within the blot; these will appear as discrete bands on the autoradiogram (F), where their position reflects their length (in kilobases, or kb).*

nation sites, and control signals—regions of genes (generally to the 5' side of coding information) that are important for hormone responsiveness or that control and coordinate differential gene expression.

Complementarity between DNA strands is the basis for many study techniques. Isolated single strands of DNA will rejoin (or *reanneal*) with complete or relative fidelity depending on the environmental conditions chosen, the length of the strands, and the match between the sequences on each strand. One of the most useful applications of this principle is detection of specific DNA sequences by using the so-called Southern blotting technique [17]. As shown in Fig. 4-5, double-stranded DNA fragments are separated on the basis of length by gel electrophoresis, denatured into single strands, and transferred to a binding and support sheet of nitrocellulose. Another DNA sequence (the *probe*, labeled in vitro with either a radioisotope or a dye tag) can then be tested for complementarity to the immobilized fragments. If there is specific base match (the specificity, or homology, again depending on the reaction conditions chosen), a discrete signal will be seen, corresponding to the size of the hybridizing fragment in the original mixture. As indicated in Fig. 4-5, this approach permits detection of changes as small as a single base if the appropriate test sequence and reaction conditions are available. Current diagnostic DNA methods make extensive use of this approach, and applications will be discussed later in this chapter.

GENE ISOLATION STRATEGIES

Unique Overproduction of a Single or Limited Species

One approach to gene isolation is based on enrichment of the mRNA molecules that code for a specific product. Either by demonstration of overproduction (such as on an electrophoretic gel) or by removal of contaminating mRNAs, the mRNA is purified. This process is based on several features. First, many (thousands of) different proteins are generally produced by a given cell. Many of these may serve "housekeeping" functions and may be common to most cells of the organism. By hybridizing mRNAs (or recombi-

Fig. 4-6. *Cloning strategy beginning with a specific mRNA molecule. Reverse transcriptase (A), beginning with oligo dT primer, produces single-stranded cDNA. The mRNA is removed (B), and the cDNA is made double stranded using a DNA polymerase derivative and a nuclease to remove the "hairpin turn" at the end (C). Oligonucleotide "linkers" (D) containing restriction enzyme sites (the sites of Eco RI are shown) are attached to the ends of the duplex cDNA. The fragment is then attached to complementary sites and ligated into a suitable cloning vector DNA molecule—usually with antibiotic resistance for a marker (E). The resulting recombinant molecule (F) is introduced into a bacterial host cell for amplification (G). Maniatis et al. See [10].*

nant DNA molecules containing the same sequences—so-called complementary DNAs, or cDNAs, made using the enzyme *reverse transcriptase* and the mRNA template) from a specialized cell against a group of sequences expressed in most cells (for example, in lens cells versus fibroblasts), one can find a population of mRNAs enriched for products unique to or overproduced by the specialized cell. This smaller population of RNAs (or their cDNA complements) can then be separated and characterized individually, since considerable purification has been achieved.

For instance, one may translate various species in the enriched mixture and analyze the protein products. If an antibody is available against a specific protein, it should react with the product of a specific clone. Alternatively, enzyme activity, an unusual amino acid composition, or some other distinguishing feature could be used for identification. As shown in Fig. 4-6, the cDNA, inserted into a plasmid or phage vector (thereby having been cloned), can be propagated independently in bacteria for further characterization such as sequencing or for possible use as a gene probe.

Several examples of this approach have already been useful in ophthalmology. Lens cells are enriched for mRNAs for crystallins, which reflect the significant proportion of crystallins among lens proteins. This enrichment permitted the isolation

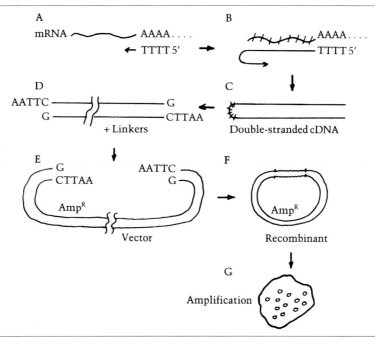

of crystallin mRNAs and led to the discovery of an entire family of crystallin-related genes in several species [2, 3].

A second example involves the acute-phase reactant amyloid A. When mice are presented with an acute-phase stimulus (such as intraperitoneal endotoxin), they respond with hepatic synthesis of large quantities of amyloid A and other acute-phase proteins. This enrichment led to clones of mouse amyloid A genes [12]. To obtain the human amyloid A genes, it was possible to use hybridization methods based on the known amino acid homology between mouse and human amyloid A proteins (which must reflect underlying coding sequence similarity). As shown in Fig. 4-7, it was possible to use a cloned mouse amyloid gene to search for homologous human DNA sequences. A "DNA library" was used which contained recombinant lambda bacteriophages each of which contained a specific human genome fragment [9]. When 10^5 of these recombinants were studied, every sequence of the human genome had been examined at least once. By adjustment of hybridization conditions, it was possible to isolate human counterparts to the mouse amyloid A genes [16]. These fragments provide reagents for the study of amyloid A fibrillar aggregation in the cornea in lattice corneal dystrophy.

Fig. 4-7. *Detection of appropriate recombinant bacteriophage in a "library" by colony hybridization [1]. Individual bacteriophage members of the library contain separate fragments of the entire DNA of interest. All phage are grown on a bacterial culture plate, and their DNA is transferred to a nitrocellulose sheet. Cloned probe DNA sequences are then used to find homologous sequences on the filter. The autoradiogram permits localization of the appropriate library bacteriophage, which can then be purified and amplified.*

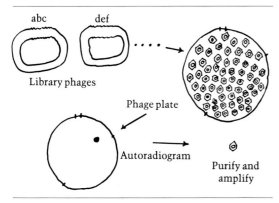

Known Protein with At Least Partial Amino Acid Sequence Determined

This approach is based on the known triplet sequences of all transfer RNA (tRNA) codons. While many amino acids have more than a single codon and corresponding tRNA (degeneracy of the code), species differ in codon usage. Thus it is possible to design a linear array of bases coding for several contiguous amino acids of the protein desired; the amino acids can be chosen to minimize the redundancy of codons encountered. As Figure 4-8 shows, a single-stranded oligomer of DNA can then be made using a DNA synthesizer; this oligomer will correspond to codons for the amino acids in a short region of the protein and should be able to hybridize to the corresponding region of cellular DNA or mRNA containing the gene. As the figure indicates, this single-stranded oligomer can then be the template for forming a double-stranded segment of DNA in a bacterial plasmid vector which can then be used to screen a phage library to obtain the entire gene.

Clearly, the longer the length of homology the better the hybridization will be with the oligomer. Generally five or more amino acid equivalents (i.e., at least 15 bases) will be needed to maximize homology and minimize cross-reaction with other sequences. Automated DNA synthesizers are now available to expedite synthesis of the desired oligomers. This approach has been used to isolate genes for neuropeptides and several other molecules for which only the sequences—or fragment(s) of the sequences—are known, and that, for technical reasons, may not be available in large quantities. An example is the isolation of the gene for bovine rhodopsin using an oligomer of 15 bases to anneal with mRNA from bovine retinal cells [14]. As more protein sequences are determined (especially with methods that can use only small amounts of protein), this method of gene isolation will become more widely used. It will be especially useful in the study of specialized tissues such as the eye and nervous system in which protein quantities may be limited.

Specific Antibody Available for Protein Product

When sufficient quantities of proteins are available, they can be used as antigens to make specific antibodies. In at least some cases, the antibodies can then be used to immunoprecipitate nascent polypeptides as they are being synthesized on ribosomes, since the entire protein is not necessarily required for antigenicity. As Fig. 4-9 indi-

A	Ser	Val	His	Tyr	Asp	Primary sequence
B	UCU	GUA	CAC	UAC	GAU	Codons
C	TCT	GTA	CAC	TAC	GAT	Oligonucleotide
D	AGA TCT	CAT GTA	GTG CAC	ATG TAC	CTA GAT	Double-stranded DNA

E

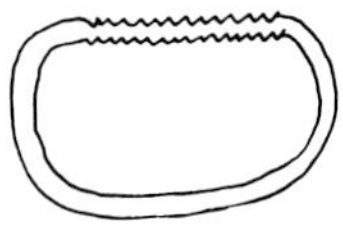

Recombinant probe

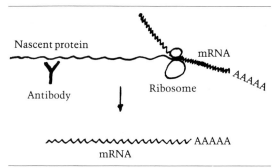

Fig. 4-8. *Strategy for gene isolation beginning with a known amino acid sequence of a protein. The short pentapeptide sequence (A) is converted into a set of possible RNA codons (B), and the corresponding deoxyoligonucleotide (C) is synthesized in vitro. The double-stranded DNA sequence is prepared (D) and attached to an amplification vector, usually through oligonucleotide linkers, to form a recombinant DNA probe (E). The probe can then be used for library screening to find the entire gene sequence. The specificity of this approach depends on the length of the amino acid sequence and the redundancy of its corresponding codons.*

cates, this technique can provide a unique population of ribosomes from which the mRNA can then be isolated. Once a specific mRNA is available, the methods outlined in Figs. 4-6 and 4-7 should be applicable with the synthesis of cDNA for hybridization to a suitable library.

Fig. 4-9. *Immunoprecipitation of nascent polypeptide and its associated ribosomes and mRNA by using an antibody reacting with the protein being synthesized. The mRNA can be recovered and should be specific (or, at least, highly enriched) for the gene of interest. The strategy shown in Fig. 4-6 can then be used to obtain corresponding DNA clones.*

Nascent protein

Antibody

mRNA

Ribosome

AAAAA

mRNA

A more recently developed method also exploits the specificity of antibodies for nascent proteins. As shown in Fig. 4-10, the antibody is immobilized on a filter, and clones of chromosomal DNA are prepared that differ from the standard DNA library by being under the control of a transcriptional promoter or start signal. When protein synthesis is induced for a series of clones, the immobilized antibody can react wherever its antigen (the nascent polypeptide) is being produced [18]. The clone or clones of interest are then isolated and purified. While such a method involves the initial preparation of suitable clones, such a library can be a permanent resource for use with many antibodies.

Determining Cosegregation of Phenotypes and DNA Markers

The approach of determining cosegregation is based on clinical or laboratory identification of mendelian factors important to the eye or eye disease. Fortunately, many of these are already cataloged [11]. The other requirement is a series of cloned fragments of chromosomal DNA with known chromosomal positions that are polymorphic (i.e., show various lengths in different persons). These fragments have been called *restriction fragment length polymorphisms* (RFLPs) [5]. The goal then becomes systematic screening of affected individuals (as well as unaffected members of the kindred) to determine if there is cosegregation of the mendelian trait with any RFLP. The question is which RFLP is found most frequently in affected members of a kindred and, conversely, is absent in unaffected relatives. At least in theory, this should permit progressive localization of the trait first to

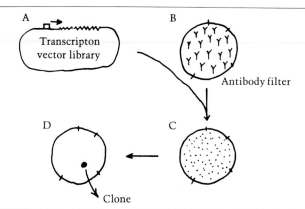

Fig. 4-10. *Specific DNA gene isolation based on antibodies to the protein product. In this case the library is constructed to permit transcription of the cloned DNA. The antibodies react with the protein and permit detection of the appropriate clone [18].*

the chromosome, then to a region, and finally to the actual DNA base sequence affected, although this final step may involve considerable work.

The most significant feature of this method is that detailed understanding of the biology or biochemistry of the trait is not required to determine its segregation pattern. This is a particularly appealing feature for many disorders of the eye and nervous system in which pathophysiology is poorly understood and dominant pedigrees are prominent. It presents the possibility of explaining the pathophysiologic nature of some mendelian traits indirectly through first identifying the gene involved.

An example of the potential of such an approach was the discovery of a DNA marker cosegregating with the mendelian dominant disorder Huntington's chorea. Here a neurologic disorder of unknown cause was found related to a specific DNA fragment change on chromosome 4 [8]. While the actual DNA segment of the gene was not identified, the chromosomal area of interest was immediately localized. Subsequently cloning strategies can further delineate the actual molecular change in the disease. Even without identifying the precise molecular defect, such DNA markers are clinically useful in prenatal and presymptomatic diagnosis and population studies.

Ophthalmology presents many challenges to which these techniques could be applied. An RFLP has been associated with an X-linked form of retinitis pigmentosa [4]. This work took advantage of the growing amount of molecular map data for the X chromosome. Another prominent target is the recognized association of a visible chromosomal change with retinoblastoma [13]. Here there

is actually more information than in Huntington's chorea since a chromosomal region has already been identified. As more markers become cataloged, they should be able to provide linkage references for most chromosomal regions. Detailed mapping (and, probably, the precise identification of the actual genetic lesions) will in general require extensive molecular biologic manipulation, but clinically useful information may be gained before all molecular details have been determined.

An important consideration in such studies is the value of extended pedigree information. Having several generations of affected and unaffected persons available for study greatly increases the power of segregation analysis. In fact, weak linkage (in which the marker is a long chromosomal distance from the genetic lesion) may be missed if only small isolated pedigrees are analyzed. In the Huntington's chorea study, the existence of a very large kindred (with hundreds of affected members) was probably critical in finding the linkage. For this reason, large kindreds will always be particularly good sources of linkage data and are most likely to advance these studies. Since ophthalmology has an especially rich array of mendelian dominant disorders that are not necessarily life-threatening, extensive pedigrees (often with particularly informative extensions to third and fourth generations) should be available. Animal models that permit the requisite length of pedigree for segregation analysis can also often be developed.

APPLICATIONS

Precise definitions of genetic changes in humans will be very useful clinically. The first obvious application is in the diagnosis of defined mendelian disorders of the eye and nervous system. So enigmatic in their physiologic basis and so important in their aggregate impact on ophthalmologic practice, these disorders (especially the dominant ones) frequently present a diagnostic challenge. The ability to establish diagnoses efficiently, unequivocally, and early should be of great importance to physicians and patients and should minimize delays.

Diagnostic applications are not limited to symptomatic individuals, however. A very useful application will be in presymptomatic or prenatal diagnosis. The techniques could provide concrete risk assessments and, possibly, permit early presymptomatic treatment. Particularly with the high (50%) recurrence risks for autosomal dominant disorders, the value to physicians and patients could be considerable.

Since counseling must be based on knowledge of risk and prognosis, the availability of diagnostic data based on precise genetic techniques will help patient treatment. While the natural histories of many mendelian disorders are reasonably well known, they are of little value unless they can be applied to specific cases.

Genetic markers may be developed that are useful as indicators of risk in common disorders—especially those with some sort of familial aggregation. Such problems as glaucoma could be managed wisely if persons at high risk could be identified earlier. An important contribution of molecular markers may be expected in such frequently encountered diseases—to help define relative risks in asymptomatic persons.

A final area of significant future contribution should be physiology. Molecular biology should identify specific proteins and DNA regions that contribute to visual biology in ways not currently recognized. Better appreciation should develop of molecules present in the eye in amounts so small as to make them undetectable by other means. The complex relations between the eye and the rest of the nervous system will undoubtedly be clarified as molecular dissection identifies specific neuropeptides and cell surface markers. Developmental changes in the eye also should be attributable to the contributions of individual genes at different stages. Such understanding may help explain developmental defects or lead to more rational prevention. All of these developments will depend critically on continuing interactions between clinical observations and laboratory studies.

REFERENCES

1. Benton, W. D., and Davis, R. W. Screening lambda-gt recombinant clones by hybridization to single plaques in situ. *Science* 196:180, 1977.
2. Bhat, S. P., and Piatigorsky, J. Molecular cloning and partial characterization of crystallin cDNA sequences in a bacterial plasmid. *Proc. Natl. Acad. Sci. U.S.A.* 76:3299, 1979.
3. Bhat, S. P., et al. Chicken lens crystallin DNA sequences show at least two crystallin genes. *Nature* 284:234, 1980.
4. Bhattacharya, S. S., et al. Close genetic linkage between X-linked retinitis pigmentosa and a restriction fragment length polymorphism identified by recombinant DNA probe L1.28. *Nature* 309:253, 1984.
5. Botstein, D., et al. Construction of a genetic linkage map in man using restriction fragment length polymorphisms. *Am. J. Hum. Genet.* 32:314, 1980.
6. Danna, K. J., Sack, G. H., Jr., and Nathans, D. Studies of SV40 DNA: VII. A cleavage map of the SV40 genome. *J. Mol. Biol.* 78:363, 1973.
7. Efstratiadis, A., et al. The structure and evolution of the human β-globin gene family. *Cell* 21:653, 1980.
8. Gusella, J. F., et al. A polymorphic DNA marker genetically linked to Huntington's disease. *Nature* 306:234, 1983.
9. Lawn, R. M., et al. The isolation and characterization of linked δ- and β-globin genes from a cloned library of human DNA. *Cell* 15:1157, 1978.
10. Maniatis, T., Fritsch, E. F., and Sambrook, J. *Molecular Cloning.* Cold Spring Harbor, N.Y.: Cold Spring Harbor Lab., 1982.
11. McKusick, V. A. *Mendelian Inheritance in Man* (6th ed.). Baltimore: Johns Hopkins Press, 1983.
12. Morrown, J. F., et al. Induction of hepatic synthesis of serum amyloid A protein and actin. *Proc. Natl. Acad. Sci. U.S.A.* 78:4718, 1981.
13. Murphree, A. L., and Benedict, W. F. Retinoblastoma: Clues to human oncogenesis. *Science* 223:1028, 1984.
14. Nathans, J., and Hogness, D. S. Isolation, sequence analysis, and intron-exon arrangement of the gene encoding bovine rhodopsin, *Cell* 34:807, 1983.
15. Sack, G. H., Jr. The use of restriction endonuclease *Hpa*-1 in the analysis of the genome of simian virus 40. Johns Hopkins University Ph.D. Dissertation, 1974.
16. Sack, G. H., Jr. Molecular cloning of human genes for serum amyloid A. *Gene* 21:19, 1983.
17. Southern, E. M. Detection of specific sequences among DNA fragments separated by gel electrophoresis. *J. Mol. Biol.* 98:503, 1975.
18. Young, R. A., and Davis, R. W. Yeast RNA polymerase II genes: Isolation with antibody probes. *Science* 222:778, 1983.

5

Ocular Ultrastructure in Inborn Lysosomal Storage Diseases

Jacques Libert
Kenneth R. Kenyon

Progress in understanding human inborn errors of metabolism has been especially rapid in the field of lysosomal diseases, of which more than 50 varieties have now been identified. Electron microscopy contributed greatly to the study of these disorders, from the basic definition of lysosomal storage to more sophisticated clinicopathologic findings leading to diagnostic approaches. The concept of lysosomal disease developed from the observation by Hers in 1965 that the storage material within hepatocytes of a patient with Hurler's syndrome appeared inside lysosomelike intracytoplasmic vacuoles [26]. Ultrastructural studies of other clinically affected tissues, including the eye, extended this interpretation. Systematic ultrastructural studies of clinically unaffected tissues then demonstrated the widespread expression of the lysosomal overloading, leading to the concept of generalized storage diseases. New screening approaches, such as skin and conjunctival biopsies, were developed.

Well-defined deficiencies of hydrolytic enzymes have been recognized in most of these disorders. A single enzyme defect usually explains the accumulation of a variety of undigested substrates in one homogeneous cell population, because each acid hydrolase is specific for one molecular linkage or radical rather than for a particular molecule. Moreover, the accumulation of simple molecules may initiate secondary enzyme inhibitions and more complex cellular dysfunctions. Although the same enzyme is deficient in all cells of the body, lysosomal storage may vary greatly from one cell type to another, with effects ranging from negligible accumulation to severe swelling. Thus, in a tissue made up of diverse cell types,

an even wider spectrum of heterogeneous molecules may accumulate. This variability is believed to be related to the rate at which the incriminated substrates are incorporated and to the life spans of the different cells.

The idea that one abnormal gene produces one primary enzyme deficiency was accepted until recently. The demonstration of partial enzyme defects and multiple enzyme deficiencies, however, initiated new research into the pathophysiology of metabolic diseases. Progress in cell fractionation, purification methods, and immunoprecipitation permitted enzymes to be viewed not only as catalysts of metabolism but as macromolecules in their particular intracellular compartments with subtle cellular processes governing their synthesis, packaging, transport, and incorporation into the lysosomal system. Defects in their translational processing have been elucidated. Molecular differences in enzyme processing have been found in various clinical subtypes of single inborn errors. Nonenzymatic activating or stabilizing proteins have been discovered. Finally, enzyme receptors have been identified, and a wide range of promising approaches is now available to the biochemist who wishes to delineate new diseases or engage in molecular genetic engineering.

As the wide variety and increasing complexity of enzymatic abnormalities become apparent, earlier classifications of inborn errors of metabolism, based on clinical observations and simple biochemical considerations, are becoming obsolete. New classifications, however, require further information on mechanisms underlying lysosomal metabolism. Many reviews and reports have described the classic diseases and their ocular

Table 5-1. *Clinical Ocular Manifestations of Inborn Lysosomal Storage Diseases*

Disease	Conjunctiva	Cornea	Retina	Optic nerve	Oculomotor
Mucopolysaccharidoses					
MPS I-H (Hurler)	−	+	+	+	−
MPS I-S (Scheie)	−	+	+	+	−
MPS II (Hunter)	−	−	+	+	−
MPS III (Sanfilippo)	−	−	+	+	−
MPS IV (Morquio)	−	+	−	+	−
MPS VI (Maroteaux-Lamy)	−	+	−	+	−
MPS VII (Sly)	−	+	−	−	−
Macular corneal dystrophy	−	+	−	−	−
Mucolipidoses					
ML I type 1	−	−	+	−	+
ML I type 2	+	+	+	−	+
ML II	−	+	−	−	−
ML III	−	+	−	−	−
ML IV	−	+	−	−	−
Oligosaccharidoses					
Fucosidosis	+	−	+	−	−
Mannosidosis	−	−	−	−	−
Aspartylglycosaminuria	−	−	−	−	−
Lipidoses					
GM$_1$ gangliosidosis	+	+	+	+	+
GM$_2$ gangliosidosis type I (Tay-Sachs)	−	−	+	+	+
GM$_2$ gangliosidosis type II (Sandhoff)	−	−	+	+	+
Fabry's disease	+	+	+	−	−
Metachromatic leukodystrophy	−	−	+	+	+
Mucosulfatidosis	−	+	+	+	+
Krabbe's disease	−	−	−	+	+
Gaucher's disease	−	−	+	−	+
Niemann-Pick disease type A	−	−	+	+	+
Niemann-Pick disease type B	−	−	−	−	−
Niemann-Pick disease type C	−	−	−	−	−
Ophthalmoplegic lipidosis	−	−	−	−	+
Farber's disease	−	−	+	−	−
Wolman's disease	−	−	+	−	−
Ceroid lipofuscinoses					
Hagberg-Santavuori type	−	−	+	+	+
Jansky-Bielschowsky type	−	−	+	+	+
Spielmeyer-Vogt disease	−	−	+	+	+
Kufs' disease	−	−	−	−	−
Miscellaneous					
Cystinosis	+	+	+	−	−
Glycogenosis type II (Pompe)	−	−	−	−	−

Table 5-2. *Histopathologic Ocular Involvement in Inborn Lysosomal Storage Diseases*

Disease	Conjunctiva	Cornea	Retina	Optic nerve
Mucopolysaccharidoses				
MPS I-H (Hurler)	+	+	+	+
MPS I-S (Scheie)	+	+	+	+
MPS II (Hunter)	+	+	+	+
MPS III (Sanfilippo)	+	+	+	+
MPS IV (Morquio)	+	+	+	+
MPS VI (Maroteaux-Lamy)	+	+	+	+
MPS VII (Sly)	NA	+	NA	NA
Macular dystrophy	−	+	−	NA
Mucolipidoses				
ML I type 1	+	+	+	NA
ML I type 2	+	NA	NA	NA
ML II	+	+	+	+
ML III	+	+	NA	NA
ML IV	+	+	NA	NA
Oligosaccharidoses				
Fucosidosis	+	+	+	+
Mannosidosis	+	+	NA	NA
Aspartylglycosaminuria	+	NA	NA	NA
Lipidoses				
GM_1 gangliosidosis	+	+	+	+
GM_2 gangliosidosis type I (Tay-Sachs)	+	+	+	+
GM_2 gangliosidosis type II (Sandhoff)	+	+	+	+
Fabry's disease	+	+	+	+
Metachromatic leukodystrophy	+	−	+	+
Mucosulfatidosis	+	+	+	+
Krabbe's disease	+	−	−	+
Gaucher's disease	+	−	NA	NA
Niemann-Pick disease type A	+	+	+	+
Niemann-Pick disease type B	+	NA	NA	NA
Niemann-Pick disease type C	+	NA	NA	NA
Ophthalmoplegic lipidosis	+	NA	+	−
Farber's disease	+	−	+	NA
Wolman's disease	NA	NA	+	NA
Ceroid lipofuscinoses				
Hagberg-Santavuori type	+	+	+	+
Jansky-Bielschowsky type	+	+	+	+
Spielmeyer-Vogt disease	+	+	+	+
Kufs' disease	−	−	+	+
Miscellaneous				
Cystinosis	+	+	+	NA
Glycogenosis type II (Pompe)	+	+	+	+

NA = information not available.

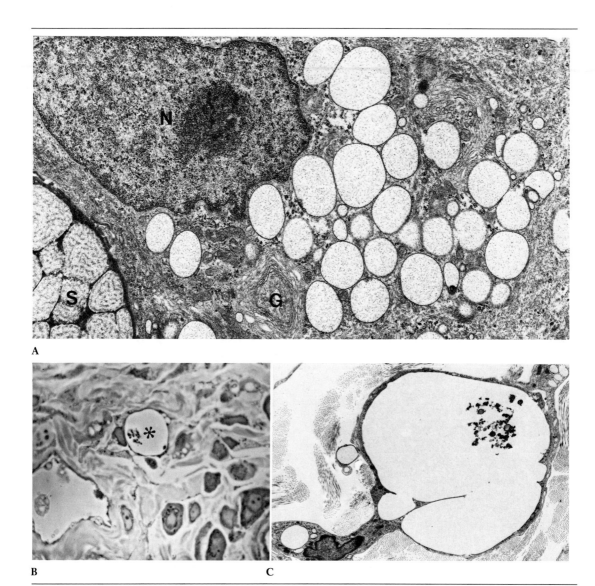

Fig. 5-1. *Conjunctiva. A. Mucopolysaccharidosis II (Hunter's syndrome). In an intermediate epithelial cell, many fibrillogranular vacuoles are localized in the perinuclear area and are closely associated with the Golgi complex (G). Some secretion granules (S) are evident in an adjacent goblet cell. (N = nucleus.) (×16,000 before 18% reduction.) B. Mucopolysaccharidosis I-H (Hurler's syndrome). Finely vacuolated connective tissue cells and grossly ballooned histiocytes (asterisk) are evident in the* *hypercellular subepithelial layer of the stroma. (Phase contrast, paraphenylenediamine, ×1,000 before 18% reduction.) C. Mucopolysaccharidosis I-H (Hurler's syndrome). In this severely ballooned histiocyte, or "gargoyle cell," a single immense storage vacuole (diameter ~15 μm) has displaced the nucleus and other organelles. However, no clinical sign results from this huge swelling. (×4,700 before 18% reduction.) (B, C, from K. R. Kenyon et al. [31].)*

alterations. We have chosen a more synthetic approach, dealing with clinicopathologic correlations between the appearance of clinical signs (Table 5-1) and the morphology of affected tissues (Table 5-2) [9, 15, 16, 28, 36].

CONJUNCTIVA

Conjunctival cells are usually involved in lysosomal storage diseases (Fig. 5-1). Inclusions containing material with typical ultrastructural architecture often have a typical repetition among the different cell components of the tissue. Electron microscopic study of the inclusions provides one of the best approaches to morphologic diagnosis [37, 66]. However, clinical manifestations are unusual and limited essentially to refractive crystals and vascular tortuosities.

Refractive crystals, corresponding to cystine crystals within stromal fibroblasts [68], may be observed in the conjunctiva of patients with cystinosis (Fig. 5-2). Similar crystals may be found in smears of lacrimal secretions, and may contribute to the patients' constant conjunctival irritation and photophobia.

Aneurysms and tortuosities of the blood capillaries and venules have been observed in the conjunctivae of patients afflicted with lysosomal diseases such as fucosidosis, mucolipidosis (ML)

I, GM_1 gangliosidosis, Fabry's disease, and a new disorder with a still unknown enzyme defect. In all these diseases, massive overloading of the lysosomal system occurs in the capillary and venous endothelial cells, with a relative sparing of arterioles. The disorganization of the cellular architecture of the vessel walls is believed to induce a loss of mechanical resistance against blood pressure and to be responsible for the clinically observed vascular abnormalities (Figs. 5-3 and 5-4) [44].

CORNEA

Keratocytes often present ultrastructural signs of overloading in inborn lysosomal disorders, whereas epithelial and endothelial cells are less frequently affected. Since corneal transparency requires a highly ordered configuration of stromal collagen bundles, extensive swelling of the keratocytes and the presence of extracellular material result in clinically evident opacities and haziness. In clinically clear corneas, keratocytes show only a few small inclusions; cloudy corneas display severely ballooned keratocytes, whose thickness, reaching 10 μm or more, far exceeds the 200-nm dimension beyond which significant light scattering occurs [23, 24]. Keratocytes in the anterior layers of the stroma are usually more extensively affected than

Fig. 5-2. *Conjunctiva. A. Cystinosis. This large, needle-shaped crystal was obtained by a single scraping of the conjunctival secretions. (×300 before 10% reduction.) B, C. Cystinosis. Epithelial and connective tissue cells contain polygonal crystalline* *profiles that represent the cystine-containing lysosomes as shown by phase-contrast (B) and electron (C) microscopy. (B, paraphenylenediamine, ×800 before 10% reduction; C, ×15,000 before 10% reduction.)*

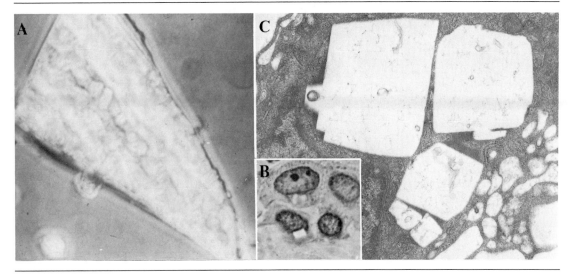

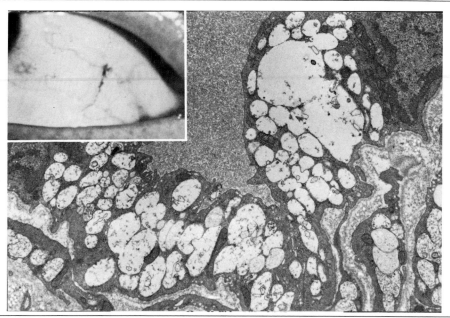

Fig. 5-3. *Conjunctiva in GM₁ gangliosidosis. The lysosomal storage of mucopolysaccharide-like material is very impressive in conjunctival blood capillary endothelial cells. This process disorganizes the normal cytoarchitecture and is supposed to induce a mechanical weakness of the vessel walls and later the tortuosities and aneurysms that may characterize the ophthalmologic picture of the disease (inset). (×10,000.)*

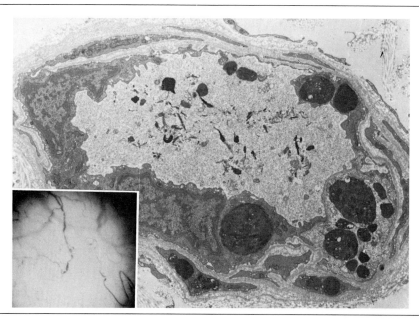

Fig. 5-4. *Conjunctiva in Fabry's disease. In addition to the severe overloading evident within the blood capillary endothelial cells, cytoplasmic rupture with embolization of lamellar lipids in the capillary lumen may further explain the formation of conjunctival aneurysms (inset). A similar phenomenon within the central retinal artery may account for the thromboembolic accidents that have been reported in the course of the disease. (×10,000 before 20% reduction.) (From J. Libert, M. Tondeur, and F. Van Hoof. The use of conjuntivial biopsy and enzyme analysis in tears for the diagnois of homozygotes and heterozygotes with Fabry disease. In D. Bergsma, A. J. Bron, and E. Cotlier (Eds.),* The Eye and Inborn Errors of Metabolism. *New York: Alan R. Liss for the National Foundation March of Dimes, BD:OAS 12(3) 221-239, 1976.*

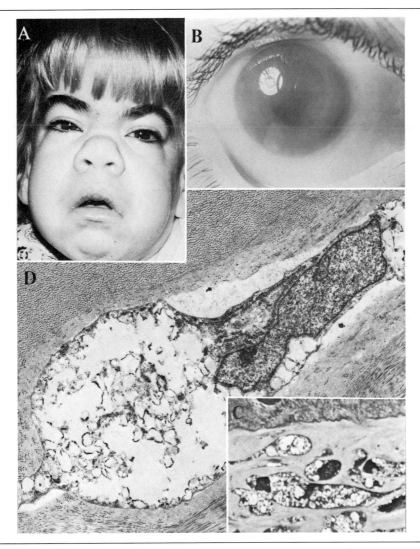

Fig. 5-5. *Cornea in mucopolysaccharidosis (MPS) VI (Maroteaux-Lamy syndrome). Coarse facies (A) and corneal clouding (B) are constant features in MPS VI. By phase-contrast microscopy (C), several ballooned keratocytes markedly disturb the general architecture of the anterior corneal stroma and disorganize* *Bowman's layer (×1,000). By electron microscopy (D), a huge swelling of the keratocyte by mucopolysaccharide-like material disrupts the regular arrangement of the collagen fiber bundles. (×8,000.) (From K. R. Kenyon et al. [33].)*

those in the posterior layers. In the most severe cases, Bowman's layer often seems to be disorganized and infiltrated with engorged histiocytes, extracellular storage material, and cytoplasmic debris. Descemet's layer is usually unaffected. Epithelial and endothelial cells, though usually involved in mucopolysaccharidosis (MPS) and GM₁ gangliosidosis, are not believed to contribute significantly to clouding (Fig. 5-5). Similarly, despite marked involvement of epithelial and endothelial

cells, no corneal clouding appears in the neuronal ceroid lipofuscinoses, Pompe's disease, fucosidosis, Niemann-Pick disease, or Sanfilippo's syndrome (MPS III), because keratocyte involvement is mild (Figs. 5-6 and 5-7). Light scattering by affected keratocytes explains the subtle stromal opacities in MPS II and VII, ML I and II, and mucosulfatidosis; the severe ground-glass clouding in MPS I-H, I-S, IV, and VI, GM₁ gangliosidosis, and ML III; and the nodular opacities in macular

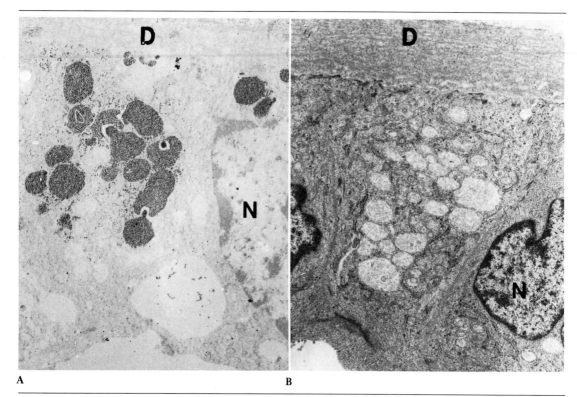

A   B

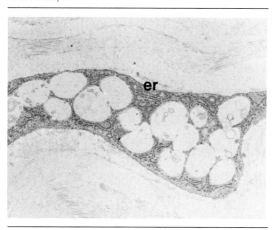

Fig. 5-7. *Cornea in mucopolysaccharidosis I-H (Hurler's syndrome). Keratocytes are already severely affected in fetus aged 24 weeks at the time of abortion after prenatal diagnosis of the disease. The well-developed rough endoplasmic reticulum (er) is characteristic of fetal cells. (×6,000 before 28% reduction.)*

Fig. 5-6. *Cornea. Endothelial cells of the fetal cornea display numerous lysosomes that contain innumerable granules of glycogen (A) in Pompe's disease, or a fibrillogranular reticulum (B) in Sanfilippo's disease type A (MPS IIIA). This involvement remains clinically silent for the entire course of the disease. (D = Descemet's membrane; N = nucleus.) (A, silver proteinate, ×12,000; B, routine lead citrate and uranyl acetate, ×12,000.) (A, from J. Libert et al. [40].)*

corneal dystrophy. In all these diseases the storage lysosomes observed within keratocytes contain mucopolysaccharide. Neither complex lipid nor glycogen storage within corneal stroma has ever been reported to induce haziness.

There are some similarities between corneal and conjunctival involvement, as the affected corneal and conjunctival cells always display identical storage lysosomes. There is no quantitative correlation, however; very severe ballooning of conjunctival cells may accompany mild keratocytic involvement, as in the case of MPS III [11, 29].

Keratocyte involvement fails to explain corneal opacity in four diseases. In cystinosis a relatively small number of crystalline structures with needlelike or rectangular profiles, located within

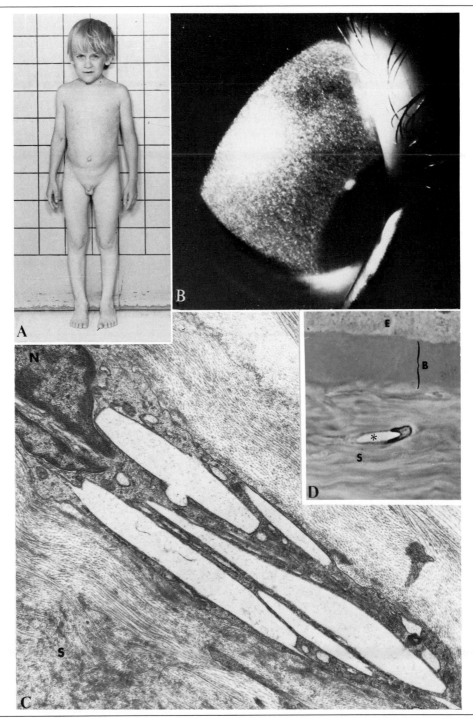

Fig. 5-8. *Cornea in infantile cystinosis. Short stature and fair complexion characterize the clinical appearance of nephropathic cystinosis patients (A). At slit-lamp examination fine shining crystals seem to be dispersed throughout the whole corneal surface (B). Electron (C) and phase-contrast (D) microscopy reveal lysosomal inclusions with geometric and often needlelike shapes. They are never large enough to disturb the regular arrangement of stromal collagen fibers, but their crystalline nature produces significant light scattering by multiple reflection, diffraction, and spectral decomposition. (N = nucleus; S = stroma; E = epithelium; B = Bowman's layer.) (C ×18,000 before 11% reduction; D, ×800 before 11% reduction.) (B, C, D, from K. R. Kenyon and J. A. Sensenbrenner, Electron microscopy of cornea and conjuntivia in childhood systinosis, Am. J. Ophthalmol. 73:718, 1972. Published with permission from the American Journal of Ophthalmology. Copyright by the Ophthalmic Publishing Company.)*

keratocytes, produce a remarkable glistening image in which polychromatic refractile dots are dispersed throughout the stroma, with a slight predilection for the periphery (Fig. 5-8). Wong and colleagues demonstrated these inclusions to be cystine storage lysosomes [68]. They are presumably responsible for the photophobia and reduced vision that characterize cystinosis patients.

The second disease is Fabry's disease, in which dustlike haziness and whorl-like corneal opacities are typical. Corneal opacities have been described in patients as young as 6 months. In a series of 25 patients followed for 10 years from childhood to puberty, we found that the opacities often appeared in those aged 7 to 10 years, in both hemizygotes and heterozygotes [43]. However, vortex dystrophy may be absent in adults with biochem-

ically proven Fabry's disease. Although keratocytes are affected in this disease, dystrophy seems to be related exclusively to the deposit of sphingolipid inclusions at the epithelial level (Fig. 5-9) [67]. Visual acuity is unaffected by the corneal pathology.

The third exception is ML IV, in which extreme overloading in corneal epithelial cells contrasts with the relative sparing of keratocytes. Corneal scraping immediately improves corneal clarity in ML IV [30, 51] but not in other (Fig. 5-10)

Fig. 5-9. *Cornea in Fabry's disease. Typical vortex dystrophy (A) is related to the involvement of epithelial cells, whose cytoplasm displays many dense inclusions (B). At high magnification (C) lamellar lipids are seen to be the principal contents of the storage lysosomes. (B, ×20,000 before 20% reduction; C, ×90,000 before 20% reduction.)*

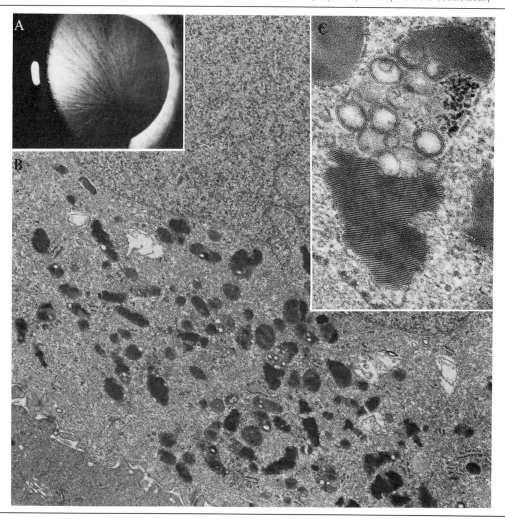

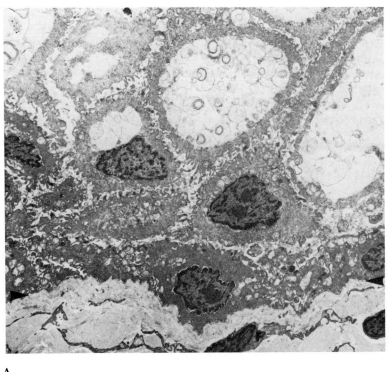

A

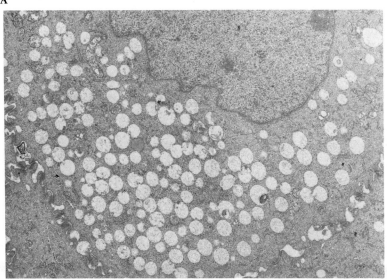

B

Fig. 5-10. *Cornea. A. Mucolipidosis IV. Epithelial cells present striking abnormalities, beginning with a mild involvement of the basal layer with small, lamellar, lipid-containing lysosomes. When the lysosomes progress to the apical layers, they accumulate a large amount of fibrillogranular material. They appear as large confluent balloons, containing isolated lamellar rings within a clear mucopolysaccharide-like material. The stromal keratocytes are little affected by the pathologic process. (×5,500 before 20% reduction.) (From K. R. Kenyon, et al. Mucolipidosis IV: Histopathology of conjunctiva, cornea, and skin. Arch. Ophthalmol. 97:1106, 1979. Copyright 1979, American Medical Association.) B. GM₁ gangliosidosis. The epithelial cells are filled with relatively small, clear inclusions that show stored acid mucopolysaccharides. (×10,000 before 20% reduction.)*

lysosomal storage diseases. A few days after epithelial healing, however, the cornea again appears cloudy. Corneal grafting is therefore inappropriate treatment in ML IV, since the host's replacement of donor corneal epithelium brings renewed clouding. Grafting is, however, an excellent procedure in mild phenotypes of lysosomal diseases such as MPS I-S, ML III, and macular corneal dystrophy; in these diseases grafts remain transparent, and the dystrophy may recur only after several years as host keratocytes containing the abnormal genome infiltrate the donor cornea.

The fourth exception is macular corneal dystrophy, which, although considered an MPS with only localized expression, may in fact result from a totally different pathophysiologic mechanism [34]. Keratocytes are the site of intralysosomal storage of a dense fibrillar material with the same histochemical characteristics as proteoglycans [34]. In macular corneal dystrophy, unlike the systemic mucopolysaccharidoses, abnormal material is deposited between the collagen fibers in the corneal stroma, and the posterior layer of Descemet's membrane contains numerous vacuoles, resulting in a honeycombed appearance. Extra-

cellular accumulation within the stroma may follow distintegration of affected cells, although more severe swelling of the keratocytes in the mucopolysaccharidoses does seem to induce as much extracellular deposition. The deposits within Descemet's membrane clearly have a different origin and almost certainly reflect a functionally abnormal corneal endothelium (Fig. 5-11).

LENS

Lens opacities have been reported in mannosidosis, Fabry's disease, and Niemann-Pick disease.

Fig. 5-11. *Cornea in macular corneal dystrophy. A. Moderate corneal clouding involves a diffuse haze extending to the limbus with dense stromal opacities more evident centrally. Endothelial cells and stromal keratocytes stain intensively for acid mucopolysaccharides. B. Guttate excrescences (asterisks) of Descemet's membrane (DM) are numerous. (Colloidal iron, ×800 before 10% reduction.) C. By electron microscopy endothelial cells (En) are seen to contain storage lysosomes. The posterior portion of Descemet's membrane is honeycombed by fine granular material and small vesicles; the anterior portion appears unaffected. Keratocytes (K) show marked storage. (×3,000 before 10% reduction.)*

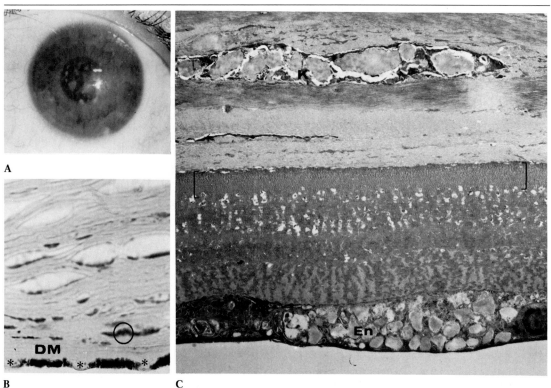

A

B

C

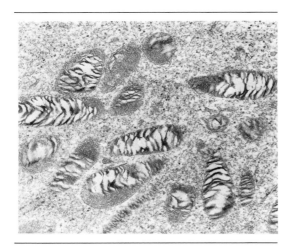

Fig. 5-12. *Lens in Niemann-Pick disease. Anterior epithelial cells contain numerous lamellar inclusions whose disrupted configuration is characteristic of Niemann-Pick disease. (×32,000 before 28% reduction.)*

Condensations of the anterior and posterior cortical sutures, discrete stellate cataracts, and octopus and spokelike opacities have frequently been documented [14, 53, 56, 60]. Lysosomal inclusions in the anterior epithelium and in stromal fibers, such as those evident in Niemann-Pick disease (Fig. 5-12), may explain this clinical picture [45, 56].

IRIS AND CILIARY BODY

Although fibroblasts, muscle fibers, capillary endothelial cells, ciliary nerves, and macrophages may be affected by lysosomal storage disorders, these lesions do not induce clinical symptoms; even the absence of pupillary reflexes in terminal stages of sphingolipidoses and ceroid lipofuscinoses result from blindness rather than from local changes.

Ciliary epithelium is markedly involved in MPS, GM_1 gangliosidosis, Niemann-Pick disease, metachromatic leukodystrophy, fucosidosis, and ceroid lipofuscinoses (Fig. 5-13). This involvement, together with the abnormalities of trabecular endothelium, may explain the glaucoma crises described in MPS (Fig. 5-14). It may also participate in the development of cataracts, described above, by modification of the composition of aqueous humor, although this possibility should be investigated further.

Abnormalities of pigmented cells, to be detailed

later, are responsible for the transparent iris that characterizes Chédiak-Higashi syndrome, a rare form of pseudoalbinism (Fig. 5-15) [39].

VITREOUS

No clinical or histopathologic abnormalities have been described in the vitreous of patients affected with inborn lysosomal diseases. However, a particular finding, white spots scattered in an arcuate distribution around the posterior pole, has been correlated with the deposit of foamy histiocytes on the vitreoretinal interface in Gaucher's disease [8, 64, 65].

RETINA

Although lysosomal storage disorders frequently affect all retinal cells in different ways, the clinical signs can be reduced to four types: vascular tortuosities, macular cherry-red spot, pigmentary retinopathy, and pseudoalbinism.

As in the conjunctiva, capillary and vein endothelial cells may be severely affected in mucolipidosis I, fucosidosis, and GM_1 gangliosidosis, as well as Fabry's, Niemann-Pick, and Pompe's diseases. Electron microscopy reveals considerable deformation of these cells; storage lysosomes often occupy more than half the cytoplasmic volume, leaving little space for other organelles. More specifically, fibrillar elements, which are essential to the normal architecture of the endothelial cells, are profoundly disorganized or even absent in some places (Fig. 5-16). The resulting weak mechanical resistance of the vessel walls to blood pressure leads, after several years, to the characteristic tortuosities seen in all the diseases listed above, except Niemann-Pick and Pompe's, in which the patients do not survive long enough to have these clinical signs develop (44). If the course of the disease is prolonged, as in Fabry's disease, vascular alterations may produce thromboemboli in retinal veins or arteries [60, 61].

Abnormal material causes extensive swelling of ganglion cells in all the lysosomal diseases studied, except ML II [46], Krabbe's disease [6], cystinosis [57], and Chédiak-Higashi disease [39]. Under light microscopy, sudanophilia, metachromasia, periodic acid–Schiff (PAS) positivity, birefringence, or autofluorescence reveals this material to have the histochemical characteristics of mucopolysaccharides, complex lipids, or ceroid lipofuscin [4, 9, 29]. The electron micro-

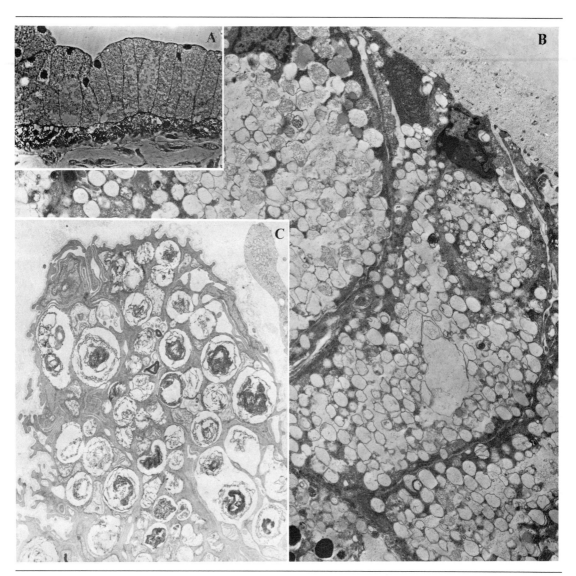

Fig. 5-13. *Ciliary body. The nonpigmented layer of the ciliary epithelium is often affected in lysosomal storage disease. By phase-contrast microscopy, marked swelling is evident in mucopolysaccharidosis III (A); it corresponds to the lysosomal storage of acid mucopolysaccharides with fibrillogranular*

appearance seen by electron microscopy (B). In Niemann-Pick disease a lamellar lipid material is associated with the fibrillogranular content (C). (A, ×300 before 20% reduction; B, ×6,000 before 20% reduction; C, ×9,000 before 20% reduction.)

scope discloses further differences that depend on the nature of the stored substance. In mucopolysaccharidoses lysosomes are distended by loose lipid membranes associated with variable proportions of a fibrillogranular reticulum [29]. In fucosidosis clear membrane-bound inclusions contain a proteinlike material without any lipid lamella [38], whereas only glycogen particles may be seen in neuron lysosomes of Pompe's disease [40]. In GM$_1$ and GM$_2$ gangliosidoses, the accu-

mulated gangliosides assume homogeneous, membranous arrays also called membranous cytoplasmic bodies (Fig. 5-17) [18, 19, 25], whereas the ceramide hexosides of Fabry's disease produce highly ordered, complex geometric architectures [13, 67]. In contrast, poorly defined inclusions with loose lamellar whorls are evident in type A Niemann-Pick disease, and irregularly stained membranous profiles within a granular matrix are seen in metachromatic leukodystrophy [45, 47]. In cer-

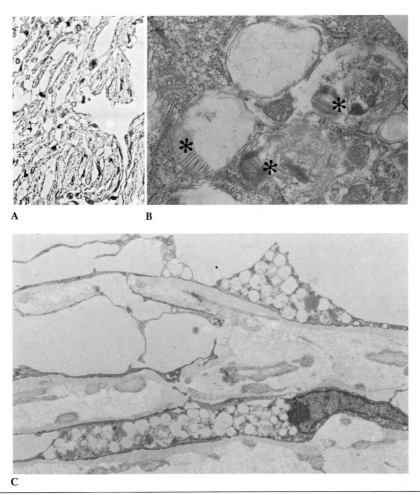

C

Fig. 5-14. *Trabecular meshwork in mucopolysaccharidosis III (Sanfilippo's syndrome). Trabecular endothelial cells show a marked accumulation of lysosomal acid mucopolysaccharides (A and C). At high magnification the stored material appears to be composed of variable proportions of fibrillogranular material and lamellar lipids (B, asterisks). (A, ×500 before 20% reduction; B, ×60,000 before 20% reduction; C, ×3,000 before 20% reduction.)*

oid lipofuscinoses so-called fingerprint, curvilinear, or snowball patterns predominate (Fig. 5-18) [20, 21, 41, 62].

Although lysosomal storage within retinal ganglion cells is frequent, the well-known clinical sign of the macular cherry-red spot has been described only in ML I, GM_1 and GM_2 gangliosidoses, Niemann-Pick disease, metachromatic leukodystrophy, and Farber's disease. This contrast phenomenon results from massive complex lipid deposition in all the retinal ganglion cells. As the number of neurons between the periphery and the perifoveal area increases, the thickening of the affected layer masks the choroidal vasculature by a white or grayish ring-shaped haze centered on the neuron-free fovea, through which the normal red color of the choroid stands out [9]. In gangliosidoses the macular cherry-red spot, also called Tay's spot, is an early and constant symptom. In ML I, it appears much later, in the second decade of life [48], and is compatible with fairly good vision in the early stages, though visual acuity gradually decreases during the course of the disease. In one case the cherry-red spot faded, coinciding with a marked visual loss, when the patient reached the age of 20 [55]. In Niemann-Pick disease and metachromatic leukodystrophy, the cherry-red spot is an inconstant and sometimes very late symptom [45, 47]. The spot has never

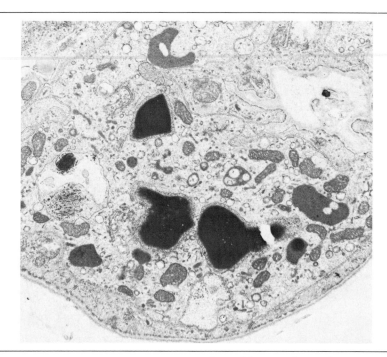

Fig. 5-15. *Posterior iris epithelium in Chédiak-Higashi syndrome. The pigment epithelium contains no normal melanosomes but displays large, very dense formations with a geographic profile and limited by a single membrane. Even at the highest magnifications, no ultrastructural detail could be seen in their dark, homogeneous matrix. (×7,000 before 20% reduction.) (From J. Libert et al. [39].)*

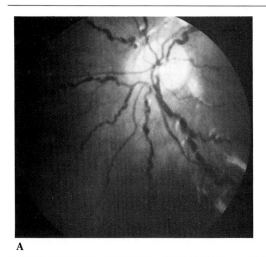

A

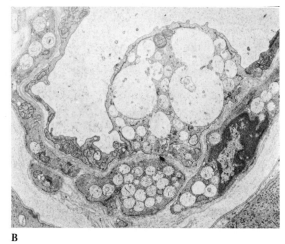

B

Fig. 5-16. *Retina in fucosidosis. A considerable swelling of retinal capillary endothelial and mural cells disorganizes the fibrillar elements that compose the cytoarchitecture of their cytoplasm (B). This process is responsible for a weak mechanical resistance against blood pressure and for the formation of the venous tortuosities (A). (×7,000 before 20% reduction.)*

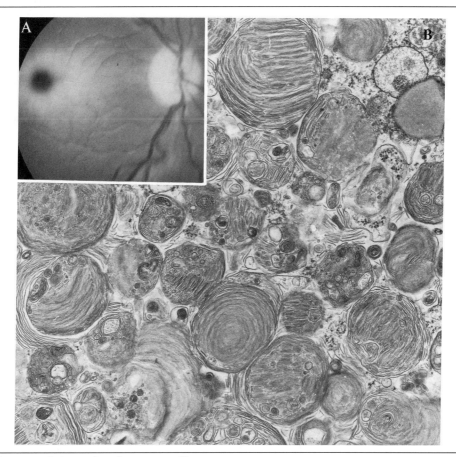

Fig. 5-17. *Retina in GM₁ gangliosidosis. As in all gangliosidoses, retinal ganglion cells are filled by glycolipids in the form of membranous cytoplasmic bodies with lamellae displaying complex parallel or concentric arrangement (B). This massive storage in the numerous ganglion cells surrounding the foveolar area explains the development of the typical cherry-red spot (A). (×30,000 before 20% reduction.)*

been described in mucopolysaccharidoses, fucosidoses, Pompe's disease, or the ceroid lipofuscinoses, although microscopy often discloses severe neuronal damage.

Three factors probably account for these differences in the appearance of the macular cherry-red spot. The first is the extent of the storage process, since more severely affected neurons, as in gangliosidoses, will produce earlier symptoms than do less severely affected neurons, as in metachromatic leukodystrophy. The second factor is the optic characteristics of the accumulated material. Indeed, it is conceivable that lysosomal swellings of the same intensity will have different expressions depending on the particular reflection and absorption indices of the intralysosomal material (Figs. 5-19 and 5-20). Third, mechanical or biochemical perturbations of the cytoplasmic metabolism may result in degeneration of the ganglion cells with histologically apparent thinning and gliosis of the inner layers of the retina. Such a phenomenon would explain the fading of the cherry-red spot reported in the final stage of ML I [55]. Moreover, the degeneration may sometimes be accelerated by the accumulation of toxic components, as in ceroid lipofuscinoses, in which peroxidation products have demonstrated toxicity against brain and retinal tissues [2, 71]. In these disorders the destructive process may develop more rapidly than the storage process, so no macular cherry-red spot appears, and then the ganglion cell loss accounts for an ascending mechanism of optic atrophy.

Müller and ganglion cells are often affected together. The substances accumulated in the two

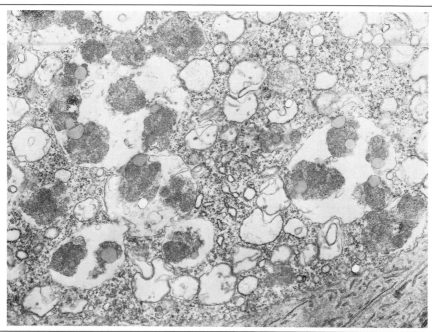

Fig. 5-18. *Retina in Kufs' disease, an adult form of ceroid lipofuscinosis. Although ganglion cells present large inclusions with granular and curvilinear material associated with neutral lipid droplets, the retina always remains clinically normal in this disease. (× 10,000 before 20% reduction.)*

cell types display the same histochemical characteristics but usually look different under the electron microscope [36, 45, 47]. These lesions may participate in the formation of the cherry-red spot but do not seem to produce other consequences. Bipolar cells contain abnormal material only in rare cases, and no clinical signs result from their involvement. The perikaryon and the myoid portions of the photoreceptors present storage lysosomes in mucopolysaccharidoses, fucosidosis, ML II, Sandhoff's, Tay-Sachs, Niemann-Pick, and Pompe's diseases, as well as in the ceroid lipofuscinoses (Fig. 5-21) [5, 7, 38, 40, 41, 45, 46]. If the retinal pigment epithelium is spared, as in fucosidosis, ML II, and Pompe's disease, these isolated lesions have no clinical consequences, but if it is involved together with photoreceptors, both structures participate in the development of the pigmentary retinopathy.

Pigmentary retinopathy is a prominent feature of several mucopolysaccharidoses and the ceroid lipofuscinoses. The lesions of the ganglion cells do not seem to be directly responsible for the photoreceptor degeneration. Not only are the bipolar cells generally well preserved, but the dystrophic process of the retina rather resembles the specific pattern described in dominantly inherited retinitis pigmentosa (Fig. 5-22) [35]. Morphologic findings suggest that progressive dystrophy is in-

itiated by the massive overloading of the pigment epithelial cells by a fibrillogranular material in the mucopolysaccharidoses and by granular, curvilinear, or fingerprint structures in the ceroid lipofuscinoses. Indeed, early evidence of lysosomal storage is found in the photoreceptor–pigment epithelium complex of fetuses affected with MPS III [7]. Observations of retinal tissue from different types of MPS have disclosed severely affected pigment epithelium and atrophic photoreceptors, even in the absence of pigmented cell proliferation or typical pigmentary retinopathy [63; J. Libert, unpublished observation].

Since the pigment epithelial cells have active catabolism and play an essential role in the renewal of photoreceptors [70], it is not surprising that their massive lysosomal overloading leads ultimately to degeneration of the photoreceptors and thinning of the outer nuclear layer. Light and electron microscopy reveal subsequent active multiplication of pigmented cells. These cells detach from the basal membrane, and as they begin to migrate toward the degenerating retina, they acquire the appearance of macrophages that

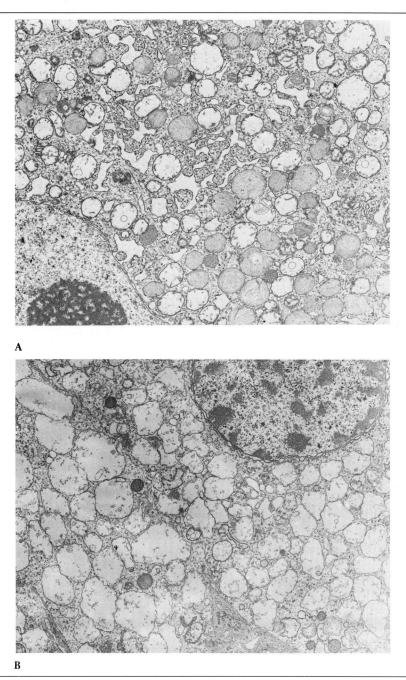

A

B

Fig. 5-19. *Retina. Although ganglion cells display a similar number of lysosomal inclusions in both cases, the child affected with metachromatic leukodystrophy (A) presented with a macular cherry-red spot, whereas the child affected with fucosidosis (B) had a normal macula. This difference is probably related to the optic character of the accumulated material. (×11,000 before 20% reduction.) (A, from J. Libert et al., Ocular findings in metachromatic leukodystrophy: an electron microscopic and enyzyme study in different clinical and genetic variants, Arch. Ophthalmol. 97:1495, 1979, Copyright 1979, American Medical Association; B, from J. Libert, Ultrastructure oculaire, J. Fr. Ophtalmol. 7:519, 1984.)*

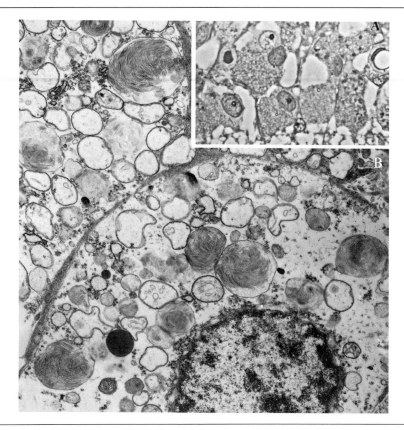

Fig. 5-20. *Retina in mucopolysaccharidosis IIIA. A. With phase-contrast microscopy, paraphenylenediamine stain resolves a fine vacuolation of the ganglion cells. (×1,000 before 20% reduction.) B. Electron microscopy identifies intracytoplasmic inclusions as lysosomes containing* predominantly whorled membranous lamellar material with less fibrillogranular substance. (×13,000 before 20% reduction.) (From M. A. Del Monte et al., Histopathology of Sanfilipo's syndrome, Arch. Ophthalmol. *101:1255, 1983. Copyright 1983, American Medical Association.)*

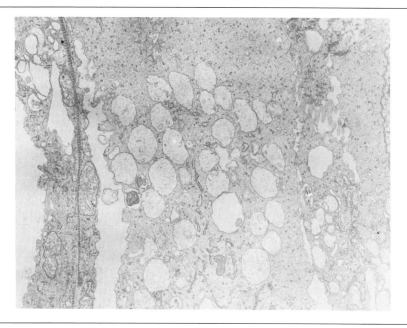

Fig. 5-21. *Retina in fucosidosis. The myoid portion of the photoreceptors displays numerous lysosomal inclusions, which remain clinically silent in this* disease since the retinal pigment epithelium is not involved in the storage process. (×11,000 before 20% reduction.) (From J. Libert [38].)

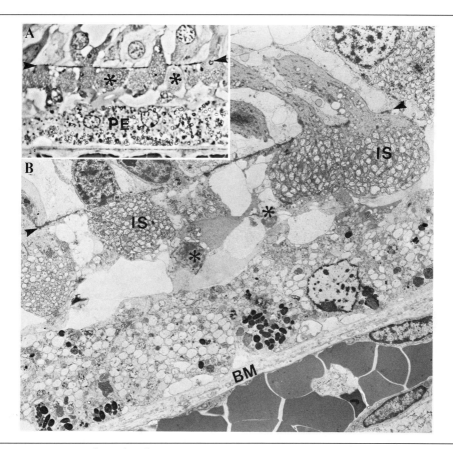

Fig. 5-22. *Retina in mucopolysaccharidosis IIIA. A. By phase-contrast microscopy, reduction of photoreceptor cell nuclei, swelling of cone inner segments (asterisks), absence of outer segments, and maintenance of pigment epithelial layer (PE) are particularly evident. (× 800 before 20% reduction.) B. Electron microscopy confirms close apposition of photoreceptor inner segments (IS) to pigment epithelial cells, with only rare outer-segment remnants interposed (asterisks). The pigment epithelial cells are filled with fibrillogranular inclusions. Bruch's membrane (BM) and the choroidal vessels remain unaffected. (× 3,000 before 20% reduction.) From M. A. Del Monte et al., Histopathology of Sanfilipo's syndrome, Arch. Ophthalmol. 101:1255, 1983. Copyright 1983, American Medical Association.)*

contain both storage material and melanin residues (Fig. 5-23). Though found throughout the retina, these cells are particularly numerous around the retinal vessels, possibly because of their affinity for oxygen. This confluence of pigmented cells creates the ophthalmoscopically visible resemblance to bone corpuscles (Fig. 5-23) [11, 20, 21, 29, 33, 36, 41, 63].

Pseudoalbinism, reported in cystinosis and in Chédiak-Higashi syndrome, must also be considered a consequence of pigment epithelial abnormalities. In pseudoalbinism pigmented melanosomes are present although abnormal; in true albinism they are absent. Histopathologic and ultrastructural examination of eyes from children afflicted with cystinosis show degeneration of the pigment epithelium characterized by moderate, localized thickening, areas of depigmentation, or zones of cellular thinning, with a generalized accumulation of cystine crystals within distended lysosomes [17, 57]. The pigment alterations, preferentially localized between the equator and ora serrata and in the perimacular area, explain the yellow mottling of the macular region and patchy depigmentation of the periphery that are classically described in infantile cases [69]. Fibroblasts and histiocytes of the choroid and the anterior uvea are greatly swollen by inclusions containing polymorphous crystalline profiles. The neurosensory retina remains unaffected [17, 57].

The lesions in Chédiak-Higashi syndrome seem rather different; ultrastructural studies show a

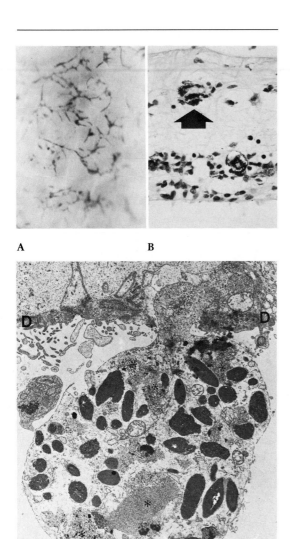

A   B

C

Fig. 5-23. *Retina. A, B. Mucopolysaccharidosis IIIA. A. Retinal pigmentary degeneration is prominent in the midperiphery where intraretinal pigmentation assumes bone corpuscle configurations. B. In the peripheral retina migratory pigment epithelial cells have assumed perivascular configurations (arrow), and photoreceptors are nearly absent. (H&E, ×200 before 20% reduction.) (From M. A. Del Monte et al., Histopathology of Sanfilipo's syndrome,* Arch. Ophthalmol. *101:1255, 1983. Copyright 1983, American Medical Association.) C. Late infantile ceroid lipofuscinosis (Jansky-Bielschowsky syndrome). Metaplastic cells, probably derived from the retinal pigment epithelium, migrate in the direction of the retina, and by diapedesis cross the*

severe disturbance of melanogenesis in the retinal pigment epithelium and uveal melanocytes. Many cells are completely depigmented; others display very few melanosomes, polyphagosomes, or giant amorphous melanin granules. Contrary to what is usually observed in lysosomal storage diseases, no massive overloading or phagocytosis is seen in pigment epithelial cells. Many connective tissue cells in the uveal tract, conjunctiva, and ocular muscles display marked lysosomal storage of granulolamellar material, and it is proposed that dysfunctions of both the lysosomes and the melanosomes arise from the same (as yet undiscovered) pathophysiologic mechanism. In patients with Chédiak-Higashi syndrome one also sees profound alterations of the photoreceptors, with undifferentiated cytoplasm instead of the normal superposition of regular discs in outer segments (Fig. 5-24) [39]. These histopathologic lesions confirm the hypothesis of a tapetoretinal abnormality suggested by the clinicians who noted the albinoid fundus, low vision, nystagmus, and flat electroretinogram in patients with Chédiak-Highashi syndrome [58].

CHOROID

Although choroidal histiocytes and fibroblasts, choriocapillary endothelial cells, ciliary nerve axons, and Schwann's cells are often involved in generalized lysosomal storage, clinical symptoms related to these abnormalities have never been reported, except in the case of pseudoalbinism described in the previous section.

OPTIC NERVE

Optic atrophy has been noted in many lysosomal storage diseases. This symptom may result from pathophysiologic mechanisms related to destruction of retinal neurons, lysosomal dysfunction within the optic nerve cells, or indirect consequences of the disease, such as glaucoma or hydrocephalus. In many cases several mechanisms produce the clinical picture.

desmosome line (D) that marks the outer limiting membrane. These cells contain typical melanosomes at different stages of maturity and large lysosomes with curvilinear profiles (asterisks). The outer portions of photoreceptors are atrophic, and only fine cytoplasmic processes of Müller cells occupy the space separating the retina from the degenerating RPE. (×8,000 before 20% reduction.) (From J. Libert et al. [41].)

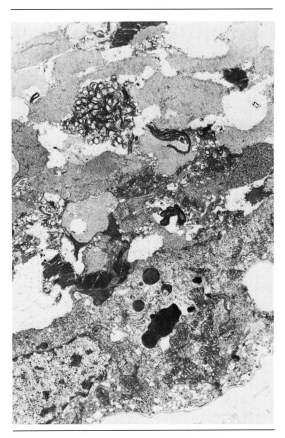

Fig. 5-24. *Retina in Chédiak-Higashi syndrome. The outer portions of photoreceptors appear as undifferentiated cytoplasmic processes in which irregular lamellar structures resemble very abnormal remnants of rod cells. No phagocytic image can be shown within the RPE cells, which have no normal melanosomes and display only large polygonal inclusions that contain a very dense homogeneous material. (×8,000 before 33% reduction.) (From J. Libert et al. [39].)*

Leukodystrophies are the best example of disorders in which the ocular pathology begins within the optic nerve. The severe demyelination of the optic nerve in Krabbe's disease is characterized by abundant multinucleated globoid cells, whose lysosomes are swollen by a sparse, granular material containing innumerable twisted tubules. The retina, by contrast, shows only a few secondary changes with moderate atrophy of the nerve fiber and ganglion cell layers and no sign of lysosomal storage [6, 12]. Ultrastructural studies of the brain and eyes of fetuses afflicted with this disease demonstrate that the lesions appear first within the white matter of the spinal cord and later in all myelinated areas of the brain and peripheral nerves [49]. The histopathology of metachromatic leukodystrophy is more complex, with both optic atrophy and ganglion cell abnormalities (Fig. 5-25). Intracytoplasmic storage and myelin destruction, however, seem much more marked in the optic nerve; degeneration of the myelin sheaths is paralleled by accumulation of myelin whorls, dense homogeneous or granular material, membranous structures, and by the typical herringbone and honeycomb patterns of sulfatides within the lysosomes of the remaining glial cells [10, 47]. Ultrastructural studies of fetuses disclose evidence of sulfatide storage within lysosomes of the glial cells before the beginning of myelination and before the appearance of intraneuronal storage [50]. Biochemical studies also demonstrate that the disease involves primarily the myelin metabolism. Perhaps neuronal storage within the retina results from axonal transport of soluble sulfatides in cytosol from the degenerating optic nerve to the lysosomal system of the neuronal cytoplasm [47].

Optic atrophies described in the ceroid lipofuscinoses probably result from the loss of retinal ganglion cells, rather than from the mild lysosomal storage observed within the optic nerve glial cells [20, 21, 41, 59]. In gangliosidoses and Niemann-Pick disease, optic atrophy is histopathologically nonspecific. Lysosomal storage within retinal neurons is followed by cellular loss, thinning, gliosis, and disorganization of the inner layers and demyelination and gliosis of the optic nerve, with massive accumulation of complex lipids within astrocytes and oligodendrocytes [5, 9, 25, 45]. Ultrastructural studies of fetal eyes revealed early involvement of ganglion cells of the retina and glial cells of the optic nerve [1, 27]; whether optic atrophy was initiated in the retina or in the optic nerve could not be determined.

The causes of optic atrophy are even more complex in the mucopolysaccharidoses and GM_1 gangliosidosis (Fig. 5-26). In addition to marked storage within ganglion and glial cells, extensive vacuolization of the connective tissue cells within the nerve sheaths may result in compression atrophy [5, 29]. Glaucoma may also develop, particularly in MPS I-S, and contribute to optic nerve damage. Some patients suffer from acute or chronic hydrocephalus, probably related to involvement of the meninges, and the impaired cerebrospinal fluid outflow results in progressive optic atrophy [22].

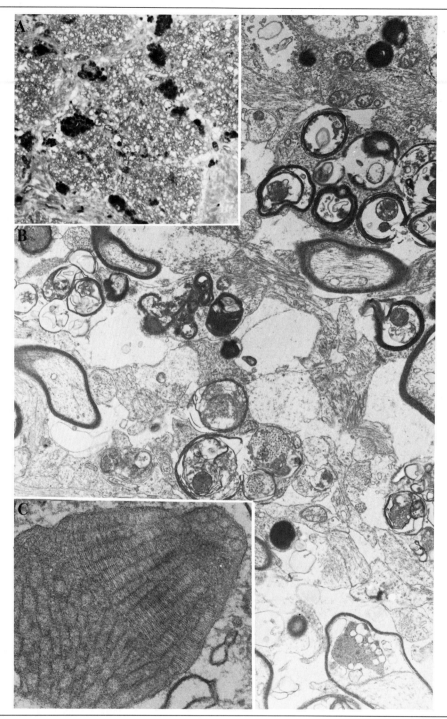

Fig. 5-25. *Optic nerve in metachromatic leukodystrophy. A. Toluidine blue stains metachromatically the numerous sulfatide inclusions of the glial cells. (×400 before 11% reduction.) B. Optic atrophy is very evident by electron microscopy. Few axons remain intact. Some of them show different stages of degeneration, but most have disappeared and are replaced by proliferating glial cells, which contain myelin debris and pleomorphic lysosomal inclusions. Myelin sheaths are also profoundly disorganized and fragmented. (×10,000 before 11% reduction.) C. At high magnification typical sulfatide inclusions are represented by honeycomb and herringbone patterns. (×100,000 before 11% reduction.) (B, from J. Libert et al., Ocular findings in metachromatic leukodystophy: an electron microscope and enzyme study in different clinical and genetic variants, Arch. Ophthalmol. 97:1495, 1979, Copyright 1979, American Medical Association.)*

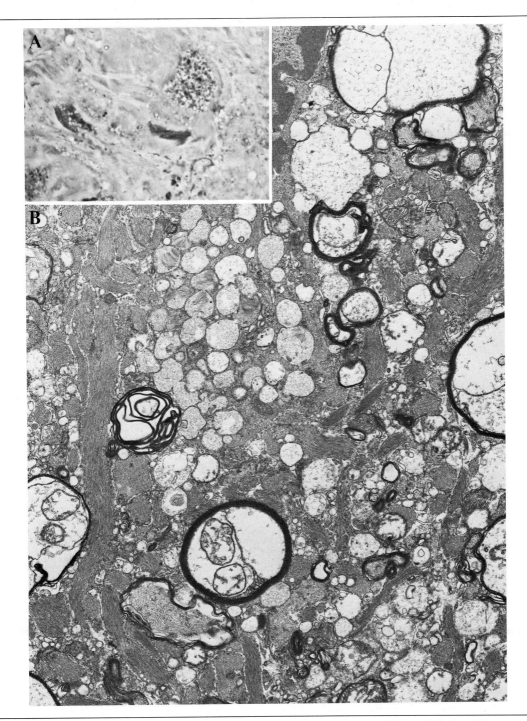

Fig. 5-26. *Optic nerve. A. Mucopolysaccharidosis I-H. The sheaths of the optic nerve are infiltrated with ballooned histiocytes containing many mucopolysaccharide inclusions. (×800.) B. GM₁ gangliosidosis. Axonal loss and glial proliferation are evident, as is stored mucopolysaccharide-like material associated with some lamellar structures within glial cells. (×10,000).*

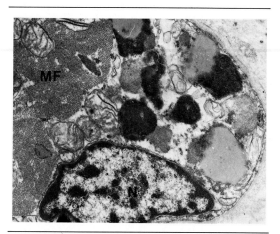

Fig. 5-27. *Oculomotor muscle. As in other neuronal ceroid lipofuscinoses, involvement of extraocular muscle fibers is a rule in Kufs' disease. Lysosomes are distended by a dense macular material in curvilinear and fingerprint patterns. (N = nucleus, MF = myofibrils.) (×14,000 before 28% reduction.)*

OCULAR MOVEMENTS

Oculomotor muscles are often involved in lysosomal storage disease. Pompe's disease affects muscle principally, with lysosomal and intracytoplasmic accumulation of glycogen. Numerous lysosomal vacuoles are seen in the periphery of the fibers in the mucopolysaccharidoses, fucosidosis, and GM_1 gangliosidosis. Lipid-containing inclusions are evident in Niemann-Pick disease. Ceroid lipofuscin, which accumulates within muscle fibers in all forms of ceroid lipofuscinosis, is of diagnostic importance in Kufs' disease, in which conjunctiva and skin are inconstantly affected (Fig. 5-27). However, these abnormalities never seem to produce clinical signs, probably because they are masked by neurologic involvement.

Nystagmus has often been reported in the sphingolipidoses. Although sometimes related directly to the disease, it is usually the typical pendular nystagmus of patients who became blind early in life, either from retinal degeneration or optic atrophy. Progressive oculomotor disintegration paralleling general neurologic deterioration has also been described in the sphingolipidoses.

More specific supranuclear disorders occur in chronic lipidoses. They affect the horizontal gaze in juvenile Gaucher's disease and the vertical gaze in type C Niemann-Pick disease and in juvenile ophthalmoplegic lipidosis (also called sea-blue histiocytosis) [3, 42, 52, 54]. These supranuclear ophthalmoplegias are characterized by inability to move the eyes voluntarily or to follow an object either horizontally or vertically, although the integrity of the gaze pathways is shown by the full range of movements generated by oculovestibular testing using the "doll's-eye" maneuver. Histopathologic studies of the brain demonstrate widespread lysosomal storage in deep neurons and particularly in the subthalamic region and reticular formation [42]. These lesions probably interrupt the pathways descending from the frontal and occipital cortices, which are concerned with the control of voluntary movements and visual fixation.

CONCLUSIONS

Ocular signs are part of the general findings in most inborn lysosomal diseases. These signs are related to physical mechanisms in the cornea and lens and to metabolic or toxic mechanisms in the retina and optic nerve. The ocular changes often present early symptoms and suggest the diagnosis as the clinical course is just beginning. Ophthalmologists can easily confirm the diagnosis by ultrastructural study of a conjunctival biopsy and enzyme analyses of tears.

As no treatment exists for these disorders, the only approach is prevention based on early screening. The risk for a couple of heterozygotes of having an affected child is 1 in 4 in autosomal recessive transmission, and the risk for a mother is 1 in 2 of having an affected boy with Hunter's disease or an affected child, male or female, with Fabry's disease, two diseases with X-linked transmission. Because people have children during a relatively short period of their lives, early recognition of a first affected child is essential to allow time for genetic counseling and to prevent the birth of another affected child. It is important to seek ocular signs very carefully in these cases, so that parents may avoid repetition of the profound trauma of the life of an abnormal child whose condition deteriorates progressively and irreversibly until an early death.

REFERENCES

1. Adachi, M., Schneck, L., and Volk, B. W. Ultrastructural studies of eight cases of fetal Tay-Sachs disease. *Lab. Invest.* 30:102, 1974.

2. Armstrong, D., and Koppang, N. Histochemical Evidence of Lipid Peroxidation in Canine Ceroid-Lipofuscinosis: Relationship to Cytotoxicity. In D. Armstrong, N. Koppang, and J. A. Rider (Eds.), *Ceroid-Lipofuscinosis (Batten's Disease)*. Amsterdam: Elsevier, 1982. P. 159.

3. Arsénio-Nunes, M. L., and Goutières, F. Morphological diagnosis of Niemann-Pick disease type C by skin and conjunctival biopsies. *Acta Neuropathol. [Suppl.] (Berl.)* 7:204, 1981.

4. Beckerman, B. L., and Rapin, I. Ceroid lipofuscinosis. *Am. J. Ophthalmol.* 80:73, 1975.

5. Brownstein, S., et al. Sandhoff's disease (G_{M2} gangliosidosis type 2): Histopathology and ultrastructure of the eye. *Arch. Ophthalmol.* 98:1089, 1980.

6. Brownstein, S., et al. Optic nerve in globoid leukodystrophy (Krabbe's disease). *Arch. Ophthalmol.* 96:864, 1978.

7. Ceuterick, C., et al. Sanfilippo A disease in the fetus: Comparison of pre- and postnatal cases. *Neuropädiatrie* 11:176, 1980.

8. Cogan, D. G., et al. Fundal abnormalities of Gaucher's disease. *Arch. Ophthalmol.* 98:2202, 1980.

9. Cogan, D. G., and Kuwabara, T. The sphingolipidoses and the eye. *Arch. Ophthalmol.* 79:437, 1968.

10. Cogan, D. G., Kuwabara, T., and Moser, H. Metachromatic leucodystrophy. *Ophthalmologica* 160:2, 1970.

11. Del Monte, M. A., et al. Histopathology of Sanfilippo's syndrome. *Arch. Ophthalmol.* 101:1255, 1983.

12. Emery, J. M., Green, W. R., and Huff, D. S. Krabbe's disease: Histopathology and ultrastructure of the eye. *Am. J. Ophthalmol.* 74:400, 1972.

13. Font, R. L., and Fine, B. S. Ocular pathology in Fabry's disease: Histochemical and electron microscopic observations. *Am. J. Ophthalmol.* 73:419, 1972.

14. Franceschetti, A. T. Fabry disease: Ocular manifestations. *Birth Defects* 12(3):195, 1976.

15. François, J. Ocular manifestations of the mucopolysaccharidoses. *Ophthalmologica* 169:345, 1974.

16. François, J. Ocular manifestations of inborn errors of carbohydrate and lipid metabolism. *Bibl. Ophthalmol.* 84:I–VII, 1, 1975.

17. François, J., et al. Cystinosis: A clinical and histopathologic study. *Am. J. Ophthalmol.* 73:643, 1972.

18. Garner, A. Ocular pathology of GM_2 gangliosidosis–type 2 (Sandhoff's disease). *Br. J. Ophthalmol.* 57:514, 1973.

19. Goebel, H. H., Fix, J. D., and Zeman, W. Retinal pathology in GM_1 gangliosidosis, type II. *Am. J. Ophthalmol.* 75:434, 1973.

20. Goebel, H. H., Fix, J. D., and Zeman, W. The fine structure of the retina in neuronal ceroid-lipofuscinosis. *Am. J. Ophthalmol.* 77:25, 1974.

21. Goebel, H. H., Zeman, W., and Damaske, E. An ultrastructural study of the retina in the Jansky-Bielschowsky type of neuronal ceroid-lipofuscinosis. *Am. J. Ophthalmol.* 83:70, 1977.

22. Goldberg, M. F., Scott, C. I., and McKusick, V. A. Hydrocephalus and papilledema in the Maroteaux-Lamy syndrome (mucopolysaccharidosis type VI). *Am. J. Ophthalmol.* 69:969, 1970.

23. Goldman, J. N., and Benedek, G. B. The relationship between morphology and transparency in the non-swelling corneal stroma of the shark. *Invest. Ophthalmol.* 6:574, 1967.

24. Goldman, J. N., et al. Structural alterations affecting transparency in swollen human cornea. *Invest. Ophthalmol.* 7:501, 1968.

25. Harcourt, R. B., and Dobbs, R. H. Ultrastructure of the retina in Tay-Sachs's disease. *Br. J. Ophthalmol.* 52:898, 1968.

26. Hers, H. G. Inborn lysosomal diseases. *Gastroenterology* 48:625, 1965.

27. Howes, E. L., Jr., et al. Ocular pathology of infantile Niemann-Pick disease: Study of fetus of 23 weeks' gestation. *Arch. Ophthalmol.* 93:494, 1975.

28. Kenyon, K. R. Ocular Ultrastructure of Inherited Metabolic Diseases. In M. F. Goldberg (Ed.), *Genetic and Metabolic Eye Disease*. Boston: Little, Brown and Co., 1974. Pp. 139–185.

29. Kenyon, K. R. Ocular manifestations and pathology of systemic mucopolysaccharidoses. *Birth Defects* 12(3):133, 1976.

30. Kenyon, K. R., et al. Mucolipidosis IV: Histopathology of conjunctiva, cornea, and skin. *Arch. Ophthalmol.* 97:1106, 1979.

31. Kenyon, K. R., et al. The systemic mucopolysaccharidoses: Ultrastructural and histochemical studies of conjunctiva and skin. *Am. J. Ophthalmol.* 73:811, 1972.

32. Kenyon, K. R., and Sensenbrenner, J. A. Electron microscopy of cornea and conjunctiva in childhood cystinosis. *Am. J. Ophthalmol.* 78:68, 1974.

33. Kenyon, K. R., et al. Ocular pathology of the Maroteaux-Lamy syndrome (systemic mucopolysaccharidosis type VI): Histologic and ultrastructural report of two cases. *Am. J. Ophthalmol.* 73:718, 1972.

34. Klintworth, G. K. Current concept of macular corneal dystrophy. *Birth Defects* 18 (6):463, 1982.

35. Kolb, H., and Gouras, P. Electron microscopic observations of human retinitis pigmentosa, dominantly inherited. *Invest. Ophthalmol.* 13:487, 1974.

36. Libert, J. Les maladies lysosomiales de stockage et la rétine. *J. Fr. Ophtalmol.* 1:699, 1978.

37. Libert, J. Diagnosis of lysosomal storage diseases by the ultrastructural study of conjunctival biopsies. *Pathol. Annu.* 15 (Part 1):37, 1980.

38. Libert, J. La fucosidose: Ultrastructure oculaire. *J. Fr. Ophtalmol.* 7:519, 1984.

39. Libert, J., et al. Ocular findings in Chédiak-Higashi disease: A light and electron microscopic study of two patients. *Birth Defects* 18(6):327, 1982.

40. Libert, J., et al. Ocular ultrastructural study in a fetus with type II glycogenosis. *Br. J. Ophthalmol.* 61:476, 1977.

41. Libert, J., et al. Les céroide-lipofuscinoses: Ultrastructure oculaire et diagnostic par biopsie conjonctivale. *Arch. Ophtalmol. (Paris)* 37:613, 1977.

42. Libert, J., et al. Ultrastructural Studies in Ophthalmoplegic Dystonic Lipidosis. In A. Huber and D. Klein (Eds.), *Neurogenetics and Neuro-Ophthalmology.* Amsterdam: Elsevier, 1981. P. 317.

43. Libert, J., Tondeur, M., and van Hoof, F. The use of conjunctival biopsy and enzyme analysis in tears for the diagnosis of homozygotes and heterozygotes with Fabry disease. *Birth Defects* 12(3):221, 1976.

44. Libert, J., and Toussaint, D. Tortuosities of retinal and conjunctival vessels in lysosomal storage diseases. *Birth Defects* 18(6):347, 1982.

45. Libert, J., Toussaint, D., and Guiselings, R. Ocular findings in Niemann-Pick disease. *Am. J. Ophthalmol.* 80:991, 1975.

46. Libert, J., et al. Ocular findings in I-cell disease (mucolipidosis type II). *Am. J. Ophthalmol.* 83:617, 1977.

47. Libert, J., et al. Ocular findings in metachromatic leukodystrophy: An electron microscopic and enzyme study in different clinical and genetic variants. *Arch. Ophthalmol.* 97:1495, 1979.

48. Lowden, J. A., and O'Brien, J. S. Sialidosis: A review of human neuroaminidase deficiency. *Am J. Hum. Genet.* 31:1, 1979.

49. Martin, J. J., et al. Fetal Krabbe leukodystrophy: A morphologic study of two cases. *Acta Neuropathol. (Berl.)* 53:87, 1981.

50. Meier, C., and Bischoff, A. Sequence of morphological alterations in the nervous system of metachromatic leucodystrophy: Light- and electronmicroscopic observations in the central and peripheral nervous system in a prenatally diagnosed foetus of 22 weeks. *Acta Neuropathol (Berl.)* 36:369, 1976.

51. Merin, S., et al. The cornea in mucolipidosis IV. *J. Pediatr. Ophthalmol.* 13:289, 1976.

52. Miller, J. D., McCluer, R., and Kanfer, J. N. Gaucher's disease: Neurologic disorder in adult siblings. *Ann. Intern. Med.* 78:883, 1973.

53. Murphree, A. L., et al. Cataract in mannosidosis. *Birth Defects* 12(3):319, 1976.

54. Neville, B. G., et al. A neurovisceral storage disease with vertical supranuclear ophthalmoplegia, and its relationship to Niemann-Pick disease: A report of nine patients. *Brain* 96:97, 1973.

55. Rapin, I., et al. The cherry-red spot–myoclonus syndrome. *Ann. Neurol.* 3:234, 1978.

56. Robb, R. M., and Kuwabara, T. The ocular pathology of type A Niemann-Pick disease: A light and electron microscopic study. *Invest. Ophthalmol.* 12:366, 1973.

57. Sanderson, P. O., et al. Cystinosis: A clinical, histopathologic, and ultrastructural study. *Arch. Ophthalmol.* 91:270, 1974.

58. Santino, D., and Scialfa, A. Un caso di sindrome di Béguéz-César-Steinbrinck-Chédiak-Higashi (albinismo universale incompleto con albinoidismo oculare, epatosplenomegalia, inclusioni leucocitarie atipiche) con grave compromissione dell' elettroretinogramma. *Ann. Ottal.* 92:793, 1966.

59. Schochet, S. S., Font, R. L., and Morris, H. H., III. Jansky-Bielschowsky form of neuronal ceroid lipofuscinosis: Ocular pathology of the Batten-Vogt syndrome. *Arch. Ophthalmol.* 98:1083, 1980.

60. Sher, N. A., Letson, R. D., and Desnick, R. J. The ocular manifestations in Fabry's disease. *Arch. Ophthalmol.* 97:671, 1979.

61. Sher, N. A., et al. Central retinal artery occlusion complicating Fabry's disease. *Arch. Ophthalmol.* 96:815, 1978.

62. Tarkkanen, A., Haltai, M., and Merenmies, L. Ocular pathology in infantile type of neuronal ceroid-lipofuscinosis. *J. Pediatr. Ophthalmol.* 14:235, 1977.

63. Topping, T. M., et al. Ultrastructural ocular pathology of Hunter's syndrome: Systemic mucopolysaccharidosis type II. *Arch. Ophthalmol.* 86:164, 1971.

64. Ueno, H., et al. Clinical and histopathological studies of a case with juvenile form of Gaucher's disease. *Jpn. J. Ophthalmol.* 21:98, 1977.

65. Ueno, H., et al. Electron microscopic study of Gaucher cells in the eye. *Jpn. J. Ophthalmol.* 24:75, 1980.

66. Van Hoof, F., et al. The assay of lacrimal tear enzymes and the ultrastructural analysis of conjunctival biopsies: New techniques for the study of inborn lysosomal diseases. *Metab. Ophthalmol.* 1:165, 1977.

67. Weingeist, T. A., and Blodi, F. C. Fabry's disease: Ocular findings in a female carrier—A light and electron microscopic study. *Arch. Ophthalmol.* 85:169, 1971.

68. Wong, V. G., et al. Intralysosomal cystine crystals in cystinosis. *Invest. Ophthalmol.* 9:83, 1970.

69. Wong, V. G., Lietman, P. S., and Seegmiller, J. E. Alterations of pigment epithelium in cystinosis. *Arch. Ophthalmol.* 77:361, 1967.

70. Young, R. W., and Bok, D. Participation of the retinal pigment epithelium in the rod outer segment renewal process. *J. Cell Biol.* 42:392, 1969.

71. Zeman, W. Batten disease: Ocular features, differential diagnosis and diagnosis by enzyme analysis. *Birth Defects* 12(3):441, 1976.

6

Animal Models of Metabolic Eye Diseases

Gustavo Aguirre
Lawrence Stramm
Mark Haskins
Peter Jezyk

Many of the genetic diseases thus far described in animals affect the eye. In some cases the diseases are primary to the eye, and no abnormalities have been found in extraocular tissues. In others the ocular lesions are the result of a more generalized metabolic defect expressed systemically as well as in the eye. It is the purpose of this chapter to describe the ocular manifestation in animals of these generalized metabolic abnormalities. We have selected to review diseases occurring in domestic rather than laboratory species (i.e., rodents and lagomorphs) because this is an area that has received little attention in the past. There has recently been a very rapid growth in the field of veterinary medical genetics, with many new disorders being described; however, the information on the ocular manifestations of these diseases has not been compiled and generally is not readily available to the medical ophthalmologist.

Current intensive animal production and breeding practices have resulted in an increased frequency of inherited diseases. Inbreeding and linebreeding, coupled in some cases with artificial insemination, superovulation, and embryo transfer methods, can increase the gene frequencies of the recessively inherited diseases. For example, the gene frequency of mannosidosis in New Zealand cattle has reached 5 percent [57], while the gene frequency of retinal degeneration in Abys-

sinian cats in Sweden is so high that 89 percent of the population is either affected or carries this recessive gene [85]. Increasing awareness and interest in the inherited metabolic diseases, in some cases because of their economic impact on the livestock industry, has led to improved screening and identification methods [53, 57]. This in turn has resulted in the recent identification of previously unrecognized metabolic diseases in animals.

Because inherited metabolic diseases that occur in humans and animals often affect the same metabolic pathway, animals can serve as models of the human diseases. Some of these animal models have been described recently, and only limited information is available on the ocular lesions and their application to ophthalmic research. These are thus models in the process of development. Other ocular diseases have been defined in far greater detail in animals than have their counterparts in humans. These can perhaps be described as animal diseases in search of a human model.

Regardless of the situation, studies of animal models of inherited metabolic diseases offer new perspectives for investigating disease mechanisms in the eye. Diseased animals can usually be bred in sufficient numbers to allow sampling of tissues at various stages of disease, thereby characterizing the evolution of the disease and differentiating the primary abnormality from the secondary manifestations of the disease. They also can be used to investigate therapeutic modalities that may be later applied to similar diseases in human beings.

In this review the inherited metabolic abnor-

Supported in part by National Eye Institute Grants EY-1244, EY-5199, and EY-1538; National Institute of Arthritis and Metabolic Diseases Grant AM-25759; National Institutes of Health University of Pennsylvania Genetics Center Grant GM-20138; the British Retinitis Pigmentosa Society; and the Charles E. Goetz Teaching and Research Fund.

malities of domestic animals will be presented according to the following classification:

Disorders of carbohydrate metabolism
Disorders of amino acid metabolism
Disorders of lysosomal enzymes
Other diseases

DISORDERS OF CARBOHYDRATE METABOLISM

Diabetes Mellitus

Diabetes mellitus occurs spontaneously in the dog and, less frequently, in the cat. The disease in dogs has been shown to be inherited in the keeshond breed [74] and is suspected of being inherited in other breeds [93]. Experimental diabetes mellitus in the dog has been readily produced and was analogous, both clinically and pathologically, to the spontaneous disease [28].

The most commonly reported ocular complication of spontaneous diabetes in the dog was cataracts. Initially, there was vacuolation of the lens fibers in a circumferential pattern in the equatorial cortex; the vacuoles extended with the newly formed lens fibers into the superficial anterior and posterior cortical regions, coalesced, and opacified the superficial cortical fibers. The process was continuous and, in dogs, rapid. Progressive opacification of the lens fibers ultimately resulted in a complete mature cataract. Treatment of diabetes mellitus with insulin may have retarded the rate of progression, but complete cataracts still developed in most dogs within 1 year of diagnosis and initiation of medical treatment. In contrast to the dog, cataracts have been seldom recognized or reported in diabetic cats.

It is not known why cataracts developed in diabetic dogs but not cats. The level of aldose reductase activity in the lens has been shown to regulate the rate of cataractogenesis in experimental diabetes. That is, high levels of activity, as in the rat and the degu, preferentially favored the sorbitol pathway and the development of cataracts; very low activity levels, as present in mice, prevented the development of diabetic cataracts [121]. It is possible that an analogous situation occurs in the dog and cat.

Alternatively, cataracts may have developed in dogs because their medical management did not favor the exact control of blood sugar. In most diabetic dogs, isophane insulin suspension (NPH insulin) has been used; however, this form of insulin is short acting, and most dogs are controlled to allow some glycosuria. When protamine zinc (PZ) or lente insulin dosage was individually adjusted to prevent significant glycosuria, blood sugar levels were more rigidly controlled and cataracts seldom formed [45].

In laboratory studies of spontaneous or induced diabetes mellitus in the dog, retinopathy, consisting of small capillary aneurysms and neovascularization, has been reported [28]. New vessel growth occurred primarily intraretinally rather than extending and proliferating into the retinal surface or vitreous. These laboratory studies, however, contrasted with clinical observations, which have failed to demonstrate proliferative or background retinopathy in spontaneously diabetic animals.

Glycogen Storage Diseases

Generalized glycogen storage disease that resembled Pompe's disease (type II glycogenosis) in humans histologically, histochemically, or both has been described in a cat [102], Corriedale sheep [81], Lapland dog [125], and two breeds of cattle—shorthorn [51] and Brahma [90]. It was only in cattle and, to a lesser extent, the dog that the diseases were adequately characterized and deficiency of acid α-glucosidase was confirmed [50, 124]. Ocular lesions were observed in both cattle [23] and dogs [125].

In cattle the disease was inherited as a simple autosomal recessive trait. Although affected animals were clinically normal at birth, there was increased muscle glycogen deposition and deficient activity of acid α-glucosidase [51]. Deficient enzyme activity was confirmed in lymphocytes, liver, kidney, skeletal and cardiac muscles [50], spinal cord, and occipital cortex [23]. Animals heterozygous for the disease showed reduced levels of acid α-glucosidase activity but no clinical signs or excessive accumulation of tissue glycogen [51].

Two clinical forms that were recognized in affected animals derived from a single, inbred family of cattle [51] have been compared to the infantile and childhood forms of the human disease. In both there was early onset, rapid progression, and death within the first 18 months of age. In the "infantile form" of the disease, affected cattle died from cardiac failure, whereas animals with the "childhood form" had clinical signs related to disease of the skeletal muscles. A late-onset adult form of the disease, analogous to acid maltase deficiency in humans, has not been recognized in cattle.

Ocular changes were observed in affected cattle as young as 1 month of age. Retinal ganglion cells as well as cells in the inner nuclear layer were swollen and vacuolated and contained a material that was periodic acid–Schiff (PAS) positive and diastase sensitive (Fig. 6-1A). The photoreceptor layer, however, was normal. These results were similar to those reported for human type II glycogenosis [33]. Optic nerve glia were markedly distended and had a peripheral foamy cytoplasm with a central PAS-positive, diastase-sensitive material. In longitudinal sections these glial cells

Fig. 6-1. *Glycogenosis type II, cattle. A. Retinal ganglion cells (*arrows) *are swollen and vacuolated. (×640.) B. Rows of swollen and vacuolated glial cells are present along the pial septa of the optic nerve. (×250.) (From R. D. Cook et al. [23].)*

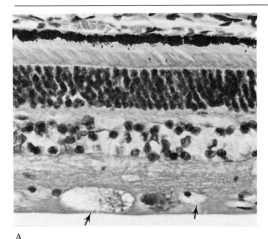

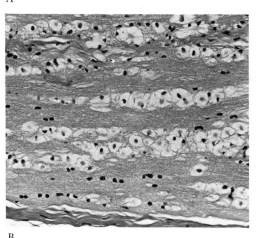

B

were oriented in rows between the nerve fibers (Fig. 6-1B). In general glycogen was present in both neurons and glia, either free in the cytoplasm or within membrane-bound structures with glycogen granules of different densities. It is surprising that no distinct neurologic deficits were attributed to the extensive intracellular glycogen storage in both retinal and central nervous system (CNS) neurons [23].

Lafora's Disease

Lafora's disease, a distinct member of the group of familial progressive myoclonus epilepsies, has been reported in the dog [49]. Complex glycoproteins accumulate in neurons and other cell types [49], and the disease has been considered to be a disorder of carbohydrate metabolism [129]. A specific biochemical defect has not been determined.

In both humans and dogs, basophilic, spherical, laminated inclusions (Lafora's bodies) were found in CNS and retinal neurons (Fig. 6-2). The inclu-

Fig. 6-2. *Lafora's disease, dog. Multiple inclusions (*arrows) *in retinal ganglion cells (A) and occipital cortex neurons (B) of a 3-year-old affected dog. (×375.) (From J. M. Holland et al., Lafora's disease in the dog. Am. J. Pathol. 58:509, 1970.)*

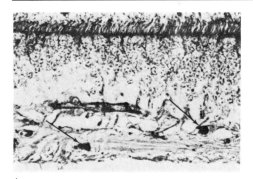

A

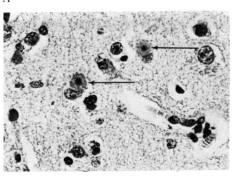

B

sions were present in morphologically normal neurons, or they coalesced into masses that obliterated the nucleus.

DISORDERS OF AMINO ACID METABOLISM

Tyrosinemia

Congenital oculocutaneous tyrosinemia has been described in the dog [75]. The disease was analogous to tyrosinemia type II (Richner-Harnhart syndrome) in humans and shared many of the clinical features of a similar hereditary disease of mink [36]. In the affected dog there was deficient activity of tyrosine aminotransferase in both the cytosolic and mitochondrial fractions of liver homogenates [54]. Serum and urine tyrosine levels were 20 to 30 times higher than normal, and metabolites of tyrosine were identified in the urine.

Superficial neovascular keratitis and cataracts were present in the affected dog when first examined at 16 weeks of age. These lesions were associated with plantar and nasal ulcerations. With time the neovascularization diminished, but the cornea remained opacified (Fig. 6-3A). The cutaneous lesions progressed: Plantar hyperkeratosis and erosions worsened, there was a loss of nails and ulcerations of the skin at the nail fold area, and additional epithelial defects appeared throughout the body. Mental retardation, present in some humans with tyrosinemia type II [18, 35], could not be evaluated in the dog.

A peripheral corneal and conjunctival biopsy specimen from the affected dog showed subepithelial and anterior stromal blood vessels in the cornea but little evidence of active inflammation. In some areas collagen fibers were of random diameter and poorly oriented; in others the collagen lamellae were normal. Although neither intracellular nor extracellular crystals were observed in the corneal epithelium or stroma, the stromal keratocytes had a dilatated rough endoplasmic reticulum and a greater than normal accumulation of cytoplasmic filament bundles. Examination of the eyes after death showed a keratitis limited to the outer half of the cornea. Blood vessels were present in the affected stroma, and there was diffuse epithelial disease. In the best-preserved areas, the epithelial layer was only four cells thick and lacked prominent basal and wing cell layers. In most areas, however, the epithelium was only one or two layers thick (Fig. 6-3B). With the exception of the lens, which showed cataractous changes,

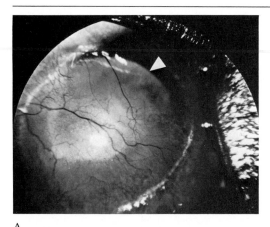

A

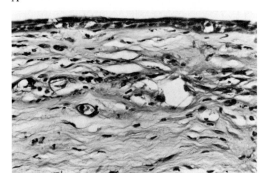

B

Fig. 6-3. *Tyrosinemia type II, dog. A. Superficial keratitis and corneal opacification. Arrowhead indicates temporal pupillary border. B. Note anterior stromal vascularization, disorientation of stromal lamellae, and epithelial thinning. (×235.)*

no other abnormalities were found in the ocular tissues.

Gyrate Atrophy of the Choroid and Retina

Hereditary diseases of the visual cells and retinal pigment epithelium (RPE) that cause retinal degeneration and blindness occur in a number of animal species [2]. In most the diseases are specific to the retina, and extraocular manifestations have not been found. It is only in the cat that a generalized defect of ornithine metabolism that is similar to gyrate atrophy of the choroid and retina in humans has been recognized.

In a cat affected with gyrate atrophy, ornithine-δ-aminotransferase (OAT) activity in tissues (liver, kidney, and skeletal muscles) and cultured fibroblasts was undetectable using either high or low pyridoxine concentrations. The activities of other mitochondrial matrix enzymes were, in general, similar to normal levels [117, 118]. This deficiency in OAT activity was associated with a 60-fold increase in plasma ornithine (1,318 mM) and overflow ornithinuria. This concentration was at the upper limit of values in humans with gyrate atrophy [113].

Histologically, there was extensive neuroretinal and pigment epithelial damage and loss. Pigment epithelial and photoreceptor cells were missing; the inner retinal layers came into close apposition with the tapetal or choroidal layers, depending on retinal location. Preservation of inner retinal integrity was variable. In the nontapetal zone adjacent to the disc, an extremely thin, disorganized, and gliosed neural retina was present, whereas the tapetal zone of the posterior pole had distinct inner nuclear, plexiform, and nerve fiber layers (Fig. 6-4A). More peripherally, inner retinal layer organization was completely lost (Fig. 6-4B). Atrophy of the choriocapillaris and small choroidal vessels was also prominent. A distinct choriocapillaris layer was not present between the atrophic retina and choroid. Only isolated segments of choriocapillaris remained. The vascular and RPE atrophic changes were specific to the disease, as they are rarely observed in cats with either hereditary or sporadic retinal atrophy.

In general the clinical and biochemical abnormalities found in the affected cat are analogous to gyrate atrophy of choroid and retina in humans. As in humans, in the cat the major clinical abnormalities were limited to the eyes, specifically the retina and choriocapillaris. However, the uniformity of the ophthalmoscopic appearance of degeneration in the affected cat differed from the scalloped, sharply demarcated lesions characteristic of humans with gyrate atrophy. The affected cat also did not have cataracts, which appear to be present in most affected humans by the third decade [113].

DISORDERS OF LYSOSOMAL ENZYMES

The Gangliosidoses

GM$_1$ GANGLIOSIDOSIS

GM$_1$ gangliosidosis has been reported in Siamese and mixed breed cats [10, 14, 29, 84], Friesian cattle [27, 104], and dogs [99]. In these species the disease was characterized clinically by progressive neurologic deterioration, appeared to follow an autosomal recessive inheritance pattern, and resulted from a deficiency of the lysosomal hydrolase β-galactosidase. In general, affected animals showed an increased content of ganglioside GM$_1$ in the cerebral cortex [27, 29, 99, 103]. Visceral storage, with or without accompanying organomegaly, was observed in affected cats and dogs but not in cattle, and resulted from the accumulation of glycolipids and glycopeptides (Table 6-1).

In affected animals neurons in the brain, spinal cord, and autonomic ganglia were distended by the accumulation of membrane-bound inclusions; in severely affected neurons these inclusions resembled the membranous cytoplasmic bodies (MCBs) found in humans [29, 84, 99, 103]. In Siamese cats other membrane-bound inclusions were present in less-affected neurons; these

Fig. 6-4. *Gyrate atrophy, cat. A. In posterior pole pigment epithelial and photoreceptor layers are lost, but inner retinal layers are preserved. (INL = inner nuclear layer; IPL = inner plexiform layer; NFL = nerve fiber layer.) B. More peripherally, a prominent ganglion cell (arrow) is present in the gliosed and disorganized neuroretina located adjacent to the tapetum lucidum (TL). (×575.) (From D. L. Valle et al. [117].)*

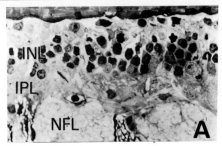
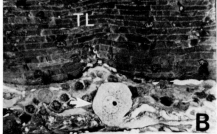

Table 6-1. *Gangliosidoses in Domestic Animals*

Feature	GM$_1$ gangliosidosis	GM$_1$ gangliosidosis	GM$_1$ gangliosidosis	GM$_2$ gangliosidosis	GM$_2$ gangliosidosis	GM$_2$ gangliosidosis
Species	Cat	Cattle	Dog	Cat	Dog	Pig
Age at clinical onset	3–4 months	3 months	5 months	1–2 months	6 months	3 months
Inheritance	AR	AR	AR	AR	AR	AR
Enzyme deficiency	β-Galactosidase	β-Galactosidase	β-Galactosidase	β-Hexosaminidases A and B	NR	β-Hexosaminidase A (partial)
Neuronal storage	Ganglioside GM$_1$	Ganglioside GM$_1$	Ganglioside GM$_1$	Ganglioside GM$_2$	Ganglioside GM$_2$	Ganglioside GM$_2$
Hepatic storage	Glycolipids and glycopeptides	–	Glycolipids and glycopeptides	Glycolipids	–	–
Corneal opacities	+	–	–	+	–	–
Lenticular storage	+	–	–	NR	NR	NR
Retinal ganglion cell storage	+	+	+	+	+	+
References	10–12, 29, 84	27, 103, 104	99	24	63–65	71, 72, 94

AR = autosomal recessive; NR = not reported; + = present; – = absent.

inclusions contained a dense amorphous material surrounded by laminated structures as well as irregular lamellar structures appearing as membranous whorls [29].

Corneal and lenticular storage was reported only in the affected mixed breed cats. Fine granular opacification of the posterior cornea was observed [84]. The corneal endothelium was heavily vacuolated, and in some instances the cells were distended by the accumulation of inclusions. Keratocytes, especially those in the anterior and posterior regions, contained numerous empty vacuoles. A granular deposit was also noted in the anterior subcapsular epithelium of the lens, a finding not reported in humans.

Retinal ganglion cell storage was reported in the three different species affected with GM_1 gangliosidosis [10, 84, 99, 104]. Clinically this was evident in cats and cattle as numerous intraretinal white to pale gray spots, which probably resulted from protuberances of the inner limiting membrane caused by retinal ganglion cell distention (Fig. 6-5A). Histologically, the retinal ganglion cells and, to a lesser extent, amacrine cells of cattle were swollen, and the cytoplasm had accumulated numerous MCBs (Fig. 6-5B) [104]. These structures probably resulted from storage of ganglioside GM_1 and other glycolipids and differed from the clear vacuolated corneal inclusions that contained water-soluble polysaccharides.

Retinal ganglion cell storage occurred in the different types of GM_1 gangliosidosis in animals, but the macular cherry-red spot so characteristic of some of these human diseases was not observed. It must be noted, however, that these animal species lack a fovea, a foveal avascular zone, and the high ganglion cell density that is normally present in the perifoveal region. Thus a cherry-red spot would not occur.

Although the same enzyme deficiency was present and similar substrates accumulated in the human and animal diseases, the distribution and severity of disease, particularly the visceral involvement, differed. This complicates a direct analogy between the animal disease and the clinical subtype of the human disease [12]. Most of the animal diseases, however, share many of the features of human GM_1 gangliosidosis type II.

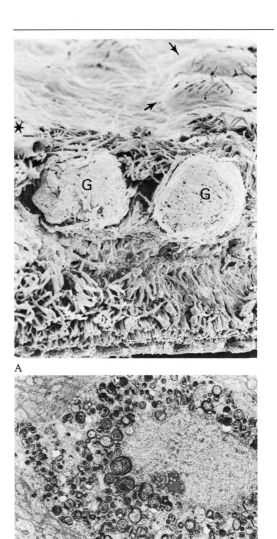

A

B

Fig. 6-5. *GM_1 gangliosidosis, cattle. A. Scanning electron microscopy discloses bulges (*arrows*) in the internal limiting membrane (*asterisk*) that result in distension of retinal ganglion cells (G). (×705.) B. A retinal ganglion cell is distended with membranous cytoplasmic bodies. (×4,285.) (From B. J. Sheahan, W. J. C. Donnelly, and T. D. Grimes [104].)*

GM₂ GANGLIOSIDOSIS

In humans a variety of disorders result from storage of ganglioside GM_2. These recessively inherited lysosomal storage diseases, often referred to as familial amaurotic idiocy, result from a deficiency of one or both isozymes (A and B) of hexosaminidase [88]. In Tay-Sachs disease (GM_2 gangliosidosis type I) hexosaminidase A is deficient; deficiency of both hexosaminidase A and B results in Sandhoff's disease (GM_2 gangliosidosis type II). The juvenile disease (type III) results from a partial deficiency of the A isozyme. GM_2 gangliosidosis has been described in mixed breed cats [24], Yorkshire swine [72, 94, 100], German shorthaired pointers [63, 65], and English setters [39]. In general, affected animals showed early onset of neurologic signs with progressive deterioration and death at a young age (Table 6-1).

The feline disease resulted from a deficiency of both the A and B forms of hexosaminidase, and heterozygotes exhibited intermediate levels of enzyme activity [24]. In the CNS there was storage of material in neurons and perivascular glial cells. Ganglioside content was increased two- to threefold, with ganglioside GM_2 levels accounting for 38 to 44 percent of total gangliosides. Visceral storage of glycolipids was evident in the liver, kidney, splenic macrophages, vascular endothelium, and smooth muscle cells.

Affected animals exhibited corneal opacities. Retinal neurons accumulated inclusions and became distended. The histopathologic lesions, glycolipid storage, and deficiency of both major forms of hexosaminidase were similar to findings in human GM_2 gangliosidosis type II (Sandhoff's disease).

In Yorkshire swine GM_2 gangliosidosis resulted from a partial deficiency of the A form of hexosaminidase [71]. Total brain ganglioside content was two to three times higher than normal, most of which was ganglioside GM_2. Neurons in the brain, spinal cord, and peripheral nerves were affected; their cytoplasm appeared foamy and diffusely vacuolated, and in the older pigs MCBs were present. Glial cells in the cerebral cortex were also affected. However, there was no evidence of wallerian degeneration, demyelination, or amyelination.

Visual impairment was not observed in these animals, perhaps because of their short life span [71]. The only reported ocular lesion was the presence of numerous gray-white spots, presumably distended ganglion cells, scattered diffusely throughout the retina. The morphology of the cytoplasmic inclusions and the degree of neuronal involvement were similar to those in GM_2 gangliosidosis types I and II. The late age of onset,

lack of macrencephaly, the moderate increases in brain gangliosides, and the partial, rather than complete, deficiency of hexosaminidase A were features in common with juvenile GM_2 gangliosidosis (type III) of humans.

In German shorthaired pointers with GM_2 gangliosidosis, ganglioside GM_2 content of the cerebral cortex was increased fivefold. Most of the CNS neurons, including the retinal ganglion cells, were affected [64]. The accumulation of granular material in the cytoplasm was related to cellular enlargement, neuronal degeneration, and necrosis. By electron microscopy the granular inclusions appeared as MCBs having a concentric structure. The histopathologic lesions, particularly the degree of neuronal involvement, appeared to be intermediate between type I and type III GM_2 gangliosidosis of humans. The disease in dogs differed from Sandhoff's disease (type II) in that it was not associated with visceral storage in histiocytes.

The Mucopolysaccharidoses

The mucopolysaccharidoses are a group of genetic diseases resulting from defective degradation of glycosaminoglycans (GAG) [83]. In both humans and other animals, each syndrome has a characteristic combination of clinical signs, tissue storage and urinary excretion of GAG, and a specific lysosomal enzyme deficiency. The general clinical characteristics include dysostosis multiplex, facial dysmorphism, corneal clouding, hepatosplenomegaly, urinary excretion of GAG, and metachromatic granules in blood leukocytes. The lysosomal enzyme deficiency results in neuronal storage of GAG in some of the human and animal diseases; in humans this is accompanied by mental retardation, a condition difficult to assess in other animals. Animal models of mucopolysaccharidosis (MPS) I (cat [42, 46] and dog [105, 106]), MPS VI (Siamese cat [4, 43, 55]), and MPS VII (dog [44]) have been characterized; their features are summarized in Table 6-2. Other apparent mucopolysaccharide storage disorders have been identified in dogs, but the enzymatic changes have not been defined conclusively [45].

The enzyme deficient in each of the animal mucopolysaccharidoses has been identified (Table 6-2) and appeared to be analogous to those in humans. The catabolic pathways, the accumulation of substrates, and the corresponding phenotypic expression of the disease appeared to be

Table 6-2. *Mucopolysaccharide Storage Diseases in Domestic Animals*

Species (breed)	Disease	Enzyme deficiency	Inheritance	Urinary GAG excreted	Corneal clouding	Facial dysmorphism, skeletal deformities	GAG storage in CNS neurons	Alder-Reilly bodies	Visceral GAG storage	Analogous Human Disease	References
Cat (Domestic shorthair)	MPS I	α-L-Iduronidase	AR	Dermatan SO$_4$, heparan SO$_4$	+	+	+	–	+	MPS I, Hurler phenotype	42, 46
Dog (Plott hound)	MPS I	α-L-Iduronidase	AR*	Dermatan SO$_4$ > heparan SO$_4$	+	+	+	–	+	MPS I, Hurler-Scheie phenotype	105, 106
Cat (Siamese)	MPS VI	Arylsulfatase B	AR	Dermatan SO$_4$	+	+	–	+	+	Maroteaux-Lamy syndrome	4, 43, 55, 122
Dog (Mixed breed)	MPS VII	β-Glucuronidase	AR*	Chondroitin 4 and/or 6 SO$_4$ > dermatan SO$_4$	+	+	+	+	+	β-Glucuronidase deficiency, severe phenotype	44

*Inheritance not proved conclusively.
GAG = glycosaminoglycans; CNS = central nervous system; MPS = mucopolysaccharidosis; AR = autosomal recessive.

similar in humans and animals. Some subtle differences, however, were present. Arylsulfatase B, the enzyme deficient in MPS VI, has been reported to be a monomer in humans and a dimer in cats. Two different subtypes of feline MPS VI, both similar in phenotype, result from mutations causing very severe structural alterations in the enzyme molecule. In one, the residual arylsulfatase is in a monomeric form, the activity of which could be increased by dimerization with sulfhydryl compounds such as cystamine [122]. In the second type there is an inactive dimeric enzyme [45].

Diffuse corneal clouding was present in animals affected with MPS (Fig. 6-6A). In MPS VI granular opacities were located in the deeper corneal layers of young animals but were distributed evenly throughout the stroma in older animals (Fig. 6-6B). In MPS I (cats and dogs) and MPS VII (dogs), granular corneal clouding was also prominent [4, 42, 105, 106]. This clouding interfered with examination of anterior and posterior segment structures; iris and fundus detail appeared hazy, as if viewed through ground glass. Ophthalmo-

scopic abnormalities of the retina, however, were not evident, and the animals appeared clinically visual. The electroretinogram (ERG) of cats affected with either MPS I or MPS VI had rod- and cone-mediated responses that were normal in waveform but reduced in amplitude (Fig. 6-7). Since visual cell degeneration did not occur in these animal diseases, we hypothesize that altered electrical conductivity of the outer ocular tunics, resulting from stromal storage of GAG, caused the observed reductions in ERG amplitudes.

Corneal opacification resulted from distention of stromal keratocytes, which accumulated intracytoplasmic inclusions and caused the secondary distortion of the corneal lamellae (Fig. 6-6D). By

Fig. 6-6. *Mucopolysaccharidoses. Corneal granular opacities are present in animals with MPS VII (A, dog) and MPS VI (B, cat). C. MPS VI in cat. Keratocytes contain electron-lucent (asterisk) and granular (arrowhead) cytoplasmic inclusions. (×12,000.) D. MPS I in cat. The inclusions cause keratocyte distention and lamellar disorientation. Endothelial cells contain numerous small vacuolated inclusions but are not hypertrophied. (×500.)*

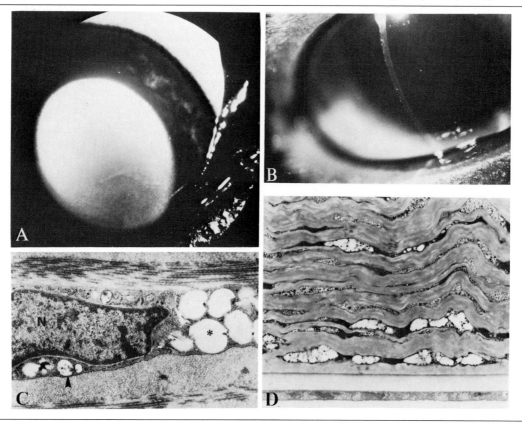

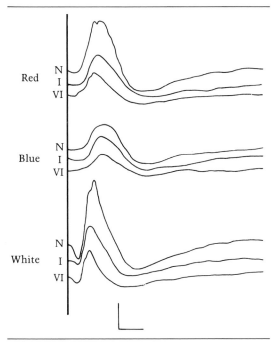

Red N
I
VI

Blue N
I
VI

White N
I
VI

Fig. 6-7. *Mucopolysaccharidoses. Dark-adapted electroretinograms (ERG) from normal cats (N) and cats affected with MPS I (I) and MPS VI (VI) in response to red, blue, and white light. The waveforms and implicit times of ERG from the affected animals are normal, but the amplitudes are reduced. Vertical line at left indicates onset of 20-msec stimulus; vertical calibration mark = 100 μv; horizontal mark = 50 msec.*

electron microscopy these inclusions appeared as membrane-bound electron-lucent vacuoles, although in some a faint granular matrix remained (Fig. 6-6C). The electron-lucent vacuoles probably represented secondary lysosomes whose GAG content was leached during tissue processing [115]. The opacified corneal stroma showed no accumulation of the extracellular material described in MPS VI and MPS I of humans [67] or edema. The absence of edema was surprising in MPS I–affected cats, because there was extensive accumulation of vacuolated inclusions in the endothelial layer (Fig. 6-6D). Thus endothelial cells appeared to function normally in spite of morphologic evidence of disease.

Vacuolated inclusions characteristic of the mucopolysaccharidoses were present in most ocular tissues of affected animals. Their distribution is summarized in Table 6-3. In neuroectoderm-derived tissues from MPS VI–affected cats, there was a difference in disease severity that was cor-

related with the spatial position of the cells within the eye, the degree of pigmentation, or both. The nonpigmented ciliary epithelia showed accumulation of vacuolated inclusions and cellular hypertrophy, but the pigmented epithelial cells remained normal. In contrast, the ciliary epithelium in MPS I–affected dogs and cats was diseased regardless of pigmentation (Fig. 6-8). The pattern of disease distribution present in ciliary epithelia of animals with MPS I and MPS VI was similar to that reported for humans with the analogous diseases [68].

The RPE of MPS VI–affected cats showed abnormalities that were qualitatively similar to those of the ciliary epithelium. Nonpigmented RPE cells became affected earlier in the disease and to a greater extent than did pigmented cells (Fig. 6-9A and B). Accumulation of numerous vacuolated inclusions with subsequent hypertrophy occurred only in nonpigmented RPE cells. The inclusions were of four types: electron-lucent, granular, lamellar, and mixed; the electron-lucent and granular classes predominated (see Fig. 6-11B). The hypertrophied cells occurred singly or in clusters that gave the appearance of a monolayer of hypertrophied RPE cells. The accumulation of intracytoplasmic vacuoles altered the normal distribution of organelles within the RPE cells. The nucleus was found basally, while other organelles were generally displaced to the periphery.

In the RPE of MPS VI–affected cats, cells at the posterior pole were more severely affected than those at the periphery. This spatial distribution of abnormalities was not concentric to the optic disc but extended for a greater distance in the superior and temporal meridians. The heavily pigmented peripheral RPE adjacent to the ora serrata remained unaffected.

Storage within the RPE cells was a feature of feline but not human MPS VI. This may represent a species-specific phenomenon, perhaps related to the lack of pigment in the RPE overlying the tapetal zone of the cat, since the heavily pigmented peripheral RPE of affected cats always remained normal. Alternatively, these differences may have resulted from the improved preservation of the feline tissues that were used in our studies. When affected feline eyes were fixed in formalin and embedded in paraffin, as the MPS VI–affected human eyes had been [68], little or no RPE pathology was observed.

In feline and canine MPS I, inclusions were uniformly distributed throughout the RPE monolayer (Fig. 6-9C, D, and E). The inclusions in the

Table 6-3. *Ocular Tissues Affected by Mucopolysaccharide Storage Diseases* in Domestic Animals*

Disease characteristic	MPS I, cat	MPS I, dog†	MPS VI, cat	MPS VII, dog
Animal age (yr)	1–3	1.5	0.5–5	1.2
Cornea and sclera				
Epithelium	−/+	NR	−	−
Keratocytes	+ +	+ +	+ +	+ +
Stromal extracellular material	−	NR	−	−
Endothelium	+/+ +	NR	−	+
Sclerocytes	+ +	+ +	+ +	+ +
Conjunctiva				
Epithelium	+	NR	+/−	NR
Stromal cells	+	A	+ +	NR
Trabecular meshwork	+/+ +	NR	+	+
Iris				
Epithelium (posterior)	+	−	−	NR
Stromal cells	+ +	A	+ +	+ +
Ciliary body				
Pigmented epithelium	+	A	−	+/−
Nonpigmented epithelium	+ +	A	+ +	+/+ +
Stromal cells	+/+ +	A	+/+ +	+/+ +
Choroidal fibroblasts	+/+ +	+/+ +	+/+ +	+/+ +
Tapetum lucidum	−	−	−	NR
Neuroretina				
Photoreceptor degeneration	−	−	−	+
Pyknotic photoreceptor nuclei	−	NR	+	NR
Perivascular glia	+ +	+/−	−	NR
Ganglion cells	−	NR	−	NR
Pigment epithelium				
Nonpigmented	+	+	+ +	+
Pigmented	+	+/−	− (peripheral) +/+ + (posterior pole)	+
Vitrous macrophages	+ +	+ +	+ +	NR
References	42, 45, 46	45, 105, 106	4, 43	44, 45

*Unless indicated, disease characterized by accumulation of vacuolated inclusions visible by light and/or electron microscopy.
†Canine MPS I retinal tissues provided by R. Munger, D.V.M.
MPS = mucopolysaccharidosis; NR = not reported; − = not affected; + = mildly affected; + + = moderately to severely affected; A = affected but severity not described.

cat RPE were membrane bound and contained a homogeneous granular matrix (see Fig. 6-11D). These filled the cell cytoplasm but did not result in hypertrophy. Because the staining characteristics of the MPS I inclusions were similar to those of the RPE cytoplasm, disease in the RPE layer was not readily apparent by light microscopy. In canine MPS VII, RPE hypertrophy was observed, but the ocular disease has not yet been fully characterized (Fig. 6-9F).

The preservation of neuroretinal structure and function in animals with MPS I and MPS VI was surprising. In spite of the extensive RPE involvement in MPS VI, there was no evidence of concurrent retinal disease. Accumulation of intracytoplasmic inclusions was restricted to the RPE. Although outer segments appeared disoriented when adjacent to massively hypertrophied RPE cells, their internal lamellar organization was preserved (Fig. 6-10). Phagosomal inclusions, indicative of RPE participation in the rod outer segment renewal process, were evident. In fact, rod

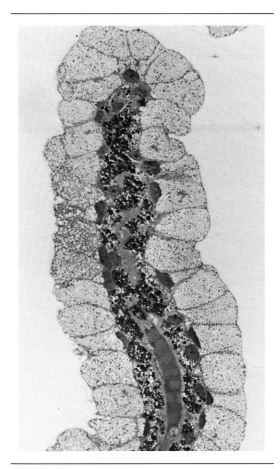

Fig. 6-8. *Mucopolysaccharidosis I, cat. Longitudinal section of a ciliary process. The nonpigmented epithelial cells are swollen, and the cytoplasm is replete with numerous vacuolated inclusions that displace the nuclei apically. The pigmented epithelial cells, although compressed, still accumulate vacuolated inclusions. (×640.)*

outer segment renewal rates were normal when studied both early and late in the disease. It was therefore apparent that MPS VI–affected RPE cells, in spite of their massive hypertrophy, were still able to maintain their photoreceptor supportive functions. The hypothesis that RPE hypertrophy per se results in visual cell death and neuroretinal degeneration thus appears to be an oversimplification [26].

Similarly, neuroretinal integrity in MPS I–affected dogs and cats was also preserved in spite of concurrent RPE disease [42, 105]. The only abnormality thus far observed in the affected cats' neuroretinas was the accumulation of vacuolated inclusions within perivascular glial cells in the outer plexiform layer capillaries. In contrast to human MPS I (Hurler phenotype) in which pigmentary degeneration of the retina occurs, the MPS I–affected animals did not show retinal degeneration. This may represent a species difference in the expression of the metabolic disease.

Retinal degeneration did occur in canine MPS VII. In preliminary studies, a 50 percent reduction in outer nuclear layer width was noted (see Fig. 6-9F). The exact mechanism of degeneration in the disease has not been defined.

The expression of the RPE disease and the factors that modify it are amenable to study using in vitro techniques. Primary cultures of affected RPE in MPS I (cat and dog) and MPS VI (cat) showed normal growth characteristics and remained well differentiated. Cultures derived from eyecup preparations appeared morphologically normal except for the presence of the inclusions characteristic of the diseases. In MPS VI the same four classes of cytoplasmic inclusions accumulated in nonpigmented RPE cells and, in some cases, resulted in cellular hypertrophy (Fig. 6-11A and B). Pigmented RPE cells remained normal or minimally affected in culture (Fig. 6-12). In MPS I the inclusions in cultured RPE cells had a homogeneous granular matrix and were similar to those found in vivo; cellular hypertrophy did not occur, and pigmented and nonpigmented RPE cells were equally affected (Figs. 6-11C–E and 6-13).

Selected lysosomal enzyme activities have been measured in primary cultures of normal and diseased RPE (Table 6-4). Activities of arylsulfatase A and B were normally several times higher in cultured RPE than in peripheral blood leukocytes, liver, and cultured fibroblasts. In contrast, normal α-L-iduronidase activity in RPE was similar to levels present in other tissues. In MPS VI arylsulfatase B activity was reduced to 4 percent of normal, while arylsulfatase A and α-L-iduronidase activities were unchanged. This low level of residual enzyme activity in cultured RPE cells was similar to that found in other tissues of MPS VI–affected cats and humans. The RPE of MPS VI heterozygote animals showed arylsulfatase B activity intermediate between affected and control values. As heterozygote tissues, including cultured RPE, remained structurally normal in spite of a significant reduction in arylsulfatase B activity, it is apparent that the level of this enzyme must be reduced below some critical point before the disease is expressed morphologically. In primary cultures of RPE from MPS I–affected dog or cats, there was no detectable α-L-iduronidase ac-

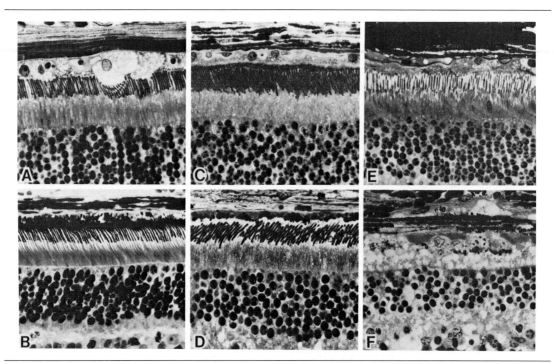

Fig. 6-9. *Mucopolysaccharidoses. Retinal sections from the tapetal (A, C, E; pigment epithelium not pigmented) and nontapetal (B, D, F; pigment epithelium pigmented) zones of animals with mucopolysaccharide storage disorders: A, B = cat, MPS VI; C, D = cat, MPS I; E = dog, MPS I; F = dog, MPS VII. Nonpigmented RPE becomes massively hypertrophied in MPS VI (A), but pigmented RPE remains normal (B). Intracytoplasmic inclusions accumulate in MPS I RPE, but cells are not hypertrophied (C, D, E); the inclusions are more apparent in nonpigmented cells (C, E). Visual cell degeneration and loss of outer nuclear layer nuclei occur only in MPS VII (F). (×325.) (Tissue sections of MPS I in dog courtesy of R. Munger, D.V.M.)*

tivity. Both MPS I (cat, dog) and MPS VI were expressed biochemically and morphologically in primary cultures of RPE cells, and the in vitro findings matched the essential features of the in vivo disease.

In addition to studies of RPE cells from the entire monolayer, it has been possible to isolate and culture RPE cells from specifically defined regions of the eye, which has allowed more critical investigations of diseases, such as MPS VI, with a regional or spatial distribution. We found that in cultures initiated from nonpigmented regions of the eye, the disease was expressed morphologically by the accumulation of vacuolated inclusions and hypertrophy, but cultures from pigmented areas remained normal (Fig. 6-14). One possibility for this variation is regional differences in residual activity of arylsulfatase B; that is, higher levels of this enzyme in pigmented cells would prevent disease expression. We have found, however, that the arylsulfatase B activity levels were equally deficient in pigmented and nonpigmented RPE cultures, which suggests that differences in disease severity cannot be explained purely by differences in residual enzyme activity. A possible explanation currently under investigation is the lack of uniformity in GAG metabolism by different regions of the RPE monolayer.

Defects in Glycoprotein Degradation

MANNOSIDOSIS

Mannosidosis is a recessively inherited deficiency of the acidic A and B forms of α-D-mannosidase, which results in intracellular storage of mannose-rich glycopeptides, glycoproteins, and oligosaccharides. In humans the ocular lesions include superficial corneal opacities, posterior cortical lens opacities in a wheel-like or spoke pattern, pallor or graying of the optic disc with blurring of the disc margin, and esotropia [6, 79]. A deficiency of α-mannosidase has been described in cattle [60, 78] and in cats [17, 45, 119] (Table 6-5).

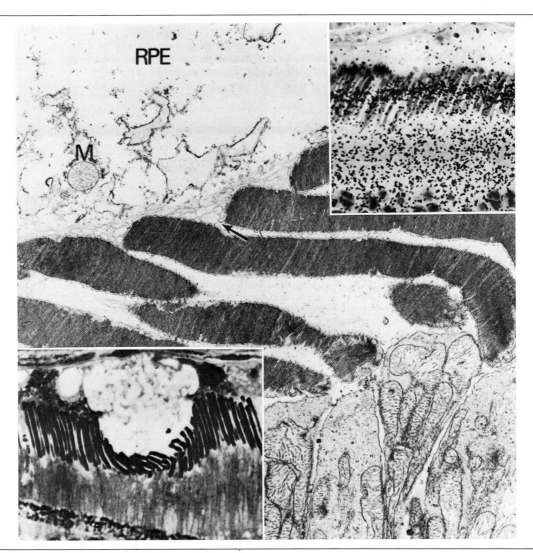

Fig. 6-10. *Mucopolysaccharidosis VI, cat. Focal disarray of photoreceptor outer segments opposite a massively hypertrophied nonpigmented RPE cell (lower inset). The internal lamellar organization of the outer segments is normal (main figure). Outer segment renewal, as indicated by displacement of band of radioactivity 3 days after intravitreous injection of ^{3}H-leucine, is normal opposite nonpigmented diseased (right) and pigmented normal (left) RPE (upper inset). The RPE cytoplasm appears empty because of coalescence of electron-lucent vacuolated inclusions (main figure). Mitochondrion (M) and apical microvilli (arrow) are normal. (×11, 740; insets ×1,000.) (Reprinted in part from G. Aguirre, L. Stramm, and M. Haskins, Feline mucopolysaccharidosis VI: General ocular and pigment epithelial pathology. Invest. Ophthalmol. Vis. Sci. 24:991, 1983.)*

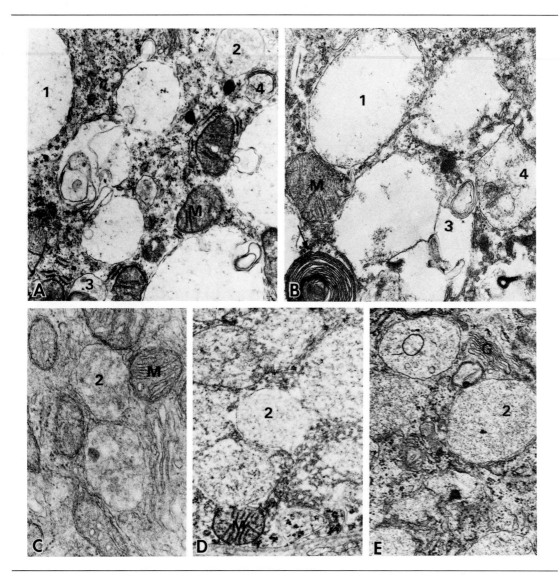

Fig. 6-11. *Mucopolysaccharidoses. Inclusions accumulating within the RPE in feline MPS VI in vitro (A) are similar to those observed in vivo (B) and can be divided into four classes: (1) electron-lucent, (2) granular, (3) lamellar, and (4) mixed.*

Homogeneous granular inclusions (2) predominate in MPS I–affected RPE from cats (C, in vitro; D, in vivo) and dogs (E, in vitro). (M = mitrochondrion.) (A, ×18,468; B, ×19,415; C, ×18,322; D, ×18,678; E, ×24,290.)

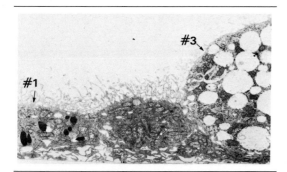

Fig. 6-12. *Mucopolysaccharidosis VI, cat. Massive hypertrophy of nonpigmented RPE cell (#3) is associated with the accumulation of vacuolated inclusions. Nearby pigmented cell (#1) is not hypertrophied and appears normal. Fourteen-day-old culture was initiated from an eyecup preparation and contained both pigmented and nonpigmented cells. (×2,675.)*

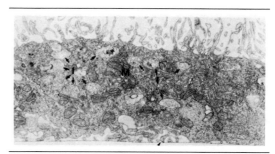

Fig. 6-13. *Mucopolysaccharidosis I, cat. After 14 days in culture, RPE cells are polarized with respect to the culture plate surface (arrowhead), and prominent microvilli are present apically. Homogeneous granular inclusions are limited by a single membrane (arrows I) and are distinct from mitochondria (M). (×6,160.)*

Table 6-4. *Enzyme Activities in Primary Cultures of RPE* Cells from Animals with Mucopolysaccharidosis*

Tissue	Arylsulfatase B (nmol/hr)	Arylsulfatase A (nmol/hr)	α-L-Iduronidase (nmol/hr)
Normal RPE, cat	595 ± 195	1253 ± 926	15.7 ± 4.7
Normal fibroblasts, cat	112 ± 89	290 ± 199	ND
MPS I RPE, cat	ND	ND	0
MPS I RPE, dog†	ND	ND	0
MPS VI RPE, cat	22 ± 59	1059 ± 371	16.2
MPS VI fibroblasts, cat	6 ± 6	509 ± 154	ND
MPS VI RPE, cat heterozygote	141 ± 72	735 ± 154	ND

*Retinal pigment epithelium enzymatically dissociated from entire eyecups containing pigmented and nonpigmented cells. Confluent 14-day-old cultures.
†Tissue provided by R. Munger, D.V.M., and R. Shull, D.V.M.
MPS = mucopolysaccharidosis; ND = not done.

Aberdeen Angus and Murray Grey calves affected with the disease exhibited a deficiency of the acid form of α-mannosidase [48] with subsequent accumulation of mannose-containing and *N*-acetylglucosamine–containing oligosaccharides. Affected calves were undersized and in generally poor condition. Abnormalities included progressive incoordination, ataxia, fine head and body intention tremors, and moderate hydrocephalus. Death usually occurred within the first year of life [60]. Histologically, neuronal vacuolation was present throughout the spinal cord and brain. Most vacuoles appeared electron lucent, although they often contained a moderate amount of amorphous electron-dense material and occa-

sionally fibrillar membranous fragments. Spheroidal swellings were common in the proximal portions of Purkinje axons, deep cerebellar nuclei, and the distal extremities of long axons. No myelin deficiency was observed; demyelination appeared to be associated with neuronal necrosis and degeneration. Vacuoles were also present in macrophages, fixed reticuloendothelial cells, and exocrine epithelial cells. Malformation of lumbar vertebrae and severe vacuolation of hepatocytes, both prominent in the human disease, were not observed. A systematic study of the eye in bovine mannosidosis has not been reported. Lenticular changes have not been observed with the naked eye [58]; the only ocular abnormality reported to

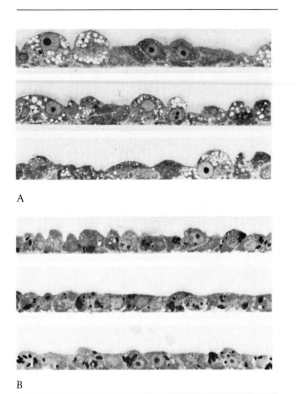

A

B

Fig. 6-14. *Mucopolysaccharidosis VI, cat. Fourteen-day-old cultures of RPE cells initiated from superior equatorial (A) and inferior equatorial (B) regions of the eye. A. Note marked accumulation of vacuolated inclusions and hypertrophy in cells from nonpigmented regions. B. Minimal to no disease is present in cells from pigmented regions. (×500.)*

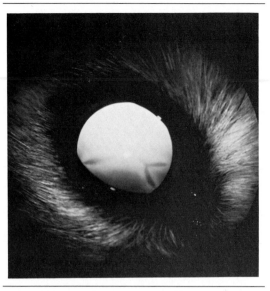

Fig. 6-15. *α-Mannosidosis, cat. Stromal opacities result in diffuse but slight corneal stippling. Posterior Y suture lines are opaque.*

Table 6-5. *Mannosidoses and Fucosidosis in Domestic Animals*

Disease finding	Mannosidosis, cat	Mannosidosis, cattle	Mannosidosis, goat	Fucosidosis, dog*
Inheritance	AR	AR	AR	AR?
Enzyme deficiency	α-Mannosidase	α-Mannosidase	β-Mannosidase	α-Fucosidase
Substrate accumulating	Mannose-rich oligosaccharides	Mannose and glucosamine oligosaccharides	Mannose and glucosamine oligosaccharides	Fucose-containing oligosaccharides
Facial dysmorphism	±	−	+	+
Visceral storage	+	+	+	+
Neuronal storage	+	+	+	+
Myelin deficiency	+	−	+	+
Corneal opacities	+	−	−	−
Lenticular opacities	+	−	−	−
Retinal ganglion cell storage	+	+	+	−
RPE storage	+	NR	NR	+
References	45, 119	60	47, 61, 62	41, 45, 66

AR = autosomal recessive; + = present; − = absent; RPE = retinal pigment epithelium; NR = not reported.
*Tissues provided by W. R. Kelly.

date has been the vacuolation of retinal ganglion cells [60].

Persian cats and a domestic shorthaired cat affected with α-mannosidosis were retarded in growth and exhibited mild tremors, ataxia, and hepatomegaly [17, 45]. Cytoplasmic vacuolation was prominent in pancreatic acinar cells, hepatocytes, and neurons of the central nervous system. The cerebral cortex was more severely affected in the feline than the bovine disease, and a marked myelin deficiency was observed in the cerebral white matter of the cats [45, 119].

In one Persian cat with α-mannosidosis, ophthalmologic examination showed gray, granular fundus lesions in the area centralis and in a band extending temporally and nasally [45]. The lenses contained numerous small vacuoles along the suture lines, and the corneas had a fine, diffuse stromal stippling (Fig. 6-15).

In the cornea vacuolation of the endothelium and stromal keratocytes was present; the vacuolation was most prominent in the posterior stroma. Vacuolated inclusions were also present in sclerocytes, choroidal fibroblasts, the iridic stroma, and the nonpigmented ciliary epithelium (Fig. 6-16). Moderate vacuolation of retinal ganglion cells was found. The retinal pigment epithelium was severely affected; accumulation of

Fig. 6-16. *α-Mannosidosis, cat. Posterior iris stromal fibroblasts are distended with vacuolated inclusions of various sizes. (×800.)*

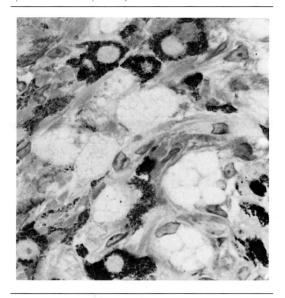

numerous inclusions resulted in a foamy appearance of the cytoplasm and cellular hypertrophy. There was no difference in disease severity between pigmented and nonpigmented RPE cells. The photoreceptors were normal. The ultrastructure of the vacuolated inclusions accumulating within ocular tissues has not been characterized.

Another form of mannosidosis, involving a recessively inherited deficiency of β-mannosidase, has been reported in Nubian goats (Table 6-5) [47, 62]. The enzyme deficiency resulted in the accumulation of mannose and glucosamine-enriched oligosaccharides in visceral and neural tissues with concomitant urinary spillover. Affected animals exhibited marked neurologic impairment, severe abduction of the forelimbs, head tremors, facial dysmorphism, carpal contractures, and deafness. Vacuolation was present in the brain and spinal cord neurons, and a marked deficiency of myelin was observed in the cerebral cortex, cerebellar folia, and brain stem. Perivascular cuffing by phagocytes in the cerebral cortex and cerebellar white matter has also been observed [47]. Vacuolation of visceral tissue, especially in the kidney, pancreas, and mesenteric lymph nodes, was prominent.

Affected goats exhibited ocular oscillations resembling pendular nystagmus, small pupils, and partial prolapse of the nictitating membrane [61]. No abnormalities of the retina or optic disc were apparent on clinical examination, and vision appeared unimpaired. Histologically, the ganglion cells of the retina were vacuolated. No human deficiency of β-mannosidase has been reported; thus this is one animal disease in search of a human model.

FUCOSIDOSIS

Fucosidosis has been described in English springer spaniels, in which α-L-fucosidase activity was reduced to 1.2 percent of normal [41, 66]. The disease has been found in males and females; obligate heterozygotes had intermediate enzyme activities suggestive of autosomal recessive inheritance (Table 6-5). Affected dogs exhibited progressive ataxia, proprioceptive deficits, dysphagia, and wasting. Some animals were visually impaired—the pupils were dilated, and a pupillary light reflex deficit was present [41].

On postmortem examination, marked bilateral enlargement of the vagi in the cervical area was present. There was CNS vacuolation and enlargement of most neurons and neuroglial cells, most

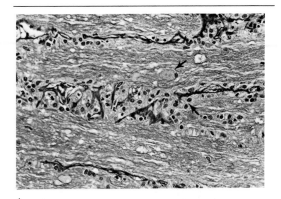

A

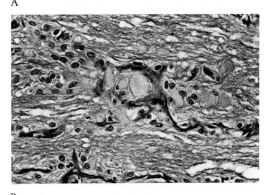

B

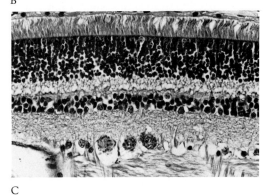

C

Fig. 6-17. *α-Fucosidosis, dog. A, B. Astrocytes (arrows) in the pial septa of the optic nerve are distended, and the cytoplasm is foamy and granular. (A, ×150; B, ×250.) C. Retinal pigment epithelium is uniformly enlarged, and the cytoplasm has a foamy and granular appearance. These changes are not striking in the paraffin-embedded tissue. (×250.) (Tissues courtesy of W. R. Kelly, D.V.M.)*

prominently in the cerebral cortex but less severely through the medulla. Most of the vacuoles appeared empty, although some contained amorphous material. The histochemical characteristics of the neuronal vacuoles were similar to those observed in humans [66]. Widespread vacuolation of epithelial and mesenchymal cells was also present in many visceral organs.

Ocular lesions were limited to the RPE and optic nerves. The optic nerves were thickened by an increased number of astrocytes present in the orbital and laminar (pre- and postlaminar) regions of the nerve. These astrocytes had a foamy, granular cytoplasm that distended the cell and, in most cases, displaced the nucleus to the periphery (Fig. 6-17A and B). Distended astrocytes were located adjacent to small vessels in the pial septa as well as between axons in the nerve proper.

The RPE was uniformly enlarged throughout the monolayer in both pigmented and nonpigmented areas (Fig. 6-17C). The cells had a granular, foamy homogeneous cytoplasm. Visual cells and other retinal neurons were normal. Since canine rhodopsin is fucosylated and since the RPE participates in the outer segment renewal process by the lysosomal degradation of phagocytized outer segment discs, storage within the RPE of fucose-containing oligosaccharides would be expected [3]. The long-term effects of this storage on the viability of visual cells is unknown, because most affected animals have died at a comparatively young age.

The Lipidoses

GLOBOID CELL LEUKODYSTROPHY

A recessively inherited disease of mice (twitcher mouse) and dogs (cairn terrier, West Highland white terrier) shares many of the clinical and biochemical features of globoid cell leukodystrophy (GCL, Krabbe's disease) in humans [30, 52, 112]. The disease has also been described in the cat [56] and sheep [96].

A deficiency of galactosyl ceramidase has been confirmed in GCL-affected humans, mice, dogs, and sheep [52, 96, 112]. The enzyme catalyzes the formation of ceramide from galactosyl ceramide. In spite of the catabolic block, there is no abnormal accumulation of galactosyl ceramide, the major natural substrate of the missing enzyme [112]. Recent studies have proposed that psychosin (galactosyl sphingosine) is the substrate that accu-

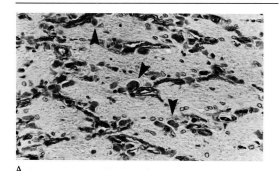

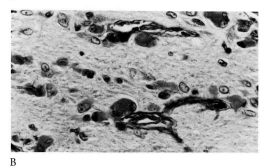

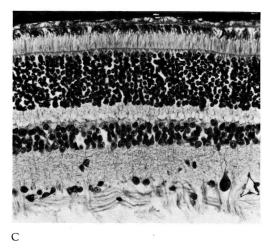

Fig. 6-18. *Globoid cell leukodystrophy, dog. A. Retrolaminar optic nerve shows the accumulation of globoid cells (*arrowheads*) along the vascular septa. (×190.) B. Higher magnification of A. Perivascular globoid cells have a foamy cytoplasm with eccentric nuclei. (×380.) C. Juxtapapillary retina, including ganglion cell and nerve fiber layers, is normal. (×300.) (Tissues courtesy of J. T. McGrath, V.M.D.)*

mulates. Elevated levels of psychosin have been found in the brain, especially the white matter, of humans, mice, and dogs with GCL. Psychosin is also a substrate of galactosyl ceramidase and is chemically and metabolically related to galatosyl ceramide. Destruction of the myelin-generating cells and axons results from psychosin accumulation within these cells, as this compound is highly cytotoxic and selectively kills the cells within which it accumulates [52].

In affected dogs neurologic deficits appeared between 2 and 7 months of age; the disease was progressive, and death usually occurred within 2 to 3 months. Neurologic abnormalities included paralysis of the pelvic limbs or cerebellar signs. Visual deficits and blindness were present later in the disease [30]. Ophthalmoscopic abnormalities have not been reported in dogs or in the other animal species affected with globoid cell leukodystrophy.

The hallmark of GCL is the globoid cell, a foamy PAS-positive macrophage that can occasionally be multinucleate; globoid cells accumulate perivascularly in regions of white matter destruction (Fig. 6-18A and B). Early in the disease, globoid cells were found adjacent to nerve fibers having axonal swelling and dilated myelin sheaths. As the white matter was lost, it was replaced by these macrophages; eventually, extensive white matter destruction resulted in marked astrocytosis [30]. By electron microscopy, two types of intracytoplasmic tubular inclusions were found in canine globoid cells. One was large, slightly arched, angular in cross-section, and more distinctive than the other, slender twisted tubules that appeared round in cross-section [31].

In dogs the optic nerves showed severe demyelination and axonal degeneration. Only a few myelin sheaths remained in severely affected areas. By approximately 6 months of age, optic nerve involvement was more extensive at the chiasm than near the disc [76]. The number of globoid cells in the optic nerve was proportional to the extent of demyelination [76]. They were present in the immediate retrolaminar portion of the nerve (Fig. 6-18A and B), where they were in close association with the perivascular spaces of the pial septa. They have not been found, however, in the prelaminar portion of the nerve. Retrograde axonal degeneration with secondary loss of ganglion cells has not been reported (Fig. 6-18C). It is likely that these changes would develop in affected animals having a longer survival.

Two other disorders of lysosomal enzymes with neurologic manifestations, Niemann-Pick disease and Gaucher's disease, have been identified in domestic animals. Niemann-Pick disease type A has been described in the dog [16] and Siamese cat [126], and a deficiency of sphingomyelinase activity has been confirmed biochemically. In the Siamese cat the disease is presumed to be recessive, as obligate heterozygotes have intermediate levels of enzyme activity.

The affected kittens had anisocoria and an abnormally pale iris color. All were apparently blind by 5 months of age. Histologically, foam cells were found singly or in small aggregates within the iris. In some retinal ganglion cells there was a loss of Nissl substance accompanied by cytoplasmic vacuolation. These changes increased in severity with time [110].

Isolated cases of Gaucher's disease have been identified in sheep [77] and the dog. In the dog large amounts of glucocerebroside accumulated in the liver and brain, but the retina was normal histologically and pingueculas were not present [40]. More recently, a deficiency of glucocerebrosidase has been confirmed in canine Gaucher's disease [120].

OTHER DISEASES

Neuronal Ceroid Lipofuscinosis

The neuronal ceroid lipofuscinoses in humans are a group of diseases divided into four distinct syndromes based on clinical and pathologic criteria: the infantile, late infantile, juvenile, and adult forms. Each form has a complex of eponyms [128], although they are often broadly grouped as Batten's disease. These diseases are characterized broadly by dementia, visual loss (except for the adult form), ataxia, seizures, and premature death and have as a common denominator the accumulation of autofluorescent lipopigments in neurons and other cells [59].

Neuronal ceroid lipofuscinosis (NCL) has been reported in cattle [101], cats [38], sheep [8, 37, 59] and several breeds of dog [5, 25, 70, 97]. With the exception of one dog having clinical and neuropathologic disease analogous to the adult form of NCL (Kufs' disease), most cases reported were similar to the late infantile and juvenile forms of the disease (Table 6-6). Only in the English setter [70] and South Hampshire sheep [59] models has

the disease been well defined and have breeding colonies been established.

In both the sheep and the dog (English setter), the diseases were inherited as autosomal recessive traits and clinical signs were associated with the progressive accumulation of lipopigments within neurons and other cells throughout the body. Animals remained normal for several months after birth (Table 6-6). Visual deficits, blindness, and neurologic abnormalities (dullness, incoordination, twitching of head muscles, and later convulsions) developed subsequently and became more severe with time. Death occurred by approximately 2 years of age. Although blindness was a major clinical finding early in both sheep and English setters, the cause of blindness differed. In sheep early visual loss was due to brain atrophy. Later there was retinal vascular attenuation observed ophthalmoscopically and a progressive reduction in ERG amplitudes with time. This reduction, however, was not uniform for rod- and cone-mediated responses. The amplitude of the rod-mediated b wave was lower than normal at 20 weeks of age and fell rapidly and monotonically until the rod ERG was nearly extinguished by 66 weeks of age (Fig. 6-19). In contrast, the cone-mediated response remained stable, although slightly lower in amplitude than normal, until 52 weeks of age; the amplitude then rapidly decayed [37]. Pigment epithelial function, as determined by the azide response, remained normal even in blind, terminal cases [58].

The selective functional preservation of the cone system in sheep with NCL was also evident morphologically. Early in the disease rod inner segments, especially in the central retina, were shorter than normal and contained disoriented and degenerating lamellar discs. The diseased rods degenerated, the outer nuclear layer became reduced in width, and short, broad cone inner segments appeared prominent (Fig. 6-20). Cones eventually degenerated, but loss of inner retinal neurons has not been noted [37].

In English setters, on the other hand, no ophthalmoscopic abnormalities have been found by us or reported by others. Berson and Watson have reported a 30 to 40 percent reduction in the amplitudes of the rod- and cone-mediated ERG responses and a mild elevation in the a and b wave thresholds [13], a finding that we have also confirmed (Fig. 6-21). They suggested that the decreased amplitude resulted from a decreased light transmission through the retina secondary to the lipopigment accumulation within ganglion cells.

Table 6-6. *Neuronal Ceroid Lipofuscinoses in Domestic Animals*

Species (breed)	Analogous human disease	Inheritance	Age at onset of clinical signs		Ophthalmoscopic findings		Pathologic findings		References
			Neurologic	Visual	Lesions	stage	Neural	Retinal	
Sheep (South Hampshire)	Late infantile	Recessive	9–12 mo	9–12 mo	Retinal vessel attenuation	Late in disease	Neuronal lipopigment storage with secondary atrophy of brain and thinning of gyri	Lipopigment storage, loss of cells and their nuclei; rod degeneration > cone degeneration	8, 37, 58, 59
Dog (English setter)	Juvenile	Recessive	14–18 mo	14–18 mo	Absent	All stages	Lipopigment storage from birth; neuronal loss and brain atrophy	Lipopigment storage; no visual cell loss	1, 8, 33, 34, 70, 86
Dog (dachshund)	Adult	Unknown	3 yr	Vision normal	Retina normal	All stages	Lipopigment storage in cerebellar Purkinje cells and other CNS neurons	—	25

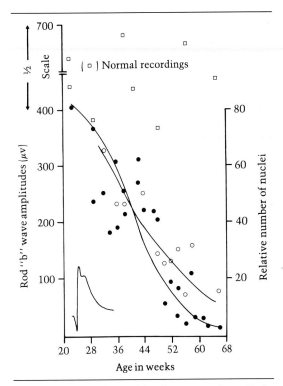

Fig. 6-19. *Neuronal ceroid lipofuscinosis, sheep. Rod-dominant b wave amplitudes in normal (□) and affected (●) sheep relative to age and number of outer nuclear layer nuclei (○). Lower inset shows characteristic normal rod-dominant ERG. (From R. J. Graydon and R. D. Jolly, Ceroid-lipofuscinosis (Batten's disease). Invest. Ophthalmol. Vis. Sci. 25:294, 1984.)*

This hypothesis, however, has been questioned and an alternative pathophysiologic mechanism proposed to account for the electrophysiologic abnormalities [82]. In dogs with very advanced disease, the decrease in amplitude and eventual disappearance of the c wave has been noted, together with a reduction of the standing potential change with illumination [87]. However, no degeneration of the retinal or pigment epithelial cell layers was found [33, 34, 70, 86]. It is probable therefore that the visual deficits and blindness observed in affected dogs early in the disease are central rather than retinal in origin.

In the early stages of both diseases, autofluorescent lipopigment inclusions accumulated within retinal neurons [37, 86]. In the dog inclusions were found in all retinal layers including the RPE [34, 86], and one report suggested that specific inclusion morphologies were characteristic of each retinal layer [86]. However, the significance of the differing morphologies of inclu-

sions found in canine retina and brain, as well as in human tissues with the different forms of NCL, is unknown [32, 70]. The association between neuronal lipopigment storage and cell death is also unknown. It is obvious that in the affected humans and sheep, visual cell degeneration occurred, at least coincidentally, with the storage of lipopigments. Such is not the case in the dog. The proper interpretation of these results and formulation of a pathogenetic mechanism awaits the definitive biochemical characterization of these diseases.

Based on the ultrastructural studies to date, it appears that the neuronal ceroid lipofuscinoses do not represent a primary lysosomal storage disorder. Early in the disease in dogs, focal areas of cytoplasmic condensation occurred in affected neurons; these areas were further condensed by autophagy into secondary lysosomes containing the undigested lipopigments [70]. The pigments extracted from the livers and brains of affected dogs were ceroid that was physicochemically identical to ceroid extracted from the brains of similarly affected human patients [108, 109]. Recent studies have suggested that lipid peroxides from the cyclo-oxygenase-prostaglandin, lipoxygenase-leukotriene pathways were the likely source of the autofluorescent lipopigment [107].

It has been proposed that the autofluorescent lipopigments accumulate as a result of polyunsaturated fatty acid peroxidation from a paraphenylenediamine peroxidase deficiency. This enzyme was reported to be deficient in the leukocytes of affected humans and English setters as well as in the retina and RPE of the affected dogs [7, 9, 92]. This appealing hypothesis has the additional benefit of defining the sequence of pathologic changes in a manner that seems analogous for both the human disease and the animal model. Questions have been raised as to the validity of this hypothesis, and alternate pathogenetic mechanisms are currently under investigation in different laboratories. Present studies are concerned with abnormalities in dolichol and retinoid metabolisms [128] and with deficiencies in a heme-dependent peroxidase [107]. To date, the biochemical defect in the NCL has not been demonstrated conclusively.

Chédiak-Higashi Syndrome

The Chédiak-Higashi syndrome (CHS) has been reported in humans [111, 116], Persian cats [73, 95], cattle [91], mice [127], mink [80], and a whale

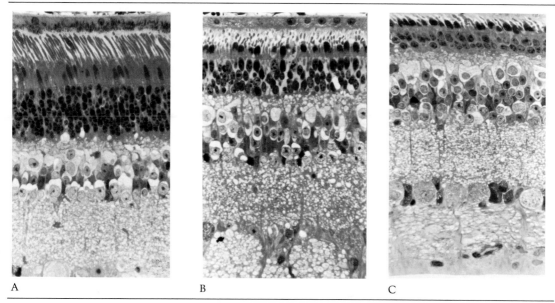

A   B   C

Fig. 6-20. *Neuronal ceroid lipofuscinosis, sheep. A. Normal. B. Affected animals, 48 weeks old. C. Affected animals, 66 weeks old. There is a progressive loss of visual cells and their nuclei. Preservation of cones and inner retinal layer is striking. (×150.) (From R. J. Graydon and R. D. Jolly, Ceroid-lipofuscinosis (Batten's disease).* Invest. Opthalmol. Vis. Sci. *25:294, 1984.)*

Fig. 6-21. *Neuronal ceroid lipofuscinosis, dog. Dark-adapted electroretinograms from normal (N) and affected (A) English setters in response to scotopically balanced blue and red stimuli and white light. The responses recorded from the affected animal are of normal waveform but of lower amplitude. Vertical line at left indicates onset of 20-msec stimulus; vertical calibration mark = 100 μv; horizontal mark = 50 msec.*

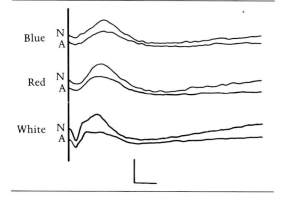

[114]. Clinically the disease is characterized by partial albinism, generalized lymphadenopathy, hematologic abnormalities, hepatosplenomegaly, and frequent pyogenic infections. The biochemical basis for this autosomal recessive disease has not been determined; however, a microtubule defect in affected humans and mice that was correctable with cyclic guanosine monophosphate (cGMP), cholinergic agents, or ascorbate has been identified [15, 89].

The ocular manifestations have been quite similar in the affected species and have included photophobia and pale irides. Hypopigmentation of the fundus was associated with a red fundus reflex in cats, cattle, mink, and mice [20]. In humans and cats congenital bilateral cataracts [73, 98] and spontaneous horizontal nystagmus [20, 116] have also been reported. The congenital cataracts in affected cats, however, segregated independently of the CHS gene and appeared to be the result of another inherited disorder [19].

A number of melanin abnormalities, including abnormal size, shape, color, and distribution and the presence of melanin-containing macrophages within the eye have been observed in CHS-affected cattle, cats, mink, and mice [22]. Pigmented intraocular structures, such as the iris, ciliary epithelium, choroid, and retinal pigment epithelium were hypopigmented. The degree of ocular pigmentation varied from species to species, with CHS cattle being the most ocularly hypopigmented while ocular structures in the CHS mouse contained considerably more melanin [22].

The amount of melanin was significantly decreased in older animals, implying a gradual depigmentation process. Clumping and enlargement of remaining melanin granules was observed in these structures and resulted in diluted pigmentation. Giant lysosome-like organelles with an abnormal lipoprotein content were present in most types of granule-containing cells; these enlarged granules appeared to result from fusion of smaller ones. In the cat the RPE inclusions were PAS positive and exhibited yellow autofluorescence with ultraviolet illumination, indicating possible lipofuscin content [69]. By electron microscopy the inclusions contained membrane fragments, melanosomes, electron-dense material, and structures resembling premelanosomes. Phosphatase activity was present in the secondary lysosomes, and weak activity was demonstrated in the huge residual bodies. Degeneration of the choroidal tapetum lucidum began in cats by 8 weeks of age and was complete by 1 year [21].

The expression of CHS in the animal species appears to be quite similar to that in the human patients. The main difference is the lack of an accelerated phase of the disease in animals. In humans this accelerated phase consists of hepatosplenomegaly, lymphadenopathy, pancytopenia, and widespread organ infiltration with mononuclear cells and usually results in death.

REFERENCES

1. Aguirre, G. Unpublished data, 1976.
2. Aguirre, G. Criteria for development of animal models of diseases of the eye. *Am. J. Pathol.* 105:187, 1981.
3. Aguirre, G., and O'Brien, P. Canine rod outer segment renewal using ^{3}H-fucose: Reduced renewal rates in PRCD affected miniature poodles. *Invest. Ophthalmol. Vis. Sci.* 25(Suppl.):17, 1984.
4. Aguirre, G., Stramm, L., and Haskins, M. Feline mucopolysaccharidosis VI: General ocular and pigment epithelial pathology. *Invest. Ophthalmol. Vis. Sci.* 24:991, 1983.
5. Appleby, E. C., Longstaffe, J. A., and Bell, F. R. Ceroid-lipofuscinosis in two saluki dogs. *J. Comp. Pathol.* 92:375, 1982.
6. Arbisser, A. I., et al. Ocular findings in mannosidosis. *Am. J. Ophthalmol.* 82:465, 1976.
7. Armstrong, D., Dimmitt, S., and van Wormer, D. E. Studies in Batten disease: I. Peroxidase deficiency in granulocytes. *Arch. Neurol.* 30:144, 1974.
8. Armstrong, D., Koppang, N., and Jolly, R. D. Ceroid-lipofuscinosis. *Comp. Pathol. Bull.* 12:2, 1980.
9. Armstrong, D., et al. Studies on the retina and the pigment epithelium in hereditary canine ceroid-lipofuscinosis: I. The distribution of enzymes in the whole retina and pigment epithelium. *Invest. Ophthalmol. Vis. Sci.* 17:608, 1978.
10. Baker, H. J., et al. Neuronal GM$_1$ gangliosidosis in a Siamese cat with β-galactosidase deficiency. *Science* 174:838, 1971.
11. Baker, H. J., et al. The gangliosidoses: Comparative features and research applications. *Vet. Pathol.* 16:635, 1979.
12. Baker, H. J., et al. Feline Gangliosidoses as Models of Human Lysosomal Storage Diseases. In R. J. Desnick, D. F. Patterson, and D. G. Scarpelli (Eds.), *Animal Models of Inherited Metabolic Diseases.* New York: Liss, 1981.
13. Berson, E. L., and Watson, E. L. Electroretinograms in English setters with neuronal ceroid lipofuscinosis. *Invest. Ophthalmol. Vis. Sci.* 19:87, 1980.
14. Blakemore, W. F. GM$_1$ gangliosidosis in a cat. *J. Comp. Pathol.* 82:179, 1972.
15. Boxer, L. A., et al. Correction of leukocyte function in Chédiak-Higashi syndrome by ascorbate. *N. Engl. J. Med.* 295:1041, 1976.
16. Bundza, A., Lowden, J. A., and Charlton, K. M. Niemann-Pick disease in a poodle dog. *Vet. Pathol.* 16:530, 1979.
17. Burditt, L. J., et al. Biochemical studies of a case of feline mannosidosis. *Biochem. J.* 189:467, 1980.
18. Charlton, K. H., et al. Pseudodendritic keratitis and systemic tyrosinemia. *Ophthalmology* 88:355, 1981.
19. Collier, L. L. Personal communication, 1984.
20. Collier, L. L., Bryan, G. M., and Prieur, D. J. Ocular manifestations of the Chédiak-Higashi syndrome in four species of animals. *J. Am. Vet. Med. Assoc.* 175:587, 1979.
21. Collier, L. L., King, E. J., and Prieur, D. J. Tapetal degeneration in cats with Chédiak-Higashi syndrome. *Curr. Eye Res.* 4:767, 1985.
22. Collier, L. L., Prieur, D. J., and King, E. J. Ocular melanin pigmentation anomalies in cats, cattle, mink, and mice with Chédiak-Higashi syndrome: Histologic observations. *Curr. Eye Res.* 3:1241,1984.
23. Cook, R. D., et al. Changes in nervous tissue in bovine generalised glycogenosis type II. *Neuropathol. Appl. Neurobiol.* 8:95, 1982.
24. Cork, L. C., et al. GM$_2$ ganglioside lysosomal storage disease in cats with β-hexosaminidase deficiency. *Science* 196:1014, 1977.
25. Cummings, J. F., and deLahunta, A. An adult case of canine neuronal ceroid-lipofuscinosis. *Acta Neuropathol. (Berl.)* 39:43, 1977.
26. del Monte, M. A., et al. Histopathology of Sanfilippo's syndrome. *Arch. Ophthalmol.* 101:1255, 1983.
27. Donnelly, W. J. C., Sheahan, B. J., and Rogers, T. A. GM$_1$ gangliosidosis in Friesian calves. *J. Pathol.* 111:173, 1973.
28. Engerman, R., et al. Ocular complications. *Diabetes* 31(Suppl. 1):82, 1982.
29. Farrell, D. F., et al. Feline GM$_1$ gangliosidosis: Bio-

chemical and ultrastructural comparisons with the disease in man. *J. Neuropathol. Exp. Neurol.* 32:1, 1973.

30. Fletcher, T. F., and Kurtz, H. J. Animal model for human disease: Globoid cell leukodystrophy, Krabbe's disease. *Am. J. Pathol.* 66:375, 1972.

31. Fletcher, T. F., Lee, D. G., and Hammer, R. F. Ultrastructural features of globoid-cell leukodystrophy in the dog. *Am. J. Vet. Res.* 32:177, 1971.

32. Goebel, H. H., Fix, J. D., and Zeman, W. The fine structure of retina in neuronal ceroid-lipofuscinosis. *Am. J. Ophthalmol.* 77:25, 1974.

33. Goebel, H. H., Köhnecke, B., and Koppang, N. Ultrastructural Studies on the Retina in Human and Canine Neuronal Ceroid-Lipofuscinosis and Other Lysosomal Disorders. In E. Cotlier, I. H. Maumenee, and E. R. Berman (Eds.), *Genetic Eye Diseases.* New York: Liss, 1982.

34. Goebel, H. H., Koppang, N., and Zeman, W. Ultrastructure of the retina in canine neuronal ceroid lipofuscinosis. *Ophthalmic Res.* 11:65, 1979.

35. Goldsmith, L. A. Tyrosinemia and Related Disorders. In J. B. Stanbury et al., (Eds.), *The Metabolic Basis of Inherited Disease* (5th ed.). New York: McGraw-Hill, 1983.

36. Goldsmith, L. A., Thorpe, J. M., and Marsh, R. F. Tyrosine aminotransferase deficiency in mink (*Mustela vison*): A model for human tyrosinemia II. *Biochem. Genet.* 19:687, 1981.

37. Graydon, R. J., and Jolly, R. D. Ceroid-lipofuscinosis (Batten's disease). *Invest. Ophthalmol. Vis. Sci.* 25:294, 1984.

38. Green, P. D., and Little, P. B. Neuronal ceroid-lipofuscin storage in Siamese cats. *Can. J. Comp. Med.* 38:207, 1974.

39. Hagan, L. O. Lipid dystrophic changes in the central nervous system in dogs. *Acta Pathol. Microbiol. Scand.* 33:22, 1953.

40. Hartley, W. J., and Blakemore, W. F. Neurovisceral glucocerebroside storage (Gaucher's disease) in a dog. *Vet. Pathol.* 10:191, 1973.

41. Hartley, W. J., Canfield, P. J., and Donnelly, T. M. A suspected new canine storage disease. *Acta Neuropathol. (Berl.)* 56:225, 1982.

42. Haskins, M. E., et al. The pathology of the feline model of mucopolysaccharidosis I. *Am. J. Pathol.* 112:27, 1983.

43. Haskins, M. E., et al. The pathology of the feline model of mucopolysaccharidosis VI. *Am. J. Pathol.* 101:657, 1980.

44. Haskins, M. E., et al. Beta-glucuronidase deficiency in a dog: A model of human mucopolysaccharidosis VII. *Pediatr. Res.* 18:980, 1984.

45. Haskins, M., et al. Unpublished data, 1984.

46. Haskins, M. E., et al. Alpha-L-iduronidase deficiency in a cat: A model of mucopolysaccharidosis I. *Pediatr. Res.* 13:1294, 1979.

47. Healy, P. J., et al. β-Mannosidase deficiency in Anglo-Nubian goats. *Aust. Vet. J.* 57:504, 1981.

48. Hocking, J. D., Jolly, R. D., and Batt, R. D. Deficiency of α-mannosidase in Angus cattle. *Biochem. J.* 128:69, 1972.

49. Holland, J. M., et al. Lafora's disease in the dog. *Am. J. Pathol.* 58:509, 1970.

50. Howell, J. M., Dorling, P. R., and Cook, R. D. Generalised glycogenosis type II. *Comp. Pathol. Bull.* 15:2, 1983.

51. Howell, J. M., et al. Infantile and late onset form of generalised glycogenosis type II in cattle. *J. Pathol.* 134:267, 1981.

52. Igisu, H., and Suzuki, K. Progressive accumulation of a toxic metabolite in genetic leukodystrophy. *Science* 224:753, 1984.

53. Jezyk, P. F., Haskins, M. E., and Patterson, D. F. Screening for Inborn Errors of Metabolism in Dogs and Cats. In R. J. Desnick, D. F. Patterson, and D. G. Scarpelli (Eds.), *Animal Models of Inherited Metabolic Diseases.* New York: Liss, 1982.

54. Jezyk, P. F., Haskins, M. E., and Patterson, D. F. Naturally-occurring Models of Inborn Errors of Metabolism: Definition of the Enzymatic Defects. *Proceedings of the 4th International Congress on Clinical Enzymology.* In press, 1985.

55. Jezyk, P. F., et al. Mucopolysaccharidosis in a cat with arylsulfatase B deficiency: A model of Maroteaux-Lamy syndrome. *Science* 198:834, 1977.

56. Johnson, K. H. Globoid leukodystrophy in the cat. *J. Am. Vet. Med. Assoc.* 157:2057, 1970.

57. Jolly, R. D. Mannosidosis and its control in Angus and Murray Grey cattle. *N. Z. Vet. J.* 26:194, 1978.

58. Jolly, R. D. Personal communication, 1984.

59. Jolly, R. D., et al. Ovine ceroid-lipofuscinosis: A model of Batten's disease. *Neuropathol. Appl. Neurobiol.* 6:195, 1980.

60. Jolly, R. D., and Thompson, K. G. The pathology of bovine mannosidosis. *Vet. Pathol.* 15:141, 1978.

61. Jones, M. Z., et al. Caprine β-mannosidosis: Clinical and pathological features. *J. Neuropathol. Exp. Neurol.* 42:268, 1983.

62. Jones, M. Z., and Lane, R. A. Caprine oligosaccharide storage disease. *J. Biol. Chem.* 256:5181, 1981.

63. Karbe, E. GM$_2$ Gangliosidose und andere neuronal Lipodystrophien mit Amaurase beim Hund. *Arch. Exp. Veterinarmed.* 25:1, 1971.

64. Karbe, E. Animal model of human disease: GM$_2$ gangliosidoses (amaurotic idiocies) types I, II, and III. *Am. J. Pathol.* 71:151, 1973.

65. Karbe, E., and Schiefer, B. Familial amaurotic idiocy in male German shorthair pointers. *Vet. Pathol.* 4:223, 1967.

66. Kelly, W. R., et al. Canine α-L-fucosidosis: A storage disease of springer spaniels. *Acta Neuropathol. (Berl.)* 60:9, 1983.

67. Kenyon, K. R., et al. The systemic mucopolysaccharidoses: Ultrastructural and histochemical studies of conjunctiva and skin. *Am. J. Ophthalmol.* 7:811, 1972.

68. Kenyon, K. R., et al. Ocular pathology of the Mar-

oteaux-Lamy syndrome (systemic mucopolysaccharidosis VI). *Am. J. Ophthalmol.* 73:718, 1972.

69. King, E. J., Collier, L. L., and Prieur, D. J. Lysosomes and residual bodies in the retinal pigment epithelium of cats with Chédiak-Higashi syndrome. *Invest. Ophthalmol. Vis. Sci.* 25(Suppl.):210, 1984.

70. Koppang, N. Canine ceroid-lipofuscinosis: A model for human neuronal ceroid-lipofuscinosis and ageing. *Mech. Ageing Dev.* 2:421, 1973/74.

71. Kosanke, S. D., Pierce, K. R., and Bay, W. W. Clinical and biochemical abnormalities in porcine GM_2 gangliosidosis. *Vet. Pathol.* 15:685, 1978.

72. Kosanke, S. D., Pierce, K. R., and Read, W. K. Morphogenesis of light and electron microscopic lesions in porcine GM_2 gangliosidosis. *Vet. Pathol.* 16:6, 1979.

73. Kramer, J. W., Davis, W. C., and Prieur, D. J. The Chédiak-Higashi syndrome of cats. *Lab. Invest.* 36:559, 1977.

74. Kramer, J. W., et al. Inherited, early onset, insulin-requiring diabetes mellitus of keeshond dogs. *Diabetes* 29:558, 1980.

75. Kunkle, G. A., et al. Tyrosinemia in a dog. *J. Am. Anim. Hosp. Assoc.* 20:615, 1984.

76. Kurtz, H. J., and Fletcher, T. F. The peripheral neuropathy of canine globoid-cell leukodystrophy (Krabbe-type). *Acta Neuropathol. (Berl.)* 16:226, 1970.

77. Laws, L., and Saal, J. R. Lipidosis of the hepatic reticuloendothelial cells in a sheep. *Aust. Vet. J.* 44:416, 1968.

78. Leipold, H. W., et al. Mannosidosis in Angus calves, *J. Am. Vet. Med. Assoc.* 175:457, 1979.

79. Letson, R. D., and Desnick, R. J. Punctate lenticular opacities in type II mannosidosis. *Am. J. Ophthalmol.* 85:218, 1978.

80. Lutzner, M. A., Tierney, J. H., and Benditt, E. P. Giant granules and widespread cytoplasmic inclusions in a genetic syndrome of Aleutian mink: An electron microscopic study. *Lab. Invest.* 14:2063, 1965.

81. Manktelow, B. W., and Hartley, W. J. Generalized glycogen storage disease in sheep. *J. Comp. Pathol.* 85:139, 1975.

82. Massof, R. W., and Johnson, M. A. Prereceptor light absorption in setters with neuronal ceroid lipofuscinosis. *Invest. Ophthalmol. Vis. Sci.* 20:134, 1981.

83. McKusick, V. A., and Neufeld, E. F. The Mucopolysaccharide Storage Diseases. In J. B. Stanbury et al. (Eds.), *The Metabolic Basis of Inherited Disease* (5th ed.). New York: McGraw-Hill, 1983.

84. Murray, J. A., Blakemore, W. F., and Barnett, K. C. Ocular lesions in cats with GM_1 gangliosidosis with visceral involvement. *J. Small Anim. Pract.* 18:1, 1977.

85. Narfström, K. Hereditary progressive retinal atrophy in the Abyssinian cat. *J. Hered.* 74:273, 1983.

86. Neville, H., et al. Studies on the retina and the pigment epithelium in hereditary canine ceroid lipofuscinosis: III. Morphologic abnormalities in retinal neurons and retinal pigmented epithelial cells. *Invest. Ophthalmol. Vis. Sci.* 19:75, 1980.

87. Nilsson, S. E. G., et al. Studies on the retina and pigment epithelium in hereditary canine ceroid lipofuscinosis: IV. Changes in the ERG and standing potential of the eye. *Invest. Ophthalmol. Vis. Sci.* 24:77, 1983.

88. O'Brien, J. S. The Gangliosidoses. In J. B. Stanbury et al. (Eds.), *The Metabolic Basis of Inherited Disease* (5th ed.). New York: McGraw-Hill, 1983.

89. Oliver, J. M. Impaired microtubule function correctable by cGMP and cholinergic agonists in the Chédiak-Higashi syndrome. *Am. J. Pathol.* 85:395, 1976.

90. O'Sullivan, B. M., et al. Generalised glycogenosis in Brahman cattle. *Aust. Vet. J.* 57:227, 1984.

91. Padgett, G. A., et al. The familial occurrence of the Chédiak-Higashi syndrome in mink and cattle. *Genetics* 49:505, 1964.

92. Patel, V., et al. *p*-Phenylenediamine-mediated peroxidase deficiency in English setters with neuronal ceroid-lipofuscinosis. *Lab. Invest.* 30:366, 1974.

93. Patterson, D. F. A Catalog of Genetic Disorders of the Dog. In R. W. Kirk (Ed.), *Current Veterinary Therapy* (7th ed.). Philadelphia: Saunders, 1980.

94. Pierce, K. R., et al. Animal model of human disease GM_2 gangliosidosis: Porcine cerebrospinal lipodystrophy. *Am. J. Pathol.* 83:419, 1976.

95. Prieur, D. J., and Collier, L. L. Chédiak-Higashi syndrome of animals. *Am. J. Pathol.* 90:533, 1978.

96. Pritchard, D. H., Napthine, D. V., and Sinclair, A. J. Globoid cell leucodystrophy in polled Dorset sheep. *Vet. Pathol.* 17:399, 1980.

97. Rac, R., and Giesecke, C. T. Lysosomal storage disease in Chihuahuas. *Aust. Vet. J.* 51:403, 1975.

98. Ratta, L. A., Hliba, E., and Yantorno, C. E. Sindrome de Chédiak-Higashi-Steinbrinck: Estudio hematologico y ultraestructural. *Sangre (Barc.)* 22:263, 1977.

99. Read, D. H., et al. Neuronal-visceral GM_1 gangliosidosis in a dog with β galactosidase deficiency. *Science* 194:442, 1976.

100. Read, W. K., and Bridges, C. H. Cerebrospinal lipodystrophy in swine: A new model in comparative pathology. *Pathol. Vet.* 5:67, 1968.

101. Read, W. K., and Bridges, C. H. Neuronal lipodystrophy: Occurrence in an inbred strain of cattle. *Pathol. Vet.* 6:235, 1969.

102. Sandstrom, B., Westman, J., and Öckerman, P. A. Glycogenosis of the central nervous system in the cat. *Acta Neuropathol. (Berl.)* 14:194, 1969.

103. Sheahan, B. J., and Donnelly, W. J. C. Enzyme histochemical and ultrastructural alterations in the brains of Friesian calves with GM_1 gangliosidosis. *Acta Neuropathol. (Berl.)* 30:73, 1974.

104. Sheahan, B. J., Donnelly, W. J. C., and Grimes, T. D. Ocular pathology of bovine GM_1 gangliosidosis. *Acta Neuropathol. (Berl.)* 41:91, 1978.

105. Shull, R. M., et al. Morphologic and biochemical studies of canine mucopolysaccharidosis I. *Am. J. Pathol.* 114:487, 1984.
106. Shull, R. M., et al. Canine α-L-iduronidase deficiency: A model of mucopolysaccharidosis I. *Am. J. Pathol.* 109:244, 1982.
107. Siakotos, A. New findings in the biochemistry of purified blood components and tissues in canine neuronal-retinal ceroidosis. In preparation, 1985.
108. Siakotos, A. N., et al. The Morphogenesis and Biochemical Characteristics of Ceroid Isolated from Cases of Neuronal Ceroid-Lipofuscinosis. In B. W. Volk and S. M. Aronson (Eds.), *Sphingolipids, Sphingolipidoses and Allied Disorders.* New York: Plenum, 1972.
109. Siakotos, A. N., et al. Procedures for isolation of two distinct lipopigments from human brains: Lipofuscin and ceroid. *Biochem. Med.* 4:361, 1970.
110. Snyder, S. P. Personal communication, 1984.
111. Spencer, W. H., and Hogan, M. J. Ocular manifestations of Chédiak-Higashi syndrome. *Am. J. Ophthalmol.* 50:1197, 1960.
112. Suzuki, K., and Suzuki, Y. Galactosylceramide Lipidosis: Globoid Cell Leukodystrophy (Krabbe's Disease). In J. B. Stanbury et al. (Eds.), *The Metabolic Basis of Inherited Disease* (5th ed.). New York: McGraw-Hill, 1983.
113. Takki, K., and Simmell, O. Gyrate atrophy of the choroid and retina with hyperornithenemia (HOGA). *Birth Defects* 12:373, 1976.
114. Taylor, R. F., and Farrell, R. K. Light and electron microscopy of peripheral blood neutrophils in a killer whale affected with Chédiak-Higashi syndrome. *Fed. Proc.* 32:882, 1973.
115. Topping, T. M., et al. Ultrastructural and ocular pathology of Hunter's syndrome: Systemic mucopolysaccharidosis type II. *Arch. Ophthalmol.* 86:164, 1971.
116. Valenzuela, R., and Morningstar, W. A. The ocular pigmentary disturbance of human Chédiak-Higashi syndrome. *Am. J. Clin. Pathol.* 75:591, 1981.
117. Valle, D. L., et al. Gyrate atrophy of the choroid and retina in a cat. *Invest. Ophthalmol. Vis. Sci.* 20:251, 1981.
118. Valle, D., Jezyk, P., and Aguirre, G. Gyrate atrophy of the choroid and retina. *Comp. Pathol. Bull.* 15:2, 1983.
119. Vandevelde, M., et al. Hereditary neurovisceral mannosidosis associated with α-mannosidase deficiency in a family of Persian cats. *Acta Neuropathol. (Berl.).* 58:64, 1982.
120. van de Water, N. S., Jolly, R. D., and Farrow, B. R. H. Canine Gaucher disease: The enzymic defect. *Aust. J. Exp. Biol. Med. Sci.* 57:551, 1979.
121. Varma, S. D. Aldose Reductase and Etiology of Diabetic Cataracts. In J. A. Zadunaisky and H. Davson (Eds.), *Current Topics in Eye Research.* New York: Academic, 1980.
122. Vine, D. T., et al. Enhancement of residual arylsulfatase B activity in feline mucopolysaccharidosis VI by thiol-induced subunit association. *J. Clin. Invest.* 69:294, 1982.
123. Walvoort, H. C. Unpublished data, 1984.
124. Walvoort, H. C., Slee, R. G., and Koster, J. F. Canine glycogen storage disease type II: A biochemical study of an acid α-glucosidase deficient Lapland dog. *Biochim. Biophys. Acta* 715:63, 1982.
125. Walvoort, H. C., et al. Canine glycogen storage disease type II: A clinical study of four affected Lapland dogs. *J. Am. Anim. Hosp. Assoc.* 20:279, 1984.
126. Wenger, D. A., et al. Niemann-Pick disease: A genetic model in Siamese cats. *Science* 208:1471, 1980.
127. Windhorst, D. B., and Padgett, G. The Chédiak-Higashi syndrome and the homologous trait in animals. *J. Invest. Dermatol.* 60:529, 1973.
128. Wolfe, L. S., and NgYing Kin, N. M. K. Batten Disease: New Research Findings on the Biochemical Defect. In E. Cotlier, I. H. Maumenee, and E. R. Berman (Eds.), *Genetic Eye Diseases.* New York: Liss, 1982.
129. Yanoff, M., and Fine, B. S. *Ocular Pathology: A Text and Atlas* (2nd ed.). Philadelphia: Harper & Row, 1982. P. 549.

7

Ocular Pharmacogenetics

William H. Havener

One might reasonably expect such a title as Ocular Pharmacogenetics to encompass a set of biologic reactions entirely unique to the eye. However, on due consideration, we will realize that the eye is a diagnostic window because it exhibits the typical behavior of all the ectodermal and mesodermal tissues of the entire body. Only endoderm is not present in the eye. Hence, pharmaceuticals will exhibit exactly the same effects on the enzymes, hormones, and other biochemically active tissue components of the eye as in other parts of the body. Strictly speaking, therefore, no such thing as "ocular" pharmacogenetics exists.

The eye does possess unique structures and functions, which are subject to genetic aberrations. Of these inherited disorders, very few are remediable by medical therapy. The dramatic exception is glaucoma. Obviously, we know of many types of glaucoma, each of which may have a somewhat different form of treatment. These variations (for example, narrow-angle vs. open-angle glaucoma) could perhaps be described as ocular pharmacogenetics, but traditionally the term *ocular pharmacology* is used to describe compilation of these different forms of treatment. So we will exclude traditional details of glaucoma therapy from this chapter. However, by far the most important aspect of ocular pharmacogenetics is the corticosteroid response in glaucoma; therefore this will be presented in some detail. (Be aware that those hypotheses to be presented are incompletely established.)

GLAUCOMA

If we consider only ocular disease and exclude inherited conditions that affect mainly other portions of the body, glaucoma and its response to corticosteroid therapy is by far the most significant pharmacogenetic relationship. Extensive studies document this relationship, which is easily verified by every ophthalmologist in routine practice. The biochemical basis for the response, its genetics, and the practical clinical implications follow.

Biochemical Basis of Corticosteroid Effect on Ocular Pressure

Living cells that respond to corticosteroids do so by means of specific receptor molecules capable of competitively binding various analogs of steroid molecules. Therefore, corticosteroid-sensitive cells can be detected and measured by the use of radioactive corticosteroids. A typical sensitive cell may contain as many as 60,000 corticosteroid receptor molecules. To obtain a uniform cell population for such studies, tissue culture methods are used to propagate a sufficient number of cells. Radiolabeling techniques applied to as few as 500,000 such cells can identify the relative affinities of these receptors and can differentiate their location in cytoplasm or nucleus. For example, the receptor affinity of dexamethasone is twice that of hydrocortisone and four times that of progesterone. This corresponds to the greater corticosteroid activity of dexamethasone and the corticosteroid antagonist activity of progesterone, which may act by partially blocking the receptors.

Methods of separating cell nuclei from the cytoplasm by means of centrifugation permit demonstration that 60 percent of the corticosteroid receptors are located in the nucleus and only 40 percent in the cytoplasm. Exposure of the cell to corticosteroids in physiologic concentrations results in radioactive labeling of the cytoplasmic receptors. Within 30 minutes, two-thirds of these labeled receptors have migrated to the nucleus. One current concept of the mechanism of corticosteroid action is that the corticosteroid-receptor complex associates with the nuclear chromatin and transmits the functional message regulating the appropriate synthesis of effector molecules. The corticosteroid response presumably changes the quality and quantity of the cellular products, such as enzymes, mucopolysaccharides, and collagen. With respect to intraocular pressure, these responses may alter the rate of aqueous production or the permeability of the outflow channels. Both the ciliary body and the trabecular meshwork contain cells that demonstrate presence of specific corticosteroid receptors. Therefore both areas are capable of being influenced by corticosteroid therapy [16, 18, 19].

Another mechanism by which corticosteroid effect on the ciliary body could change outflow facility may be lysosome stabilization. Lysosomal glycosidase activity in the ciliary body and aqueous humor is decreased by systemic administration of hydrocortisone in rabbits. These enzymes break down mucopolysaccharides and may function to maintain normal permeability of the outflow pathways [9]. The concept of lysosomal stabilization by corticosteroids is well established. This stabilization occurs by a strengthening of the membrane wall enclosing the lysosome. The wall becomes bimolecular in composition as a result of the joining of protein and lipid molecules. Hence the release of lysosomal enzymes is inhibited. This is the reason for the well-known clinical effect of corticosteroids, namely, a reduction of inflammatory damage to tissue.

Lysosomal stabilization within the trabecular meshwork itself should be even more effective at that location than the remote effect from the ciliary body. It has been suggested that the goniocytes (trabecular meshwork cells) are not all identical but are derived from the multiplication of original cells to form a number of clones of the original goniocytes [3]. These clones may differ genetically in their corticosteroid responsiveness or in other factors predisposing to glaucoma. Because of local variations in the populations of these clones, the glaucomatous responsiveness of the individual would also be variable and would not follow the usual well-defined patterns of mendelian recessive or dominant inheritance; nor would the two eyes be identical in their degree of glaucoma [3].

I am unaware of any experimental proof of the presence of such different clones of goniocytes.

However, the lymphocytes of glaucomatous patients can be differentiated from those of normal persons on the basis of corticosteroid inhibition of lymphocyte activation by phytohemagglutinins and theophylline [20].

Inheritance of Corticosteroid Ocular Hypertensive Response

The concepts of the inheritance of glaucoma continue to change. Originally, the observation of familial incidence of the disease and the statistical bias resulting from the reporting of more obvious extensive pedigrees led to the conclusion that "chronic simple glaucoma" was dominantly inherited.

Discovery of the corticosteroid hypertensive response permitted recognition of an ocular hypertensive characteristic affecting one-third of the entire population. A much smaller group, only 5 percent, develop a more severe pressure rise resulting in the ocular damage of glaucoma. These findings were interpreted to mean that open-angle glaucoma is a recessive trait carried by one-third of the population and manifesting overt glaucoma only in the homozygous state. Subsequently, this monogenic concept was challenged because of inconsistent statistical findings. For example, only 65 percent of monozygotic twins show the same corticosteroid-induced ocular pressure response [14]. Of 87 children of glaucomatous parents, only 34 percent showed a corticosteroid response, whereas all should have been heterozygotes according to the theory of recessive inheritance [3]. This discrepancy may indicate that the inheritance of glaucoma is actually multifactorial.

Before discarding the concept of recessive inheritance, one should consider the numerous explanations for pedigree variability. The concept of penetrance, for example, states that some 50,000 separate genes modify the characteristics of an individual and help to determine the effect of the single suspect gene. No one would question the dominance of von Recklinghausen's neurofibromatosis just because the severity of the condition is so variable. The corticosteroid hypertensive response is not constant—it is only 73 percent reproducible in the same individual [12]. Furthermore, this response is dose related, increasing with the potency and dosage of the corticosteroid [10].

Practical Implications

Knowledge of the corticosteroid responsiveness of various categories of eye disease is helpful in guiding our routine decisions as to therapy. Since the overwhelming majority of patients with open-angle glaucoma are corticosteroid responsive, we will try to avoid corticosteroid use here. For example, allergy to glaucoma medications is not rationally treated by corticosteroids; rather, discontinue the offending medication. Inquire as to improper corticosteroid use in patients with poorly controlled glaucoma. Do not inject repository corticosteroids. The frequent requirement for corticosteroid treatment after intraocular lens implantation is a relatively strong contraindication to this procedure in patients with poorly controlled glaucoma.

The incidence of corticosteroid hypertensive response is about one-third in the general population, in secondary glaucoma [1], in contusion angle glaucoma, and in pigmentary glaucoma [21]. Therefore, these disorders can be treated alike insofar as the judgment for corticosteroid therapy is concerned. A positive dexamethasone pressure response did not occur in 17 patients with early postoperative glaucoma after cataract surgery. Hence surgical factors, rather than genetic predisposition, are responsible for early postoperative pressure rises.

A high corticosteroid pressure response was found in 20 percent of patients with nontraumatic rhegmatogenous retinal detachments (5% would be expected). Furthermore, 53 percent had a cup/disc ratio greater than 0.3 (18% expected). These figures were obtained *after* exclusion from the study group of any patient with recognizable open-angle glaucoma [15]. Practically, this means that corticosteroid therapy will cause glaucoma in 1 of every 5 retinal detachment patients. Furthermore, this supports my conviction that "miotic-induced detachment" is nothing more than a genetic coincidence of detachment, glaucoma, and cataract [6].

Obviously, this practical clinical wisdom as to when to avoid corticosteroids and when to use them with caution and frequent pressure monitoring will remain valid regardless of whether open-angle glaucoma is dominant, recessive, multifactorial, or due to sensitive clones of goniocytes.

PRINCIPLES OF PHARMACOGENETICS

During my residency I learned that atropine dilated rabbit eyes only poorly and transiently. Further evaluation of this finding revealed that the resourceful little beasts could munch contentedly on belladonna vines and fruits that would kill a human being 100 times the size of the rabbit. Even more intriguing was the revelation that not all rabbits can do this. Only the possessors of the genetic trait of manufacturing atropine esterase are protected against the fatal consequences of accidentally nibbling on a tasty but poisonous piece of succulent vegetation. You need read no further than this paragraph to perceive the two most important facts about pharmacogenetics. First, pharmacologic facts about one species are not necessarily true about another species. Second, pharmacologic facts about an individual within a species are not necessarily true about another individual of the same species.

Mode of Action of Pharmacogenetic Phenomena

A disclaimer is necessary. All differences in drug reactions are not necessarily due to genetic factors. Certainly many environmental and other influences affect drug responses. These influences include biologic interactions, immunologic status, biorhythms, diet, exercise, age, and spontaneous variability. Even in the same individual, marked perturbations in drug concentrations result from different routes of administration, the presence of other drugs or normal biologic materials, or various physiologic states.

Recognized pharmacogenetic variations may be mediated via absorption, transport, biotransformation, and excretion mechanisms [2]. These phenomena occur with the aid of proteins and enzymes with selective binding sites that may enhance delivery, retention, inactivation, or destruction of various drugs and biologic substances. The presence, characteristics, and amount of such proteins are governed by genetic coding. In the eye active transport mechanisms are known to affect the concentrations of many substances, including antibiotics, amino acids, prostaglandins, glycosides, vitamins, and immunoglobulins. Multiple mechanisms, acting throughout the body, are available to implement the different responses that have been categorized as pharmacogenetics.

Pharmacogenetic Evaluation in Twins

Twin studies, as expected, have shown drug metabolism to be more alike in monozygotic twins than in dizygotic twins. Many pitfalls exist in twin studies and permit erroneous conclusions as to the respective importance of genetics and environment. Also, the consequences of a given metabolic finding may not necessarily be the obvious and apparent first clinical prediction. An especially good reference for the reader interested in the evaluation of twin studies is the review by Vesell [17].

Meticulous care in the planning of twin studies and very sophisticated data processing demonstrate that genetic factors are a primary cause of the large interindividual variations in drug metabolism in normal human subjects. This statement must be followed immediately by the equally important fact that the microsomal enzymes of the liver (which are enormously important in pharmacokinetics) can easily be induced to change their activity greatly in response to many commonly used drugs and foods. Unless these environmental factors are exquisitely controlled, the value of a twin study is severely diluted. Furthermore, no patient is ever in a basal pharmacogenetic state, since the effects of environment (past and present disease, medications, food, and all other external factors) have certainly modified his or her responses.

To illustrate the virtual certainty of a genetic basis for variations in drug metabolism, twin studies of variance were undertaken by a formula in which a value of 0.00 would indicate no hereditary and complete environmental influence; a value of 1.00 would indicate complete hereditary and no environmental influence. Both monozygotic and dizygotic twins were studied. Since monozygotic twins are genetically identical, their theoretical value would be 1.00. Dizygotic twins share approximately half their genes and have a theoretical value of 0.50. The metabolism of a number of common and important drugs was studied, and the results are stated in Table 7-1. The close approximation between these actual values and the theoretical values of 1.00 and 0.50 are highly significant and verify the presumption of pharmacogenetic influence. That is, variances between monozygotic twins reflect only environmental factors, whereas variances between dizygotic twins are due to both environmental and genetic differences.

Assay Techniques

Study of drug responses has been greatly extended by the development of effective assays of blood levels of drugs. Blood level studies are not commonplace in the clinical treatment of individual patients and are invaluable in the study of genetic responses.

The Complexity of Pharmacogenetics

The statement that glucose 6-phosphate dehydrogenase (G6PD) deficiency is the most common human enzyme abnormality leads to the false conclusion that we now know a single specific fault responsible for a disease. Actually, at least 130 different G6PD variants that can be differentiated by enzymatic, immunologic, physical, and functional characteristics are known to exist. G6PD deficiency is not due to reduced concentration of the normal enzyme but invariably results from the production of molecular variants that differ in their affinity for the various other molecules involved in the specific enzymatic activity of this substance [7]. This molecular complexity should come as no surprise to anyone who knows that there are over 100 different forms of the simple molecule H_2O. These result from different combinations of the various valences and isotopes of its constituent atoms.

The laboratory tests used to study enzyme variants may have inherent deficiencies. For example, the study of pseudocholinesterase-deficient sera is usually done with a substrate of benzoylcholine for reasons of technical convenience. However, this assay confirms the presence of an atypical pseudocholinesterase in only 70 percent of patients exhibiting prolonged apnea after use of succinylcholine. Development and use of a new assay using a substrate of succinyldicholine detected a atypical enzyme in 90 percent of the apneic patients. By means of these enzyme assays it is possible to identify patients who are homozygous for the abnormal enzyme, heterozygous, or homozygous for the normal enzyme [5].

The Importance of Pharmacogenetics

Biologic differences in individuals are so enormous that a lifesaving drug for one person will be

Table 7-1. *Heritability of Pharmacokinetic Variations in Monozygotic and Dizygotic Twins*

Drug	Heritability value*	
	Monozygotic	Dizygotic
Antipyrine	0.98	0.47
Phenylbutazone	0.99	0.33
Bishydroxycoumarin	0.97	0.66
Ethanol	0.98	0.38
Halothane	0.88	0.36

*See text for explanation of heritability values.

fatal to another. (Consider epinephrine, given by injection to a patient suffering a severe anaphylactic reaction with bronchospasm or to a patient with acute coronary vessel insufficiency.) My message is that we cannot, as ophthalmologists, divorce ourselves from knowledge of the reactions of the entire body to potent drugs. Even when drugs are used only as eyedrops, sufficient absorption may occur to result in systemic toxicity. (Witness the timolol maleate response of a patient with pulmonary decompensation.) Hyperreactivity, idiosyncrasy, or unresponsiveness to drugs are extremely common individual variants and require consideration in our everyday practice. Do not be skeptical! Only recall, for instance, that because of the melanin pigment sink, you daily use more than twice as much of mydriatic, cycloplegic, and miotic drugs to achieve the same effect in a black patient as in a blond Scandinavian. Conversely, a retinotoxic drug such as chloroquine is selectively retained and toxic in the pigment epithelium of a dark brunette, yet is almost harmless to an albino.

Human Biochemical Faults

We tend to forget the immense biochemical complexity of each individual. (I know I do.) On some idle weekend, leaf through the 2,032 pages of *The Metabolic Basis of Inherited Disease,* the simply massive and unbelievably detailed masterwork edited by Stanbury and colleagues [16A]. Having reviewed the known complexity of human biology, reflect for a moment on the much larger amount of unknown detail. If this experience does not fill you with true awe and wonder, you are either too young to understand or too old to care.

Let me present only a skeleton review of this exceptional book, intended to refresh your memories of a subject that you may have last considered in depth while you were a medical student. Your inherited characteristics depend on 23 pairs of chromosomes, which are composed of perhaps 50,000 individual pairs of genes. As if this were not sufficiently complicated, each gene can itself vary in molecular composition or stereotaxic configuration. Exchange of only a single atom in this intricate array can and does change the biochemical responses of the resulting human being. You have seen that no two snowflakes in the history of the world have been exactly alike; consider how much more complex you are than is a snowflake!

A genetic syndrome may result from change of a single gene. An accepted concept is that a single gene endows the organism with the presence of a single specific enzyme; for example, homogentisic acid oxidase. Absence of this enzyme results in the accumulation of homogentisic acid, which is the basis of alkaptonuria.

Genetic syndromes are clinically identifiable because of a variety of look-alike characteristics. At first recognition such a syndrome seems to be a single fault. With detailed analysis we find that malfunction of a variety of genes, perhaps involved in a sequential chain of biochemical reactions, can cause the apparently same clinical syndrome. Another type of variant is due to alleles, which are slight differences in the chemical structure of the same gene. For example, ophthalmologists are aware that a number of different variants of retinitis pigmentosa exist; hematologists know of more than 100 different hemoglobin molecules.

Identification of the precise fault responsible for a genetic abnormality may infrequently permit its correction. For example, the progress of galactose cataracts can be arrested or even reversed by avoidance of dietary lactose from an early age. The Kayser-Fleischer ring of Wilson's disease can be removed by penicillamine treatment to remove copper from the body. This treatment is, of course, indicated to prevent or reverse central nervous system and hepatic disease, since the corneal ring is of no consequence except for its diagnostic value.

Idiosyncratic reactions to drugs are very common and necessitate careful evaluation of the history of such drug intolerances, with respect to both the individual patient and the family. Presumably a very high proportion of adverse drug reactions occur on this basis. As examples, G6PD deficiency predisposes millions of persons to hemolytic anemia on exposure to a large variety of drugs and foodstuffs. Prescription of barbiturate sedatives or alcoholic elixirs causes attacks of acute porphyria. Pseudocholinesterase-deficient individuals suffer prolonged apnea when anesthetized with the aid of succinylcholine chloride. A number of anesthetic agents precipitate malignant hyperthermia.

SPECIFIC EXAMPLES

From the legions of metabolic derangements that are known or suspected, the examples to be presented will be chosen on the basis of ocular significance, high prevalence and therefore sufficient importance to justify recognition by all physicians, or theoretical significance.

Albinism

Deficiency or absence of melanin on the basis of recessive inheritance is one of the most obvious genetic faults.

Because of the absence of melanin binding, albino eyes are more responsive to many of our commonly used ophthalmic drugs, including all cycloplegics, mydriatics, and miotics. Hence, lower concentrations will be therapeutically effective in albinos than in darkly pigmented patients.

Albino skin is vulnerable to sunlight damage, which causes skin cancer. Sunscreen lotions such as 5% para-aminobenzoic acid are useful. Fortunately these individuals are photosensitive and spontaneously prefer to avoid excessive light.

The popular use of albino animals in research is especially inappropriate and improper in drug testing. Melanin acts as a drug receptor for many chemicals, thereby causing profound differences in responses between pigmented and albino animals. Uptake, retention, and attainable concentrations of drugs are markedly affected. Data from drug tests in albino animals simply cannot be extrapolated to human beings. Eye researchers should be particularly hesitant to use albino animals since their visual system is grossly abnormal. Not only the eye itself, but also the visual pathways are atypical.

An extraordinary feature of albinism is that many more nerve fibers from the temporal retina *cross* to the opposite side in the optic chiasm instead of being uncrossed as normally occurs. This occurs in many animals, including the guinea pig, rat, rabbit, mink, ferret, Siamese cat, chinchilla, and tiger, as well as in albino humans. Lack of retinal pigment appears to be the feature associated with the abnormal crossing characteristic. The affected individual has defective binocular vision. Differences between albino and pigmented animals also include changes in the auditory system, the digestive tract, the liver, psychological behavior, skin, and autonomic nervous system.

Malignant Hyperthermia

Malignant hyperthermia is an autosomal dominant trait affecting 1 in 20,000 persons. It is precipitated by various anesthetics, including halothane [17]. Recognition of the condition may be by the realization that the anesthetized patient is becoming obviously hot. At this point, survival is at stake and emergency treatment with ice baths and dantrolene sodium is necessary.

Far better is detection of the condition by a family history of serious or fatal reactions during anesthesia. Supported by this knowledge, the physician may pretreat with dantrolene sodium, choose local anesthesia rather than general (not certainly safe), and have cooling mechanisms ready for instant use.

The sensitivity of response of biopsied muscle tissue to caffeine is a fairly reliable test for malignant hyperthermia. Muscle tissue from affected individuals is highly sensitive to caffeine alone or to the combination of caffeine and halothane. Unaffected family members are frequently sensitive to the combined effect of caffeine and halothane but not to caffeine alone. Normal muscle tissue is less responsive to either stimulus. This test suggests that at least two gene characteristics are active in the transmission of malignant hyperthermia, which behaves like an autosomal dominant trait [8].

Familial Hypercholesterolemia

Unlike most of the exotic and rare recessive gene faults that fascinate us, the heterozygote status of dominant familial hypercholesterolemia has a frequency of 1 in 500 persons. It is probably the most common single gene disease. All heterozygotes, even at the youngest age, manifest hypercholesterolemia. Arcus juvenilis of the peripheral cornea is found in most patients by the age of 30 years. Palpebral xanthelasma may also be transmitted independently of hypercholesterolemia.

Coronary heart disease affects half of heterozygotes 50 years of age; 25 percent of these will die a coronary death within 4 years. Cardiovascular damage is the reason that this very common genetic trait is of great importance. Five percent of heterozygous men have already had a myocardial infarction by age 30.

Cholesterol is an essential part of all cell membranes. Cells can produce their own cholesterol but preferentially obtain it from serum, outside the cell. Serum cholesterol is transported by a carrier, low-density lipoprotein (LDL). LDL delivers its cholesterol to LDL receptor molecules on the cell surface. LDL receptors vary in number in accordance with the current cell need for cholesterol. A single cell may have as many as 50,000 LDL receptors. The LDL receptors are clustered in coated pits, which are small cavities in the cell wall. The cell ingests the cholesterol-laden LDL by phagocytosing the coated pit, which closes over to become a cholesterol-filled vesicle. This process occurs very rapidly, half of the surface receptor–bound LDL being ingested every 5 minutes. When sufficient cholesterol exists within the cell, biofeedback stops cholesterol biosynthesis within the cell, stops production of LDL receptors, and activates cholesterol storage enzymes.

The fault in familial hypercholesterolemia is a reduced number of LDL receptors. Heterozygotes have a 50 percent deficiency of LDL receptors; homozygotes have none at all. The obvious consequence of this is that excess cholesterol-laden LDL remains in the plasma, and the cells are constantly biosynthesizing more endogenous cholesterol.

Therapy for hypercholesterolemia includes cholestyramine and nicotinic acid, which can lower LDL cholesterol levels by 30 percent. The mechanism of action of the nicotinic acid is unknown. The cholestyramine is an exchange resin that binds bile acids. The cellular response to the resultant cholesterol decrease is to make more LDL receptors (the deficiency of which is the cause of familial hypercholesterolemia).

The ophthalmologic implications of all this are that recognition of arcus juvenilis and xanthelasma permit detection of persons at high risk of being heterozygotes for familial hypercholesterolemia. If laboratory testing confirms a high cholesterol level, cholestyramine therapy may be helpful. Dietary avoidance of exogenous cholesterol will lower lipid levels somewhat, but not nearly to normal levels.

Familial Type III Hyperlipoproteinemia

High cholesterol serum levels also occur in patients with abnormal apoprotein E, a normal remnant of broken-down lipoprotein carriers. Apoprotein E causes the liver to cleanse the blood of lipoprotein remnants. The abnormal remnant escapes liver uptake, resulting in high blood lipid levels. Scavenger cells bind the lipids, resulting in localized deposits, such as in xanthomas and atheromas.

About 1 in 100 European whites are homozygous for this trait, which is recessive with poor expressivity. One must simultaneously suffer from other inherited or environmental effects (e.g., obesity, diabetes mellitus, hyperthyroidism, other lipid metabolic traits), or else cholesterol levels will be normal.

This condition is included as an example of a number of other causes of elevated cholesterol besides familial hypercholesterolemia. There are many specific inherited disorders of lipid metabolism.

Wilson's Hepatolenticular Disease

Unknown transport disorders in Wilson's disease, a recessive condition, cause a deficiency in ceruloplasmin, one of the copper transport proteins. Excessive amounts of copper accumulate in the body, causing liver and basal ganglia damage.

The Kayser-Fleischer copper ring in the peripheral Descemet's membrane is the most easily observed diagnostic sign and is found in 100 percent of these patients with neurologic complaints, in 95 percent of all recognized patients, but in only 70 percent of children with Wilson's disease presenting with acute hepatic disease. Slit-lamp examination is the most important part of the physical examination of these patients.

Because penicillamine (dosage 1–3 gm daily) is curative and can reverse both liver and basal ganglia disease, the diagnosis of acute or chronic liver disease or of basal ganglia disease must always be Wilson's disease until this possibility has been excluded. Also, examine all siblings of patients, for they have a 25 percent chance of being affected.

Copper measurement should be included in all liver biopsy studies. Since the liver is the primary excretory organ for copper, a secondary elevation of liver copper may occur in biliary obstructive syndromes.

Galactosemia

Galactitol, an alternate pathway metabolite of galactose, is formed within the lens via aldose reductase enzymatic action. The semipermeable lens capsule traps the galactitol, which increases the osmotic pressure excessively, resulting in lens hydration and cataract formation. Aldose reductase inhibitors (e.g., 3,3-tetramethyleneglutanic acid, aspirin) will prevent the development of experimental galactose cataracts. The concept of use of aldose reductase inhibitors to prevent cataracts in general is under investigation.

The neurotoxicity and brain damage of galactose is also due to galactitol-induced hyperosmolarity.

Of course, avoidance of galactose ingestion is well known to be the standard treatment for galactosemia. All of the systemic toxic effects of this disease, as well as the typical developmental cataracts, can be arrested or even partially reversed by this dietary approach. All well-informed ophthalmologists should know that baby kangaroos are deficient in galactokinase and will develop cataracts if fed cow's milk.

Alpha$_1$-Antitrypsin

Alpha$_1$-antitrypsin, a multienzyme inhibitor, is named after trypsin, for this was the substrate first used in characterizing its properties. However, the name that would best describe the most important function of this enzyme is α_1-antielastase. An ophthalmologist (or any other physician, for that matter) should be aware of this genetically determined enzyme because it provides the basis for one of the major toxic effects of the most preventable cause of all the medical problems in the United States.

Alpha$_1$-antitrypsin is genetically deficient in amount in 1 of 3,000 homozygous Americans. It is a circulating protein small enough to traverse tissue barriers, especially those of the pulmonary alveoli. In less than 0.5 msec, α_1-antitrypsin can bind and inactivate neutrophil elastase. This elastase inactivation is important because neutrophils tend to sediment in the lower portions of the lungs. Pulmonary irritation, as from smoking tobacco, greatly increases the number of defending neutrophils present within the alveoli. Smoking also destroys α_1-antitrypsin. The important consequence of all this is that emphysema is caused by alveolar destruction by neutrophil elastase acting in the absence of the protective enzyme α_1-antitrypsin. This can happen to anyone who smokes too much but is positively devastating to those unfortunate persons who are genetically deficient in this protective enzyme. Of these genetically deficient persons, 70 percent die before age 50 if they smoke, as compared to 20 percent who are nonsmokers.

Quite seriously, the caption "The Surgeon General has determined that smoking is dangerous to your health" is not printed in all tobacco ads because it is not true. *It is true.* In fact, fully half of the medical costs in our country are directly attributable to only two preventable causes—smoking and drinking.

Sickle Cell Anemia

Although only about 50,000 individuals affected by the recessive sickle cell trait reside in the United States, its characteristics of causing anemia and arterial occlusion with the severe pains of infarction (bones, spleen) are well known to lay persons and physicians alike. Severe exacerbations may occur with anesthesia, and ischemic necrosis of the eye may complicate retinal detachment repair. Exchange transfusion before anesthesia has been suggested.

Therapy is generally not very effective. Urea and cyanate reduce sickling but are not generally practicable therapeutic methods. Attention to good nutrition and hygiene is important to minimize the problems of chronic anemia and susceptibility to infection.

Glucose 6-Phosphate Dehydrogenase Deficiency

The aging normal erythrocyte becomes deficient in G6PD. In persons who suffer from a sex-linked recessive deficiency of G6PD, older red blood cells become vulnerable to hemolytic destruction if they are stressed by illness, diabetic acidosis, or certain therapeutic drugs. This destruction results in an attack of hemolytic anemia with jaundice.

Since younger erythrocytes contain more G6PD, they do not hemolyze, and the hemolytic attack spontaneously ceases within a few days (after the older cells are gone). Therefore this enzyme deficiency does not cause life-threatening anemia.

Physicians should be aware of G6PD deficiency because it is the most common inherited enzyme deficiency causing human disease. Hemolytic crises may be caused by, for example, several (not all) sulfonamides (including sulfacetamide, sulfapyridine, sulfamethoxazole, and sulfanilamide), acetanilid, primaquine phosphate and pentaquine (antimalarials), nalidixic acid, nitrofurantoin (Furadantin), methylene blue, naphthalene, and phenylhydrazine. Exposure to such drugs should be avoided in patients with a history of hemolytic anemia or neonatal icterus.

G6PD deficiency hemolysis does not occur from acetaminophen (Tylenol), phenacetin, aspirin, antazoline, ascorbic acid, chloramphenicol, chloroquine, colchicine, diphenhydramine hydrochloride (Benadryl), isoniazid, probenecid, pyrimethamine (Daraprim), quinidine, quinine sulfate, streptomycin sulfate, sulfadiazine, sulfaguanidine, sulfamerazine, sulfisoxazole, or tripelennamine.

Glucose 6-phosphate dehydrogenase deficiency (drug-induced hemolytic anemia, favism) is an x-linked incomplete dominant trait affecting up to 100 million human beings.

Fabry's Disease (α-Galactosidase A Deficiency)

For ophthalmologists Fabry's is the disease that causes whorls of gray opacities in the corneal epithelium, marked tortuosity of retinal vessels, angiokeratoma of the skin (especially perineal), and painful palms and soles. Renal failure is the most serious late complication.

Chloroquine and amiodarone cause decreased α-galactosidase A activity within lysosomes, which is presumably why these drugs also produce corneal whorls.

Diphenylhydantoin sodium therapy may be helpful in relieving the pain of Fabry's disorder.

Cystathionine β Synthase Deficiency (Homocystinuria)

Cystathionine β synthase is one of several enzymes that catalyze the reactions transforming homocysteine to cysteine, deficiencies of these resulting in abnormal renal excretion of homocysteine. The recessively inherited deficiency of this enzyme commonly causes ectopic lenses, iridodonesis, and myopia, usually noted between 3 and 10 years of age. Lens dislocation is more often downward, rather than upward as is characteristic of Marfan's syndrome; however, the direction of dislocation is not a reliable differential criterion. Marfan's zonular fibers are thin, elongated, and perhaps scanty in number. In contrast, cystathionine β synthase–deficient zonular fibers are broken, thickened, stubby remnants that remain adherent to the equator of the dislocated lens. Pupil block glaucoma may result from anterior dislocation of the lens. Cataract, optic atrophy, retinal degeneration, and retinal detachment also are encountered.

This enzyme deficiency also may cause severe skeletal faults resembling those of Marfan's syndrome, including arachnodactyly, scoliosis, tall and thin habitus, pectus excavatum or carinatum, and high-arched palate. Mental retardation and psychiatric disturbances are common. Thromboembolic disease is a life-threatening complication of cystathionine β synthase deficiency. Such thromboembolism is particularly likely after surgery. Livedo reticularis, an erythematous mottling of the skin of the extremities (especially the legs), is a vascular fault seen in perhaps half of these patients.

Treatment with pyridoxine (250 to 1,000 mg daily) and folic acid (2 mg twice weekly) supplements has frequently caused complete biochemical remission of homocystinuria. Because of the progressive and severe structural faults of bone, sinew, and especially blood vessels, such therapy is important. The effectiveness of treatment in a given individual can easily be assessed by measurement of the urinary excretion of homocysteine. Not all patients respond; at least some remaining cystathionine β synthase activity must be present if its function is to be enhanced by pyridoxine.

Search for an explanation of the abnormalities resulting from homocysteine excess suggests that the normal cross-linking of collagen is inhibited. This would explain all of the structural damage. Similar faults occur in lathyrism (sweet pea poisoning).

A low-methionine diet with cysteine supplementation is also important. This reduces the precursor of homocysteine, yet ensures the needed cysteine (lower in the metabolic pathway). The diet is gelatin based, with supplements, or may be soybean based. Identification of patients most benefited by such diets is by examination of subsequent siblings of the proband patient.

A number of patients have died from thromboembolism after cataract surgery, which should be avoided if at all possible. Vitreous hemorrhage and retinal detachment are also common complications.

The incidence of homocystinuria may be about 1 in 45,000.

Disorders of Folate Metabolism

Folates are essential nutrients derived from many leafy vegetables, for example, spinach and cabbage. Rare genetic deficiencies of folate absorption and metabolism exist.

Far more important to ophthalmologists is the recognition that antifolate drugs such as methotrexate, pyrimethamine (Daraprim) (used in treatment of toxoplasmosis), and aminopterin are potent teratogens. Severe central nervous system and skeletal damage, even fetal death, result from drug-induced folate deficiency. Antifolate medications must be strictly avoided during pregnancy and are particularly devastating during the first month, a time when the existence of the fetus may not yet be recognized.

Abetalipoproteinemia (Bassen-Kornzweig Syndrome)

The unique feature of abetalipoproteinemia, a rare recessive disorder, is the total absence of apoprotein B from the plasma. This protein is necessary for the formation of chylomicrons and can be considered as a carrier protein for fatty substances. Consequently, all plasma lipids are greatly reduced in abetalipoproteinemia. For example, cholesterol levels are usually below 50 mg/dl (less than one-fourth of normal). Since fat-soluble vitamins (A, E, K) are transported via chylomicrons, their absorption is severely compromised in abetalipoproteinemia. This results in deficiency states for these vitamins. (Vitamin D is fat soluble but is transported by an alpha globulin; therefore D deficiency states (rickets) do not develop in abetalipoproteinemia.) Hypoprothrombinemia is due to deficient vitamin K. The typical severe neuromuscular degeneration may be caused by abnormal peroxidation of myelin, occurring in the absence of protection by vitamin E. Neuropathy and myopathy associated with vitamin E deficiency are partially reversible.

Rod degeneration and night blindness result from the vitamin A deficiency. Dark adaptation measurements are markedly reduced. Pendular nystagmus is commonly present, which suggests an ocular rather than cerebellar origin. Ptosis and ophthalmoplegia occur. Atypical retinitis pigmentosa is perhaps the feature of this syndrome that is best known to ophthalmologists. Retinitis pigmentosa does not appear in clinical or experimental vitamin A deficiency. Vitamin A treatment of abetalipoproteinemia may improve dark adaptation but does not prevent the development of retinitis pigmentosa. Experimental and clinical deficiencies of vitamin E also cause changes in the retinal pigment epithelium, which suggests that a combined vitamin A and vitamin E deficiency may be responsible for the retinitis pigmentosa. Only long-term therapy with these vitamins could be expected to produce demonstrable clinical results. Only arrest of the disease is possible, since pigmentary changes signify irreversible cell death.

Plasma lipoprotein abnormalities may cause acanthocytosis, the malformation of more than half of the circulating erythrocytes, which assume a globular shape with multiple pseudopod-like projections. Red cell autohemolysis is 10 times that of normal and may be reduced by as much as 90 percent in vitro by the addition of vitamin E. This is significant and objective evidence of the efficacy of vitamin E treatment of abetalipoproteinemia.

Therapy for abetalipoproteinemia consists of continuing high-dose supplementation of vitamins A, E, and K. The dosage of vitamin E is 100 mg/kg/day. Such management may arrest the neuromuscular, retinal, and hematologic problems.

Phytanic Acid Storage Disease (Refsum's Disease)

Phytanic acid storage disease consists of retinitis pigmentosa, peripheral neuropathy, cerebellar ataxia, and elevated spinal fluid protein. It is a recessive trait caused by deficiency of phytanic acid α-hydroxylase. Homozygotes oxidize phytanic acid at less than 5 percent of the normal rate; heterozygotes at about 50 percent.

Phytanic acid is a long-chain fatty acid. The mechanism whereby it causes damage may be displacement of the straight-chain fatty acids in complex neural structures such as the photoreceptor outer segments, which are composed of high concentrations of retinoic acid (vitamin A).

Note that retinitis pigmentosa also occurs in abetalipoproteinemia, a deficiency in absorption and transport of fat-soluble vitamins such as A and E. Abetalipoproteinemia and phytanic acid storage disease are of considerable theoretical interest, for they suggest that retinitis pigmentosa may be an outer segment disorder or a retinal pigment cell fault caused by the absence of proper utilization of vitamin A.

Phytanic acid may have the lay name of *grass fat* because it is a long-chain fatty acid resulting from the metabolism of chlorophyll by ruminant animals (e.g., cows). Phytanic acid may represent as much as 10 percent of the fatty acids in bovine plasma. Nonbovine animals have only traces of phytanic acid because they do not metabolize chlorophyll and they have enough phytanic acid α-hydroxylase to destroy as much as 1,000 times their average daily intake of phytanic acid.

The treatment of this rare disease is effective and is the absolute avoidance of grass fat, the food products derived from ruminant animals—their milk, flesh, cheese, yogurt, and other products. The patient will have enormous amounts of phytanic acid stored in body fat—as much as a pound. Any cause of weight loss will mobilize the stored grass fat in far greater concentration than dietary intake, thereby causing an acute exacerbation of all symptoms. Therefore any diet cannot be permitted to result in weight loss.

Hyperornithinemia

Since amino acids are derived from protein food, limitation of protein intake is theoretically helpful in treating patients with metabolic blocks resulting in excess amounts of individual amino acids. Particular ophthalmic interest is associated with hyperornithinemia, one type of which causes gyrate atrophy of the fundus. No effective treatment is established.

Narcotic Response

Every day a surgeon is confronted with the response that in some patients apprehension and postoperative pain are dramatically alleviated by an injection of meperidine hydrochloride. We are also aware that many individuals experience such desirable and pleasant sensations from prolonged narcotic use that they become addicted, both psychologically and physically. And yet, peculiarly, when we order narcotics for pain relief, other individuals respond by turning pale and clammy and retching miserably and uncontrollably. We know that an identical response will frequently be evoked by subsequent injections of the offending narcotic. On the morning of this writing I watched a handsome, powerful, 22-year-old athlete, who underwent surgery yesterday for retinal detachment, fill a basin with vile, sour, greenish vomitus. The same thing happened last year after his other detachment operation. On both occasions the vomiting followed my attempt to relieve his discomfort with meperidine hydrochloride. (On discharge I gave him the pharmacologic advice that he should use aspirin and warm compresses for pain relief.) In 1946 the pharmacology professor told us that cats are driven mad by morphine and that dogs are tranquilized. I accept without question that differences within humans cause them to respond to narcotics in a "felinelike" or "caninelike" manner, although unfortunately I cannot recite to you the biochemical basis for the response.

Lysosomal Enzyme Disorders (Mucopolysaccharide Storage Diseases—Hurler, Hunter, Scheie, Morquio)

Mucopolysaccharide storage occurs because of the deficiency within the lysozymes of specific enzymes required to metabolize these substances.

At least 10 such specific enzymes are known, and their malfunction characterizes specific diseases.

Corneal clouding is common in these disorders. Retinal pigmentary disease is sometimes seen, as may be glaucoma. Deafness is frequent. Skeletal, joint, and tendon entrapment syndromes are characteristic. Vascular, neural, and reticuloendothelial tissues are damaged by the mucopolysaccharide deposition. The affected infant is normal but deteriorates as mucopolysaccharide accumulation worsens during life. No therapy is available.

An ophthalmologist may be the first to make the diagnosis if he encounters a "funny-looking kid" with a complaint of photophobia (owing to the corneal infiltrates).

Lysosomal enzyme disorders also include the syndromes of Farber, Niemann-Pick, Gaucher, Krabbe, Fabry, Tay-Sachs, and Sandhoff.

Hyperoxaluria

Severe renal damage results from deposition of calcium oxalate in the kideny. Oxalate deposition can occur in primary hyperoxaluria, caused by inherited enzyme deficiency, or as a result of intake of ethylene glycol antifreeze, rhubarb leaves, or methoxyflurane anesthesia (all of which are or contain oxalate precursors). The ophthalmologic interest of this condition is that crystalline masses can be seen in ocular tissues, including the retinal pigment epithelium.

Therapy is not very satisfactory but is directed toward preventing renal deposits. Magnesium and phosphate ions may be helpful, as is a high fluid intake to dilute the urine. In the genetic forms, pyridoxine may decrease the amount of endogenous oxalate formation. Prevention is the best approach—ethylene glycol is sweet tasting and will be eaten by dogs and children if not stored out of their reach.

Cholinesterase

Genetic factors may be responsible not only for vulnerability to drugs but also for resistance to adverse effects. The human response to parathion, a highly toxic insecticide, is an excellent example of this. Parathion is metabolized to paraoxon. Both molecules are toxic through their inactivation of serum cholinesterase. However, by selection of an appropriate concentration of paraoxon for incubation with human serum, one can demonstrate inactivation of cholinesterase to a very different degree, varying from 67 percent to 0 residual cholinesterase activity. This variation is due to the presence of a specific paraoxonase enzyme, the amount of which is genetically determined [4].

Atypical plasma pseudocholinesterase is an autosomal recessive trait affecting about 1 in 2,500 persons. Such individuals cannot inactivate succinylcholine chloride, a paralyzing agent commonly used in anesthesia. Consequently, their recovery from paralysis requires many hours instead of the few minutes normally expected.

Acetylation Deficiency

Systemic lupus erythematosus has been classified as an autoimmune disease in which antinuclear antibodies develop for unknown reasons. Recognition that a drug-induced lupus erythematosus–like syndrome can result from exposure to medications such as procainamide, hydralazine, practolol, isoniazid, penicillamine, and other drugs resulted in the discovery that individuals with a genetically slow acetylation rate will suffer a prolonged presence of these drugs in the body and are much more susceptible to development of the drug-induced lupus syndrome. The disease is related to the size of the dose and the duration of therapy. A positive antinuclear antibody test result developed in 50 percent of slow acetylators within 3 months of procainamide therapy, as compared to 8 months for rapid acetylators.

This leads to the question of whether acetylation deficiencies are present in spontaneous lupus. Of 13 lupus patients, 10 were slow acetylators. Approximately half of the normal population are slow acetylators. The current theory suggests that the incriminated drugs (aromatic amines or hydrazines) react with nuclear proteins to increase the immunogenicity of nuclear antigens. Presumably "spontaneous" lupus is due to exposure of susceptible individuals to such drugs. For example, the azo food dyes can be transformed to aromatic amines by the action of intestinal bacteria [13].

Cystic Fibrosis

Among U.S. whites, 1 in 2,000 live-born infants suffers from cystic fibrosis, an autosomal recessive trait. This is the most common semilethal trait. It appears to be related to plugging of glandular structures with thickened secretions, thereby occluding pulmonary, pancreatic, and other glandular structures.

From the standpoint of the ophthalmologist, low vitamin A levels may occur because of deficiencies in the specialized proteins needed for retinol carrying and retinol binding. The resulting xerophthalmia and night blindness is corrected by vitamin A. Supplemental doses of water-soluble forms of vitamins are a standard therapeutic measure because the pancreatic enzyme deficiency is well known to interfere with intestinal absorption of fat-soluble vitamins.

Xeroderma Pigmentosum

Many eye changes occur in xeroderma pigmentosum, a recessive disease in which there is inability to repair ultraviolet damage to cellular DNA. This disorder differs from porphyrin-enhanced ultraviolet damage, in which repair is normal but damage is increased.

Eyelid changes include erythema, hyperpigmentation, keratosis, papilloma, and carcinoma. Scarring can cause ectropion, entropion, or even loss of the lid. Comparable changes affect the conjunctiva, leading to dryness and symblepharon. Severe exposure keratopathy, ulceration, and scarring of the cornea occur. Even the interior of the eye can be affected, with iritis, synechiae, iris atrophy, and melanomas.

Malignancies also develop in the internal organs of the body. Microcephaly and mental retardation may be seen, as well as involvement of cerebellum and basal ganglia.

Study of xeroderma pigmentosum has disclosed much information about DNA repair, ultraviolet toxicity, pyrimidine metabolism, mutation, and carcinogenesis.

Remember to caution patients to avoid sunlight by using protective clothing and staying indoors. Outdoors they can use sunscreens such as titanium dioxide, para-aminobenzoic acid, and heavy makeup.

Other Conditions

Innumerable other conditions are of genetic interest. The commonly used behavior-modifying drugs show great individual variation in their therapeutic and adverse responses. Inability to perceive the bitter taste of phenylthiourea (phenylthiocarbamide) is an autosomal dominant trait affecting 30 percent of whites. The mechanism of action is unknown. The trait may be associated with the tendency to open-angle glaucoma. Lacrimal insufficiency (dry eyes) is genetic. Lubricants are helpful.

Pharmacogenetic variations also include vulnerability to more complex reactions such as carcinogenesis or teratogenesis, as well as to ordinary toxicity or therapeutic benefit. Nutrition is affected by genetic variations such as iron absorption or lactose intolerance. Resistance to microorganisms and allergens is also genetically determined [11].

REFERENCES

1. Becker, B. The effect of topical corticosteroid in secondary glaucomas. *Arch. Ophthalmol.* 72:769, 1964.
2. Bozler, G. Human pharmacokinetics. *Hum. Genet. [Suppl.]* 1:13, 1978.
3. François, J. Corticosteroid glaucoma, *Ann. Ophthalmol.* 9:1075, 1977.
4. Geldmacher-von Mallinckrodt, M. Polymorphism of human serum paraoxonase. *Hum. Genet. [Suppl.]* 1:65, 1978.
5. Goedde, N. W., and Agarwal, D. P. Pseudocholinesterase variation. *Hum. Genet. [Suppl.]* 1:45, 1978.
6. Havener, W. H. *Ocular Pharmacology* (5th ed.). St. Louis: Mosby, 1983.
7. Kahn, A. G6PD Variants. *Hum. Genet. [Suppl.]* 1:37, 1978.
8. Kalow, W. Malignant hyperthermia. *Hum. Genet. [Suppl.]* 1:69, 1978.
9. Kasavina, B. S., and Chesnokova, N. B. Lysosomal hydrolases of the eye tissues and the effect of corticosteroids on their activity. *Exp. Eye Res.* 16:227, 1973.
10. Kitazawa, Y. Increased intraocular pressure induced by corticosteroids. *Am. J. Ophthalmol.* 82:492, 1976.
11. Motulsky, A. G. Pharmacogenetics and ecogenetics. *Hum. Genet. [Suppl.]* 1:1, 1978.
12. Palmberg, P. F., et al. The reproducibility of the intraocular pressure response to dexamethasone. *Am. J. Ophthalmol.* 80:844, 1975.
13. Reidenberg, M. M., and Drayer, D. E. Aromatic amines and hydrazines, drug acetylation, and lupus erythematosus. *Hum. Genet. [Suppl.]* 1:57, 1978.
14. Schwartz, J. T., et al. Twin study on ocular pressure following topically applied dexamethasone: II. Inheritance of variation in pressure response. *Arch. Ophthalmol.* 90:281, 1973.
15. Shammas, H. F., Halasa, A. H., and Faris, B. M. Intraocular pressure, cup-disc ratio, and steroid responsiveness in retinal detachment. *Arch. Ophthalmol.* 94:1108, 1976.
16. Southren, A. L., et al. Nuclear translocation of the cytoplasmic glucocorticoid receptor in the iris-ciliary body of the rabbit. *Invest. Ophthalmol. Vis. Sci.* 18:517, 1979.
16A. Stanbury, J. B., et al. (Eds.), *The Metabolic Basis of Inherited Disease* (5th ed.). New York: McGraw-Hill, 1983.
17. Vesell, E. S. Twin studies in pharmacogenetics. *Hum. Genet. [Suppl.]* 1:19, 1978.
18. Weinreb, R.N., et al. Detection of glucocorticoid receptors in cultured human trabecular cells. *Invest. Ophthalmol. Vis. Sci.* 21:403, 1981.
19. Weinstein, B. I., et al. Specific glucocorticoid receptor in the iris-ciliary body of the rabbit. *Invest. Ophthalmol. Vis. Sci.* 16:973, 1977.
20. Zink, H. A., Palmberg, P. F., and Bigger, J. R. Increased sensitivity to theophylline associated with primary open-angle glaucoma. *Invest. Ophthalmol.* 12:603, 1973.
21. Zink, H. A., et al. Comparison of in vitro corticosteroid response in pigmentary glaucoma and primary open-angle glaucoma. *Am. J. Opthalmol.* 80:478, 1975.

Part Two

Genetic Determination of Clinical Eye Disease

8

Human Chromosomal Disorders and the Eye

Stephen C. Gieser
John C. Carey
David J. Apple

The three decades since the establishment of the correct number of chromosomes in humans represent an epochal period in medicine and human genetics. Rapid advances in the methodology of cytogenetics have permitted detailed study of the human chromosomal makeup. Modern banding techniques have linked specific chromosomal anomalies to several heretofore unrecognized clinical syndromes and have characterized some previously known syndromes of unclear causation.

A knowledge of chromosomal disorders is important for the ophthalmologist for reasons other than merely academic interest. The second edition of the *Birth Defects Atlas and Compendium* lists 1,005 anatomic variants, malformations, and syndromes that are inherited by a mendelian mode of transmission or caused by spontaneous mutation, chromosomal abnormality, or teratogenic agents [12]. Of these, approximately 450 involve the structure of the eye, ocular adnexa, or orbit. In many of these conditions, such as trisomy 13, the ocular abnormalities are distinctive and assist in the clinical diagnosis of the syndrome.

The diagnosis of chromosome-induced disorders is relatively straightforward in the full-blown, well-established case. However, one may encounter difficulty in the evaluation of the individual with more subtle physical variations. The ophthalmologist is frequently called on to contribute information in consultation to hospital services and is occasionally asked to participate in genetic counseling in relation to chromosomal conditions. At a minimum one should have sufficient knowledge of these disorders to permit screening of patients, to provide judgment concerning the need for cytogenetic evaluation, and to make appropriate referral of families for genetic counseling and other medical services.

The purpose of this chapter is to review the chromosomal basis of inheritance, the basic principles of clinical cytogenetics, and the numerous ocular findings occurring in chromosomal disorders. Special emphasis is placed on the alterations encountered in the common trisomy syndromes and in the chromosomal deletions and duplication syndromes of importance to the ophthalmologist.

BIOLOGIC ASPECTS OF HUMAN CHROMOSOMES

Definition of Chromosomal Disease

A distinction must be made between chromosomal abnormalities and single gene defects. As opposed to large chromosomal aberrations, single gene defects, also known as mendelian disorders, are caused by point mutations on the human genome. The mutation may be present on only one chromosome of a pair (matched with a normal gene on the partner chromosome) or on both chromosomes of a pair. In either case the cause of the defect is a single major error in an apparently single locus on the human genome.

In chromosomal disease the defect is not due to a single abnormality in the genetic blueprint but to developmental confusion arising from an excess or deficiency of whole chromosomes or chromosomal segments [20]. As we might expect, chromosomal abnormalities result in *multiple defects* since many genes are affected. Assuming that there are no less than 100,000 active genes, a change in a one percent of the chromosomes would affect at least 1,000 genes [157].

The type of defects seen in chromosomal syndromes are generally dysmorphic, that is, they cause abnormalities in the prenatal development of the structure of organs, such as colobomas or oral-facial clefts. Less medically significant defects such as oblique palpebral fissures or hypertelorism reflect variations in relative growth of the bones surrounding and comprising the orbit. Epicanthal folds form when the relative growth of the nasal bridge is less than the growth of the skin of the medial portion of the eyelid.

Some dysmorphic syndromes result when the relative growth of adjoining structures is abnormal. This changed growth pattern may reflect a change of relative dosage of the genes that affect the developing structures. Hypertelorism, for instance, could result if the genes for frontal bone growth were increased relative to those for the parietal and temporal bones. This disproportion would also result if the interval of growth for the frontal bone were increased in relation to that of the other facial bones [157]. The phenotypic aspects of chromosomal syndromes will be expanded on in the section entitled Clinical Cytogenetics.

Historical Background

More than a century has elapsed since the first detailed descriptions of the events in nuclear division in animal cells. Rudolph Virchow, the first investigator to emphasize the study of diseases at the cellular level, described the process of cellular divison in 1857 [179]. In 1879 human chromosomes were clearly illustrated in a tumor cell. Waldeyer introduced the name *chromosome* in 1888 to describe the colored bodies in the nuclei of cells [182].

Advances in science, particularly in cytogenetics, have been and continue to be at the mercy of methodology. No better example can be given than the establishment of the correct number of chromosomes in the human.

Until the 1920s the method commonly used for chromosomal analysis was based on fixation of tissue in Carnoy-Flemming's solution, preparation of microtome sections by the paraffin method, and staining with iron hematoxylin. Most of the chromosomal counts in the human were based on testicular tissue obtained from patients with tuberculosis of the epididymis or from executed criminals. Thus it seems likely that the processing of these tissues, that is, fixation, dehydration, cleaving, paraffin embedding under high temperature conditions, sectioning, staining, and often postmortem changes may have played a role in the variability of chromosomal counts obtained by different workers. At best these methods yielded mitotic figures with considerable overlapping of the chromosomes in a crowded metaphase plate, with the morphology of the chromosomes often being indistinct. Thus it is not surprising to find that Flemming, the first to describe and depict human chromosomes in 1882, thought the number of chromosomes in human somatic cells ranged from 22 to 24 [55, 56]. Flemming's figure of 22 to 24 chromosomes was accepted and "reaffirmed" repeatedly for 30 years. In 1923 Painter, an American, published a paper in *J. Exp. Zool.* indicating that the human had 48 chromosomes, an XX consitution characterizing the female and XY characterizing the male [132].

Rapid technical advances during a period beginning in the early 1950s and continuing to the present time have permitted more accurate chromosomal analysis by a wide variety of techniques. Such techniques, described under Methodology of Chromosomal Analysis, make possible an abundant in vitro growth of cultured cells undergoing active mitosis. These cells may be harvested in such a fashion as to ensure easy isolation and localization of the individual chromosomes.

In 1956 a major turning point occurred in the field of human cytogenetics when Tjio and Levan established that the normal chromosome complement of humans (the diploid number) is 46, not 48 as was previously suggested [176]. This finding did much to stimulate research into chromosome-related disease. The ensuing period can be considered an era of delineation of chromosomal disorders, that is, the correlation of chromosomal aberrations with previously recognized syndromes of unclear causation and the description of new disorders.

The important syndromes that were described in this period may be divided into two major groups: those related to the sex chromosomes, and those related to the autosomal group of chromosomes. The description of sex chromatin by Barr and Bertram did much to improve our understanding of the sex chromosome–related syndromes [6]. Ford and coauthors in 1959 showed that Turner's syndrome, a distinctive clinical disorder long considered idiopathic, was based on a deficiency of the X chromosome, with the resultant sex chromosome pattern of 45,XO [57]. Also in 1959 Lejeune and co-workers [103, 104] confirmed Waardenburg's original theory [181] that Down's syndrome has a chromosomal basis by demonstrating that individuals with Down's syndrome had trisomy 21. Jacobs and coauthors proved that Klinefelter's syndrome was based on an XXY chromosome pattern [89].

With the exception of Turner's syndrome, the sex chromosome anomalies reveal few significant eye findings and will not be considered further in this chapter.

In 1970 Caspersson and coauthors stained human chromosomes with quinacrine mustard and demonstrated a specific banding pattern for each chromosome pair [24]. The pioneer work of Caspersson's group proved to be the beginning of an explosive development in that area. Since that time numerous other staining techniques have been described that allow the visualization of differentially stained regions of the chromosomes.

In the mid-1970s Yunis [203] and other investigators introduced the technique of examining highly extended chromosomes in the prophase or early metaphase period of cell division. This method enabled these investigators to expand the number of bands seen on the banded chromosome from about 300 to over 800. The advanced degree of resolution allows the cytogeneticist to demonstrate chromosomal aberrations affecting only a very small portion of a chromosome. Since that time some previously recognized conditions of unknown causation, such as the Prader-Willi syndrome [102] and the aniridia–Wilms' tumor association [147], have been found to be due to subtle chromosomal deletions that can be detected by high-resolution banding techniques.

The application of these procedures to human chromosomes has dramatically changed the field of clinical cytogenetics. New, more subtle, chromosomal findings involving partial duplication or deficiency of every chromosome of the human complement have been subdivided according to the chromosomal segment, making phenotypic mapping of chromosomes possible.

Methodology of Chromosomal Analysis

PREPARATION OF THE METAPHASE PLATE

During the early decades of chromosomal research, several limitations prevented direct clinical applications of various laboratory techniques. Most early data were collected on animals and plants, and clinical correlations were therefore highly restricted. There were too many chromosomes in the human cell to work with easily, and not until the use of hypotonic saline was initiated was it possible to spread chromosomes sufficiently to observe them individually. The lack of asepsis before the antibiotic era and the limitations of early tissue culture media prevented optimal growth and viability of cells that were being grown to obtain chromosomes. Unlike such cells in many lower species, human somatic cells have a relatively long generation time.

The use of peripheral blood (lymphocyte) cultures was hampered by the limited mitotic activity of lymphocytes. The clinical application of the lymphocytic culture method (which is among the least expensive, most convenient, and least traumatic) could not be perfected until an agent causing increased mitotic activity was discovered. Phytohemagglutinin, when added to the culture, solved this problem. Also, before the introduction of colchicine, an agent that terminates the process of mitosis during metaphase, there was no way to control timing of the stages of cell division.

Besides lymphocyte cultures, chromosomes can be studied in other tissues that contain proliferating cells, such as fibroblasts from a skin biopsy or amniocytes in amniotic fluid. Examples of situations in which these other tissues are needed for chromosomal study include the investigation of a deceased infant with multiple congenital anomalies or the prenatal diagnosis of a chromosomal disorder by amniocentesis.

The principles of chromosomal analysis may be illustrated by a description of several basic steps commonly used in most techniques designed to obtain metaphase plates and karyotypes (modified from Arakaki and Sparkes [4]):

1. Peripheral capillary blood is collected by venipuncture or lancet finger puncture, usually in a heparinized pipet.
2. The blood sample is inoculated into a suitable culture medium (prefabricated microculture systems are commercially available) containing nutrient media, antibiotics, and phytohemagglutinin. The latter substance is a mucopolysaccharide material extracted from kidney beans that has mitosis-stimulating potential, that is, it induces mitosis in an increased number of cells per sample. This ensures a higher percentage of metaphase plates.
3. The culture is incubated for 72 hours.
4. Colchicine is added to the media 4 to 6 hours

before harvesting. The colchicine produces a "metaphase arrest," thus permitting accumulation of sufficient metaphase plates. This ensures the highest possible yield of mitotic figures (and therefore of individually reproducible chromosomes) at the optimal stage for photographic analysis.

5. The cells are harvested by obtaining a cell sediment by centrifugation. Hypotonic saline is added to the cell sediment. The influx of fluid into the relatively hypertonic intracellular compartment of each leukocyte leads to extensive swelling and eventual rupture of the cell.

6. The cell suspension is air-dried, and rupture of the swollen nuclei is induced. This rupture produces a spreading and dispersion of individual chromosomes, which are now readily isolated individually at the point of metaphase.

7. The microslide is stained with any suitable nuclear stain, and satisfactory metaphase plates are photographed under oil immersion.

8. Chromosomal counts and evaluation of chromosomal aberrations may be carried out from simple observations of the metaphase plate. In many instances, however, the preparation of a standardized map, or *karyotype*, is essential for full evaluation of the total pattern. Photographic prints of metaphase plates are made. Individual chromosome images are then cut from the print and arranged in a standard systematized fashion, forming a karyotype (Fig. 8-1).

Before 1970 solid staining was the only staining method available. Since that time several special techniques have been developed for staining chromosomes in banded patterns [151]. More detailed descriptions of these various staining methods are available in reviews by Yunis [204] and Miller [119].

Q-BANDING

Q-banding was the first staining method utilized in human cytogenetics to produce banded patterns on the chromosomes. Caspersson and his colleagues found that when chromosomes are stained with quinacrine mustard or related compounds and examined by fluorescein microscopy, each pair stains in a specific pattern of bright and dim bands (Q-bands; see Fig. 8-33B) [24]. This method has disadvantages in clinical usage in that the fluorescent preparations fade and are thus not permanently available. In addition, fluorescent microscopy is not generally available.

Fig. 8-1. *A normal male G-banded karyotype, showing 22 pairs of autosomes, one X chromosome, and one Y chromosome (46,XY). The faded appearance of one of the chromosome 22s is artifactual. (Courtesy of K. van Dyke.)*

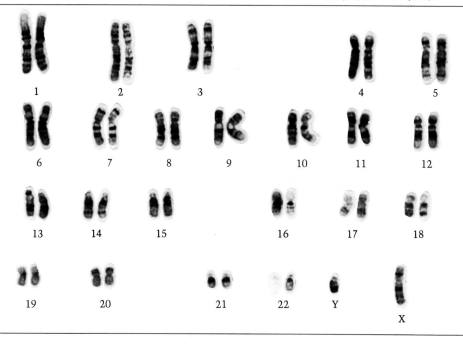

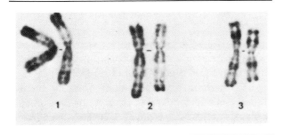

Fig. 8-2. *R-banding, chromosomes 1, 2, and 3. Note that the dark and light bands are the reverse of those on the usual G-banded karyotype shown in Fig. 8-1. (Courtesy of the National Foundation, March of Dimes.)*

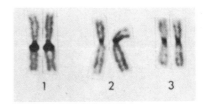

Fig. 8-3. *C-banding, chromosomes 1, 2, and 3. Notice the prominent staining of the centromere regions. (Courtesy of the National Foundation, March of Dimes.)*

G-BANDING

In G-banding, a widely used technique, chromosomes are treated with trypsin, which denatures chromosomal protein, and then stained with Giemsa stain. The chromosomes take up stain in a pattern of dark- and light-staining bands (G-bands), with the dark bands corresponding to the Q-bands (Fig. 8-1). This technique permits permanent chromosomal preparations.

R-BANDING

If the chromosomes receive a heat pretreatment and then Giemsa staining, the resulting dark- and light-stained bands (R-bands) are the reverse of those produced by Q- and G-banding. This method is particularly useful for examining the ends of chromosomes, which are lightly stained by G-banding (Fig. 8-2).

C-BANDING

C-banding specifically stains the centromere regions and other regions containing constitutive heterochromatin, that is, the secondary constrictions of chromosomes 1, 9, and 16 (Fig.8-3). This method also stains the heterochromatin in the distal segment that forms part of the normal constitution of several chromosomes as distinguished from facultative heterochromatin (which makes up the inactive X chromosome in female somatic cells).

NOR STAINING

NOR staining uses ammoniacal silver to stain the nucleolar organizing regions, that is, the secondary constrictions (stalks) of the satellited acrocentric chromosomes (e.g., chromosomes 13, 14, and 15).

G-11 BANDING

G-11 banding is a modification of Giemsa banding at high pH. This stain preferentially stains the secondary constriction of chromosome 9, the distal segment of the long arm of the Y chromosome, and the pericentromeric area of chromosome 20. G-11 banding is particularly useful for demonstrating common normal variants (polymorphisms) of chromosome 9.

HIGH-RESOLUTION BANDING

High-resolution banding involves the staining of extended chromosomes from prophase or early metaphase with Giemsa (Fig. 8-4). This technique can detect subtle deletions unseen with conventional G-banding.

The Karyotype

Each human cell contains a total of 46 chromosomes. Meiosis, which occurs in each parent during spermatogenesis and oogenesis, reduces the number of chromosomes in the germ cell to a total of 23, the haploid number (n). Fertilization of haploid gametes restores the total number to 46 chromosomes (diploid [$2n$]) in the offspring (the zygote). Of the total of 46 chromosomes, 22 pairs (44) are autosomes. The two remaining chromosomes are the sex chromosomes (XX in females, XY in males).

To determine the karyotype, the chromosomes are photographed as previously described and are arranged serially in descending order according to their lengths. They are further subclassified according to the position of their centromeres. When

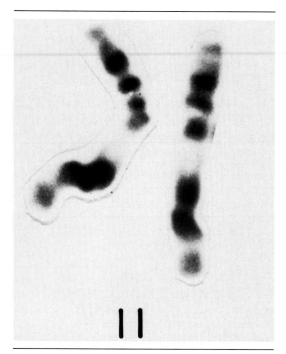

Fig. 8-4. *High-resolution study of chromosome 11. Note the additional bands that can be seen compared to chromosome 11 on a regular G-banded karyotype (Fig. 8-1).*

one looks at chromosomes on a karyotype, the replicated chromosome with joined chromatid pairs is seen.

Chromatid is the term applied to each of the two components of a chromosome formed at metaphase, when each chromosome divides lengthwise into two equal portions. Each chromatid retains its attachment to its mirror image by way of the centromere. The *centromere* is defined as the nonstaining portion of the chromosome, where the individual chromatids are joined at a constriction. The location of the centromere along the length of the chromatid varies as follows:

1. Metacentric (mesocentric) chromatids are joined by the centromere midway between the ends of the chromosome (e.g., chromosomes 1, 2, and 3; see Fig. 8-1).
2. Submetacentric chromosomes characteristically contain a centromere that is positioned off-center, dividing the chromosome into a *short arm*, called p, and a *long arm*, labeled q (e.g., chromosome 4; see Fig. 8-1).
3. Acrocentric chromosomes contain a centromere located near the distal or peripheral end

of the chromosome (e.g., chromosome 13; see Fig. 8-1).

The human acrocentric chromosomes (except the Y) have small masses of chromatin known as satellites attached to their short arms by narrow stalks (secondary constrictions). In metaphase spreads satellites are often seen in association; this association apparently reflects the participation of the stalks in the organization of the nucleolus.

Before the advent of banding techniques, several classifications of chromosomes in terms of karyotypic pattern were widely used. Important examples of these include the Denver classification [26], the classification of Patau [135], the London classification [27], and the Chicago classification [26–28]. In these classifications the chromosomes were grouped according to size and location of the centromere: A group (chromosomes 1–3); B group (chromosomes 4 and 5); C group (chromosomes 6–12 and X); D group (chromosomes 13–15); E group (chromosomes 16–18); F group (chromosomes 19 and 20); and G group (chromosomes 21, 22, and Y).

With the development of banding techniques, each individual chromosome could be easily identified by its own specific banding pattern [134]. Fig. 8-5 is a diagram of the individual numbered chromosomes on a standard G-banded karyotype. The short arm (p) and the long arm (q) of each chromosome are designated, and the individual G-bands are ordered by segment numbers and band numbers by the established convention.

Cytogenetic Nomenclature

With the introduction of banding techniques, a number of cytogeneticists met in Paris in 1971 to establish conventional nomenclature for human cytogenetics [134]. This conference established and numbered the individual bands on the chromosomes (Fig. 8-5) and made some changes and additions to the previously described nomenclature of the Denver and Chicago conferences. The Paris conference nomenclature is very complicated and is designed to enable the cytogeneticist to label all the clinical and functional variations in every chromosome on a given karyotype. This section will highlight the important labels useful in clinical practice. The so-called short form will be used in this presentation. The reader is referred to the proceedings of the Paris conference for a more

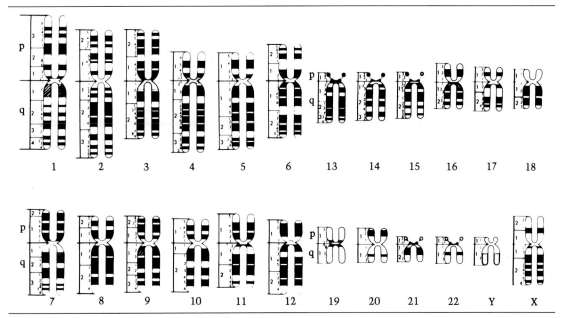

Fig. 8-5. *Diagram of chromosome bands as observed with the Q-, G-, and R-staining methods. (Courtesy of the National Foundation, March of Dimes.)*

detailed description of chromosomal nomenclature [134].

In the usual description of a chromosomal finding, the number of chromosomes in the karyotype is first specified, followed by the particular sex chromosomal designation. For example, a normal female would be 46,XX and a normal male 46,XY. Any extra or missing chromosomes are then noted—for example, 47,XY, +21 would indicate trisomy 21 (Down's syndrome). Structural rearrangements or abnormalities are designated by the appropriate symbols, many of which are listed in Table 8-1. Representative examples of chromosomal disorders commonly encountered in clinical practice are listed in Table 8-2.

One should note that the terminology of partial trisomies for a chromosomal segment (usually caused by an unbalanced translocation) is complex. In this chapter the abbreviation *dup* (duplication) will be used to refer to a partial trisomy for the designated segment. For example, dup 3p refers to a partial trisomy of the short arm of chromosome 3.

A band on a chromosome is defined as a region that can be distinguished from a neighboring region on the basis of a difference in staining intensity. Dark bands on G-banding are designated as G positive, while light-staining or white bands

are designated as G negative. R-banding (or reverse banding) has the opposite designations. Each arm of the chromosome is divided into segments numbered 1, 2, 3, or 4, moving distally from the centromere. Each individual band in the segment then is numbered (see Fig. 8-5). In the numerical notations of a chromosomal band, the first number indicates the segment on the short or long arm, while the second number designates the individual band. For example, on the long arm of chromosome 13, the second light-staining G-band (from the centromere moving distally) would be band 14 (see Fig. 8-5).

In 1978 a new conference was convened and resulted in an international system for human cytogenetic nomenclature [11]. This conference consolidated the information from all of the previous conferences and is an up-to-date work in human cytogenetic nomenclature.

With high-resolution banding, the individual bands are further subdivided into sub-bands. These sub-bands within a major band would be designated by the usual band number, a decimal point, and then the numerical notation for the sub-band. For example, a sub-band of the major band 14 on the long arm of chromosome 13 could be 14.1, with the .1 referring to the sub-band.

For an interpretation of a chromosome report from the laboratory, one can refer to the list of accepted symbols and abbreviations used in the

Table 8-1 *Selected Symbols and Abbreviations Used in Cytogenetic Nomenclature*

Symbol	Meaning
cen	Centromere
:(colon)	A break
:: (double colon)	Breakage and reunion
, (comma)	Separates chromosome number from sex chromsome constitution; separates sex chromosome constitution from description of unusual chromosome(s)
del	Deletion
der	Derivative chromosome
dup	Duplication
fra	Fragile site
h	Heteromorphic regions of 1q, 9q, and 16q
i	Isochromosome
ins	Insertion
inv	Inversion
mar	Marker chromosome
mat	Maternal origin
mos	Mosaic
p	Short arm
pat	Paternal origin
q	Long arm
r	Ring
rob	Robertsonian translocation
/ (slash)	Separates different karyotypes in mosaics and chimeras
t	Translocation
var	Variant or heteromorphic chromosome
band 14	1 refers to segment on arm; 4 to band

Table 8-2 *Representative Notations Using Short Form of Cytogenetic Nomenclature*

46,XY	Normal male
47,XY,+13	Male with 47 chromosomes, an extra chromosome 13; trisomy 13
45,XX,t(14;21)(q11;q11)	Female with balanced robertsonian translocation involving long arms of 14 and 21 with breaks at band 11 on long arm of chromosome 14 and at band 11 on long arm of chromosome 21
46,XX,del(13)(q21)	Female with terminal deletion of 13 long arm with material below band 21 missing
46,XY,r(18)	Male with ring chromosome of chromosome 18
46,XX,t(2;8)(p13;q12)	Female with balanced reciprocal translocation involving short arm of chromosome 2 (break at band 13) and long arm of chromosome 8 (break at band 12)

more common chromosomal abnormalities (see Tables 8-1 and 8-2 and Fig. 8-5).

Classification of Chromosomal Aberrations

Abnormalities of the chromosomes may be either *numerical* or *structural* and may affect either autosomes or sex chromosomes. A given abnormality may be present in all body cells, or there may be two or more cell lines, one or more of which may be abnormal (mosaicism). In this section the more common types of chromosomal aberrations are defined (Table 8-3).

Table 8-3 *Types of Human Chromosomal Abnormalities and Common Examples*

I. Numerical alterations
   A. Involving an entire set: triploidy—69,XXX
   B. Involving individual chromosomes:
      1. Autosomal trisomy—47,XY,+21 (Down's syndrome)
      2. Double trisomy—48,XXY,+21
      3. Monosomy—45,XO (Turner's syndrome)
      4. Sex chromosomal aneuploidy—47,XXX
      5. Mosaicism (multiple cell lines from a single zygote)—46,XX/47,XY,+21

II. Structural alterations
   A. Translocations: reciprocal, robertsonian—45,XX, t(13q;14q)
   B. Deletions: terminal, interstitial, ring chromosome—del (11)(p13)
   C. Duplications: direct, inverse, isochromosome—dup (13)(q21)
   D. Inversions: pericentric, paracentric—inv (3)

NUMERICAL ABERRATIONS: ANEUPLOIDY

A deviation from the normal total number of chromosomes is termed *aneuploidy*. One may recall that in diploids (2n) the normal total count is 46. An example of an aneuploidic cell is one containing 2n + 1 chromosome, for a total of 47. *Polyploidy* is the term describing a cell containing an exact multiple of the normal diploid number, for example, 3n (69), 4n (92), and so on. The most common example of polyploidy in the human is triploidy, 69,XXX. This is the second most common chromosomal finding in spontaneous abortions and is usually lethal in the live-born infant.

Trisomy is a situation in which a particular chromosome exists in triplicate rather than in the normal paired formation, thus producing a hyperdiploid or aneuploid state (e.g., trisomy 21). In most instances, the extra chromosome results in a total count of 47 (2n + 1). In contrast, a *monosomy* is the absence of one chromosome from a normally paired group, resulting in a hypodiploid state, that is, a total of 45 chromosomes (2n − 1) (e.g., 45,XO, Turner's syndrome).

The process thought to be responsible for most instances of complete trisomy is termed *nondisjunction* (Fig. 8-6). In this process there is aberrant division of a cell during either meiosis or mitosis. During meiosis, before anaphase (the process of separation of homologous pairs of chromosomes during cell division), the chromosomes making up each pair come together before separation. If the process of anaphase is abnormal within a given pair of homologous chromosomes, both members of the pair may remain in one of the daughter cells (gametes), and the other gamete may receive none, therefore precluding the equal separation of one chromosome to each daughter cell. Fertilization of the daughter cell containing one extra chromosome (total of two) with a normal haploid daughter cell (one chromosome) produces a zygote in which the involved chromosome group is represented by three (trisomy) rather than by the normal two members.

Mosaicism refers to a situation in which multiple cell lines from a single zygote lineage are present. This is designated by separating the different cell lines by a slash. For instance, 46,XY/47,XY,+21 would refer to an individual who has some normal cells and some cells that are trisomic for chromosome 21. Trisomy 21 mosaicism is felt to arise either by nondisjunction after fertilization of the zygote during mitotic cell division or by the loss of an extra chromosome 21 in a trisomic conceptus during the early division process.

STRUCTURAL ABERRATIONS

Chromosomal breaks occur normally at a low frequency, but they may be experimentally induced by a wide variety of breaking agents (clastogens) such as ionizing radiation, some virus infections, and many chemicals. The changes in chromosomal structure resulting from breakage may be either stable (i.e., capable of passing through cell division unaltered) or unstable. The stable types include translocations, deletions, and inversions (Table 8-3). An example of an unstable type, incapable of undergoing regular cell division, is ring formation.

Translocation. Translocation is the transfer of a part of one chromosome to another chromosome. This process is initiated by a chromosomal break, in which one of the arms and the attached centromere are freed; the chromosome then undergoes a reciprocal attachment or fusion with another chromosome that has undergone a similar breakage, thus producing newly formed chromosomes. *Balanced reciprocal translocation* refers to the reciprocal interchange of material between two chromosomes (Fig. 8-7). The individual who has this rearrangement has the normal amount

Fig. 8-6. *Trisomy induction by nondisjunction. During gamete formation (meiosis), each daughter cell normally receives one member of a chromosome pair. In this example, nondisjunction of the maternal chromosome pair has occurred, leaving an extra chromosome in the daughter cell. Fertilization of this cell necessarily leads to a trisomy.*

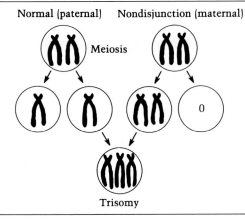

Trisomy

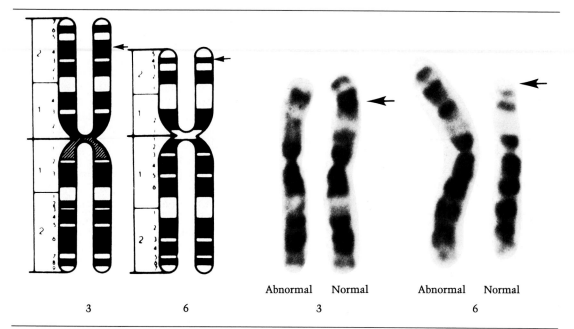

Abnormal	Normal		Abnormal	Normal
	3			6

Fig. 8-7. *Reciprocal translocation. Left, diagram of chromosomes 3 and 6. Right, photograph of chromosomes in a woman with a balanced reciprocal translocation involving the short arms of chromosomes 3 and 6. The arrows show the location of the breakpoints. Note that the short arm of the normal 3 is translocated to the short arm of chromosome 6 (see Fig. 8-8).*

of the genetic material, but it is arranged differently than in the usual state. In individuals with reciprocal balanced translocations, the segregation of chromosomes during gametogenesis may occur in such a way that the offspring will have an unbalanced translocation state.

The translocation is termed unbalanced when the new chromosomal population is characterized by an abnormal amount and arrangement of genetic material. Unbalanced translocations result in a duplication (partial trisomy) and deletion partial monosomy state in the individual. Fig. 8-7 includes a diagram of a balanced reciprocal translocation involving the short arm of chromosome 3 and the short arm of chromosome 6. Fig. 8-8 shows a partial karyotype of an individual with this aberration and of her daughter, who has an unbalanced translocation. The affected child has a partial trisomy of the short arm of chromosome 3 and a partial monosomy of chromosome 6.

Robertsonian translocations are a special type of rearrangement that occurs in acrocentric chromosomes in which the breaks are at the centromere and whole chromosome arms are exchanged. The most common robertsonian translocations in humans involve chromosomes 13 and 14 (Fig. 8-9). In this case the newly translocated chromosome that consists of the long arms of chromosomes 13 and 14 is designated as (13q;14q).

Although the major syndromes involving trisomies 13 and 21 are usually due to a nondisjunction process, the mechanism of robertsonian translocation is operative in a lesser, although significant, proportion of cases. About 5 percent of individuals with Down's syndrome have a translocation type of chromosomal abnormality resulting in an excess of the long arm of chromosome 21. In individuals who carry a balanced robertsonian translocation, the total chromosome count of the cell population is only 45 because the translocated short arms of the rearrangement are apparently lost in cell division. The chromosomal constitution of this individual then would be designated as 45,XX,t(14q;21q) (Fig. 8-10). The loss of the short arm material of acrocentric chromosomes does not appear to have a morphologic effect on development.

Tandem Duplications. Intrachromosomal duplication of the same chromosomal segment is another structural aberration, in addition to unbalanced translocation, that produces partial trisomy.

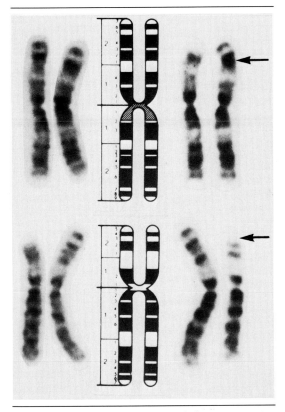

Fig. 8-8. *Reciprocal translocation of chromosomes 3 and 6 in a parent resulting in partial trisomy 3p in the child. The photographed chromosomes to the right of the diagram are those of the parent; the arrows indicate the breakpoints on the normal chromosomes 3 and 6 (see Fig. 8-7). The chromosomes to the left of the diagram are those of the offspring; note the two normal chromosome 3s (upper) and the chromosome 6 with the translocated segment of the 3 short arm (lower). The child inherited the parent's normal chromosomes 3 and 6 with the attached segment of 3.*

These defects are called *direct* when a serial rearrangement is present and *inverted* or *mirror* when the duplicated segment is reversed. For example, a direct duplication of genes ABCDEFG would be ABCDE*BCDE*FG. On the other hand, a mirror duplication of the same genes would be ABCD-E*EDCB*FG.

Deletion. Deletion is the loss of a portion of a chromosome, either terminally after a single chromosomal break, interstitially between two breaks, or as the result of an unbalanced translocation. The deleted portion is an acentric fragment, which fails to move on the spindle because it has no centromere and is eventually lost at subsequent cell division. The structurally altered chromosome lacks whatever genetic material was present in the lost fragment. One common example of deletion in humans is the short arm deletion of chromosome 4, also known as the Wolf-Hirschhorn syndrome (Fig. 8-11).

Before banding techniques were developed, a few large deletions of human chromosomes could be recognized. These included deletions on the short arm of chromosome 4 (4p−), the short arm of chromosome 5 (5p−), the long arm of chromosome 13 (13q−), the short arm of chromosome 18 (18p−), the long arm of chromosome 18 (18q−), and the long arm of chromosome 21 (21q−). With the advent of banding techniques in the early 1970s, many deletion situations that result in a large number of previously unrecognized syndromes have been described. The more important of these

Fig. 8-9. *Robertsonian translocation of chromosomes 13 and 14. Left, diagram of chromosomes 13 and 14, with small arrows indicating the breakpoints before fusion. Center, diagram of the fused 13/14 chromosome and photograph of the 13/14 translocation chromosome, abbreviated t(13q; 14q). Right, photographs of the two normal chromosomes.*

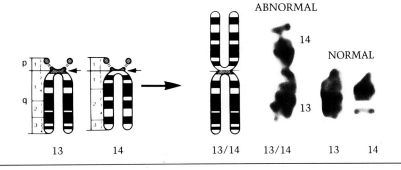

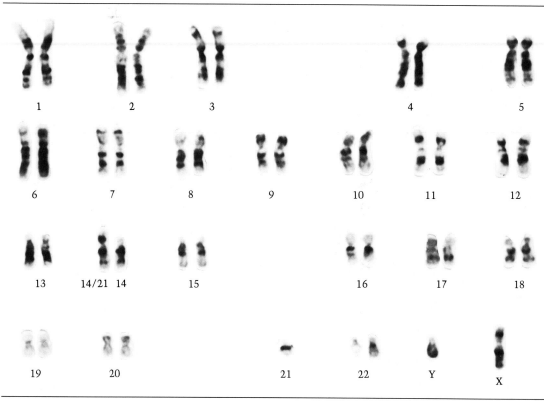

1	2	3		4	5
6	7	8	9	10	11	12
13	14/21 14	15		16	17	18
19	20		21	22	Y	X

Fig. 8-10. *G-banded full karyotype of a balanced 14/21 robertsonian translocation, abbreviated 45,XY,t(14q;21q). Note that this individual has 45 chromosomes, with the long arm of one of the 21s attached to chromosome 14 at the centromere. Since the chromosome material is balanced, this individual is phenotypically normal.*

Fig. 8-11. *Terminal deletion of the short arm of chromosome 4 (del 4p). Left, diagram of chromosome 4. Arrow shows breakpoints. Center, chromosome 4 with deletion. Right, normal chromosome 4. A deletion of the short arm of chromosome 4 produces the Wolf-Hirschhorn syndrome.*

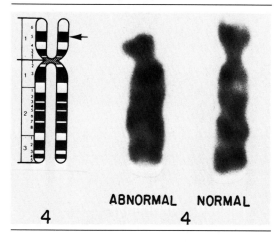

ABNORMAL   NORMAL

4   4

conditions will be described in the next section of this chapter.

A *ring chromosome* is a type of deletion in which both ends of the chromosome have been lost and the two broken ends have reunited to form a ring (Fig. 8-12). If the ring has a centromere, a ring chromosome can pass through cell division, but it may undergo alteration in structure. Ring chromosomes have been described in all human autosomes [156].

Inversion. Inversion involves breaking the chromosome at two places followed by reconstitution with inversion (rotation by 180 degrees) of the segment of the chromosome between the breaks (Fig. 8-13). For example, the genes ABC*DEF*GH would become ABC*FED*GH. If the inversion is in a single chromosome arm, it is labeled paracentric (beside the centromere). If it involves the centro-

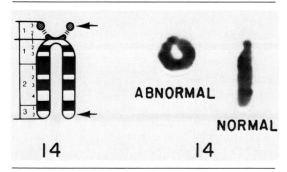

Fig. 8-12 *Ring. 14. Left, diagram of chromosome 14. Arrows indicate the location of the breaks before ring formation. Center, Ring 14. Right, normal chromosome 14.*

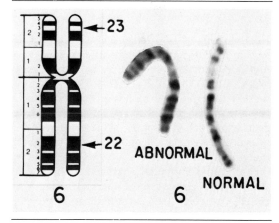

Fig. 8-13. *Pericentric inversion of chromosome 6. Left, diagram of chromosome 6 with arrows indicating the breakpoints. In this case, the segment of the chromosome between band 23 on the short arm and band 22 on the long arm inverts, resulting in the abnormal chromosome pictured in the middle. Right, normal chromosome 6. Notice that these chromosomes have more bands than the usual G-banded karyotype as a result of high-resolution banding.*

mere region, it is labeled a pericentric inversion (around the centromere).

Because inversions interfere with pairing between homologous chromosomes, crossing over may be suppressed within them. This can lead to a retention of groups of genes that can evolve as units. Usually the change in gene order produced by an inversion does not lead to an abnormal phenotype. The medical significance of inversion is for the subsequent generation. The problem arises during crossing over between a normal chromosome and one with an inversion.

For the homologous chromosomes to pair in an inversion situation, one of them must form a loop in the region of the inversion. If the inversion is pericentric, the centromere lies within the loop. If a cross-over now takes place, each of the two chromatids involved in it has both a duplication and a deficiency at the first division of meiosis. This then can lead to unbalanced gametes and thus unbalanced chromosome material in the offspring. In humans pericentric inversions have been described in chromosomes 12, 17, and 20 [36, 156]. The duplication and deficiency state in the unbalanced individual that results from an inversion of chromosome 3 is particularly important for the ophthalmologist because the children with this condition have severe ocular defects. For a more detailed description of the biology of inversions in the human, one can read the review by Daniel [36].

CLINICAL CYTOGENETICS

Approximately 1 in 160 newborn infants have a chromosomal abnormality involving either the autosomes or sex chromosomes [175]. Slightly more than half of these aberrations are due to abnormalities of the sex chromosomes (usually a full extra chromosome); the remainder involve duplication or deletion of an autosome.

With the exception of XO and the polysomy X syndromes (e.g., XXXY), sex chromosomal aneuploidy rarely produces structural defects or mental retardation. On the other hand, abnormalities of number and structure of an autosome usually induce a broad pattern of phenotypic variations, congenital malformations, and mental retardation, that is, a syndrome.

With the advent of chromosomal banding techniques in the 1970s, it soon became obvious that there was potentially an infinite number of syndromes associated with partial deletions and partial trisomies of various segments of the human chromosome. This section will overview the basic principles of phenotypic analysis in clinical practice, while the remainder of the chapter will describe the more common conditions and newly discovered disorders of interest to the ophthalmologist. Particular emphasis will be placed on the distinctive ocular alterations that occur in these disorders.

The Biology of Malformations and Phenotype Analysis in Chromosomal Disorders

Approximately 3 to 4 percent of newborn infants have at least one medically significant congenital malformation noted at birth or within the early years of life. About 10 percent of these malformation patterns have a chromosomal cause. Of the remainder, 5 percent are cause by a single-gene or mendelian disorder, 80 percent are either of unknown causation or multifactorial inheritance, and about 5 percent are due to a well-documented environmental teratogen [191].

Autosomal chromosomal aberrations are associated with consistent patterns of *multiple congenital abnormalities* that involve both medically significant malformations and minor phenotypic variations (often called minor anomalies). Although many of the physical abnormalities described in these disorders are nonspecific and occur in several of the syndromes, the entire constellation of characteristics is recognizable and allows for clinical diagnosis.

This concept of *overlapping phenotypes* is exemplified by the fact that certain congenital abnormalities occur with increased frequency in every chromosomal syndrome. For example, almost all autosomal defects are associated with mental retardation, microcephaly, and short stature. Prenatal growth deficiency of height and weight is a common feature in most autosomal disorders. Congenital heart malformations occur with increased prevalence in all of the common chromosomal syndromes. Certain ocular abnormalities such as microphthalmos, colobomas, and hypertelorism are a feature of many entities. In fact, reading a list of the findings seen in many of the chromosomal syndromes may give one the idea that the list of abnormalities is the same in every disorder. However, some clinically useful generalizatons do emerge.

FACIAL CHARACTERISTICS

Unbalanced autosomal defects produce alterations of phenogenesis and morphogenesis that are frequently subtle and not medically significant in and of themselves. These minor anomalies are especially present in the face and distal limbs. Facial morphogenesis is extremely complex and involves the differentiation of many tissues. Chromosomal defects invariably alter the physical characteristics of the facial appearance in a consistent manner, so that it is different from that of the family and ethnic background. In other words, a child with Down's syndrome more closely resembles other children with this syndrome than his or her siblings.

The overall appearance of the facial phenotype and many of the individual facial characteristics are so similar in children with chromosomal syndromes that the affected individuals will resemble each other remarkably. However, phenotypic analysis of the human face is not a skill that is taught to most physicians. In analyzing the facial gestalt, it is important to describe the individual components and to compare the features to family background and to photographs of individuals with syndromes published in the literature. Photographs of individuals of the same age should be used because the facial phenotype will change with age [41].

The minor anomalies noted in chromosomal syndromes can be divided into two types:

1. *Alterations of morphogenesis or histogenesis*, that is, true structural defects or dysplasias that are of minimal medical consequence. These are really "mild malformations" and include clearcut discontinuous findings like an iris coloboma or preauricular tag [131].
2. *Alterations of phenogenesis*, that is, the more subjective, graded features that are continuous, and without a clearly defined threshold of abnormality, are not always easy to define. Sparse eyebrows, widely-spaced eyes, and micrognathia are examples of this class of minor anomalies. Whenever possible, precise measurements should be used in defining the phenotype. Anthropometric standards for many structures of the face have been established by Farkas [53], but most of these measurements are not practical for the clinician. Such commonly used measurements are available in syndrome catalogues [41, 156].

In the evaluation of an individual with a potential syndrome the need for *precise measurement* of structures for which anthropometric standards are available cannot be overemphasized. The need for objectivity and careful measurements is best typified by the confusion surrounding the child with widely spaced eyes (Fig. 8-14). A child who has the appearance of widely spaced eyes could have either orbital hypertelorism, short palpebral fissures with blepharophimosis, primary telecanthus with displacement of the inner canthi, bilateral epicanthal folds, or a flat nasal root [43]. For this reason it is recom-

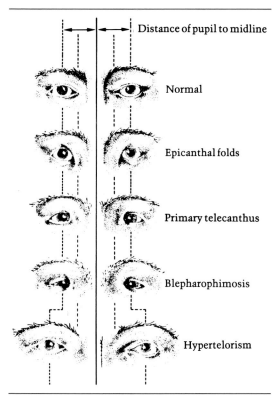

Distance of pupil to midline

Normal

Epicanthal folds

Primary telecanthus

Blepharophimosis

Hypertelorism

Fig. 8-14. *Relationship between distance from inner canthus to midline and from pupil to midline in normal individuals and in individuals with abnormalities of ocular soft tissue and ocular distance seen in many chromosomal syndromes.*

mended that when one sees a child with the appearance of widely spaced eyes, eye measurements of the inner canthal, interpupillary, and outer canthal distance should be taken and compared to reference graphs to make these distinctions [71, 164].

For instance, hypertelorism is a common feature mentioned in connection with many chromosomal syndromes. However, if one examines published photographs of children with abnormalities labeled as ocular hypertelorism, it soon becomes apparent that many of these children do not have true orbital hypertelorism (teleorbitism) but rather have primary telecanthus. Since eye measurements are rarely reported in a description of a chromosomal disorder, one cannot always objectively define the abnormality of ocular placement. Because the syndromes that are associated with telecanthus are often different from those associated with ocular hypertelorism, it is recommended that this distinction be made by

the clinician. Fig. 8-14 depicts the differences between the various alterations of ocular and canthal development. Epicanthal folds are merely redundant skin tissue that overlaps the inner canthi. Primary telecanthus or dystopia canthorum is a lateral displacement of the inner canthi, that is, a soft tissue abnormality. Ocular hypertelorism (teleorbitism) is an outward placement of the orbital structures and thus increases the interpupillary distance and produces a secondary telecanthus. A shortened palpebral fissure is an overall shortening of the fissure length, often accompanied by blepharophimosis.

The clinical usefulness of any minor anomaly depends on the degree of objective determination of the finding, its frequency in the general population, its consistency within a syndrome, and the family and ethnic comparison. The graded features that are subjective are usually of less weight in clinical decision making than the more objective findings that can be defined by standards or clear definition. Features that are uncommon in the population and not part of the child's family background are more important in deciding if a child has a syndrome than are common variants or familial features. Comparison to ethnic as well as family background assists in separating the helpful clues from the nonspecific ones.

Most of the phenotypic variations and ocular malformations reported in the chromosomal syndromes are summarized in the tables and discussions later in this chapter.

Another useful principle in the phenotypic analysis of the face is that the whole is equal to more than the sum of the individual parts. The previous discussion has emphasized the analysis of the separate components of the face. However, this is not to say that the clinical impression of the gestalt is unimportant. The facial gestalt that the clinical observer notes is made up of the individual features and the manner in which they fit together as a whole. For example, in the newborn with Down's syndrome, the individual features are nonspecific, frequent in the population, and continuous. Yet, the features as a whole present a distinctive impression and are consistent in the syndrome.

DISTINGUISHING OCULAR FEATURES

Even though there are many overlapping phenotypes and nonspecific features, the entire constellation of findings often allows for recognition.

Table 8-4 *Distinctive Ocular Features and Associated Chromosomal Abnormalities*

Ocular finding	Chromsomal abnormality
Aniridia	del (11)(p13)
Retinoblastoma	del (13)(q14)
Rieger eye malformation	dup 3p, del 4q, del 4p
Persistent hyperplastic primary vitreous	Trisomy 13
Cyclopia, cebocephaly	Trisomy 13, del 18p, triploidy
Cystic malformation of globe	del 12p

In addition, there are a few *discriminating phenotypic findings* that provide useful clues for particular conditions. Examples of some of these more distinctive abnormalities of the eye that occur in specific chromosomal syndromes are listed in Table 8-4.

The altered morphogenesis that is involved in the development of aniridia and the Rieger eye malformation may be more limited than those of coloboma and orbital displacement and thus occur in fewer entities. The presence of one of these more distinctive findings in combination with a broad pattern of defects then brings to mind a limited differential diagnosis. On the other hand, the developmental pathways that lead to an iris coloboma or hypertelorism are probably more complex and diverse; they thus involve many genes and can result from imbalance in many chromosomes. These concepts of overlapping phenotype and discriminating features are reviewed by Lewandoski and colleagues [109].

INDICATIONS FOR CHROMOSOMAL ANALYSIS

A karyotypic investigation is indicated in the following situations: (1) a recognizable chromosomal syndrome such as Down's syndrome, (2) a pattern of *multiple* malformations or phenotypic variations seen in the newborn period, (3) a stillborn infant for whom there is no known cause of fetal death, (4) ambiguous genitalia, (5) mental retardation accompanied by phenotypic variations or malformations, (6) a girl with amenorrhea and short stature (to rule out Turner's syndrome), (7) first-degree relatives of individuals who have balanced structural rearrangements (e.g., reciprocal translocations), (8) parents of children with a deletion or duplication of chromosomal material (e.g., a child with deletion of the short arm of chromosome 5), (9) couples with three or more spontaneous abortions and, (10) males with mental retardation who have a family history or the phenotypic findings of the fragile X syndrome. The fragile X syndrome will not be discussed in this review since ocular abnormalities are not a feature of this disorder.

A karyotypic analysis is *not* indicated in a person with a single congenital abnormality. Because of the association of retinoblastoma and del 13q14, a karyotypic study should be considered in an individual with retinoblastoma. However, in patients without mental retardation or other physical defects, the yield will be low.

The actual pathogenesis of the malformations involved in chromosomal syndromes is poorly understood. In trisomy situations, nondisjunction is felt to be the process that produces the extra chromosome in gametogenesis. However, the exact manner in which the extra chromosome material produces the recognizable and consistent constellation that we recognize as a syndrome has only recently been investigated.

From gene mapping studies (see Chap. 3) certain genes in the human have been assigned to certain segments of chromosomes. Investigations performed in vitro on gene dosage alterations in trisomy situations show that the gene product known to be associated with the localized gene is increased to 150 percent of normal [166]. This suggests that gene dosage effects may be an important mechanism in the altered morphogenesis that occurs in the particular syndrome. A generalized effect of developmental instability has also been alluded to as a potential mechanism in the trisomy state [20].

In regard to deletion situations, it is possible that the missing genetic material in a deleted chromosomal segment may unmask a recessive gene, making the individual essentially homozygous for a recessive disorder. In addition, the work performed on the association of retinoblastoma with a deletion of the long arm of chromosome 13 at band 14 shows that it is also possible that a deletion may bring out the effects of a dominant disorder when the gene locus is present within the deleted segment.

Epidemiology of Chromosomal Abnormalities in the Human

The precise causative factors that produce chromosomal abnormalities in the human are poorly understood. Most of the literature on the epidemiology of human chromosomal syndromes involves trisomy 21 [83]. The principal epidemiologic factor that has stood the test of time in the study of determinants of trisomy 21 (Down's syndrome) is parental age. It has been known for over 50 years that the mean maternal age of individuals with Down's syndrome is increased over that of the general population. In the last few decades data have been accumulated that indicate age-specific risks of trisomy 21 at each maternal age [83]. From these studies it is clear that as women get older the risk of having a child with trisomy 21 (and other extra chromosome situations) increases. However, because most children are born to women who are under 30, 60 percent of the children with Down's syndrome are born to younger mothers [80].

Although originally paternal age was not felt to be a factor, recent investigations have reevaluated this issue, and some have shown a paternal age effect [82]. Data on paternal age are still being accumulated, and in the future enough information may be available to provide more refined risk figures based on both parents' ages [82].

In the 1970s amniocentesis for the prenatal diagnosis of genetic disorders became available in the United States, Canada, and Europe. Because of the increased risk of trisomy 21 and other trisomies with increasing age, advanced maternal age became the most common reason for referral for amniocentesis in North America. Most centers now offer this procedure to couples when the woman is 35 years or older. Age-specific risks for a live-born with trisomy 21 at each maternal age are available when counseling a couple [83]. Amniocentesis is also indicated in couples who have had a previous child with any chromosomal abnormality regardless of parental age and when one of the parents carries a balanced translocation or other rearrangement.

Other factors have been raised as potential determinants in the risk for trisomy 21. These include parental mosaicism, preconceptual exposure to radiation, maternal thyroid autoantibodies, genetic predisposition to nondisjunction, and use of clomiphene citrate (Clomid) [83]. Harris and colleagues found that about 3 percent of the cases of couples' producing a child with trisomy 21 can be explained by paternal trisomy 21 mosaicism [76]. The evidence about the other factors is conflicting and is not clearly related to the causation of trisomy 21.

Recent studies on the origin of the extra chromosome 21 in children with trisomy 21 have shown that the extra chromosome derives from the mother about 80 percent of the time and from the father in about 20 percent of cases. These investigations are accomplished by examining Q-band and other polymorphisms of chromosome 21 in the affected child and the parents [93]. These data clearly indicate that the nondisjunction process occurs during spermatogenesis, as well as oogenesis.

Trisomy 13, trisomy 18, and XXY are also known to have a maternal age effect. No clear-cut agents or environmental exposures that produce translocations and deletions in humans are definitely agreed upon. These structural abnormalities can be lumped under the category of mutation, a process that is also poorly understood in humans. The reader is referred to the comprehensive review of the topic of mutation by Vogel and Motulsky [180].

The frequency of chromosomal abnormalities in the human is shown in Table 8-5. Actually these prevalence figures in live-born infants rep-

Table 8-5 *Prevalence of Chromosomal Aberrations Seen in Surveys of Newborns*

Abnormality	Approximate frequency
Sex Chromosome Disorders	
In 37,779 males	
XYY	1:1,000
XXY	1:1,000
Other	1:1,300
In 19,173 females	
45,XO	1:10,000
XXX	1:1,000
Other	1:3,000
Total sex chromosomal disorders	1:440
Autosomal Disorders	
Trisomy 21	1:800
Trisomy 18	1:8,000
Trisomy 13	1:20,000
Other trisomies	1:50,000
Structural rearrangements	
Balanced	1:500
Unbalanced	1:2,000
Total autosomal disorders	1:250
Total chromosomal disorders	1:160 (0.06%)

Source: Modified from J. S. Thompson and M. W. Thompson [175].

resent only a small portion of chromosomal defects in the human. Surveys of spontaneous abortions indicate that in about 50 to 60 percent of fetal deaths less than 20 gestational weeks the fetus has an unbalanced chromosomal abnormality; about 5 to 10 percent of stillborn infants (fetal deaths at greater than 20 weeks) possess a chromosomal defect [130]. From these data one can see that the occurrence of chromosomal imbalance in humans is not rare.

CLASSICAL TRISOMY SYNDROMES

The three most common autosomal trisomy syndromes—trisomy 13, 18, and 21—have been well delineated since the introduction of cytogenetics to clinical practice. Trisomy 13 will be dealt with in detail because the ocular abnormalities and pathologic changes in the globe are so distinctive. In trisomy 18, 90 percent of infants die before 1 year of age. Despite this shortened survival, this condition will be discussed because the ophthalmologist will often be called to consult on these cases in early life. In regard to trisomy 21, the ophthalmologist can play an integral part in the overall care of individuals with Down's syndrome.

Trisomy 13

Trisomy 13 is the chromosomal aberration most closely associated with severe intraocular abnormalities. Although rarely seen in the ophthalmologic clinic or office, the syndrome is observed more frequently by the pediatrician or the pathologist at necropsy. Approximately 90 percent of these children die before 12 months; 50 percent die by the age of 1 month.

Although the syndrome is rarely encountered in day-to-day practice, the ophthalmologist should have knowledge of this disorder. A detailed discussion of the numerous ocular aberrations is warranted for the following reasons:

1. Knowledgeable opinions in consultation with a pediatric service are sometimes expected.
2. The ocular findings in this syndrome are more severe and are more consistently present than those encountered in most chromosome-related syndromes.
3. The ocular findings are distinctive and occasionally may greatly contribute to the correct diagnosis.

4. The presence of the wide variety of embryonic defects observed in this syndrome renders it highly instructive as a model demonstrating the pathogenesis of various forms of congenital ocular disease.

The first known recorded case of this syndrome is attributed to Thomas Bartholin, who in 1657 described an infant with a complex of malformations now typically associated with the trisomy 13 syndrome [8]. In the prekaryote era, examples of this syndrome were often described in single case reports or in small series of cases. No unifying concept of pathogenesis was available, and the published case reports generally emphasized changes within specific organ systems corresponding to the author's particular interest. For example, the neuroscientists termed this syndrome *arhinencephalia*, based on specific brain abnormalities; vision researchers applied the term *retinal dysplasia syndrome* to describe a prominent intraocular change [143, 144, 149]; embryologists defined this disease as a *mesodermal dysplasia* to identify the defects in facial cleft fusion (cleft lip and palate). Thus because of insufficient knowledge regarding pathogenesis, varied names were applied, including, in addition to those already given, oculocerebral syndrome, encephalo-ophthalmic dysplasia [99], Reese-Blodi-Straatsma syndrome, idiopathic microphthalmos, and dyscraniopygophthangeal syndrome.

In 1960 Patau and coauthors provided one unifying pathogenetic basis to what had been a chaotic, heterogeneous, uncategorized complex of abnormalities [136]. They correlated this complex of abnormalities with a specific chromosomal abnormality based on a trisomy of the acrocentric chromosomes of the 13 to 15 group. With banding, the particular chromosome that is trisomic in this syndrome was designated as chromosome 13 (Fig. 8-15).

Estimates of the frequency of trisomy 13 vary from 1 in 4,000 [208] to 1 in 20,000 [175] live births. As in most trisomies, the frequency of trisomy 13 increases with maternal age. In a small minority of instances, Patau's syndrome may be induced not by nondisjunction, but by the mechanism of an unbalanced translocation, usually a robertsonian translocation (see Fig. 8-9) [3].

The systemic findings of this syndrome are well detailed by Smith and coauthors [163], Warkany and associates [185], Taylor [171, 172], and Mottet and Jensen [124]. It should be emphasized that the most characteristic brain abnormality, holopro-

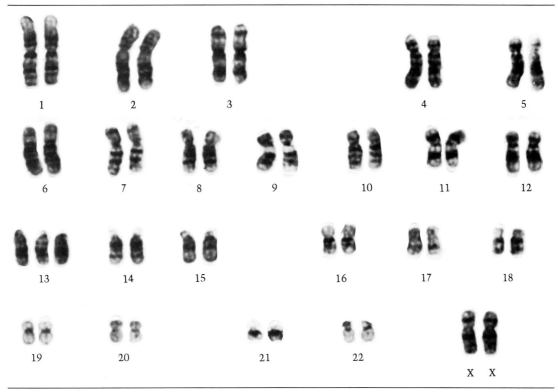

Fig. 8-15. *G-banded karyotype of trisomy 13, showing an extra chromosome 13 (47,XX, + 13). (Courtesy of K. van Dyke.)*

Fig. 8-16. *Trisomy 13. This view of the base of the brain demonstrates two commonly observed features of holoprosencephaly (arhinencephalia): (1) the absence of the olfactory nerve (first cranial nerve) and (2) fusion of the frontal lobes (F), with the absence of the midline sagittal fissure.*

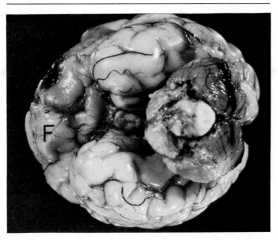

sencephaly (Fig. 8-16), represents varying degrees of aberration of formation of the forebrain. These aberrations may include formation of a single frontal lobe, abnormalities of the olfactory system (arhinencephalia), and anomalies in formation of the portion of the forebrain most related to this discussion, the optic vesicle. Anophthalmia and cyclopia would represent the most severe examples of optic anlage malformation. The pattern of malformation also includes a characteristic face, cleft lip and palate (in 60% of cases; Fig. 8-17), postaxial polydactyly (in 60% of cases; Fig, 8-18), scalp defects, and congenital heart disease (in 80% of cases). The common systemic manifestations of trisomy 13 are listed in Table 8-6.

One of the first detailed early descriptions of the ocular pathology of a case that undoubtedly represents true trisomy 13 was recorded by George Coats in 1910 (Fig. 8-19), the same ophthalmologist one associates with the well-known Coat's syndrome [30]. He demonstrated in photomicrographs the majority of the intraocular changes one typically observes in this condition. Several earlier and equally accurate reports of the ocular pathology of the trisomy 13 syndrome are also doc-

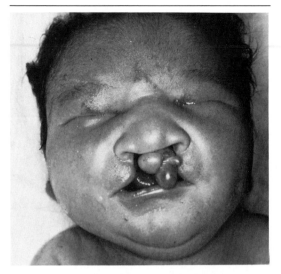

A

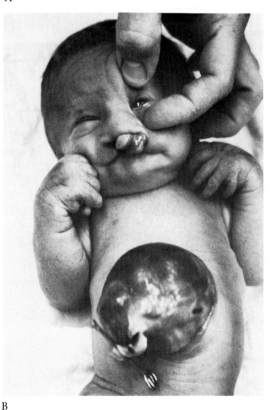

B

Fig. 8-17. *Trisomy 13. A. Cleft lip and palate are usually features of this syndrome. Note the apparent anophthalmia. (Courtesy of J. Holden, M.D., E. Anderson, M.D., and J. O'Neill.) B. Omphalocele and polydactyly associated with trisomy 13. (Courtesy of J. C. Carey, M.D.)*

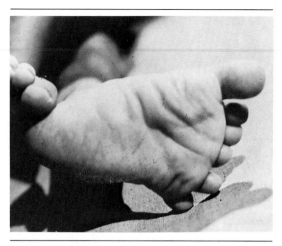

Fig. 8-18. *Polydactyly in trisomy 13.*

Table 8-6 *Systemic Manifestations of Trisomy 13*

General

 Failure to thrive; death usually within first few months of life
 Congenital cardiac defects (ventricular septal defect, patent ductus arteriosus)
 Hematologic abnormalities
 Skin hemangiomas
 Inguinal or umbilical hernia
 Cryptorchidism and abnormal scrotum in males
 Bicornuate uterus in females

Nervous system

 Holoprosencephaly (arhinencephalia), abnormal development of olfactory apparatus, abnormal fusion of frontal lobes; cyclopia represents the most extreme degree
 Mental retardation
 Wide sagittal suture and fontanelles
 Apneic spells
 Minor motor seizures
 Defective hearing

Head

 Bulbous nasal tip
 Scalp defects

Musculoskeletal

 Microcephaly
 Cleft lip and palate
 Polydactyly, rudimentary digits on hands and feet
 Simian crease
 Hyperconvex narrow fingernails
 Posterior prominence of heel

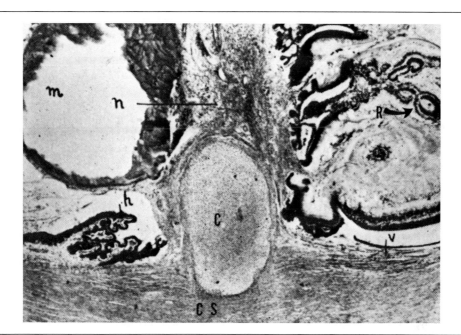

Fig. 8-19. *Trisomy 13. Photomicrograph of the limbal region of a globe studied by Coats, demonstrating that the salient pathologic features of this syndrome have been documented for decades [30]. Note the striking similarities to Fig. 8-20B. (C = cartilage within a ciliary body coloboma; CS = corneal-scleral collagen; R = rosette within area of retinal dysplasia.) (h, m, n, and v are notations from Coats's original description.)*

Table 8-7 *Ocular Manifestations of Trisomy 13*

Microphthalmos; sometimes apparent (clinical) anophthalmia

Colobomas (usually of ciliary body and iris, less commonly optic nerve); colobomas are seen in almost 100% of affected eyes

Persistent hyperplastic primary vitreous (communication of extraocular connective tissue of mesodermal origin with intraocular hyaloid system and tunica vasculosa lentis via ciliary body coloboma); sometimes pigmented

Intraocular cartilage formed in mesoderm within the ciliary body coloboma; ingrowth of uveal melanocytes into globe through the coloboma

Retinal dysplasia, including abnormal, anteriorly dislocated sensory retinal tissue formed over pars plana

Cataracts; primary aphakia (rare)

Rudimentary differentiation of angle structures

Corneal opacities; posterior corneal "ulcers" (rare)

Optic nerve hypoplasia, atrophy; occasional coloboma of the optic nerve

Cyclopia

umented in early German literature, reviewed by Dötsch [45].

Bilateral ocular involvement is present in almost 100 percent of cases of the full-blown trisomy 13 syndrome (Table 8-7). The most important clinical and histopathologic ocular findings are microphthalmos, colobomas, intraocular cartilage formation, persistent hyperplastic primary vitreous, aphakia, retinal dysplasia, and cyclopia [31, 77, 160, 200].

MICROPHTHALMOS VERSUS ANOPHTHALMIA

Individuals with trisomy 13 invariably have some degree of microphthalmos, ranging from mildly affected globes to extreme involvement (see Fig. 8-17). For years, the extreme cases were thought to represent anophthalmia. In Patau and colleagues' original case report, the globes were not found during the initial postmortem examination [136]. The researchers assumed that a state of anophthalmia existed, and the case was reported as such. However, most investigators have found that a true primary anophthalmia is seldom an inherent part of the trisomy 13 syndrome.

True anophthalmia is defined as the total absence of the original optic anlage, so that no ocular rudiments ever form. Anophthalmia was first mentioned by Lycosthenes in 1557 [113], but it was not until a century later that Bartholin provided the first medical description [8]. Numerous reports followed, with little attempt to delineate the precise nature of any intraorbital tissue. In 1963 Duke-Elder reported that the true form of anophthalmia was rare and that most cases showed some neuroectodermal derivatives in the orbit [48]. When such derivatives are present in a patient with no grossly evident eye structures, extreme microphthalmos is a more appropriate designation.

Therefore, in a vast majority of cases of trisomy 13, if not all, the true state is one of extreme microphthalmos, in which the eyes have formed and are present, although they may not be readily observed clinically [133]. However, because of a possible misinterpretation in the original description of this syndrome, anophthalmia is listed as a prominent feature of trisomy 13 in most articles and texts dealing with this subject.

COLOBOMA AND CARTILAGE FORMATION

Mottet and Jensen [124] and others have established that the anomalies associated with trisomy 13 are manifestations of retarded developmental events occurring in embryos at 5 to 6 weeks of gestation (embryo length 7–15 mm). This is precisely the period in which the embryonic optic vesicle normally is undergoing invagination of its distal and inferior margins, leading to formation of the two-layered optic cup and the ventral embryonic ocular fissure, which subsequently should close at about 6 weeks of gestation. The varied lesions seen in the affected eyes of trisomy 13 are best explained by regarding the basic defect as a deviation from the pathway of normal tissue migration and closure of the ocular fissure during this period [3].

Very small, underdeveloped eyes result from grossly abnormal, misdirected invagination of the optic vesicle and exhibit such widespread abnormalities as clinical anophthalmia (extreme microphthalmos), aplasia of the anterior segment, primary aphakia, and extensive colobomas. In most instances, however, invagination of the neuroec-

toderm and formation of the two-layered optic cup proceed along a more normal pathway up to the point of closure of the embryonic fissure. Therefore, the presence of a coloboma, characteristically involving the ciliary body and iris (Fig 8-20), is the major manifestation that apparently initiates a number of secondary changes to create the total clinical pathologic picture.

For many years investigators have noted the presence of intraocular cartilage in microphthalmic eyes (most of which we now know must have come from bona fide cases of trisomy 13). However, Cogan and Kuwabara were instrumental in emphasizing the association of intraocular cartilage deposition with the trisomy 13 syndrome [31]. Cogan and Kuwabara pointed out that cartilage was more commonly observed in severely microphthalmic eyes than in others, a phenomenon that is not surprising if one assumes that a small globe implies more retarded development and potential for more severe, qualitative intraocular aberrations.

The cartilage typically is situated within the band of fibrovascular tissue at or near the site of colobomatous defect (Fig. 8-20C). In essence the mesodermally derived fibrovascular tissue within the coloboma undergoes a cartilaginous metaplasia. One can assume that this peculiar change is brought about by a lack of proper organizing or inducing forces at the site of the coloboma, thus permitting the bizarre cellular differentiation, which is highly characteristic, if not quite diagnostic, of this syndrome. Intraocular cartilage is by no means seen only in trisomy 13 eyes. Cartilage often is formed in ciliary body tumors (diktyomas) and may even be seen in globes obtained from otherwise normal individuals [199].

Just as the lens will not develop normally if the optic vesicle (neural ectoderm) does not make contact with the surface ectoderm of the embryo, so apparently does the tissue of the ciliary region fail to develop in a controlled fashion at the site of a ciliary coloboma. Certain structures seem to be necessary for normal development of adjacent tissues; that is, the pigmented and nonpigmented layers of the ciliary body are disrupted at the site of the defect.

PERSISTENT HYPERPLASTIC PRIMARY VITREOUS AND CATARACT

In simplified terms it is attractive to speculate that a genetic aberration involving a locus somewhere along the length of one of the thirteenth

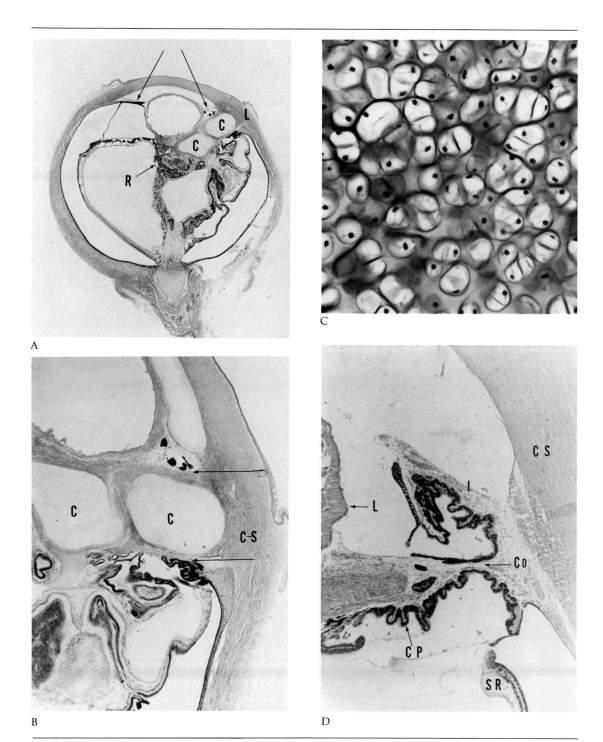

Fig. 8-20. A. Photomicrograph of a trisomy 13 globe. Note the communication between the limbal sclera (L) and the retrolental dysplastic retina (R) through a coloboma of the ciliary body and iris. The colobomatous defect contains a band of fibrovascular tissue and two nodules of cartilage (C). Arrows indicate hypoplastic iris and angle structures. (H&E, ×10.) B. High-power photomicrograph of the limbal region of A. The margins of the colobomatous defect are demarcated by the two arrows. The corneal-scleral (C-S) mesodermal collagen is continuous with intraocular mesodermal tissue, including the metaplastic cartilage (C). Note dysplastic ciliary and sensory retinal epithelium. Note also the similarity to Coats's earlier micrograph (Fig. 8-19). (H&E, ×30.) C. The hyaline cartilage of B is more readily recognized at higher magnification and consists of chondrocyte nuclei within individual compartments (lacunae). (H&E, ×350.) D. Note the very small ciliary body coloboma (Co) that divides the rudimentary iris (I) anteriorly from the ciliary processes (CP) posteriorly. The lens (L) is cataractous. Note the abnormal differentiation of pars plana epithelium into multilayered sensory retina (SR). (H&E, ×50.)

chromosomes (two are normal, one is extraneous) is responsible for initiation of, at the minimum, an iris and ciliary body coloboma, as well as other possible ocular changes. In explaining the findings further, one must recall that the eye now contains a gap or defect along the line of the former embryonic fissure (inferonasally), through which there is communication of the extraocular mesenchyme (future choroid and sclera) with intraocular mesoderm (the primary vitreous or hyaloid vascular system). This interaction of tissue at the site of the ciliary body defect seems to initiate further disruption of the intraocular contents.

In addition, the primary vitreous, including its anteriormost arborization, the tunica vasculosa lentis, commonly persists in trisomy 13, forming a retrolental fibrovascular membrane (Fig. 8-21). This membrane, well known to ophthalmologists in its complicated form as persistent hyperplastic primary vitreous (PHPV), serves to interrupt adequate growth and development of the lens. Because of pressure on the posterior lens capsule and even occasional rupture of the posterior capsule, induction of microphakia or a severe cataract may occur. Pathologically, the lenticular changes are easily recognizable as liquefaction and degeneration within the lens cortex, posterior migration of lens epithelium (recall that lens epithelium is normally present only anteriorly and equatorially), and bladder-cell formation. Bladder cells are swollen, abnormally proliferating lens epithelial cells. These cells are observed in numerous types of cataract and should not be considered characteristic of any single form of disease.

The retrolental persistent band of fibrovascular tissue, which joins the primary (hyaloid) vitreous with the mesoderm ouside the optic cup via the colobomatous gap in the ciliary body, permits a peculiar ingrowth of uveal melanocytes into the eye. During normal development of the primarily mesodermal choroid, dendritic, uveal melanocytes migrate into the differentiating choroid from the neural crest, thereby forming the pigmented cells of the choroid as well as the ciliary body and iris. This is the same general group of pigmented cells responsible for intraocular uveal nevi and melanomas and should not be confused with melanin normally present in the neuroectodermal retinal pigment epithelium. The uveal melanocytes normally remain outside or external to the optic cup, but in at least 50 percent of the cases of trisomy 13, the pigmented cells migrate inward through the cleft and become situated on the retrolental membrane. In our experience this curious phenomenon has been unique to trisomy 13;

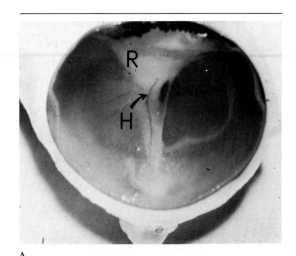

A

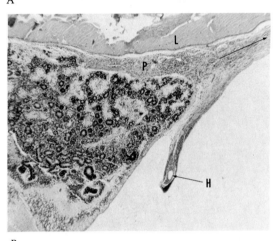

B

Fig. 8-21. *A. Gross photograph of trisomy 13 globe. The lens is completely blanketed by a funnel-shaped mass of dysplastic retina (R), which overlies the ciliary body coloboma (not evident in this plane of section). (H = persistent hyaloid vessel.) B. Same case as in A, showing the retrolental funnel-shaped mass of dysplastic retina including numerous rosettes. Interposed between the cataractous lens (L) and the dysplastic retina is a band of mesodermally derived fibrous tissue (persistent hyperplastic primary vitreous), which joins the persistent hyaloid vessel (H) posteriorly and courses toward the colobomatous defect laterally (arrow). (H&E, × 30.)*

however, one can theoretically expect this phenomenon any time such a colobomatous defect permits it, no matter what the disease.

RETINAL DYSPLASIA

Retinal dysplasia is visible grossly as a funnel-shaped, white retrolental mass (Fig. 8-21A). Because of its large size and interesting microscopic patterns, this phenomenon is probably the most frequently described and best known component of the trisomy 13 syndrome. The studies of Reese and coauthors have emphasized this aspect of the syndrome [143, 144]. In the prekaryotype era, the disease was often termed *retinal dysplasia syndrome*.

Retinal dysplasia, defined simply as abnormal growth and differentiation of embryonic retina, is best considered to be a lesion, not a disease. It is a secondary finding common to many examples of ocular maldevelopment [88]. It may result from any type of disruption of normally regulated growth of the neuroectoderm, such as may be initiated by abnormal position and function of adjacent organizer structures (in the present context, the ciliary body coloboma). Most of the dysplastic retina in the trisomy 13 syndrome is characterized by aimless retinal and ciliary epithelial overgrowth situated at, or adjacent to, the site of the coloboma.

Histopathologically, retinal dysplasia may take several forms, including rosette formation (Figs. 8-21B and 8-22) (an abortive attempt to form retinal rods and cones); aimless proliferations of ciliary epithelium, both pigmented and nonpigmented; proliferation of cords of tissue that closely resemble primitive optic cup neuroepithelium; and aberrant glial tissue formation. In addition, there occasionally appears to be an abnormal anterior displacement of sensory retina, so that the multilayered sensory retina, which has replaced the simple cuboidal epithelial layer of the pars plana, is observed near the coloboma site. Something has induced the pars plana epithelium to differentiate toward the sensory retina.

CYCLOPIA

Cyclopia is a rare congenital defect in which the two orbits have merged to form a single, centrally located cavity with one eye. The results of chromosomal analysis of 31 cases of cyclopia revealed that more than half the cases had trisomy 13 [85, 127].

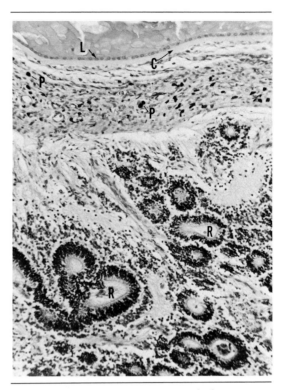

Fig. 8-22. *Trisomy 13. Photomicrograph showing retrolental tissue relationships. Note cataractous lens (L) showing posterior migration of lens epithelium and bladder-cell formation; lens capsule (C); pigmented uveal dentritic melanocytes (P) within the persistent hyperplastic primary vitreous—these cells have migrated into the globe through the colobomatous defect; and rosettes (R) within area of retinal dysplasia. (H&E, ×125.)*

Cyclopia results from an anomalous development of the ocular primordia during the first month. In most instances the two optic vesicles actually fuse; this phenomenon is correctly termed synophthalmia. True cyclopia with a solitary optic anlage is extremely rare.

Neither true cyclopia nor synophthalmia is compatible with life, because there is an associated anomalous development of midline components of the brain. There is typically a failure in the division of the telencephalon into hemispheres. In addition to the ectodermal aberrations affecting the brain and eyes, there is abnormal development of the mesodermal structures of the face, leading to a creation of a proboscis-like structure above the orbit [2, 209].

Table 8-8 *Systemic Manifestations of Trisomy 18*

General

    Death within first year of life
    Mental deficiency; delay of psychomotor
    development
    Decreased growth rate
    Cardiac abnormalities
    Cryptorchidism
    Inguinal or umbilical hernia

Musculoskeletal system

    Hypoplasia of skeletal muscle and subcutaneous
    and adipose tissue
    Prominent occiput; narrow bifrontal diameter
    Low-set, malformed ears
    Micrognathia, receding chin
    Small oral opening (microstomia) with narrow
    palatal arch
    Hypertonia with limbs in flexion; flexion
    contractures of the fingers (camptodactyly)
    Clenched hand with tendency for overlapping of
    index finger over third, fifth finger over fourth
    Short sternum
    Rocker-bottom feet
    Small pelvis with limited hip abduction
    Hypoplasia of nails, especially on fifth finger and
    toes

Source: Modified from J. Warkany, et al. [185]; and A. E. Krill. *Hereditary Retinal and Choroidal Diseases, Vol. 1: Evaluation.* New York: Hoeber Med. Div., Harper & Row, 1972.

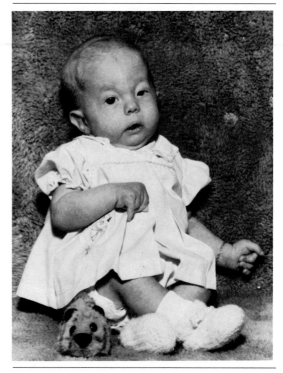

Fig. 8-23. *A 4-month-old girl with trisomy 18, 47,XX, + 18. Note the characteristic clenched fists.*

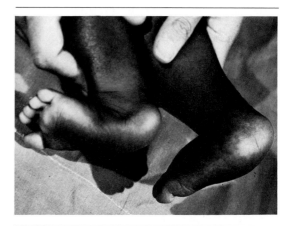

Fig. 8-24. *Rocker-bottom feet in trisomy 18.*

Trisomy 18

In 1960 Edwards and coworkers described a syndrome associated with trisomy of an E group chromosome [49]. Banded cytologic studies have demonstrated that the extra chromosome is number 18 [61]. The trisomy is probably the result of a nondisjunction in gametogenesis.

Trisomy 18 is second only to trisomy 21 as the most frequently occurring autosomal trisomy in neonates [81]. Estimates of its frequency range from 1 in 3,500 births [112] to 1 in 14,500 births [32, 74, 75]. Female infants outnumber males 3 to 1. Affected infants are often born to women of advanced maternal age and have a limited capacity for survival. Over 50 percent of these patients die within 2 months of birth, and only 1 in 10 survives the first year of life. However, some patients with trisomy 18 are reported to have lived into the second decade [81, 165].

The systemic findings (Table 8-8) are characteristic and include a prominent occiput, short palpebral fissures, small mouth, micrognathia, a short sternum, and rocker-bottom feet (Figs. 8-23 and 8-24). The hand configuration is distinctive in that the fifth finger overlaps the fourth and the second overlaps the third with hyoplastic nails.

Table 8-9 *Ocular Manifestations of Trisomy 18*

Globe
  Corneal opacities, clouding
  Microphthalmos
  Colobomas
  Cataractous changes
  Persistent hyaloid artery
  Glaucoma
  Other: blue sclera, absent retinal pigment,
  nictitating membrane, pupillary membrane,
  conjunctiva overriding the cornea, short radius of
  corneal curvature

Adnexa
  Slanted or narrow palpebral fissures
  Epicanthus
  Ptosis
  Abnormally thick lids
  Abnormally long or sparse lashes
  Inability to close lids
  Blepharophimosis

Orbit
  Shallow orbits, hypoplastic orbital ridges
  Hypertelorism, hypotelorism

Neuro-ophthalmology
  Strabismus, lateral gaze, asynergy of extraocular
  movement
  Decreased response to visual stimulus
  Nystagmus
  Anisocoria

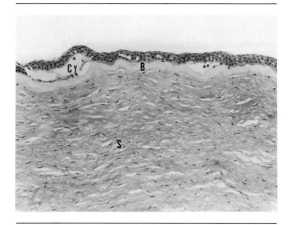

Fig. 8-25. *Trisomy 18. The corneal epithelium is irregular, and there is cystic separation (Cy) of epithelium from Bowman's membrane (B). Bowman's membrane is thickened and wrinkled, and the corneal stroma (S) shows irregularity of the lamellae. (H&E, ×150.)*

Ninety percent of affected children have congenital heart disease, especially multiple valvular abnormalities [5].

Initial reports emphasized the clinical ocular findings. In 1968 Ginsberg and co-workers presented the first comprehensive study of the ocular histopathology in trisomy 18 [65]. Subsequently, many additional ocular pathologic findings have been described (Table 8-9) [20]. Corneal anomalies are often noted (Fig. 8-25). Immaturity of the angle structures and anomalies of the ciliary process and iris are frequently described [98]. Cataractous changes in the lens have also been noted. Retinal folds are the single most common histopathologic finding. Other common retinal observations include hypopigmentation of the posterior pigment epithelium (Fig. 8-26), dysplasia, and areas of hemorrhage and gliosis [20].

Since one-third of trisomy 18 babies are born prematurely, it is important to distinguish the pathologic changes of this syndrome from those of prematurity alone [20]. For example, at birth the corneal stroma and choroid show increased cellularity. During the ninth month in the normal fetus, anterior chamber mesoderm has disappeared only up to the trabecular meshwork, and certain ciliary muscle fibers are still developing. The hyaloid system does not fully disappear until the middle of the eighth month of gestation. Exact determination of fetal age as well as a variability in ocular development may lead to difficulties in interpretation of several of the reported findings. However, the presence of colobomas or retinal dysplasia, for example, is indisputably pathologic. Incomplete angle cleavage or corneal stromal hypercellularity, on the other hand, may represent developmental findings alone.

It is of interest to compare the intraocular manifestations of trisomy 18 with those of trisomy 13, which is well known for its intraocular findings. Both syndromes are associated with microphthalmos, colobomas, retinal dysplasia, cataracts, poorly differentiated angle structures, and optic nerve hypoplasia. However, microphthalmos, retinal dysplasia, and most anomalies associated with these syndromes occur with much increased incidence and severity in trisomy 13. Colobomas, also less severe in trisomy 18, tend to affect the posterior globe in the region of the embryonic cleft in this trisomy and the anterior aspect of the globe in trisomy 18. Persistent hy-

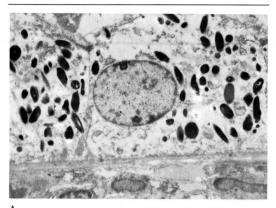

A

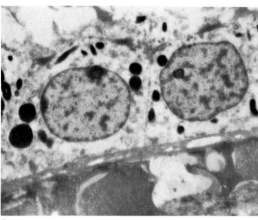

B

Fig. 8-26. *A. Trisomy 18. Transmission electron microscopic examination demonstrates an abundance of well-pigmented melanosomes in the equatorial retinal pigment epithelial cells. B. By contrast, posterior retinal pigment epithelial cells have fewer well-pigmented melanosomes. Occasional incompletely pigmented granules (arrow) are seen in these cells. (×4,914.) (Courtesy of Anne Fulton, M.D.)*

perplastic primary vitreous, intraocular cartilage, and cyclopia are found, for the most part, only in trisomy 13.

Most of these ocular manifestations are uncommon in the individual child with trisomy 18, and many are reported in only one patient, while clinically recognizable ocular involvement is the rule in trisomy 13.

Ginsberg and colleagues postulate that the basic effect of the extra chromosome in trisomy 18 may be the initiation of abnormal, widespread cellular hyperplasia and hypertrophy [65, 66]. Such phe-

nomena are seen not only within the eye (e.g., corneal epithelium and endothelium, ciliary epithelium, retinal neurons) but are likewise observed in a wide variety of extraocular sites in patients with trisomy 18. Examples of the latter include proliferation of nodules of renal blastema (embryonic kidney) and neuronal heterotopias seen in a variety of foci within the brain.

From phenotype-karyotype correlations that have been recently reported, it appears that the chromosomal segment necessary to produce Edward's syndrome (trisomy 18) involves the distal half of the long arm [177].

Trisomy 21 (Down's Syndrome)

The clinical features of Down's syndrome have been well known since John Down's original descriptions in 1866 [47]. The chromosomal basis of this condition was first theoretically predicted in 1932 by Waardenburg, an ophthalmologist [181]. This astute prediction was confirmed by Lejeune and co-workers in 1959, who verified that the basic chromosomal abnormality of Down's syndrome is an aneuploidy consisting of 47 chromsomes [103, 104].

Down's syndrome is by far the most common of the autosomal trisomy conditions, showing an incidence of 9.8 percent of 12,000 retarded children in one series, equivalent to approximately 1 in 800 births [175]. The incidence sharply increases to 1 in 32 births when the maternal age is 45 years and older [83].

More than 90 percent of persons with Down's syndrome show a characteristic trisomy 21 induced by nondisjunction of this chromosome ($2n + 1 = $ a total of 47 chromosomes). About 5 percent have a translocation of the long arm of chromosome 21, usually because of a robertsonian translocation (see Fig. 8-10). Although the genotype shows such variation, there are no significant clinical differences between the trisomy 21 and the translocations; all the affected individuals have similar abnormalities.

Based on the few cases of Down's syndrome caused by reciprocal translocations, trisomy of only the distal one-third of the long arm of chromosome 21 is all that is needed to produce the complete phenotype [170].

Systemic findings include mental retardation (IQ in the 25–70 range), short stature, hypotonia, brachycephaly, and characteristic facial phenotype (Table 8-10). The facial characteristics (Fig. 8-27) consist of a flat nasal root, epicanthal folds,

Table 8-10 *Systemic Manifestations of Down's Syndrome*

General

Two populations as regards survival, one with significant mortality the first year, the other living into adulthood

Mental deficiency (IQ 25–70); often euphoria

Small stature

Cardiac abnormalities (especially endocardial cushion defects)

Dry, rough skin

Susceptibility to stress, infection

Head

Brachycephaly

Thin cranium; delayed fontanelle closure

Frontal and perinasal sinus hypoplasia

Small nose with low nasal bridge

Small, round external ear with defective lobules

Broad lips that are irregular and fissured

Tendency toward open mouth, with a thick, roughened, protruding tongue

Dental hypoplasia

Short, thick neck (excessive skin on the nape of neck)

Trunk and extremities

Hypotonia; hyperextensible joints

Pelvic hypoplasia

Diastasis recti abdominis

Small, broad, stubby hands; incurved little finger

Characteristic dermatoglyphic findings, with altered palmar creases (simian line)

Short, broad feet with poorly developed arch, wide gap between first and second toes

Genitourinary system

Infertility

Undescended testes

Absent or defective spermatogenesis

Abnormal development of labia

Irregular menses

Ovarian hypoplasia

Gastrointestinal

Duodenal atresia

Source: Modified from J. Warkany, et al.; and A. E. Krill, *Hereditary Retinal and Choroidal Diseases, Vol. 1: Evaluation.* New York: Hoeber Med. Div., Harper & Row, 1972.

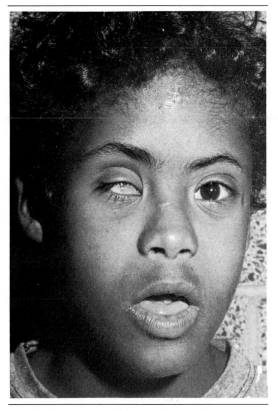

Fig. 8-27. *A 12-year-old boy with trisomy 21. Note the classic facial features, including epicanthus, flat nasal root, and short neck. The child's right eye has phthisis bulbi with corneal opacification and associated ptosis, secondary to complications of an intraocular lens implantation.*

upslanted palpebral fissures, midfacial hypoplasia, round cheeks, and a short neck. Children with Down's syndrome are often felt to have widely spaced eyes, but this is usually an illusion owing to the flat nasal root and epicanthal folds. In fact, radiographs show that children with Down's syndrome usually have orbital hypotelorism. Abnormalities of the extremities include short broad hands with a simian crease and short fifth fingers with clinodactyly. Congenital heart disease is present in about 35 percent of individuals with Down's syndrome.

Abnormalities of the eyes are common (Table 8-11). The malformations comprise a variety of nonspecific hyperplasias or hamartomas, hypoplasias, tissue defects, and heterotopias [50, 91]. Virtually every tissue may exhibit abnormalities; only the vitreous has failed to show any detectable alteration [67]. The pathologic findings are

TABLE 8-11 *Ocular Manifestations of Down's Syndrome*

General ocular and adnexal abnormalities

Mongoloid slant (palpebral fissures slant upward and outward)

Epicanthus

External hypertelorism

Narrowed interpupillary distance

Convergent strabismus

Blepharitis, blepharoconjunctivitis

Ectropion

High myopia, refractive error

Specific intraocular pathologic lesions

Cataracts (develop after age 8–10)

Brushfield's spots

Iris hypoplasia (usually peripheral iris)

Keratoconus, sometimes acute (occurs in adults)

Nystagmus

Hyperopia

Fundus anomalies

Iris coloboma

Adherent leukoma

Heterochromia iridis

Ganglion and neuroretinal hypoplasia (rare)

Source: Modified from A. E. Krill, *Hereditary Retinal and Choroidal Diseases, Vol. 1: Evaluation.* New York: Hoeber Med. Div., Harper & Row, 1972.

generally minor, and a distinctive picture has not emerged.

It is difficult to correlate the embryologic timing, incidence, or severity of the ocular and extraocular abnormalities in Down's syndrome. The type of ocular anomalies usually encountered in Down's syndrome suggests that the chromosomal anomaly affects the globe rather late in its development, that is, toward the close of the embryonic period or afterward.

Practically every ocular and adnexal lesion in Down's syndrome occurs occasionally in otherwise normal individuals or persons with other mental or physical defects. The most commonly observed or clinically significant intraocular lesions in Down's syndrome are cataracts, iris lesions, and keratoconus.

CATARACTS

The cataracts of patients with Down's syndrome are diverse and are best observed by slit-lamp biomicroscopy rather than by examination of pathologic specimens. Lens opacities are seen in 60 to 85 percent of all patients [44, 150]. They are rarely observed before the age of 8 to 10 and characteristically develop or become manifest after puberty. Lowe divided the cataracts into four main categories [111]:

1. *Arcuate opacities.* This cataract, the most distinctive type seen in trisomy 21, represents opaque lens fibers that arch around the equator of the early layers of the fetal nucleus. Such cataracts form in relation to abnormal capsulopupillary vessels, embryonic vessels that are normally transient and should begin a regression during the fourth fetal month. It follows that this type of cataract is the earliest type to be seen in Down's syndrome.

2. *Sutural cataracts.* Although such opacities are typically observed along the line of the original Y sutures formed before birth, they are seldom seen at an early age. They become manifest much later, often in the teens, and thus develop many years after the sutures are originally laid down.

3. *Flake opacities.* The nature of this type of cataract remains obscure. Many are beneath the capsule, but a certain percentage may represent excrescences of the lens capsule. The latter phenomenon is also observed in other conditions, including Lowe's and Miller's syndromes.

4. *Uncommon congenital cataracts.* Lamellar and posterior polar cataracts are occasionally observed in Down's syndrome patients.

IRIS LESIONS

In 1924 Thomas Brushfield described spots encircling the periphery of the iris in children with Down's syndrome [17]. He observed two main varieties of irides: (1) mottled or marbled, and (2) speckled with white or very light yellow pinpoint elevations clearly defined near the outer margin, generally placed at regular intervals in a ring, and appearing to be placed on the iris.

About 20 years earlier Wolfflin had described similar nodules occurring in about 10 percent of all normal individuals [198]. He described about 10 to 20 nodules in each eye, usually situated in the periphery of the iris.

Lowe noted a thinning or hypoplasia of the iris in persons with Down's syndrome and felt that this was a more prominent feature of the syndrome than Brushfield's spots [111]. Lowe stated that thinning occurred in about 95 percent of Down's syndrome children and could be found at an early age.

Donaldson analyzed irides of 180 individuals with Down's syndrome and in two cases correlated the important pathologic features with clinical photographs [46]. Histopathologically, hypoplasia of the peripheral iris was the most prominent feature. The pathologic counterpart of Brushfield's spot is less obvious but consists of increased density of the anterior stromal layer. Presumably the increased anterior stromal density not only is white itself but also may shield from view the pigmented layers of the iris. Brushfield's

Fig. 8-28. *A. Brushfield's spot of the iris. The anterior border layer (arrows) of the iris stroma shows increased density because of deposition of aggregates of stromal fibrocytes. (H&E, × 450.) B. Normal iris. The stromal cells are relatively few and loosely arranged, and there is no increase in cell density at the anterior surface. (PE = posterior iris pigment epithelium.) (H&E, × 200.)*

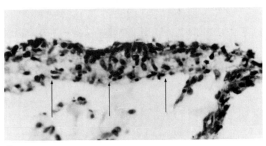

A

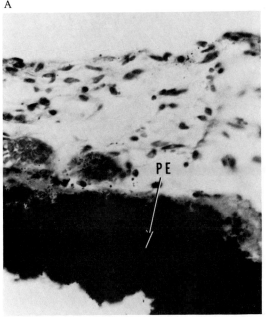

B

spot is sometimes further characterized by formation of large empty spaces (areas of rarefaction) of the iris stroma behind the dense anterior border layer (Fig. 8-28).

Brushfield's spots occur in 85 to 90 percent of persons with Down's syndrome, whereas normal individuals show an incidence of only 24 percent or less [190]. Such spots in normal persons are often termed Wolfflin-Kruckmann spots. Furthermore, the irides in Down's syndrome generally contain a greater number of spots than in normal individuals with Wolfflin-Kruckmann spots [158]. Brushfield's spots are commonly found in the midzone, whereas the spots found in normal individuals are situated more peripherally. Spotting occurs nearly as frequently in brown-eyed as in blue-eyed patients with Down's syndrome. There is no significant difference in occurrence, number, or distinctness of spots as a function of age. The IQ of the Down's syndrome individual is not correlated with the presence or absence of spots. A further distinction between the Down's syndrome iris and the iris of normal individuals rests in the marked thinning or hypoplasia of the peripheral portion of the iris in Down's syndrome; such a degree of thinning is rarely seen in the unaffected individual.

KERATOCONUS

Rados was the first to report an association between Down's syndrome and keratoconus in 1948 [142]. Since that time investigators have reported an incidence of keratoconus between 5.5 and 8 percent in individuals with Down's syndrome [34, 140].

Cullen and Butler analyzed the ocular findings of 143 patients with Down's syndrome [34]. Keratoconus was seen in 8 patients, or in 5.6 percent. In 160 control patients keratoconus occurred in only 2 percent. It is noteworthy that in only 3 of the 8 Down's syndrome patients was the simple form of keratoconus observed; 5 of the 8 demonstrated evidence of active or previous corneal hydrops (acute keratoconus). The incidence was greater in the older age groups. Acute keratoconus is a rare condition in any circumstance, and it is now well established that it is seen with far greater frequency in persons with Down's syndrome than in the general population.

Pathologically, simple keratoconus is characterized in its initial stages by fragmentation of the corneal epithelial basement membrane and fibrillation of Bowman's layer and anterior stroma

[2]. Eventual thinning of the entire corneal stroma may occur, especially at the apex of the cone. Ruptures and folds in Descemet's membrane commonly lead to a disturbance in corneal hydration, resulting either in chronic edema of the cone or in the full-blown syndrome of acute keratoconus (Fig. 8-29).

Pierce and Eustace found that acute hydrops occurs with increased frequency in keratoconus patients with Down's syndrome or other forms of mental deficiency [140]. They suggested that the ruptures in Descemet's membrane occur in patients because of eye rubbing. Boger and colleagues [13] and Coyle [33] support this idea with cases of acute keratoconus in which the patients had vigorously rubbed and poked their eyes.

FUNDUS ANOMALIES

Ophthalmoscopically, irrespective of the refractive error or the degree of skin or iris pigmentation, the fundus in individuals with Down's syndrome resembles that of blond individuals [161]. Pigmentation of the retinal pigment epithelium and choroid is scanty, and the choroidal vasculature is easily visible. A large number of retinal vessels crossing the disc margin gives it a pinker color than usual. These vessels often assume a characteristic wheel-spoke arrangement [210].

Fig. 8-29. *A. Keratoconus in trisomy 21 and Soemmering's ring cataract. B. Same case as A. Note marked corneal edema and bullous change characteristic of acute keratoconus. (H&E.) (Courtesy of L. E. Zimmerman, M.D., and the Armed Forces Institute of Pathology, Washington, D.C.)*

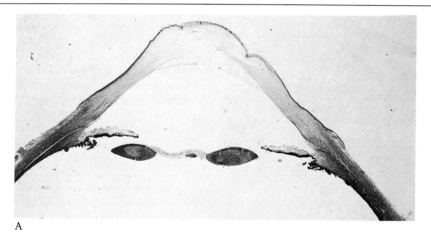

A

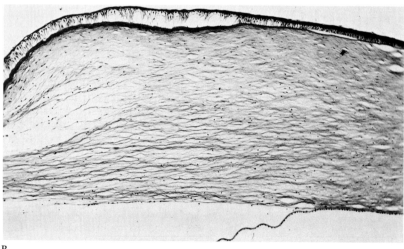

B

BLINDNESS IN TRISOMY 21

Severe visual difficulties are relatively infrequent in Down's syndrome [186]. Cullen, however, has emphasized the exceptions to this statement [35]. Of 143 Down's syndrome patients examined, 7 were bilaterally blind and 3 had one blind eye, giving a total of 17 blind eyes in 10 patients. Basically, three mechanisms are responsible for blindness in these patients:

1. Keratoconus, particularly corneal hydrops (acute keratoconus) [183].
2. Sequelae of cataracts. It is postulated that in some instances the cataracts become hypermature, with leakage of lens material, secondary uveitis, and eventual phthisis. Alternatively, a hypermature cataract may dislocate and again initiate an inflammatory process, leading to phthisis [35].
3. Occasionally, surgical failure of cataract operations. The trisomy 21 eye is apparently prone to react unfavorably to surgical interference [35].

Recurrence Risk Counseling in the Classical Trisomy Syndromes

The issues surrounding the recurrence risk for a family after the birth of a child with a complete trisomy syndrome are complicated by the limitations of available data. First, all of the existing recurrence data are in regard to trisomy 21. Second, the crude data are few, and some figures are outdated, having been obtained before 1959. Third, the data are lumped into 5-year maternal age intervals and have not been calculated for specific ages. Stene compiled the data in 1970 [169], and this reference is still cited in most reviews. When the maternal age at the birth of the affected child is under 30, the empirical risk for a second child with trisomy 21 is 1.4 percent. When the maternal age at birth of the first child is greater than 30, the empirical risk is 0.4 percent and thus similar to advanced maternal age risk for any live-born.

These data have been interpreted differently by different geneticists [83]. The limited figures would suggest a risk of 1 to 2 percent for a family in which the mother is under 30; for the family in which the woman is older than 30, the risk of having a second affected child would be the same age-specific risk as for the general population. Thus, as has been suggested by Hook, age-dependent factors may be operating for families in which the mother is younger, while in the situation of ad-

vanced maternal age, the age-dependent factors predominate [83].

There are no existing empirical risk figures for the family of the baby with trisomy 13 and 18. However, there are a few reports of families who have had two affected offspring with these trisomies [137], and there are several reports of multiple affected siblings with different trisomy conditions [83, 137, 165]. These case studies would suggest that a family who has had one child with these less common trisomies is at some increased risk to have a second affected child. Most geneticists use the above 1 to 2 percent risk figure empirically calculated for trisomy 21 and apply it to these situations as well.

In regard to recurrence risk in translocation trisomy situations, the stated risk depends on whether or not either parent has a balanced translocation. Therefore, chromosomal studies are always indicated in parents of a child who has an unbalanced translocation or duplication. If one of the parents has a balanced rearrangement, available empirical data on that translocation are utilized for estimating risk. If the parental chromosomes are normal, the risk for a second child with a de novo translocation is considered to be low but possibly increased over the general population risk. In the case of de novo 21–21 translocation producing Down's syndrome, empirical risk figures for recurrence have been calculated [168].

Amniocentesis is offered to families who have had a child with any of these chromosomal abnormalities regardless of maternal age or parental karyotypes.

CHROMOSOMAL DELETIONS AND DUPLICATIONS OF PARTICULAR IMPORTANCE TO THE OPHTHALMOLOGIST

With the advent of chromosome banding in the early 1970s, delineation of partial monosomy and trisomy syndromes has increased tremendously. At present at least one deficiency and duplication syndrome has been delineated for every autosomal chromosome.

After the introduction of high-resolution banding techniques in the mid-1970s, even more subtle deletion and trisomy situations were recognized. For the ophthalmologist the most important of these included the association of retinoblastoma with a deletion at band 14 on the long arm of chromosome 13 and the discovery that the aniridia–Wilms' tumor association was usually due

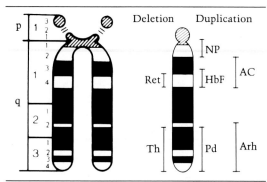

Fig. 8-30. *A phenotype-karyotype map of chromosome 13. Left, diagram of G-banded chromosome 13 for reference. Right, single-stranded schematic of chromosome 13. The brackets indicate the segments of the long arm where the particular phenotypic characteristic is mapped. The brackets on the left represent the physical characteristics that are related to deletion in that segment; brackets on the right, those related to duplication. (Ret = retinoblastoma; Th = thumb agenesis; NP = abnormal nuclear projections in neutrophils; HbF = elevated hemoglobulin F; AC = aplasia cutis of the scalp; Pd = polydactyly; Arh = arhinencephalia.)*

to a deletion of band 13 on the short arm of chromosome 11.

Phenotype-karyotype correlations have been performed for various chromosomal syndromes, implicating particular segments of the chromosome in the production of certain abnormalities. In chromosome 1, for example, three different syndromes have been described for deletions in three different portions of the long arm. Many of the abnormalities and findings of trisomy 13 have been tentatively mapped to different portions of the long arm of chromosome 13.

These karyotype-phenotype correlations are performed by cataloging the physical findings in individuals who have partial trisomies of different portions of the long arm of chromosome 13, usually as a result of balanced translocations, chromosomal duplications, or pericentric inversions. For example, the polydactyly seen in the full trisomy 13 syndrome is present in children who have a partial trisomy of the distal one-third of the long arm of chromosome 13. Individuals who have trisomy of more proximal portions of the long arm do not have polydactyly. Tentative assignments of other distinctive findings caused by duplication or deletion of chromosome 13 material are depicted in Fig. 8-30.

In this section the various deletion and dupli-

cation syndromes will be organized according to their chromosome number. For more information on the particular syndrome, one can refer to the comprehensive reviews of de Grouchy and Turleau [41], Yunis [204], and Schinzel [156]. In addition the chromosomal syndromes and their associated eye disorders were recently reviewed by Howard [86].

Parental chromosomal studies are always indicated in the parents of a child with a deletion, duplication, or other structural aberration. In addition amniocentesis should be offered to these couples in future pregnancies.

The clinical phenotype noted in cases with partial trisomies or monosomies is more variable than the classical complete trisomy syndromes. This variability is due to (1) the smaller number of reported individuals—the complete spectrum of the syndrome is not delineated, (2) the varying sizes of the duplicated or deleted segments in the reported cases because of different breakpoints, and (3) the presence of different associated chromosomal aberrations in individuals who have the unbalanced state because of a translocation.

Table 8-12 lists various ocular manifestations and the chromosomal syndromes in which they occur. This table is meant to update previous reviews [86, 96, 196, 210] and to disguise some of the particular bands associated with specific syndromes (e.g., deletion 11p13 in the aniridia–Wilm's tumor association). Note that we have not included some features in this table that were usually noted in earlier reviews: epicanthal folds, blue sclera, blocked tear ducts, and strabismus. This was done because of the nonspecificity of these features and because of their common occurrence in the general population. These particular characteristics are so nonspecific that they are rarely helpful in the overall diagnosis.

CHROMOSOME 1

DELETION OF THE LONG ARM (DEL 1Q)

Several cases of terminal or interstitial deletions of different segments of the long arm of chromosome 1 have been reported [173]. The various deleted segments fall into three groups: (1) terminal long-arm deletions of chromosome 1 usually distal to band 1q42, (2) interstitial deletions of 1q involving the middle segment of the long arm (deletion 1q24–2q32), and (3) proximal 1q deletions.

The cases with the terminal long-arm deletions

Table 8-12. *Ocular Anomalies in Chromosomal Disorders*

I. Face, adnexa
- A. Palpebral fissure, lids
  1. Upslanted: dup 3q, dup 5p, del 9p, dup 10p, del 11q23, +18, dup 20p, +21, XXXXY
  2. Downslanted: dup 2q, del 4p, dup 4p, dup 4q, del 5p, +8, r9, dup 9p, dup 10q, del 11q, dup 11p, dup 14q, dup 15q, dup 17p, +18, del 21q, dup 22p, CES, XXXXX
  3. Short, blepharophimosis: del 2p, dup 2q, del 3p25, dup 4p, dup 4q, dup 6p, dup 7q, +9, del 10p, dup 10q, dup 14q, dup 15q, +18
  4. Ptosis: del 3p25, del 4p, dup 4q, dup 10q, del 11p, r13, dup 14q, dup 17p, del 18p, +18, dup 19q, del 22q, XO
  5. Blepharochalasis: del 21q
  6. Ectropion: +21
  7. Epiblepharon: r21
  8. Telecanthus: del 1q, dup 3p, dup 3q, dup 4p, dup 4q, del 5p, r6, dup 6q, dup 9p, del 11q, dup 11q, dup 12p, dup 20p
- B. Orbit
  1. Hypertelorism: dup 3q, del 4p, del 4q31, del 5p, dup 7q, +8, dup 9p, dup 11p, del 13q, +13, dup 14q, del 18q, +18, CES, XXXXX, XXXXY
  2. Hypotelorism: dup 5p, +13, dup 14q, +21, r22
  3. Orbital hypoplasia: del 4p, del 9q, dup 9q, dup 15q, +18
  4. Enophthalmos: dup 9q, dup 9q, dup 11p, dup 16p, del 18q
- C. Eyebrows
  1. Synophrys: dup 3q, del 4p, dup 4q, del 5q, dup 10p, dup 13q
  2. Sparse: del 1q, del 4p, +13
  3. High-arched: del 9p, r9, dup 10p, dup 10q, del 12p

II. Globe
- A. General
  1. Microphthalmos, anophthalmia: del 4p, dup 4q, del 5p, dup 5q, dup 10p, dup 10q, del 13q, r13, +13, dup 13q, dup 14q, dup 16q, del 18p, del 8q, r18, +18, r21, CES, triploidy
  2. Coloboma: del 4p, dup 4p, del 5p, dup 5p, r6, dup 8p, dup 9p, dup 10p, del 11q23, r13, del 13q, +13, dup 13q, dup 14q, del 18q, CES, triploidy, XXXXX
  3. Cystic eye: del 12p
  4. Cyclopia, holoprosencephaly: dup 3p, del 13q, +13, del 18p, +18, +21, triploidy
  5. Congenital glaucoma: dup 3q, +13, dup 13q, dup 17p, del 18q, +18, +21
  6. Nystagmus: del 4p, del 5p, dup 11p, dup 17p, del 18q, +18, +21
- B. Cornea
  1. Microcornea: +13, del 18q, +18
  2. Keratoconus: del 18p, +21
  3. Corneal clouding: del 2q, del 4p, dup 4q, +8, +13, del 18p, del 18q, +18, r21
  4. Thick corneas: +18
  5. Sclerocornea: del 4p
- C. Anterior chamber, iris
  1. Brushfield's spots; +21
  2. Rieger's anomaly: dup 3p, del 4p, del 4q, +21
  3. Peters' anomaly: del 4p, +9
  4. Anirida: del 11p13, dup 13q, +13, XXXXY
  5. Corectopia: dup 3p, del 4p, dup 9p, dup 17p
- D. Lens
  1. Cataract: del 4p, del 13q, r13, +13, dup 15q, del 18p, del 18q, r18, +18, r21, +21, triploidy
  2. Aphakia: +13
- E. Persistent hyperplastic primary vitreous: +13
- F. Retina, fundus
  1. Retinal dysplasia: del 13q, +13, r18, +18, triploidy
  2. Retinoblastoma: del 13q14, +21, XXX
- G. Optic nerve
  1. Atrophy: del 5p, r6, +13, del 18q, r18
  2. Optic hypoplasia: +13, del 18q, +18

p = short arm; q = long arm; r = ring; + = full trisomy of numbered chromosome; dup = duplication or partial trisomy; del = deletion; CES = cat-eye syndrome.

appear to represent a distinctive syndrome because of the phenotypic similarity of the craniofacies. The clinical manifestations of the patients with the interstitial deletion of the middle segment are too variable and nonspecific for a recognizable pattern to be described at present. The few reported individuals with the proximal interstitial deletion have a strikingly similar constellation of findings, permitting delineation of a recognizable condition. All have prenatal and postnatal growth deficiency, mental retardation, microcephaly, ear abnormalities, small hands and feet, and abnormalities of palmar creases. The children have distinctively sparse eyebrows and upslanted palpebral fissures [173].

The different patterns of malformation that have been assigned to various segments of the long arm of the chromosome 1 are a good example of attempts at phenotype-karyotype correlation and typify the increase in the description of newer syndromes with the advent of high-resolution banding.

CHROMOSOME 3

DELETION OF THE SHORT ARM (DEL 3P)

Anomalies of chromosome 3 have usually involved duplication rather than deletion. However, at least 8 individuals with deletions, including 3 with ring chromosome 3, have been described. Breakpoints of the short arm in the nonring cases have usually involved band 25. All of the reported cases of terminal 3p deletion have involved de novo sporadic events. [78, 156].

Besides the rather nonspecific features of growth retardation, microcephaly, congenital heart disease, and mental retardation seen in most chromosome syndromes, the children with 3p deletion syndrome have a distinctively altered craniofacies. The combination of triangular face, prominent nasal bridge, micrognathia, ptosis, and blepharophimosis evoke a similar facial gestalt. The blepharophimosis in some of the children with this syndrome is particularly severe, and thus 3p deletion can be listed in the differential diagnosis of the syndromes associated with blepharophimosis [152].

DUPLICATION OF THE SHORT ARM (DUP 3P); ASSOCIATION WITH THE RIEGER EYE MALFORMATION

Partial trisomy of the distal half of the short arm of chromosome 3 appears to represent a distinctive and recognizable condition. At least 18 cases have been reported since Rethore and associates noted three siblings with this chromosomal abnormality in 1972 [146]. Prenatal and postnatal growth deficiencies are usually absent, which is unlike many chromosomal or partial trisomy situations. Psychomotor retardation was present in all the children who were alive at the time of the respective reports [114].

About 50 percent of the patients died before 2 years of age. The facial characteristics consist of low nasal root, telecanthus, a short nose with a large tip, long philtrum, prominent cheeks, and a short neck. Although most of these features are individually nonspecific, the combination is consistent and allows for a recognizable gestalt. Eighty percent of the reported patients have had congenital heart disease. In all of the reported cases thus far, the partial trisomy was due to a balanced reciprocal translocation in one of the parents. This fact emphasizes the importance of performing karyotypic analysis in the parents of children with extra or missing pieces of chromosome.

The child described by Carey and co-workers had the Rieger eye malformation with associated glaucoma [22]. In addition, one other case in the literature was noted to include corectopia, which suggests a similar anterior chamber defect [146]. The Rieger eye malformation is heterogeneous and can be a feature of several syndromes.

DUPLICATION OF THE LONG ARM (DUP 3Q)

The duplication 3q syndrome is of importance to the ophthalmologist because of its resemblance to another syndrome with ocular findings, de Lange's syndrome, and because of the high frequency of various ocular manifestations. The duplication 3q syndrome has been reported in more than 40 cases [167]. Most individuals with the syndrome have a partial trisomy of one-third to one-half of the long arm of chromosome 3.

The facial phenotype is distinctive and consists of synophrys, upslanted palpebral fissures, telecanthus, interverted nares, long prominent philtrum, downturned corners of the mouth, and micrognathia. This pattern of facial features is similar to that seen in de Lange's syndrome, which is a malformation–mental retardation syndrome of unknown causation [164]. The ocular abnormalities are varied and consist of ptosis, microphthalmos, coloboma, and cataracts. The most distinguishing ocular manifestation is infantile-onset glaucoma, sometimes with corneal clouding. Other consistent features include cleft palate, abnormal auricles, short neck, and brachyphalangia. Congenital heart disease has been present in over 50 percent of reported cases [167].

The duplication 3q syndrome has been associated with a parental translocation or a pericentric inversion in most individuals. In the 8 individuals whose duplication 3q was due to a parental inversion, a terminal deletion of the short arm of chromosome 3 at band 25 was consistently found [164]. Thus, in these children the combination of both a duplication and a deficiency of chromosome material is clearly documented. Since the children who have the duplication 3q and the deletion 3p25 have the same pattern of malformation as the children who do not have this deficiency, the clinical characteristics seen in these cases are felt to be mostly due to the excess of material rather than the deficiency. The striking blepharophimosis seen in children with a terminal deletion of the short arm of chromosome 3 is not seen in these cases.

CHROMOSOME 4

DELETION OF THE SHORT ARM (DEL 4P): WOLF-HIRSCHHORN SYNDROME

In 1965 Wolf and associates described a child who had a partial deletion of the short arm of B chromosome [197]. The child's phenotype, however, did not correspond to the cri du chat syndrome (5p−), the only B-deletion syndrome recognized at that time. Using autoradiography they were able to confirm that the abnormality was in chromosome 4 (see Fig. 8-11). At least 60 cases of the 4p monosomy syndrome have been reported since that time [195].

This condition is discussed in detail because of the high frequency and severity of ocular involvement. The life expectancy of the affected individual is not well known. Several individuals in their twenties are known. Mental retardation is profound and is probably more severe in this condition than in most chromosomal disorders. The IQ is usually below 20. Microcephaly is consistent and marked and is occasionally accompanied by a median defect of the scalp (10% of cases). The forehead is high and, when the infant cries, is marked by deep wrinkles that attest to the hypertonia of the subcutaneous muscles. The glabella is large with an occasional hemangioma. The eyebrows, sparse toward the interior, accentuate this impression of broadness. The nose is noteworthy: the edges of the nasal root are rectilinear and parallel and prolong the eyebrow line; the nasal bridge is as wide as the apex, which is square. This aspect evokes a "Greek warrior helmet" (Fig. 8-31) [41]. Preauricular pits and fuzz are common, and the corners of the mouth are downturned. The philtrum is usually short [118].

The palpebral fissures are horizontal or slanted downward and outward. True ocular hypertelorism is present, and the orbits are hypoplastic, producing the appearance of prominent eyes. The following ocular manifestations are common: ptosis or a unilateral retraction of the upper eyelid, Marcus Gunn's sign (in some cases), strabismus, corectopia, nystagmus, myopia, and obliteration of the lacrimal ducts. More severe eye malformations include colobomas and cataracts. One patient with the 4p− syndrome was also reported to have Rieger's anomaly [187].

In addition to the craniofacial alteration, skeletal, palatal, and cardiac defects are frequent. Growth retardation, distinct at birth, accentuates with age.

Cytogenetic studies show either an interstitial deletion involving the 15 to 16 band or a terminal deletion starting at band 14 of the short arm of chromosome 4 [195]. Thus, the phenotype of the Wolf-Hirschhorn syndrome is due to a deleted segment within the 4p16 segment. About 13 percent of instances of the 4p− syndrome are due to parental translocations [195].

DELETION OF THE LONG ARM (DEL 4Q)

Various patterns of phenotypic alteration associated with deletions of different segments of the long arm of chromosome 4 have been thoroughly reviewed by Mitchell and colleagues [121]. These authors conclude that deletion of the distal one-third from band 31 produces a recognizable entity consisting of growth deficiency, mental retardation, postnatal microcephaly, telecanthus, cleft palate, and micrognathia. Congenital heart disease, as with most chromosomal syndromes, is a common finding (70%). Some children have had

Fig. 8-31. *Wolf-Hirschhorn syndrome (del 4p or 4p−). This infant has ocular hypertelorism, a short philtrum, and a high nasal root.*

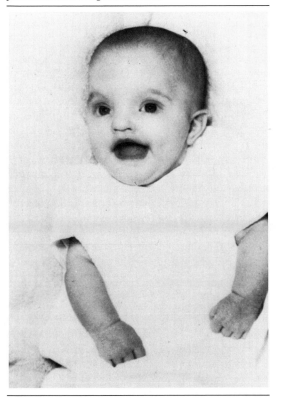

the Pierre Robin syndrome as the cause of the cleft palate. Individuals with deletions of the upper two-thirds of the long arm of chromosome 4 have variable findings, and it is difficult to clearly delineate any recognizable entities. However, Ligutič and co-workers described a child who had the Rieger eye malformation, mental retardation, missing teeth in both dentitions, and a number of other facial and limb findings [110]. The child's deletion of the long arm of chromosome 4 was interstitial and involved bands q23 to q27. Because of the combination of the ocular abnormalities and hypodontia, the authors imply that the child had Rieger's "syndrome" as part of her overall chromosomal disorder and that the autosomal dominant gene for the well-described Rieger's syndrome may be present on chromosome 4. Because the Rieger eye malformation has been noted in other chromosomal disorders, and because hypodontia is a nonspecific finding, no firm conclusion about the location of the gene for the autosomal dominant Rieger's syndrome can be made. It is more likely that the combination of features in this child caused by the deletion also happened to include the two principal characteristics of Rieger's syndrome: the anterior chamber eye defect and hypotonia. This case, however, is important because it emphasizes the heterogeneity of the Rieger eye malformation, which can occur in a number of chromosomal syndromes, and raises an interesting hypothesis. Further case reports of individuals with interstitial deletions of the middle third of the long arm of chromosome 4 will ideally establish the limits of interstitial deletion syndromes involving this chromosome.

DUPLICATION OF THE SHORT ARM (DUP 4P)

Nearly 40 cases have been reported with a duplication of the short arm of chromosome 4. The first observation of proven trisomy 4p was reported by Wilson and associates in 1970 [193]. In almost every case trisomy resulted from a parental translocation or pericentric inversion [41].

The striking feature of this syndrome is the appearance of a "boxer nose" in adults. Because of the lack of development of the nasal bones, the glabella joins the orbital ridges and hangs over the nose, accentuated by eyebrows that are extremely dense toward the nasal aspect. As the child grows, the nasofrontal angle does not develop and a round, fleshy tip persists, giving the nose its characteristic appearance.

Individuals with duplication of 4p have downslanted palpebral fissures and occasionally blepharophimosis. Microphthalmos and strabismus are also frequent findings of this syndrome [196].

Mental deficiency is in the moderate to severe range. More than one-third of the patients die in childhood, mainly as the result of infection [41].

DUPLICATION OF THE LONG ARM (DUP 4Q)

About 30 cases of partial trisomy of the 4q have been published since the first demonstrated case. The mouth is the characteristic feature of this syndrome: the upper lip is short but protruding, with pronounced philtrum pillars and sometimes a median raphe. It overlaps the lower lip, raising the median portion and producing the *cul de poule* or pursed mouth. The palpebral fissures are narrow and slanted downward and outward. Blepharophimosis, epicanthus, ptosis, and microphthalmos are often present. Mental retardation is moderate to severe with an IQ usually below 50. One-fourth of the patients die in the first year [41]. In most cases the partial trisomy is a consequence of a parental translocation.

CHROMOSOME 5

DELETION OF THE SHORT ARM (DEL 5P): CRI DU CHAT SYNDROME

The deletion of the short arm of chromosome 5 was first described by Lejeune and co-workers in 1963 in three mentally retarded children who had a particular mewing phonation that resembled a crying cat [105]. Although its exact prevalence is not established, the best estimation seems to be about 1 in 50,000 births. The syndrome has been reported in most racial groups including blacks, whites, and Asians.

The degree of developmental retardation is usually in the moderate to severe range and is inversely correlated with the size of the deletion [188, 189]. Affected children have small, soft larynges; this may explain the cry, which usually disappears with advanced age. Craniofacial characteristics include microcephaly, hypertelorism or telecanthus, rounded facies, short philtrum, and micrognathia (Fig. 8-32). True ocular hypertelorism is documented in some cases of deletion 5p, but in most cases telecanthus is present [189]. Despite the nonspecificity of the individual facial features, examination of published photographs shows a remarkable similarity in the facial phe-

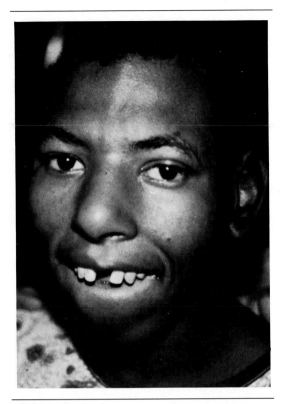

Fig. 8-32. *Cri du chat syndrome (del 5p or 5p−). This 25-year-old woman had pronounced microcephaly and a catlike cry in infancy. She has unslanted eyelid fissures and an abnormal Schirmer tear test result.*

notype of children of similar age. Hypotonia, skeletal abnormalities, and short stature are common. The individual develops a long, thin, often asymmetric face and has a characteristic stooping, shuffling gait. Premature graying of the hair may be present in the older person [15].

Considerable overlap is evident in the ocular findings in patients with chromosome deletions 4p− and 5p−. Such ocular abnormalities include epicanthal folds, hypertelorism, downslanted palpebral fissures, and cataracts. In contrast, individuals with 5p− commonly have abnormal Schirmer test results [187] and an abnormal pupillary constriction after instillation of 2.5% methacholine [84].

About 80 percent of individuals with deletion 5p have a de novo deletion. The other 20 percent possess an unbalanced translocation between the short arm of chromosome 5 and another chromosome because of a parental translocation [41]. The cases with unbalanced translocations have a greater occurrence of physical anomalies, lower

IQ, and a higher mortality. This is probably due to the presence of the concomitant partial trisomy [188].

DUPLICATION OF THE SHORT ARM (DUP 5P)

Duplication of the short arm of chromosome 5 is particularly noteworthy because of the occurrence of this condition in families who also have a child with deletion 5p (cri du chat syndrome). In the family reported by Lejeune and associates, the mother had a balanced translocation involving the short arm of chromosome 5 and chromosome 13 [106]. Children in this family thus would be at risk for two described conditions, partial trisomy of 13 or partial trisomy of distal 5p. In most individuals with duplication 5p, the unbalanced chromosome abnormality was related to a parental translocation [97].

The characteristics constellation of findings in dup 5p consists of psychomotor retardation, hypotonia, seizures, macrocephaly, scaphocephaly, hypotelorism, upslanted palpebral fissures, macroglossia, long thin fingers, and club feet. Congenital heart disease occurs with increased frequency. Ocular malformations consisting of microphthalmos or colomboma have been reported in a few individuals. Both hypertelorism and hypotelorism have been reported in this syndrome, although eye measurements are usually not available. The combination of the macroscaphocephaly and upslanted palpebral fissures contribute to the recognizable gestalt in the children [23].

CHROMOSOME 6

DUPLICATION OF THE SHORT ARM (DUP 6P)

At least 11 cases of partial trisomy of 6p have been published. In this chromosomal syndrome, the infants are very pale and show severe growth retardation. The eyes are very characteristic: The palpebral fissures are short, contracted by blepharophimosis, ptosis, or both [29]. Strabismus, with or without nystagmus, and hypotelorism have been reported in some cases. The mouth is small, and the lips are thin. Cardiac and renal malformations have been noted in some children [41].

DUPLICATION OF THE LONG ARM (DUP 6Q)

More than 10 cases of partial trisomy of the long arm of chromosome 6 have been reported [156].

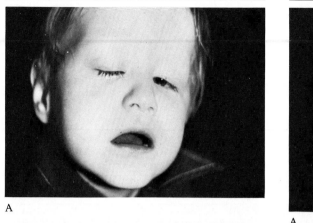

A

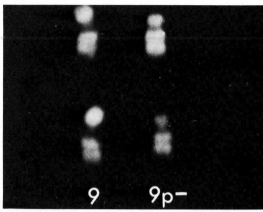

A

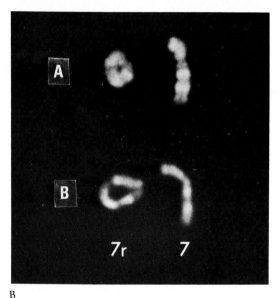

B

Fig. 8-33. *A. Ring 7. This 23-month-old boy has facial asymmetry and craniosynostosis. He is microcephalic and has bilateral ptosis. No lid fold is present on the right side. The right eye is markedly microphthalmic and turned in to the nose. The left cornea measures 10 mm. B. Ring formation of chromosome 7 is illustrated with Q-banding in two separate cells (A and B).*

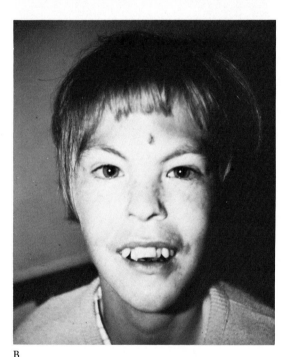

B

Fig. 8-34. *A. Deletion of a portion of the short arm of chromosome 9 shown by Q-banding. B. Deletion of short arm of chromosome 9 (del 9p or 9p−). This 20-year-old woman is microcephalic and retarded and has a prominent ridge along the metopic suture.*

In most of the children the duplication was due to malsegregation of a balanced translocation in a parent or was associated with a pericentric inversion of chromosome 6 [25]. The syndrome consists of prenatal growth deficiency, mental retardation, microcephaly, a strikingly short and webbed neck, overriding fingers, joint contractures, and internal malformations. The webbed neck is particularly unusual because it involves a webbing of skin in the anterior neck and underneath the chin. The ocular manifestations consist of telecanthus and orbital hypoplasia, which make the eyes appear prominent.

CHROMOSOME 7

RING 7 (R7)

At last 3 cases of individuals with r7 have been reported [156]. The clinical phenotype is variable, but all had growth deficiency and dysmorphic features. Ocular findings, present in 2 cases, consisted of optic atrophy and nystagmus in one and ptosis and coloboma in the other (Fig. 8-33). The breakpoints were in the terminal bands of both arms of chromosome 7 in all cases.

DUPLICATION OF THE LONG ARM (DUP 7Q)

Infants with partial trisomy of the long arm of chromosome 7 have a low birth weight, wide fontanelles, and severe mental retardation. The palpebral fissures are most often horizontal or slanted slightly downward and outward. The fissures are narrow, long, and slightly almond shaped. Hypertelorism and epicanthus are inconsistent findings. Strabismus and iridoshcisis have been reported. Affected individuals often have abnormal, low-set ears, cleft palate, micrognathia, small nose, and skeletal deformities [41, 96].

CHROMOSOME 9

DELETION OF THE SHORT ARM (DEL 9P)

Since the initial description by Alfi and colleagues in 1974 [1], at least 30 patients with deletion of the short arm of chromosome 9 have been described [156, 202]. In most of the cases the deletion has been distal to 9p21 (Fig. 8-34A). Besides moderate developmental retardation, this syndrome consists of a constellation of medically insignificant physical variations. The facial phenotype is particularly distinctive (Fig. 8-34B) and includes trigonocephaly with prominent forehead and shallow supraorbital ridges, upslanting palpebral fissures, low nasal root, anteverted nostrils, a long philtrum, and ear abnormalities. The eyebrows are sometimes pointed, and because of the orbital hypoplasia the eyeballs protrude to some degree. The neck is short and occasionally webbed, and the digits are long [207].

The upslanted palpebral fissures and supraorbital ridge hypoplasia are usually seen in any patient with premature fusion of the metopic suture and concomitant trigonocephaly. Thus the ocular findings in this syndrome are probably secondary to the craniosynostosis and by themselves are not specific. However, the combination of metopic craniosynostosis, trigonocephaly, and developmental delay should make one suspect the deletion 9p syndrome [108].

TRISOMY 9 (+9)

Besides the classical trisomy syndromes involving chromosomes 13, 18, and 21, few complete trisomy syndromes have been reported in liveborn infants. Exceptions include trisomies of complete extra chromosomes 8, 9, and 22, which have each been reported in several individuals. Most of the reported cases in these three trisomies have involved mosaicism. Trisomy 8, which has been reviewed elsewhere, will not be discussed because of the nonspecificity of the ocular findings [139]. The existence of complete trisomy 22 is controversial because of the small size of the chromosome and the difficulty in interpretation of many of the so-called trisomy 22 cases and the exact delineation of the extra chromosomes [154]. Cases of the mosaic trisomy 9 syndrome have included a variety of ocular malformations, and thus this syndrome is relevant to the ophthalmologist.

At least 18 cases of trisomy 9 have been reported; 3 of the individuals have had complete trisomy 9. More than half of the children died before 1 year of age. Developmental delay, mental retardation, feeding problems, and low birth weight are common. While many of the cases share common phenotypic features, the pattern of malformation is variable because of the high incidence of mosaicism. The most consistent facial features appear to be a bulbous nasal tip and micrognathia [95]. The most frequent ocular abnormalities consist of short palpebral fissures and microphthalmos. Ginsberg and coauthors reviewed the ocular findings of trisomy 9 and reported a case with a complete pathologic examination of the eye [70]. These findings include microphthalmos, telecanthus or hypertelorism, epicanthus, and strabismus. In the case reported by Ginsberg (Fig. 8-35), an ocular lesion involving the anterior segment that was similar to Peter's anomaly was present.

Other less consistent and variable malformations seen in the reported cases include congenital heart disease, joint contractures, cleft lip and palate, renal malformations, and primary central nervous system defects.

The most consistent facial features seen in the patients with trisomy 9 mosaicism (contour of the nasal tip and deep-set eyes) are also features of duplication 9p syndrome [156]. In addition, the trisomy 9 mosaicism syndrome shares some nonspecific features with the duplication 9q syndrome. However, many of the other abnormalities reported in trisomy 9 mosaicism are not seen in either of the two partial trisomy conditions. Therefore, some of the phenotype is due to the fact that there is full trisomy. The number of trisomy 9 cells in these cases has ranged from less than 10 percent to greater than 90 percent. This difference in the number of abnormal trisomy 9 cells may account for the wide phenotypic variation reported in the cases. Relatively precise phenotype-karyotype correlation, as has been done in the partial trisomy 13 situations, is difficult in the trisomy 9 mosaicism syndrome because of the differences in the cases and the percentage of trisomy 9 cells.

Fig. 8-35. *Trisomy 9. A. Gross photograph showing that the lens is adherent to a central corneal opacity. (×6.5.) B. Cornea is indented by an adherent lens. Thinning or dehiscence of posterior capsule (arrow) is associated with beginning extrusion of liquefied cortex. Note marked anterior displacement of hypoplastic iris and elongated ciliary processes. (H&E, ×16.) C. Nasal retina extends approximately halfway onto the pars plana. (H&E, ×35.) (Courtesy of Joseph Ginsberg, M.D.)*

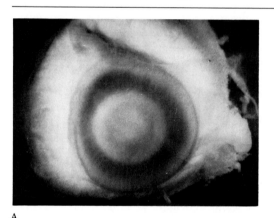

A

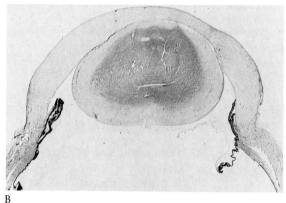

B

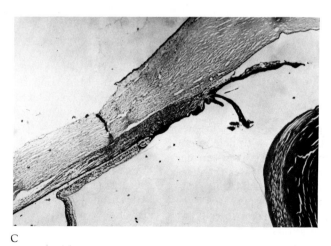

C

CHROMOSOME 10

DELETION OF THE SHORT ARM (DEL 10P)

At least 10 cases of deletion 10p have been reported in the literature. Most individuals have the break at 10p13–14. With the exception of one familial translocation, all of the cases have been sporadic terminal-appearing deletions [52].

Psychomotor retardation or developmental delay has been a consistent finding in all reported cases. Growth deficiency is variable and not always present. As with many of the other partial deletions and duplications, the most distinctive aspect of this syndrome is the recognizable facial phenotype. Most of the facial alterations in this syndrome are nonspecific, but taken together in affected children they produce a recognizable gestalt. The characteristics consist of a low nasal root, short palpebral fissures with ptosis, upturned nose, round cheeks, and a short neck. Central nervous system and cardiac malformations have been variable. The degree of palpebral fissure shortening in some of the cases has been marked and thus would make the 10p deletion syndrome a disorder in the differential diagnosis of blepharophimosis [52].

DUPLICATION IN THE LONG ARM (DUP 10Q)

The duplication of 10q syndrome is one of the most common entities reported since the advent of banding techniques. As in most reported partial trisomies, most cases have been associated with a parental rearrangement.

Marked mental and growth retardation are present within the first year of life in most of the individuals. The facial features are distinctive and consistent. They include microcephaly, broad forehead, midfacial flattening, arched and wide eyebrows, downslanting palpebral fissures, blepharophimosis, upturned nares, and a prominent upper lip. About 50 percent of individuals have a cleft palate, congenital heart disease, or both. Overlapping fingers, camptodactyly, and joint contractures are also noted in about 50 percent of cases [41].

Ocular abnormalities include blepharophimosis, ptosis, and microphthalmos. Although hypertelorism is reported in some cases, this is most probably an illusion created by the associated telecanthus and overall shortening of the palpebral fissures. This mislabeling of children as having hypertelorism when the appearance of widely spaced eyes is due to another feature has been documented in one review of this syndrome [205] and has already been emphasized in this chapter.

Duplication 10q trisomy is a severe entity, with approximately 50 percent of the patients dying before 1 year of age.

CHROMOSOME 11

DELETION OF THE SHORT ARM (DEL 11P); ASSOCIATION WITH ANIRIDIA AND WILMS' TUMOR

Aniridia is often associated with Wilms' tumor, growth and mental retardation, and genitourinary anomalies. This constellation of defects is usually accompanied by a deletion on the short arm of chromosome 11.

Aniridia is an uncommon, bilateral disorder that actually represents an iris hypoplasia rather than aplasia. A small rudimentary bud of iris is usually present [2]. Aniridia is panocular, affecting not only the iris, but the cornea, anterior chamber, lens, retina, and optic nerve as well [126].

Following Barrata's original description in 1818 [7], many reports of this disorder appeared in ophthalmic literature. The increased occurrence of Wilms' tumor in individuals who have aniridia was reported in 1953 by Brusa and Toricelli [16, 120]. In 1964 Miller and co-workers found an association of aniridia, Wilms' tumor, hemihypertrophy, and other congenital anomalies [120]. Francke and associates [58] and Smith and colleagues [162] separately described individuals with these findings who had interstitial deletion of the short arm of chromosome 11. Since that time about 20 cases of individuals with aniridia and deletion 11p have been reported [59, 63, 184]. Yunis and Ramsay were able to demonstrate with extended high-resolution banding that the deleted segment required to produce the syndrome is in band 11p13 [206].

Of the cases of del 11p reported since 1977, all have included aniridia, while Wilms' tumor has been a variable feature in the condition [63]. Six patients have had this embryonal tumor, while two have had a gonadoblastoma. In addition, as in most other chromosomal disorders, the alterations in facial morphogenesis have a similar appearance [79, 147]. Although the facial characteristics are nonspecific and not particularly distinctive, the features have been consistent. Genital abnormalities have been present in many of the males, including one child with male pseudohermaphroditism.

In 3 of the reported cases the interstitial deletion was due to a balanced reciprocal translocation in one of the parents. This resulted in a history of several affected family members in two of the pedigrees [206].

Although all of the reported cases have included aniridia, this may be a selected sample because of the increased knowledge of the chromosomal deletion in children with aniridia. Thus, it would not be surprising for some individuals to have the other features of the deletion syndrome without aniridia.

Apparently not all individuals who have the association of aniridia–Wilms' tumor have this extended pattern of malformation and the 11p13 deletion. At least two individuals of normal intelligence who have the combination of aniridia and Wilms's tumor with normal chromosomes on high-resolution study have been described [148]. These observations could be accounted for by the following explanations: (1) the deletion was present at such a microscopic level that present techniques were not able to visualize the missing segment. (2) The combination of aniridia and Wilms' tumor may have some developmental relationship in embryogenesis that involves more than one mechanism.

Because the diagnosis of the deletion 11p syndrome has genetic and prognostic implications for the family, high-resolution banded karyotyping should be considered for infants with aniridia. In addition, although the actual risk for a child with deletion 11p or with isolated aniridia to develop a Wilms' tumor is not known, yearly evaluations with renal ultrasound until age 5 are suggested.

Recently it was shown that the 11p13 band also carries the structural gene coding for catalase [63, 94]. Gene dosage studies performed in a few of the reported cases in the literature have shown deficiency of catalase activity in individuals with the 11p deletion. These investigations like those performed with esterase D in deletion 13q [166], demonstrate the potential usefulness of the study of individuals with chromosomal abnormalities in human gene mapping.

CHROMOSOME 12

DUPLICATION OF THE SHORT ARM (DUP 12P)

About 20 cases of dup 12p are known. In trisomy 12p there is marked hypertelorism and bilateral epicanthus. The palpebral fissures are horizontal. The most distinguishing features may be oxycephaly and a flat face. The nose is short, the upper lip is long, and the lower lip turns outward. In addition the infants are hypotonic and mentally retarded [156].

CHROMOSOME 13

DELETION OF THE LONG ARM (DEL 13Q); ASSOCIATION WITH RETINOBLASTOMA

Children with del 13q have severe mental retardation associated with microcephaly and arhinencephalia. Facial deformities are marked, with broad prominent nasal bridge, low-set and malformed ears, and micrognathia. These children also manifest abnormalities of the orbits and periorbital structures such as hypertelorism, antimongoloid palpebral fissures, epicanthus, and ptosis (Fig. 8-36). Short stature, congenital heart disease,

Fig. 8-36. *Deletion of the long arm of chromosome 13 (del 13q or 13q−). This 6-year-old girl has seven normal older siblings. The parents say esotropia has been present since birth. A white retinal tumor was present when her eyes were examined at age 6 years. The clinical diagnosis of retinoblastoma was confirmed by histopathologic examination of the eye.*

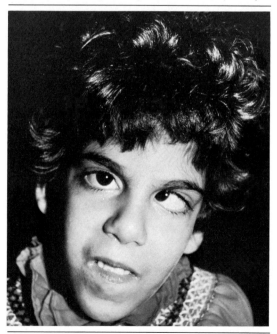

cryptorchidism, anal atresia, and absent thumbs are all associated defects [14, 72].

Of particular importance in the 13q− syndrome is the frequent association of retinoblastoma. Retinoblastoma, the most common malignant intraocular tumor in children, occurs with a high frequency among two groups of genetically predisposed individuals: those who inherit a major gene as an autosomal dominant trait and those born with a partial deletion of the long arm of chromosome 13. This latter group is particularly interesting in that a specific chromosomal anomaly consistently predisposes to a specific tumor [141].

Many reported cases have demonstrated that the chromosomal abnormalities associated with retinoblastoma are clustered on chromosome 13 [62, 100, 107, 116, 117, 123, 207]. In all cases in which G-banding or high-resolution banding were done, the aberrations were shown to be interstitial deletions involving the q14 banding region (see Fig. 8-30) [19, 51, 92, 122, 192].

François reported that several retinoblastoma patients with a small deletion manifested minimal somatic deviations and only mild mental retardation, and some manifested no congenital anomalies [60]. Therefore it is possible that very small deletions of chromosome 13 are present in more retinoblastoma patients, deletions that cannot be identified even with modern banding techniques because they are too small or are limited to a single locus [10].

Sparkes and coauthors correlated the gene for retinoblastoma with the gene for esterase D, suggesting that these two genes may be linked [166]. These investigators demonstrated that there is an esterase deficiency in the lymphocytes of retinoblastoma patients when there is a deletion on the long arm of chromosome 13, near or at the site of the retinoblastoma gene. In the case of retinoblastoma the esterase activity, which is normally 60 to 75 units, is reduced by 50 percent (to 30–35 units). In the case of trisomy 13, the amount is increased 150 percent. When there is a deletion above or below 13q14, but not involving 13q14, the amount is normal.

Howard reviewed the association of retinoblastoma with 13q deletions [87]. Five percent of individuals in a large series of karyotyped cases of retinoblastoma have a del 13q. At this point, because of the genetic implications and because the phenotypic alterations can be subtle in infancy, chromosomal studies are indicated in young children with retinoblastoma. However, Murphee and colleagues suggested that assaying esterase D levels as a screening test in infants with retinoblastoma may be more cost-effective [125]. If enzyme activity is 50 percent of normal, then the more expensive karyotype could be performed.

DUPLICATION OF THE LONG ARM (DUP 13Q)

The syndromes associated with partial trisomy of the different segments of the long arm of chromosome 13 have been reviewed by Niebuhr [129] and others [159]. Most authors have divided the conditions into (1) those caused by partial trisomy of the proximal one-third to one-half of the long arm, and (2) those caused by partial trisomy of the distal one-third to two-thirds of the long arm. Many of the physical features in these two groups of partial trisomies are overlapping and common to both conditions [129]. In comparing the patterns of abnormalities in these individuals as well as in individuals with complete trisomy 13, one can make a few generalizations about the correlation of the distinctive phenotypic findings with various segments of the long arm of chromosome 13. Since polydactyly, a common finding in full trisomy 13, is seen only in patients who have partial trisomy of the distal long arm of chromosome 13 (and not of the proximal half), duplication of the distal one-third of the long arm below band 31 must be present for this finding to occur. Using the same reasoning and comparing patients who have partial trisomies of different parts of the long arm of chromosome 13 leads to the conclusion that the increased hemoglobin F levels seen in patients with full trisomy is due to duplication of a segment around the 14 band.

Features such as ocular malformations, hemangiomas, and cleft lip cannot be located with any certainty, perhaps because the morphologic alterations involved in these abnormalities are less specific. The cyclopia malformation has not been seen in any of the cases of partial trisomy and may require trisomy 13 of the entire arm for its development. The ocular malformations associated with partial duplication of the chromosome 13 have been reviewed by Ginsberg and associates [64, 68]. Although ocular defects are common in the partial duplication situations, no straightforward phenotypic mapping of the various eye findings can be accomplished. Fig. 8-30 is a diagram depicting the phenotypic findings in both partial

13 duplication and deletion that have been assigned with reasonable certainty.

CHROMOSOME 15

DELETION OF THE LONG ARM (DEL 15Q); ASSOCIATION WITH THE PRADER-WILLI SYNDROME

The Prader-Willi syndrome consists of mental retardation, short stature, hypotonia, obesity, hypogonadism, characteristic facies, and small hands and feet [102]. Until recently no definite clue to the cause of this disorder existed, and most cases were thought to be sporadic. In 1981, using high-resolution banding, Ledbetter and colleagues reported a subtle deletion of the proximal long arm of chromosome 15 involving bands q11–13 in 4 patients with the Prader-Willi syndrome [101]. These authors also pointed out that 8 other cases of the syndrome in the literature exhibited structural abnormalities of chromosome 15 [102].

Further studies of patients with Prader-Willi syndrome have revealed that about one-half of all cases have chromosome abnormalities involving chromosome 15 detectable by high-resolution banding [102, 115]. In addition to the apparent del 15q, the other chromosome 15 abnormalities include 15:15 robertsonian translocations, reciprocal translocations involving chromosome 15 and other autosomes, and the presence of a small metacentric marker chromosome. The relationship of these various chromosome 15 aberrations to the Prader-Willi syndrome is not clear-cut. First, only one-half of patients with the syndrome have a chromosomal finding, even with high-resolution banding. Second, some of the chromosomal findings have been apparently balanced. Third, at least 3 of the cases with the metacentric marker have tetrasomy (four copies) of part of chromosome 15 (not deficiency, but excess). Although it is unlikely that these diverse chromosome 15 abnormalities are coincidental, the exact relationship of the findings to the causation of the syndrome is complex.

The ocular manifestations of the Prader-Willi syndrome are nonspecific: upslanted palpebral fissures, strabismus, and epicanthal folds.

CHROMOSOME 18

DELETION OF THE SHORT ARM (DEL 18P)

After cri du chat syndrome, the 18p− syndrome is probably the second most frequent autosomal deletion syndrome [156]. Since the first description of this condition, more than 70 cases have been reported in the literature [156]. In the majority of observations the dysmorphic features are subtle and nonspecific. Affected individuals have a mild to moderate degree of mental retardation and short stature. The facial phenotype consists of a low nasal root, ptosis, ear variations, round cheeks, and downturned corners of the mouth. Webbing of the neck is reported in some individuals, and the combination of this finding with ptosis makes the phenotype similar to Turner's and Noonan's syndromes. Besides ptosis, the ocular findings may include epicanthus, strabismus, and microphthalmos. Eccentric pupils, posterior keratoconus, corneal opacities, and cataracts have been reported in a few instances [201]. It is interesting that cyclopia, cebocephaly, and some of the defects of the holoprosencephaly developmental field complex have been seen in about 16 percent of cases. Apart from the cases that are associated with these more severe central nervous system malformations, life expectancy of individuals with 18p deletion is not diminished. This chromosomal condition is probably the second most common disorder associated with the holoprosencephaly developmental field complex (after trisomy 13).

In more than two-thirds of the patients a de novo deletion is present. The remainder of the cases have the deletion as part of a more complex chromosome abnormality or associated with malsegregation of a parental translocation [41].

DELETION OF THE LONG ARM (DEL 18Q): DE GROUCHY'S SYNDROME

The pattern of malformation associated with deletion 18q is much more distinctive and recognizable than that of the short arm deletion of chromosome 18. This condition, like 18p deletion, was also recognized in the 1960s before banding [37–40]. The facial characteristics are distinctive and consist of deep-set eyes, midfacial hypoplasia producing a secondarily prominent jaw, downturned corners of the mouth, and narrowed ear canals [128]. Microcephaly, mental retardation, and short stature are present as in most deletion syndromes. Other distinguishing features include prominent dimples over joints and long, thin, tapered fingers. Ocular malformations are common and consist of microcornea, nystagmus, congenital glaucoma, optic atrophy, and coloboma. While most cases are the result of a de novo deletion, a small number of individuals have the abnormality from a parental pericentric inversion or translocation [194].

RING CHROMOSOME (R18)

Ring chromosome 18 phenotypically resembles the 18q syndrome. Some individuals display webbing of the neck, which suggests effects of a combination of the short arm deletion and the long arm deletion. Ocular malformations are similar to those seen in deletion 18q [41].

CHROMOSOME 21

DELETION OF THE LONG ARM (DEL 21Q)

Partial monosomy of the long arm of chromosome 21 has been reported in at least 8 individuals [145]. This deletion results in mental and physical retardation, hypertonia, and microcephaly. The individuals also have marked blepharochalasis with downslanting of the palpebral fissures, a prominent nasal bridge, large ears with wide external auditory canals, micrognathia, hypospadias, and skeletal abnormalities. Cataracts were found in one case [96].

CHROMOSOME 22

CAT-EYE SYNDROME (SCHMIDT-FRACCARO SYNDROME)

The cat-eye syndrome was first recognized by Schachenmann and co-workers in 1965 [153]. The principal features of this syndrome are coloboma of the uvea and anal atresia, so affected individuals are usually recognized immediately after birth. Other characteristics include preauricular skin tags and fistulas, urinary tract abnormalities and umbilical hernias. Cardiac anomalies of many types

have also been found, including tetralogy of Fallot, anomalous pulmonary venous drainage, and single ventricles.

Ocular anomalies make up a prominent and diagnostically important part of this syndrome. The uveal colobomas with the vertically oriented iris defect give rise to the name *cat-eye syndrome* (Fig. 8-37). Unilateral or bilateral microphthalmos, hypertelorism, and antimongoloid palpebral fissures are common. Cataracts and strabismus are occasionally reported. Visual acuity is highly

Fig. 8-38. *Infant with triploidy syndrome. Note low-set ears, small nose, downturned corners of mouth, ambiguous external genitalia, and rocker-bottom feet. (Courtesy of Joseph Ginsberg, M.D.) [69].*

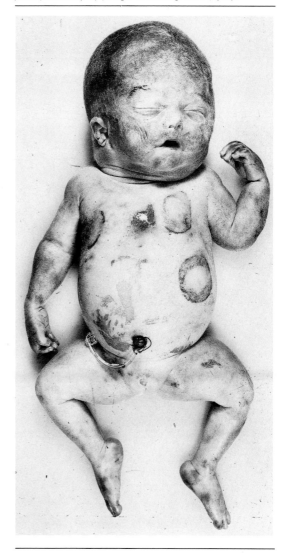

Fig. 8-37. *Bilateral colobomas seen in the cat-eye syndrome.*

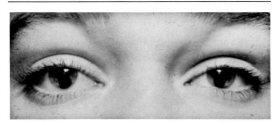

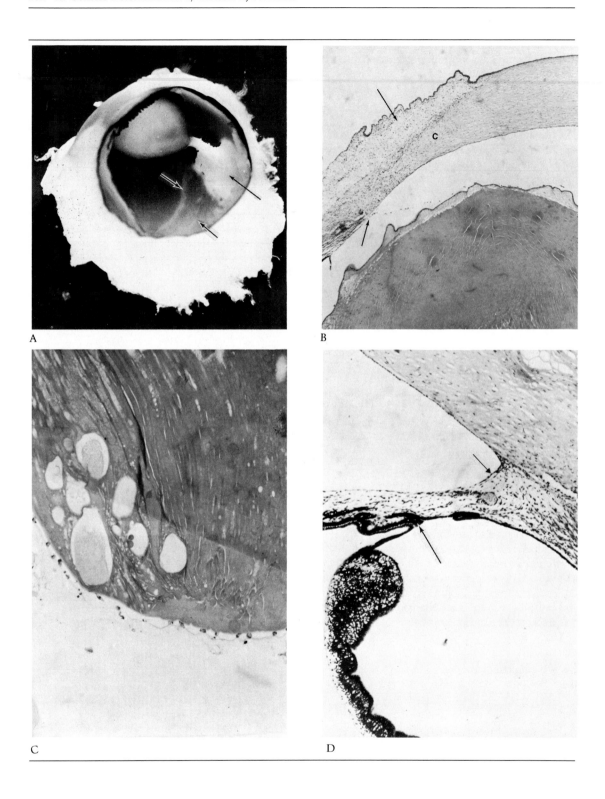

A

B

C

D

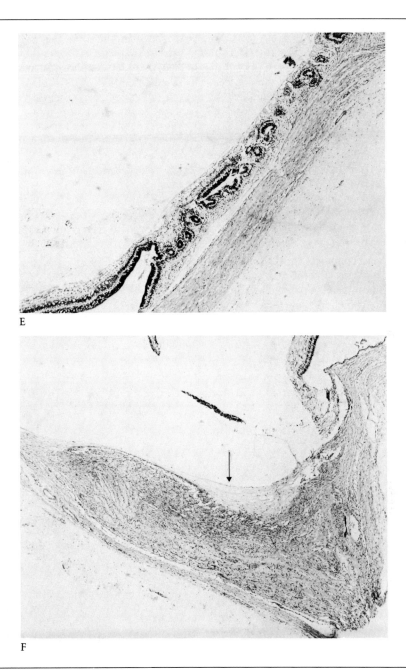

E

F

Figure 8-39. *Tripolidy. A. Gross photograph of inferior coloboma (*long arrow*), which involves the entire uvea. Retina is thickened and folded (*short arrows*) adjacent to the coloboma. (×6.5.) B. Conjunctiva (*long arrow*) is thickened and overgrown in relation to peripheral corneal thickening (C). Note coloboma of iris and ciliary body (*short arrow*). (H&E, ×45.) C. Lens exhibits advanced liquefaction with cavitation near the equator inferiorly. (H&E, ×150.) D. Iris and ciliary body insert directly into hypoplastic* trabecular meshwork. *Retina is attached to iris adjacent to heterotropic ciliary processes (*long arrow*). Corneal endothelium continues over trabecular meshwork (*short arrow*). (H&E, ×120.) E. Retina exhibits dysplastic duplication and rosettes involving nuclear layers adjacent to optic disc. (H&E, ×60.) F. A pit in the optic disc is most marked inferiorly (*arrow*). Notice absence of retina and choroid in area to the left of the arrow. (H&E, ×65.) (Courtesy of Joseph Ginsberg, M.D.[69].)*

variable, depending on the extent of the ocular abnormalities.

The karyotypic finding in this disorder is a complex one and consists of a small, extra G-like chromosome. The origin of this chromosome is controversial and has recently been discussed by Schinzel and associates [154, 155] and Guanti [73]. The most convincing evidence suggests that the marker chromosome derives from chromosome 22 and consists of an isochromosome of the short arms and proximal portion of the long arm of this acrocentric chromosome, making the individual tetrasomic for part of chromosome 22.

RING CHROMOSOME (R22)

Ring 22 has been detected in approximately 20 patients [156]. The ring 22 syndrome has a distinguishing eye finding that has been labeled doe's eyes, in which the palpebral fissures are almond shaped. The eyebrows are set low, and epicanthus is present at birth, regressing in most individuals as the child grows. Ptosis occurs in at least one-third of the cases. The nasal tip is globular, and the upper lip is thin. Mental retardation is severe. Systemic malformations are variable in frequency.

X CHROMOSOME

45,XO: TURNER'S SYNDROME

A syndrome was described by Turner in 1938, before it was known to be associated with a single sex chromosome [178]. This syndrome is characterized by females whose cells exhibit a male sex chromatin pattern. The karyotype reveals 44 autosomes but only one X chromosome. This syndrome represents the only known aneuploid condition in which an entire chromosome may be absent that is still compatible with life. The incidence is approximately 2 to 3 in 10,000 births [41].

The genetic result is believed to be due to the fertilization of a normal egg (carrying a normal X from the mother) by an abnormal sperm that is devoid of either the paternal X or Y chromosome. The offspring female thus produced is hemizygous, as is a normal male, and she will exhibit X-linked recessive traits at a greater frequency than seen in normal (XX) females [109].

Patients have a normal life span in the absence of complicating renal or cardiac disease. Affected individuals are characteristically short with tri-

angular facies, webbed necks, and a low posterior hairline. Anomalies of the maxilla, mandible, and ears are frequent. Multiple skeletal anomalies, especially of the extremities, are commonly found. Visceral anomalies most often seen include congenital heart disease (especially coarctation of the aorta) and renal anomalies (hydronephrosis, horseshoe kidney, and renal aplasia) [90]. The gonads are almost always rudimentary streaks with little evidence of function [9, 54, 57]. Secondary sex characteristics remain infantile in appearance.

Multiple ophthalmic findings have been described in association with Turner's syndrome: proptosis [18], hypertelorism, epicanthus, antimongoloid palpebral fissures, melanosis bulbi, microphthalmos, blue sclera, corneal opacities or scarring, microcornea, iris colobomas, cataracts, retinitis pigmentosa, strabismus, oculomotor nerve palsy, blepharoptosis, coloboma, tubular vision, color blindness, marked myopia or hypermetropia, Coats' disease [21], nystagmus, and congenital glaucoma. Thomas and co-workers have stated that there is no ophthalmic symptom characteristic of Turner's syndrome, but rather that this syndrome features various congenital anomalies at an increased rate [174].

TRIPLOIDY

Triploidy is one of the most commonly occurring abnormalities of fecundation in man, as about 20 percent of all spontaneous abortions have this karyotype [42]. Some triploid pregnancies do result in live births, as about 40 cases have now been reported. The karyotypes are either 69,XXX, 69,XXY, or 69,XYY. Mosaicism for a triploidy line has been described in older children [156].

In the newborn the pattern of malformation consists of growth deficiency, cranial contour abnormalities, oral-facial clefts, ear malformations, syndactyly of hands and feet, thumb hypoplasia, and genital defects (Fig. 8-38). Central nervous system malformations, congenital heart defects, and other internal abnormalities are common and severe [138]. Most infants die at birth or within a few days [156].

Ocular anomalies including retinal dysplasia, microphthalmos, anophthalmia, coloboma, lens subluxation, cataracts, and corneal clouding are found frequently. Ginsberg and colleagues detailed the various manifestations and suggested that the combination of microphthalmos, dislocated spherical lens, typical coloboma, and retinal dysplasia is highly indicative of triploidy (Fig. 8-39) [69].

REFERENCES

1. Alfi, O. S., et al. 46,del(9)(22): A new deletion syndrome. *Birth Defects* 108:27, 1974.
2. Apple, D. J., and Rabb, M. F. *Ocular Pathology: Clinical Applications and Self-Assessment* (3rd ed.) St. Louis: Mosby, 1985.
3. Apple, D. J., Holden, J. D., and Stallworth, B. Ocular pathology of Patau's syndrome with an unbalanced D/D translocation. *Am. J. Ophthalmol.* 70:383, 1970.
4. Arakaki, D. T., and Sparkes, R. S. Micro-technique for culturing leukocytes from whole blood. *Cytogenetics* 2:57, 1963.
5. Barash, B. A., Freedman, L., and Opitz, J. M. Anatomic studies in the 18-trisomy syndrome. *Birth Defects* 6(4):3, 1970.
6. Barr, M. L., and Bertram, E. G. A morphological distinction between neurones of the male and female, and the behavior of the nucleolar satellite during acclerated nucleoprotein synthesis. *Nature* 163:676, 1949.
7. Barrata, G. Observazioni pratiche sulle principal malattie degli orchi, Milano 1818 Tomo 2, 349, as cited by C. Jungke, Veber den angeborren mangel der Iris. *J. Chir. Augen-Heilkunde (Berlin)* 2:677, 1821.
8. Bartholin, T. *Historiarum Anatomicarum Rariorum.* Centuria III. Observatio 47. Amsterdam, 1657.
9. Becker, K. L., Paris, J., and Albert, A. Ovarian dysgenesis due to deletion of X chromosome. *Mayo Clin. Proc.* 38:389, 1963.
10. Benedict, W. F., et al. Patient with 13 chromosome deletion: Evidence that the retinoblastoma gene is a recessive cancer gene. *Science* 219:973, 1983.
11. Bergsma, D. S. Report of Standing Committee on Human Cytogenetic Nomenclature. *Birth Defects* 14:313, 1978.
12. Bergsma, D. S. *Birth Defects Atlas and Compendium* (2nd ed.). Baltimore: Williams & Wilkins, 1979.
13. Boger, W. P., III, Petersen, R. A., and Robb, R. M. Keratoconus and acute hydrops in mentally retarded patients with congenital rubella syndrome. *Am. J. Ophthalmol.* 91:231, 1981.
14. Bonioli, E., et al. Karyotype-phenotype correlation in partial trisomy 13. *Am. J. Dis. Child.* 135:1115, 1981.
15. Breg, W. R. Cri du Chat Syndrome. In L. I. Gardner (Ed.), *Endocrine and Genetic Diseases of Childhood.* Philadelphia: Saunders, 1969. P. 632.
16. Brusa, P., and Toricelli, C. Nefroblastoma de Wilms' ed affezioni renali congenite nella casistica dell' I.P.P.A.I. de Milano *Minerv Paediatr.* 5:453, 1953.
17. Brushfield, T. Mongolism. *Br. J. Child. Dis.* 21:241, 1924.
18. Buckley, C. A., and Cheng, H. Intraocular mela-

noma, diabetes, and Turner's syndrome: Presentation with proptosis. *Br. J. Ophthalmol.* 65:460, 1981.
19. Bundey, S. Recent views on genetic factors in retinoblastoma. *J. Med. Genet.* 17:386, 1980.
20. Calderone, J. P., et al. Intraocular pathology of trisomy 18 (Edward's syndrome): Report of a case and review of the literature. *Br. J. Ophthalmol.* 67:162, 1983.
21. Cameron, J. D., Yanoff, M., and Frayer, W C. Coats' disease and Turner's syndrome. *Am. J. Ophthalmol.* 78:852, 1974.
22. Carey, J. C., et al. Heterogeneity of the Rieger eye malformation. *Clin. Res.* 28:116A, 1980.
23. Carnevale, A., et al. A clinical syndrome associated with dup (5p). *Am. J. Med. Genet.* 13:277, 1982.
24. Caspersson, T., et al. Identification of human chromosomes by DNA-binding fluorescent agents. *Chromosoma* 30:215, 1970.
25. Chase, T. R., et al. Duplication 6q24–6qter in an infant born from a balanced paternal translocation. *Am. J. Med. Genet.* 14:347, 1983.
26. Chicago Conference: Standardization in human cytogenetics. *Birth Defects* 2(2), 1966.
27. Chicago Conference: Standardization in human cytogenetics. *Birth Defects* 2(2):12, 1966.
28. Chicago Conference: Standardization in human cytogenetics. *Birth Defects* 2(2):18, 1966.
29. Chiyo, H., et al. A 6p trisomy detected in a family with a "giant satellite." *Humangenetik* 30:63, 1975.
30. Coats, G. A case of microphthalmos: With remarks. *Ophthalmoscope* 8:702, 1910.
31. Cogan, D. G., and Kuwabara, T. Ocular pathology of the 13–15 trisomy syndrome. *Arch. Ophthalmol.* 72:246, 1964.
32. Conen, P. E., and Erkman, B. Frequency and occurrence of chromosomal syndromes: I. D-trisomy. *Am. J. Hum. Genet.* 18:374, 1966.
33. Coyle, J. T. Keratoconus and eye rubbing. *Am. J. Ophthalmol.* 97:527, 1984.
34. Cullen, J. F., and Butler, H. G. Mongolism (Down's syndrome) and keratoconus. *Br. J. Ophthalmol.* 47:321, 1963.
35. Cullen, J. F. Blindness in mongolism (Down's syndrome). *Br. J. Ophthalmol.* 47:331, 1963.
36. Daniel, A. Structural differences in pericentric inversions: Applications to a model of risk of recombinants. *Hum. Genet.* 56:321, 1981.
37. de Grouchy, J., et al. Dysmorphia complexe avec des oligophrenia: Deletion des bras courts d'un chromosome 17–18. *C. R. Séances Acad. Sci.* 256:1028, 1963.
38. de Grouchy, J., et al. Chromosome 17–18 en anneau et malformations congenitales chez un fille. *Ann. Genet. (Paris)* 27:189, 1963.
39. de Grouchy, J., et al. Deletion partielle des bras longs du chromosome 18. *Pathol. Biol. (Paris)* 12:579, 1964.
40. de Grouchy, J. Chromosome 18: A topologic approach. *J. Pediatr.* 66:414, 1965.
41. de Grouchy, J., and Turleau, C. *Clinical Atlas of*

Human Chromosomes (2nd ed.). New York: Wiley, 1984.

42. Delhanty, J. D. A., Ellis, J. R., and Rowley, P. T. Triploid cells in a human embryo. *Lancet* 1:1286, 1961.

43. DeMyer, W. Median facial malformations and their implications for brain malformations. *Birth Defects* 11(7):155, 1975.

44. Dhareshwar, S. S., Gokarn, V. V., and Ambari, L. M. Cataracts in Down syndrome (letter). *Indian Pediatr.* 19:642, 1982.

45. Dötsch, A. Anatomische Untersuchung eines Falles von Mikrophthalmus congenitus bilateralis. *Albrecht von Graefes Arch. Klin. Exp. Ophthalmol.* 48:49, 1899.

46. Donaldson, D. D. The significance of spotting of the iris in mongoloids: Brushfield's spot. *Arch. Ophthalmol.* 65:26, 1961.

47. Down, J. L. H. Observations on ethnic classifications of idiots. *Clin. Lect. Rep. Lond. Hosp.* 3:259, 1866.

48. Duke-Elder, S. Anophthalmos and Extreme Microphthalmos. In S. Duke-Elder (Ed.), *System of Ophthalmology.* St. Louis: Mosby, 1963, Vol. 3, p. 416.

49. Edwards, J. H., et al. A new trisomic syndrome. *Lancet* 1:787, 1960.

50. Eissler, R., and Longenecker, L. P. The common eye findings in mongolism. *Am. J. Ophthalmol.* 54:398, 1962.

51. Ejima, Y., et al. Possible inactivation of part of chromosome 13 due to 13qXp translocation associated with retinoblastoma. *Clin. Genet.* 21:357, 1982.

52. Elstner, C. L., et al. Further delineation of the 10p deletion syndrome. *Pediatrics* 73:670, 1984.

53. Farkas, L. G. *Anthropometry of the Hand and Face.* New York: Elsevier, 1981.

54. Ferguson-Smith, M., et al. Clinical and cytogenetical studies in female gonadal dysgenesis and their bearing on the cause of Turner's syndrome. *Cytogenetics* 3:355, 1964.

55. Flemming, W. Beitraege zur Kenntniss der Zelle und ihrer Lebenserscheinungen. III. *Arch. Mikroskop. Anat.* 20:1, 1882.

56. Flemming, W. *Zellsubstanz, Kern and Zelltheilung.* Leipzig: Vogel, 1882.

57. Ford, C. E., Jones, K. W., and Polani, P. E. A sex-chromosome anomaly in a case of gonadal dysgenesis (Turner's syndrome). *Lancet* 1:711, 1959.

58. Francke, U., et al. Interstitial del (11p) as a cause of the aniridia–Wilms' tumor association: Band localization and a heritable basis. *Am. J. Hum. Genet.* 30:81A, 1978.

59. Francke, U., Holmes, L. B., and Riccardi, V. M. Aniridia—Wilms' tumor association: Evidence for specific deletion of 11p13. *Cytogenet. Cell Genet.* 24:185, 1979.

60. François, J. The significance of genetic research in ophthalmology. *Birth Defects* 18(6):3, 1982.

61. Fulton, A. B., et al. Retinal anomalies in trisomy 18.

Abrecht Von Graefes Arch. Klin. Exp. Ophthalmol. 213:195, 1980.

62. Gallie, B. L., and Phillips, R. A. Multiple manifestations of the retinoblastoma gene. *Birth Defects* 18(6):689, 1982.

63. Gilgenkrantz, S., et al. Association of del(11)(p 15.1p12), aniridia, catalase deficiency, and cardiomyopathy. *Am. J. Med. Genet.* 13:39, 1982.

64. Ginsberg, J., and Perrin, E. V. D. Ocular manifestations of 13–14 trisomy: Report of a case with clinical, cytogenic, and pathologic findings. *Arch. Ophthalmol.* 74:487, 1965.

65. Ginsberg, J., Perrin, E. V., and Sueoka, W. T. Ocular manifestations of trisomy 18. *Am. J. Ophthalmol.* 66:59, 1968.

66. Ginsberg, J., et al. Ocular pathology of trisomy 18. *Ann. Ophthalmol.* 3:273, 1971.

67. Ginsberg, J., et al. Further observations of ocular pathology in Down's syndrome. *J. Pediatr. Ophthalmol. Strabismus* 17:166, 1980.

68. Ginsberg, J., et al. Ocular abnormality associated with partial duplication of chromosome 13. *Ann. Ophthalmol* 13:189, 1981.

69. Ginsberg, J., Ballard, E. T., and Soukup, S. Pathologic features of the eye in triploidy. *J. Pediatr. Ophthalmol. Strabismus* 18:48, 1981.

70. Ginsberg, J., Soukup, S., and Ballard, E. T. Pathologic features of eye in trisomy 9. *J. Pediatr. Ophthalmol. Strabismus* 19:37, 1982.

71. Goodman, R. M., and Gorlin, R. J. *Atlas of the Face in Genetic Disorders* (2nd ed.). St. Louis: Mosby, 1979.

72. Grace, E., et al. The 13 q – deletion syndrome. *J. Med. Genet.* 8:351, 1971.

73. Guanti, G. The aetiology of the cat eye syndrome reconsidered. *J. Med. Genet.* 18:108, 1981.

74. Hamerton, J. L., et al. Chromosome studies in a neonatal population. *Can. Med. Assoc. J.* 106:776, 1972.

75. Hamerton, J. L., Canning, N., and Ray, M. Cytogenetic survey of 14,609 newborn infants: I. Incidence of chromosomal abnormalities. *Clin. Genet.* 8:223, 1975.

76. Harris, D. J., et al. Parental trisomy 21 mosaicism. *Am. J. Hum. Genet.* 34:125, 1982.

77. Heimann, K. Histopathologische Augenveranderungen beim D_1-(13–15) Trisomie-Syndrom. *Buch. Augenarzt.* 50:66, 1968.

78. Higginbottom, M. A second patient with partial deletion of the short arm of chromosome 3. *J. Med. Genet.* 19:71, 1981.

79. Hittner, H. M., Riccardi, V. M., and Francke, U. Aniridia caused by a heritable chromosome 11 deletion. *Ophthalmology (Rochester)* 86:1173, 1979.

80. Holmes, L. B. Genetic counseling for the older pregnant woman: New data and questions. *N. Engl. J. Med.* 298:1419, 1978.

81. Hook, E. B., et al. Trisomy 18 in a 15-year-old female. *Lancet* 2:910, 1965.

82. Hook, E. B., et al. Paternal age and Down syndrome in British Columbia. *Am. J. Hum. Genet.* 33:123, 1981.

83. Hook, E. B. Epidemiology in Down Syndrome. In S. M. Pueschel and J. E. Rynders (Eds.), *Down Syndrome: Advances in Biomedicine and the Behavioral Sciences.* The Ware Press, 1982.

84. Howard, R. O. Ocular abnormalities in the cri du chat syndrome. *Am. J. Ophthalmol.* 73:949, 1972.

85. Howard, R. O. Chromosomal abnormalities associated with cyclopia and synophthalmia. *Trans. Am. Ophthalmol. Soc.* 75:505, 1977.

86. Howard, R. O. Classification of chromosomal eye syndromes. *Int. Ophthalmol.* 4(1–2):77, 1981.

87. Howard, R. O. Chromosome errors in retinoblastoma. *Birth Defects* 18(6):703, 1982.

88. Hunter, W. S., and Zimmerman, L. E. Unilateral retinal dysplasia. *Arch. Ophthalmol.* 74:23, 1965.

89. Jacobs, P. A., et al. Evidence for the existence of a human "super female." *Lancet* 2:423, 1959.

90. Jacobs, P. A., et al. Abnormalities involving the X chromosome in women. *Lancet* 1:1213, 1960.

91. Jaeger, E. A. Ocular findings in Down's syndrome. *Trans. Am. Ophthalmol. Soc.* 78:808, 1980.

92. Johnson, M. P., et al. Retinoblastoma and its association with a deletion in chromosome #13: A survey using high-resolution chromosome techniques. *Cancer Genet. Cytogenet.* 6:29, 1982.

93. Juberg, R. C., and Mowrey, P. N. Origin of nondisjunction in trisomy 21 syndrome. *Am. J. Med. Genet.* 16:111, 1983.

94. Junien, C., et al. Regional assignment of catalase (CAT) gene to band 11p13: Association with the aniridia–Wilms' tumor–gonadoblastoma (WAGR) complex. *Ann. Genet. (Paris)* 23:165, 1980.

95. Katayana, K. P., et al. Clinical delineation of trisomy 9 syndrome. *Obstet. Gynecol.* 56:665, 1980.

96. Keith, C. G. *Genetics and Ophthalmology.* Edinburgh: Churchill Livingstone, 1978.

97. Khodr, G. S., et al. Duplication (5p13–pter): Prenatal diagnosis and review of the literature. *Am. J. Med. Genet.* 12:43, 1982.

98. Kolbert, G. S., and Seelenfreund, M. Sclerocornea, anterior cleavage syndrome, and trisomy 18. *Ann. Ophthalmol.* 2:26, 1970.

99. Krause, A. C. Congenital encephalo-ophthalmic dysplasia. *Arch. Ophthalmol.* 36:387, 1946.

100. Kusnetsova, L. E., et al. Similar chromosomal abnormalities in several retinoblastomas. *Hum. Genet.* 61:201, 1982.

101. Ledbetter, D. H., et al. Deletions of chromosome 15 as a cause of the Prader-Willi syndrome. *N. Engl. J. Med.* 304:325, 1981.

102. Ledbetter, D. H., et al. Chromosome 15 abnormalities and the Prader-Willi syndrome: A follow-up report of 40 cases. *Am. J. Hum. Genet.* 34:278, 1982.

103. Lejeune, J., Turpin, R., and Gautier, M. Le mongolisme: Premier exemple d'aberration autosomique humaine. *Ann. Genet. (Paris)* 1:41, 1959.

104. Lejeune, J., Gautier, M., and Turpin, R. Étude des chromosomes somatiques de neufs enfants mongoliens. *C. R. Séances Acad. Sci.* 248:1721, 1959.

105. Lejeune, J., et al. Trois cas de délétion partielle du bras court d'un chromosome 5. *C. R. Séances Acad. Sci.* 257:3098, 1963.

106. Lejeune, J., et al. Ségrégation familiale d'une translocation 5–13 déterminant une monsomie et une trisomie partielle due bras court du chromosome 5: Maladie due "cri du chat" et sa "réciproque." *C. R. Séances Acad. Sci.* 258:5767, 1964.

107. Lele, K. P., Penrose, L. S., and Stallard, H. B. Chromosome deletion in a case of retinoblastoma. *Ann. Hum. Genet.* 27:171, 1963.

108. Lewandoski, R. C., and Yunis, J. J. New chromosome syndromes. *Am. J. Dis. Child.* 129:515, 1975.

109. Lewandoski, R. C., Jr., and Yunis, J. J. Phenotypic Mapping in Man. In J. J. Yunis (Ed.), *New Chromosomal Syndromes.* New York: Academic, 1977.

110. Ligutić, I., et al. Interstitial deletion 4q and Rieger syndrome. *Clin. Genet.* 20:323, 1981.

111. Lowe, R. The eyes in mongolism. *Br. J. Ophthalmol.* 33:131, 1949.

112. Lubs, H. A., and Ruddle, F. H. Chromosomal abnormalities in the human population: Estimation of rates based on New Haven newborn study. *Science* 169:495, 1970.

113. Lycosthenes. *Prodigiorum al Ostentorum Chronicon.* Basal, 1557.

114. Martin, N. J., and Steinberg, B. G. The dup(3)(p25–pter) syndrome: A case with holoprosencephaly. *Am. J. Med. Genet.* 14:767, 1983.

115. Mattei, J. F., Mattei, M. G., and Giraud, F. Prader-Willi and chromosome 15. *Hum. Genet.* 64:356, 1983.

116. Mehes, K., and Bajnoczky, K. Unusually early dividing chromosomes 13–15 in a child with retinoblastoma and 13q deletion. *Hum. Genet.* 61:78, 1982.

117. Michalová, K., Kloucek, F., and Musilová, J. Deletion of 13q in two patients with retinoblastoma, one probably due to 13q– mosaicism in the mother. *Hum. Genet.* 61:264, 1982.

118. Miller, O. J., et al. Partial deletion of the short arm of chromosome number 4 (4q–): Clinical studies on five unrelated patients. *J. Pediatr.* 77:792, 1970.

119. Miller, O. J. Chromosomal Basis of Inheritance. In A. E. H. Emery and D. L. Rimoin (Eds.), *Principles and Practice of Medical Genetics.* New York: Churchill Livingstone, 1983.

120. Miller, R. W., Fraumeni, J. F., and Mannin, M. D. Association of Wilms' tumor with aniridia, hemihypertrophy and other congenital anomalies. *N. Engl. J. Med.* 270:922, 1964.

121. Mitchell, J. A., et al. Deletions of different segments of long arm of chromosome 4. *Am. J. Med. Genet.* 8:73, 1981.

122. Motegi, T. High rate of detection of 13q14 deletion mosaicism among retinoblastoma patients (using more extensive methods). *Hum. Genet.* 61:95, 1982.

123. Motegi, T., et al. Retinoblastoma in a boy with a de novo mutation of a 13/18 translocation: The assumption that the retinoblastoma locus is at 13q141, particularly at the distal portion of it. *Hum. Genet.* 60:193, 1982.

124. Mottet, N. K., and Jensen, H. The anomalous embryonic development associated with trisomy 13–15. *Am. J. Clin. Pathol.* 43:334, 1965.

125. Murphree, A. L., et al. Recent developments in the genetics and treatment of retinoblastoma. *Birth Defects* 18(6):681, 1982.

126. Nelson, L. B., et al. Aniridia: A review. *Surv. Ophthalmol.* 28:621, 1984.

127. Neu, R. L., Grant, J. F., and Gardner, L. I. A case of cyclopia with D trisomy. *Am. J. Obstet. Gynecol.* 127:212, 1977.

128. Neu, R. L., and Takashi, K. Partial Deletion of Long Arm of Chromosome 18 and Deletion of Short Arms of Chromosome 18. In L. I. Gardner (Ed.), *Endocrine and Genetic Diseases of Childhood.* Philadelphia: Saunders, 1969. P. 655.

129. Niebuhr, E. Partial Trisomies and Deletions of Chromosome 13. In J. J. Yunis (Ed.), *New Chromosomal Syndromes.* New York: Academic, 1977.

130. Opitz, J. M. Study of the malformed fetus and infant. *Pediatr. Rev.* 3:57, 1981.

131. Opitz, J. M. What the pediatrician should know about developmental anomalies. *Pediatr. Rev.* 3:267, 1982.

132. Painter, T. S. Studies in mammalian spermatogenesis: II. The spermatogenesis of man. *J. Exp. Zool.* 37:291, 1923.

133. Pap, Z., et al. Hochgradiger Mikrophthalmus beim Patau-Syndrom. *Klin. Monatsbl. Augenheilkd.* 173:342, 1978.

134. Paris Conference, 1971. *Birth Defects* 3(7), 1972.

135. Patau, K. The identification of individual chromosomes, especially in man. *Am. J. Hum. Genet.* 12:250, 1960.

136. Patau, K., et al. Multiple congenital anomaly caused by an extra autosome. *Lancet* 1:790, 1960.

137. Pauli, R. M., Pagon, R. A., and Hall, J. G. Trisomy 18 in sibs and maternal chromosome 9 variant. *Birth Defects* 14(6C):297, 1978.

138. Penrose, L. S., and Delhanty, J. D. A. Triploid cell cultures from a macerated foetus. *Lancet* 1:1261, 1961.

139. Pfeiffer, R. A. Trisomy 8. In J. J. Yunis (Ed.), *New Chromosomal Syndromes.* New York: Academic, 1977.

140. Pierce, D., and Eustace, P. Acute keratoconus in mongols. *Br. J. Ophthalmol.* 55:50, 1971.

141. Pruett, R. C., and Atkins, L. Chromosome studies in patients with retinoblastoma. *Arch. Ophthalmol.* 82:177, 1969.

142. Rados, A. Conical cornea and mongolism. *Arch. Ophthalmol.* 40:454, 1948.

143. Reese, A. B., and Blodi, F. C. Retinal dysplasia. *Am. J. Ophthalmol.* 33:23, 1950.

144. Reese, A. B., and Straatsma, B. R. Retinal dysplasia. *Am. J. Ophthalmol.* 45:199, 1958.

145. Reisman, L. E., et al. Anti-mongolism: Studies in an infant with a partial monosomy of the 21 chromosome. *Lancet* 1:394, 1966.

146. Rethore, M. O., et al. Trisomie pour la partie distale du bras court du chromosome 3 chez trois germains. *Ann. Genet. (Paris)* 15:159, 1972.

147. Riccardi, V. M., et al. Chromosomal imbalance in the aniridia–Wilms' tumor association: 11p interstitial deletion. *Pediatrics* 61:604, 1978.

148. Riccardi, V. M., et al. Wilms' tumor with aniridia, iris dysplasia and apparently normal chromosomes. *J. Pediatr.* 100:254, 1982.

149. Ricks, R. M., and Riffenburgh, R. S. Retinal dysplasia. *Arch. Ophthalmol.* 72:637, 1964.

150. Robb, R. M., and Marchevsky, A. Pathology of the lens in Down's syndrome. *Arch. Ophthalmol.* 96:1039, 1978.

151. Sanchez, O., and Yunis, J. J. New Chromosome Techniques and Their Medical Applications. In J. J. Yunis (Ed.), *New Chromosomal Syndromes.* New York: Academic, 1977.

152. Saul, R. Blepharophimosis syndromes. *Genet. Clin.* 1:23, 1982.

153. Schachenmann, G., et al. Chromosomes in coloboma and anal atresia. *Lancet* 2:290, 1965.

154. Schinzel, A. Incomplete trisomy 22. *Hum. Genet.* 56:269, 1981.

155. Schinzel, A., et al. The "cat-eye syndrome": Dicentric small marker chromosome probably derived from a no. 22 tetrasomy (22pter–q11) associated with a characteristic phenotype. *Hum. Genet.* 57:148, 1981.

156. Schinzel, A. *Catalogue of Unbalanced Chromosome Aberrations in Man.* New York: de Gruyer, 1984.

157. Schmickel, R. D. The genetic basis for ophthalmological disease. *Surv. Ophthalmol.* 25:37, 1980.

158. Schmidt, I. The Wolfflin spots on the iris. *Am. J. Optom.* 48:573, 1971.

159. Schutten, H. J., Schutten, B. T., and Mikkelson, M. Partial trisomy of chromosome 13: Case report and review of literature. *Ann. Genet. (Paris)* 21:95, 1978.

160. Sergovich, F., et al. The D trisomy syndrome: A case report with a description of ocular pathology. *Can. Med. Assoc. J.* 89:151, 1963.

161. Sherk, M. C., and Williams, T. C. Disc vascularity in Down's syndrome. *Am. J. Optom. Physiol. Opt.* 56:509, 1979.

162. Smith, A. C. M., Sujansky, E., and Riccardi, V. M. Aniridia, mental retardation, and genital abnormality in 2 patients with 46,XY,11p−. *Birth Defects* 13:257, 1977.

163. Smith, D. W., et al. The D₁ trisomy syndrome. *J. Pediatr.* 62:326, 1963.

164. Smith, D. W. *Recognizable Patterns of Human Malformation* (3rd ed.). Philadelphia: Saunders, 1982.

165. Soudek, D., McCreary, B., and Larayap, P. Trisomies 21 and 18 in two sibs: Another case. *J. Pediatr.* 87:326, 1975.

166. Sparkes, R. S., et al. Gene for hereditary retinoblastoma assigned to human chromosome 13 by linkage to esterase D. *Science* 219:971, 1983.

167. Steinbach, P., et al. The dup (3q) syndrome: Report of eight cases and review of the literature. *Am. J. Med. Genet.* 10:159, 1981.

168. Steinberg, C., et al. Recurrence rate for de novo 21q21q translocation Down syndrome: A study of 112 families. *Am. J. Med. Genet.* 17:523, 1984.

169. Stene, J. Detection of higher recurrence risk for age-dependent chromosome abnormalities with an application to trisomy G. *Hum. Hered.* 20:112, 1970.

170. Summitt, R. L. Chromosome 21: Specific Segments That Cause the Phenotype of Down Syndrome. In F. F. de la Cruz and P. S. Gerald (Eds.), *Trisomy 21 Research Perspectives*. Baltimore: University Park Press, 1981.

171. Taylor, A. I. Patau's, Edwards', and cri du chat syndromes: A tabulated summary of current findings. *Dev. Med. Child Neurol.* 9:78, 1967.

172. Taylor, A. I. Autosomal trisomy syndromes: A detailed study of 27 cases of Edwards' syndrome and 27 cases of Patau's syndrome. *J. Med. Genet.* 5:227, 1968.

173. Taysi, K., Sekhon, G. S., and Hillman, R. E. A new syndrome of proximal deletion of the long arm of chromosome 1: 1q21–23–1q25. *Am. J. Med. Genet.* 13:423, 1982.

174. Thomas, C., Cordier, J., and Reny, A. Les manifestations ophthalmologiques du syndrome du Turner. *Arch. Ophtalmol.* 29:5565, 1969.

175. Thompson, J. S., and Thompson, M. W. *Genetics in Medicine* (3rd ed.). Philadelphia: Saunders, 1980.

176. Tjio, J. H., and Levan, A. The chromosome number of man. *Hereditas* 42:1, 1956.

177. Turleau, C., and de Grouchy, J. Trisomy 18qter and trisomy mapping of chromosome 18. *Clin. Genet.* 12:361, 1977.

178. Turner, H. H. A syndrome of infantilism, congenital webbed neck, and cubitus valgus. *Endocrinology* 23:566, 1938.

179. Virchow, R. Uber die Theilung der Zellenkerne. *Virchows Arch. [Pathol. Anat.]* 11:89, 1857.

180. Vogel, R., and Motulsky, A. G. *Human Genetics: Problems and Approaches*. New York: Springer, 1979.

181. Waardenburg, P. J. *Das Menschliche Auge und Seine Erbanlangen*. The Hague: Nijhoff, 1932.

182. Waldeyer, W. Karyokinesis and its relation to the process of fertilization. *Q. J. Micr. Sci.* 30:159, 1888. (Translation by W. B. Benham, *Arch. Mikr. Anat.* 32:1, 1890.)

183. Walsh, S. Z. Keratoconus and blindness in 469 institutionalized subjects with Down syndrome and other causes of mental retardation. *J. Ment. Defic. Res.* 25:243, 1981.

184. Warburg, M., et al. Aniridia and interstitial deletion of the short arm of chromosome 11. *Metab. Pediatr. Ophthalmol.* 4:97, 1980.

185. Warkany, J., Passarge, E., and Smith, L. B. Congenital malformation in autosomal trisomy syndromes. *Am. J. Dis. Child.* 112:502, 1966.

186. Warshowsky, J. A visual screening of a Down's syndrome population. *J. Am. Optom. Assoc.* 52:605, 1981.

187. Wilcox, L. M., Bercovitch, L., and Howard, R. O. Ophthalmic features of chromosome deletion 4p− (Wolf-Hirschhorn syndrome). *Am. J. Ophthalmol.* 86:834, 1978.

188. Wilkins, L. E., Brown, J. A., and Wolf, B. Psychomotor development in 65 home-reared children with cri-du-chat syndrome. *J. Pediatr.* 97:401, 1980.

189. Wilkins, L. E., et al. Clinical heterogeneity in 80 home-reared children with cri du chat syndrome. *J. Pediatr.* 102:528, 1983.

190. Williams, R. D. B. Brushfield spots and Wolfflin nodules in the iris: An appraisal in handicapped children. *Dev. Med. Child. Neurol. [Suppl.]* 23:646, 1981.

191. Wilson, J. G., and Fraser, F. C. *Handbook of Teratology*, Vol. 1. New York: Plenum, 1977.

192. Wilson, L., et al. Cytogenetic analysis of a case of "13q− syndrome" (46,XX,del 13) using banding techniques. *J. Pediatr. Ophthalmol. Strabismus* 17:63, 1980.

193. Wilson, M. G., et al. Inherited pericentric inversion of chromosome no. 4. *Am. J. Hum. Genet.* 22:679, 1970.

194. Wilson, M. G., et al. Syndromes associated with deletion of the long arm of chromosome 18 [del(18q)]. *Am. J. Med. Genet.* 3:155, 1979.

195. Wilson, M. G., et al. Genetic and clinical studies in 13 patients with the Wolf-Hirschhorn syndrome [del(4p)]. *Hum. Genet.* 59:297, 1981.

196. Wilson, W. A., Alfi, O. S., and Donnell, G. N. Ocular findings in cytogenetic syndromes. *Ophthalmology (Rochester)* 86:1184, 1978.

197. Wolf, U., et al. Deletion on short arms of a B-chromosome without "cri du chat" syndrome. *Lancet* 1:769, 1965.

198. Wolfflin, E. Ein klinischer Beitrag sur Kentniss der Structur der Iris. *Arch. Augenheilkd.*, 1902.

199. Yanoff, M., and Font, R. L. Intraocular cartilage in a microphthalmic eye of an otherwise healthy girl. *Ophthalmology* 81:238, 1969.

200. Yanoff, M., Frayer, W. C., and Scheie, H. G. Ocular findings in a patient with 13–15 trisomy. *Arch. Ophthalmol.* 70:372, 1963.

201. Yanoff, M., Rorke, L. B., and Niederer, B. S. Ocular and cerebral abnormalities in chromosome 18 deletion defect. *Am. J. Ophthalmol.* 70:391, 1970.

202. Young, R. S., et al. Two children with de novo del (9p). *Am. J. Med. Genet.* 14:751, 1983.

203. Yunis, J. J. High resolution of human chromosomes. *Science* 191:1268, 1976.

204. Yunis, J. J. (Ed.). *New Chromosomal Syndromes.* New York: Academic, 1977.

205. Yunis, J. J., and Lewandoski, R. C. Partial Duplication 10q and Duplication 10p Syndromes. In J. J. Yunis (Ed.), *New Chromosomal Syndromes.* New York: Academic, 1977.

206. Yunis, J. J., and Ramsay, N. K. C. Familial occurrence of the aniridia–Wilms tumor syndrome with deletion 11p13–14.1. *J. Pediatr.* 96:1027, 1980.

207. Yunis, J. J., Zuniga, R., and Ramirez, E. Retinoblastoma, gross internal malformations and deletion 13q 14–13. *Hum. Genet.* 56:283, 1981.

208. Zellweger, H. Cytogenetic aspects of ophthalmology. *Surv. Ophthalmol.* 15:77, 1970.

209. Zimmer, E. Z., et al. Cyclopia with trisomy D. *Eur. J. Obstet. Gynecol.,* reproduced in *Biology* 13:215, 1982.

210. Zion, V. M. Chromosomal Disorders. In T. D. Duane (Ed.), *Clinical Ophthalmology,* Vol. 5. Philadelphia: Harper & Row, 1979.

Ocular Defects in Craniofacial Syndromes

Samuel Pruzansky
Marilyn T. Miller

The association of ophthalmic pathology with craniofacial syndromes merits attention for several reasons. The skull is a community of bones, of diverse phylogenetic origin and variable developmental patterns, that together relate to several functions. If, in the course of development, one member is affected adversely, other parts of the community will inevitably suffer. Thus if the bony orbit is distorted in its size or shape or is arrested in its growth, the development of the eye and its adnexa, essential to normal vision, may be altered. Conversely, primary defects in the eye may induce developmental abnormalities in the bony orbit.

In genetic counseling it is important to distinguish between an abnormality of the eye as an isolated finding and a similar defect in association with one of several syndromes. For example, congenital cataracts may be associated with trisomy (13–15); Hallermann-Streiff, Conradi's, Pierre Robin, Lowe's, Rothmund-Thomson, and Down's syndromes; and anhidrotic ectodermal dysplasia (see Chaps. 8, 13, and 19). The recurrence risks for congenital cataract depend on the clinical entity with which it is associated.

In a clinical atlas that catalogues congenital facial anomalies with neurologic defects, Aita lists a wide range of orbital-ocular defects in a number of syndromes that include craniofacial syndromes, defects of the first and second branchial arches, generalized metabolic defects, chromosomal defects, syndromes of dwarfism, neurocutaneous diseases, primary neurologic or muscular defects, and other unclassifiable entities. [2]. As

Supported in part by Core Grant EY-1792 from the National Eye Institute, Bethesda, Maryland.

the mere enumeration of ocular defects in this atlas occupies nearly four pages, it is clear that we must limit our discussion to a few selected entities, referring the reader to other sources for a comprehensive evaluation.

Concurrent with a consideration of the human condition, it is worthwhile to note the existence of animal models for the study of genetic disorders involving the eye (see Chap. 6). In a study of inherited skeletal disorders in animals, Grüneberg has observed that, since it is possible to study malformations in animals stage by stage in their developmental making, significant insights can be gained into their pathogenesis [28]. He also points out that gene effects on the morphologic level are almost without exception manifold or pleiotropic. Simply stated, genes tend to produce syndromes. There are two probable mechanisms by which this effect occurs. One mechanism involves coordinated gene actions in different parts of the body. A second mechanism may be likened to a domino effect, in which one malformation induces secondary and tertiary changes. For example, gross derangement in the bony orbit may alter the relationship of the globe to the ocular muscles and lids, producing strabismus, refractive errors, or both.

It is in this context that we wish to consider a few examples out of a wide array of craniofacial anomalies. Our purpose is threefold:

1. To consider certain disorders of the eye that are probably secondary to defects in the craniofacial skeleton, in which the onset and severity of the pathologic condition may be age dependent and relate to developmental changes in contiguous structures.

2. To consider certain craniofacial syndromes in which the eye and the adjacent facial skeleton are commonly and characteristically malformed from birth onward. This group differs from the preceding in that the severity of the malformation remains essentially unchanged as the child grows older. In this category, as in the preceding, an appreciation of the regional pathology is essential as a rational basis for multidisciplinary treatment planning, with appropriate priorities and planned sequences.

3. To alert the ophthalmologist to certain craniofacial syndromes that ordinarily do not come within his or her purview but that represent high risks for a wide variety of nonspecific disorders. Increasing numbers of such clinical entities are being identified as a result of the growing interest in congenital anomalies and the development of birth defect clinics and centers for genetic study.

There are many schemes by which craniofacial malformations may be classified. One useful method of clinical assessment has been proposed by Mustardé; it reflects a surgical reconstruction orientation [47]. The first category in this scheme includes a group of deformities in which the soft tissues themselves may or may not be abnormal, but in which the primary deformity involves the facial skeleton. The second category comprises obvious soft tissue abnormalities as well as definite and well-organized underlying deformities of the orbital bones. The third category consists of deformities involving primarily the soft tissues, with the focus on the eyelids. In this final category there are no or minimal underlying bony abnormalities. This chapter considers only the second and third groups.

CRANIOSYNOSTOSIS SYNDROMES

The development of the skull is partly influenced by the development of the brain. The intracranial pressure of the growing contents keeps the sutures open, allowing the skull to increase in volume. From birth to 2 years of age, intracranial volume is nearly tripled, closely paralleling the increase in brain weight [61].

Postnatal growth of the eye parallels that of the brain, and the eye attains its adult size at a much earlier age than the body as a whole. From birth to maturity, the body increases 21-fold in volume, while the eye increases less than threefold, and

70 percent of this increment is attained by the age of 4. The period of greatest growth for the eye is up to the age of 3; growth is most pronounced during the first year of life [17]. Volume of the orbits is more than doubled during the first year and is nearly quadrupled by 6 to 8 years of age. By adulthood, orbital volume is more than five times the size at birth [17].

These facts make evident the consequences of arrested or distorted growth of the craniofacial complex on the development and function of the eye. The resulting ophthalmopathy not only challenges therapeutic skills but also presents the clinical investigator with an extraordinary experiment of nature.

Visual loss is by far the most serious ophthalmologic problem in craniosynostosis patients. It may exist at birth or occasionally develop in later years. It is usually, but not always, bilateral and may occur as a complication of reconstructive orbital surgery.

The most frequent causes of visual loss are acquired types of ocular disease, such as optic atrophy and corneal damage, and result from abnormalities in the adnexal, orbital, or skull structures or from amblyopia secondary to strabismus or anisometropia.

If a crucial group of cranial sutures are stenosed, increased intracranial pressure may occur with ensuing papilledema and, if not reversed, ultimately optic atrophy (Fig. 9-1). In 1886 von Graefe noted the association between an abnormal skull,

Fig. 9-1. *Craniofacial dysostosis (Crouzon's disease). Severe optic atrophy with 20/400 visual acuity in better eye in 12-year-old boy.*

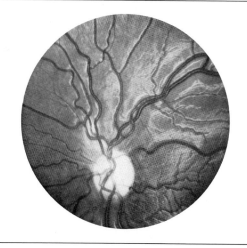

increased intracranial pressure, and poor visual function [62]. This combination has been repeatedly observed in subsequent reports of craniosynostosis syndromes [1, 4–9, 12, 18, 23, 29, 32, 38, 49]. It has been proposed that compression of the vascular supply to the optic nerve occurs in some situations from a sudden change in intracranial pressures [34]. Kinking of the optic nerve also may be a factor. These proposed local causes of atrophic optic disc changes may best explain why some patients clinically demonstrate a marked difference in degree of optic nerve involvement between the two eyes or lack a documented stage of papilledema.

Although the relative importance of all the factors that may produce optic nerve damage is not proved, there appears to be no question that the conditions that predispose to increased intracranial pressure are the most significant risk factors for subsequent nerve damage. Optic atrophy is infrequent in children if only the sagittal suture is involved or if suture closure is unilateral, as seen in plagiocephaly [4, 27, 32]. It is frequent if multiple sutures are affected, especially if the coronal suture is one that is synostotic.

Although any patient with premature closure of certain specific sutures may show signs and symptoms of optic nerve damage, a very high incidence of 80 percent has been reported by Bertelsen in Crouzon's disease, although many of the patients had not been identified at an early age [7]. These profound visual defects often necessitate special schooling for the patient and counseling for the family. Families with Crouzon's disease may demonstrate a wide range of suture and optic nerve involvement, even with therapeutic intervention. The common finding of optic atrophy in patients with Crouzon's disease may suggest periods of increased intracranial pressure at some phase of development; however, the number of children with mental retardation is surprisingly quite low. Conversely, the percentage of mentally retarded patients is significantly higher in Apert's disease, yet the incidence of optic nerve disease is lower, which indicates a somewhat unclear correlation of optic nerve disease, increased intracranial pressure, and mental retardation. Computed tomography (CT) may prove to be an invaluable tool for characterizing better the course of optic nerve disease and providing information on other anatomic factors that may cause or contribute to optic nerve damage.

Craniectomy prevents or alleviates some of the neurologic complications in these patients and also improves the shape of the developing skull. If increased intracranial pressure can be eliminated at a fairly early stage of papilledema, little residual visual impairment may ensue.

The proptosis caused by anatomic factors in the craniosynostosis syndromes differs from exophthalmos secondary to tumors and pseudotumors in patients with orbits of normal size and shape. However, both may cause similar ophthalmic symptoms and complications. Proptosis resulting from a reduced volume of the bony orbital space in premature synostosis of the cranial and midfacial sutures is produced by many factors: (1) arrested growth of the maxilla, which reduces the length of the orbital floor; (2) shortened anterior cranial base; (3) depressed planum sphenoidale; (4) forward displacement of the greater wing of the sphenoid bone; and (5) lateral expansion of the ethmoidal air cells. Proptosis is often a more prominent feature in Crouzon's disease than in Apert's disease and may occur in a number of less common craniosynostosis syndromes or in isolated craniosynostosis. However, unlike many causes of exophthalmos, if severe proptosis is not present at birth, progression is usually slow, and frequent monitoring of the cornea for warning symptoms will prevent serious complications in most cases.

The severity of the exophthalmos is variable even in one syndrome type and may become more severe as the child gets older, owing to the disturbed growth pattern. The midface hypoplasia contributes to the prominent appearance of the globe (Fig. 9-2). Often there is a disparity between Hertel exophthalmometry readings and the clinical impression, in which a more prominent appearance of the globes is noted than the measured amount would suggest. This method may not be valid in these conditions, as it assumes that the bony orbital rims are not involved in the pathologic process.

The lids may not afford adequate protection for the globe, with the result of corneal exposure and drying, punctate keratitis, and ensuing pain and conjunctival hyperemia. If these problems are not adequately treated, corneal ulceration with possible perforation of the globe and further damage to the eye and vision may result (Fig. 9-3). Corneal sensation may be diminished by repeated insults to the cornea, or on occasion diminished sensation may represent a primary pathologic condition. Reconstructive surgery around the orbit has been noted to result in transient or permanent decrease in corneal sensitivity with potential sec-

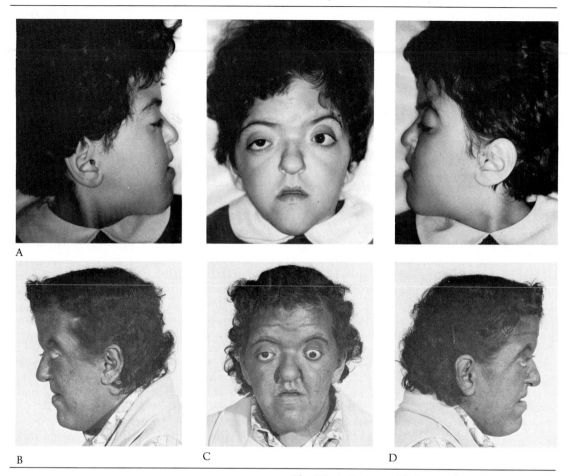

A

B   C   D

Fig. 9-2. *A. Patient with Apert's disease at age 7 years 11 months. B–D. Same patient at age 16.*

ondary corneal ulceration. Either situation intensifies the keratitis.

On the basis of a significant number of family studies, an autosomal dominant inheritance has been demonstrated for craniofacial dysostosis, or Crouzon's disease. However, a significant number of sporadic cases are encountered. Most Apert's disease cases are sporadic, although a few reported studies of familial occurrence suggest an autosomal dominant gene. An advanced male parental age effect has been suggested as an causal factor.

A few patients have such severe proptosis that conservative management is not sufficient to prevent corneal damage. When there is persistent exposure, a tarsorrhaphy (usually laterally) may be indicated (see Fig. 9-3). This may be done as a temporary or a permanent measure, depending on the plan for long-term management of the facial deformity in the patient. It is usually desirable to avoid surgery to the eyelids if extensive recon-

structive surgery is planned in the near future, unless the cornea has undergone recurrent episodes of severe damage. At times the tarsorrhaphy itself greatly improves the appearance by narrowing the abnormally wide palpebral fissure. Unfortunately, permanent tarsorrhaphies often have not been successful in this group of patients because of the constant mechanical force on the sutured lids owing to the small volume of the orbit.

The extreme proptosis observed in some patients, which Tessier refers to as exorbitism [57], can result in luxation of the eyeball. Sherne explained this tendency on the basis that the plane of action of the orbicularis muscle may be behind the globe, thereby reversing its normal effect and propelling the eye forward [53].

Craniofacial syndromes have been particularly

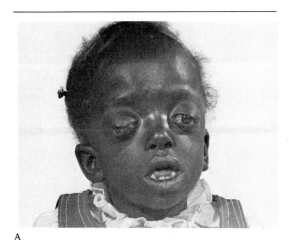

A

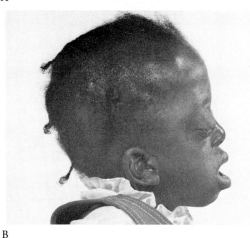

B

Fig. 9-3. *Craniofacial dysostosis (Crouzon's disease) in 6-year-old girl. Note severe proptosis and tarsorrhaphies.*

interesting from the standpoint of ocular motility because the majority of severely affected patients not only have obvious strabismus but also a very characteristic type of ocular movement disturbance. The observed ocular motility pattern is generally predictable, especially in Apert's and Crouzon's diseases. The type of disturbed movement noted in these patients may be secondary to mechanical factors induced by abnormal bony anatomy and may result from changes in ocular muscle size or location.

Abnormal ocular alignment and movement have been described repeatedly in the literature in Apert's and Crouzon's diseases [16, 24, 27, 35, 40–42, 45, 46, 63]. The deviation in the primary position varies from esotropia to exotropia, al-

though exotropia has been the most common finding and has occurred in over 50 percent of our patients. The most consistent finding, however, has been the presence of a V pattern—an exotropia in the up position and straight eyes or esotropia in the down position that produces a V configuration [51]. There is also an associated overaction of the inferior oblique muscle in most patients (Fig.9-4). Another finding in many patients is a limitation of movement in the field of action of the superior rectus and superior oblique muscles on monocular and binocular testing [24, 27, 33, 40–42, 51, 63]. This prototype pattern (V) of ocular muscle imbalance is not unique to patients with these craniofacial anomalies and is present in many patients without bony abnormalities. What is unparalleled is the number of patients who manifest this abnormality.

It is tempting to attribute the changes in mechanical action of the muscle to a disturbance in the normal relationship between the origin and the insertion of the muscles, as suggested by many authors. Urrets-Zavalía and colleagues [59, 60] have noted the presence of an A or V phenomenon in various ethnic groups with different facial development, particularly involving malar bones, and Zaki and Kenney [67] have felt that the position of the bony orbital walls affects the type of strabismus in nonsyndrome patients [32].

Gobin [24] and Morax [45, 46] suggest that the hypoplastic maxilla in craniosynostosis patients contributes to an alteration of mechanical forces of the inferior oblique muscle and an enhancement of its effect with corresponding diminished action of the superior oblique. Inferior oblique overaction may occur unilaterally in patients with plagiocephaly [52]. Reconstructive surgery on patients with Apert's and Crouzon's diseases has not routinely resolved the V pattern [9, 11, 43]. However, this does not necessarily negate the mechanical argument, as a muscle may continue to overact, even when the cause of its overaction has been removed.

A somewhat unexpected but well-documented factor in the vertical ocular muscle imbalance in craniosynostosis patients is an abnormal insertion or structure of the muscle. A number of case reports have noted the apparent absence of a vertical-acting muscle at the time of surgery [13, 42, 46, 65]. Diamond and co-workers reported extraocular muscle anomalies (primarily of the inferior and superior rectus muscle) in 42 percent of their patients with craniofacial dysostosis [16]. More information in this area is being accumulated from

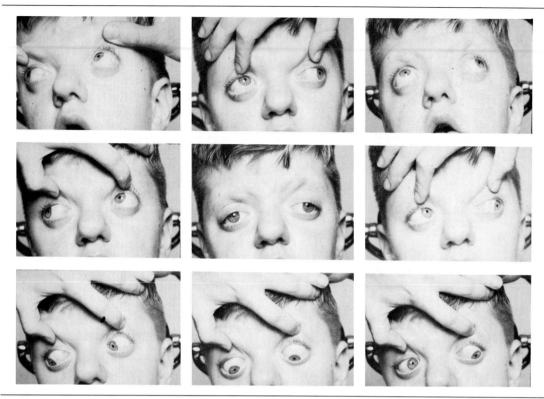

Fig. 9-4. *Patient with Apert's disease demonstrating typical abnormal eye motility. Note "V" exotropia, overacting inferior obliques, and underacting superior obliques.*

CT findings. Orbital high-resolution CT with small cuts (1–1.5 mm) shows these changes in location or size of extraocular muscles. Axial, coronal, and sagittal projections are useful in obtaining an accurate estimate of the degree of abnormality. Repositioning of the gantry to −15 provides good visualization of the course of the inferior rectus in a sagittal cut; however, if sagittal cuts cannot be obtained, computer reformation may be used to acquire this information [36]. Coronal sections may be direct or reformed. Patients with gross limitation of movement are most likely to demonstrate CT scan abnormalities, and if ocular motility surgery is contemplated, this type of evaluation is indicated to plan the appropriate surgical procedures and alternative procedures if the ocular muscles cannot be located [36].

Prevention and Treatment

Since brain growth is particularly active during the first 2 years of life (the brain increases from 350 gm at birth to about 800 gm at 2 years of age), the inhibiting mechanical effect of a fused skull becomes obvious. For these reasons, early recog-

nition of craniostenosis followed by craniectomy in selected cases, particularly those involving the coronal complex, becomes essential during the first few months of life to prevent visual loss and skull deformity. Alterations in cranial shape toward the normal as a result of craniectomy have been demonstrated by radiography by Bertelsen [7] and by the more precise methods of roentgenocephalometry in our center [31, 51].

Presumably, early intervention through craniectomy may prevent the compensatory deformations in the skull base that act to reduce orbital volume and distort its shape and position.

In addition to monitoring the structures of the optic nerve and treating corneal exposure problems, attention should be given to some of the simple but frequent ocular complications observed in these patients. Patients with craniofacial syndromes show an increased incidence of abnormalities such as astigmatism, paralytic deviations, and structural anomalies, but the treatment differs only slightly from that of the more routine strabismus in nonsyndrome patients. Correction of refractive errors, fundus evaluation, and amblyopia therapy remain the important modes of treatment and evaluation. When possible these should be done concurrently with the evaluation and treatment of the patient's other problems. If ocular muscle surgery appears necessary, the decision should be arrived at through consultation with the craniofacial team to establish appropriate priorities, communicate surgical risks, and arrive at an integrated treatment plan. There are, however, exceptions, especially in children for whom reconstructive surgery is not planned until late childhood.

Corrective eye muscle surgery is often appropriately delayed in these patients primarily because (1) repair of other deformities may be of higher priority for improving the patient's functional and cosmetic problems; (2) their may be an increased risk with the use of anesthetics, especially in younger children, because of anomalies of the respiratory system; and (3) corrective plastic surgery in the orbital areas may alter the degree or type of ocular deviation. This last factor has not been as significant in craniosynostosis patients is in patients with more severe types of hypertelorism, but changes occasionally occur because of neurologic damage or restricted movement secondary to scar tissue formation [9, 10, 42].

Clinical interest in craniofacial synostosis has been quickened recently, largely as a result of the work of Paul Tessier of Paris, whose patient and innovative research has made it possible to mobilize the facial bones, particularly those of the orbit. By advancing the oribital floor, the grossly exophthalmic eye can be contained within the greatly deepened orbital cavities [57].

Ocular complications after major reconstructive surgery are potentially serious. Direct or indirect damage to the neurologic pathways of the eye can result in permanent visual loss. Although blindness has been reported in a few cases, it has been a rare complication [9, 11]. In a combined report of 683 cases, Whitacker and colleagues found only 2 patients who sustained permanent visual loss [66]; David and associates reported a severe visual complication in 12 of 75 cases [15].

Other potentially vision-threatening sequelae are corneal damage after surgery from bandages rubbing the eyes, exposure caused by incomplete protection by the lids, and orbital edema. At times corneal damage may be asymptomatic and may go undetected for a period of time if a transient or permanent decreased corneal sensation exists postoperatively.

The ptosis so frequently noted after craniofacial surgery in craniosynostosis patients appears to result more from mechanical factors owing to stretching than from neurologic damage [12, 37, 58]. Tessier advocates levator resection for this type of ptosis [58]. Since the levator muscle is often normal from a neuromuscular standpoint, resection may have more of an effect than in cases of congenital ptosis.

MANDIBULOFACIAL DYSOSTOSIS

Mandibulofacial dysostosis has been selected as an example in which the adnexa of the eye and the adjacent facial skeleton are commonly and characteristically malformed from birth onward. Insofar as we have been able to determine, the severity of the malformation remains essentially unchanged as the child grows older, in contrast to the situation in craniofacial synostosis.

Mandibulofacial dysostosis, also known as Treacher Collins or Franceschetti syndrome, was first described by Thompson in 1846, according to Gorlin and coauthors [26]. Credit for its discovery is also shared by Berry; however, the most extensive reviews were published by Franceschetti and his co-workers Zwahlen and Klein [20, 21]. Mandibulofacial dysostosis is characterized by bilateral involvement of facial structures including malar and mandibular hypoplasia, microstomia, coloboma in the outer third of the lower lid, and external and middle ear anomalies (Fig. 9-5).

In the severe form the zygomatic bone is underdeveloped and may also be absent. According to Mustardé the zygomatic arch and temporalis muscle may be absent, and a fissure in the maxilla and a defect in the lower margin of the orbit are often present [47]. Hypoplasia of the supraorbital rim also has been observed.

In about 50 percent of the patients the lateral canthus is displaced downward, producing the characteristic antimongoloid slant. At times there is an illusion of a slant produced by the lower lid coloboma [50]. Deficiency in the cilia medial to the lid coloboma also may occur, as may a number of low-incidence anomalies such as iridic coloboma and absent lower lacrimal puncta and meibomian glands [26]. The syndrome is inherited as an autosomal dominant trait with incomplete penetrance and variable expressivity.

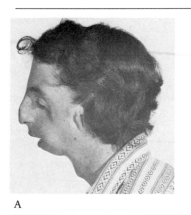
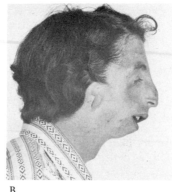
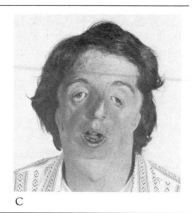

A   B   C

Fig. 9-5. *Eighteen-year-old man with classic features of mandibulofacial dysostosis.*

In a retrospective and prospective study of 17 patients with mandibulofacial dysostosis in our clinic, 7 patients were noted to have horizontal strabismus, primarily (5 of 7) exotropia [44]. Although Urrets-Zavalía [59] observed A and V patterns in patients with mongoloid and antimongoloid slants of the fissures, we did not find a preponderance of any one pattern. Our most surprising observation in these patients was the predilection for astigmatic correction. Cylindrical corrections greater than two diopters were noted in 14 of 34 eyes, with the axis of the cylinder usually located at 140 to 180 degrees or 0 to 40 degrees [44]. It could be speculated that the frequent astigmatic corrections were induced by the changes in the soft (e.g., coloboma) and bony structures around the globe, as noted by Cuttone and colleagues in animal experiments in which upper lid colobomas were produced in rabbits and changes in astigmatic correction were observed [14].

Surgical Reconstruction

As Mustardé [47] and Tessier [58] have pointed out, surgical reconstruction begins with building up the deficient zygoma and re-forming the orbital floor and supraorbital ridge. Both sides are dealt with at the same time, and shaped iliac bone grafts are introduced by a direct approach. Canthoplasties are performed only after the lateral, inferior, and superior borders of the orbits have been reconstructed.

Anterior osteotomy of the mandible and genioplasty with subsequent rhinoplasty can produce satisfactory cosmetic results. To our knowledge, the changes in eye motility after such reconstruction have not been documented.

SYNDROMES WITH HIGH RISK FOR EYE MALFORMATIONS

Clefts of the Lip, Palate, and Face; Deafness Syndromes

Clefts of the lip or palate, or both, constitute one of the most common malformations in humans. The incidence seems to be dependent on racial factors: It is higher in Japanese and American Indians than in whites and is lowest in American blacks [22]. Among whites the incidence is approximately 1 in 600, though underreporting must be considered in evaluating estimates of population frequency [39].

It has long been recognized that patients with facial clefts may have associated malformations. In 1942 Fogh-Anderson estimated that at birth 10 percent of children with facial clefts showed severe associated malformations [19]. The weight of cumulative evidence gathered since then suggests a much higher figure. As increasing numbers of such children come under surveillance by multidisciplinary teams in medical centers, previously undetected malformations, both major and minor, are identified. In addition attention has been drawn to the frequency with which clefts are associated with a variety of syndromes [64].

In a review of facial clefting and its syndromes, Gorlin and associates described several syndromes that included the eye [25]. Among these were clefts in association with ankyloblepharon filiforme adnatum, ectrodactyly and atresia of the lacrimal puncta, Wildervanck's syndrome, retinal detachment observed in hereditary progressive arthro-ophthalmopathy as described by Stickler and coauthors [55] (see Chap. 15), and a variety of other entities.

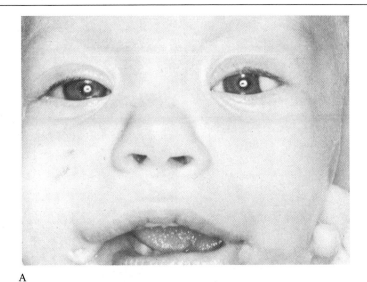

A

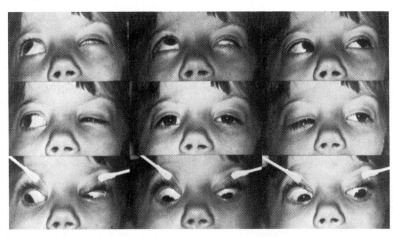

B

Fig. 9-6. *Goldenhar variant of hemifacial microsomia. A. Child's appearance in infancy with severe left ear deformity, macrostomia, mouth cleft, and limbal dermoid in left eye. B. Same child at age 8 years with bilateral Duane's syndrome. (From M. T. Miller, Ocular Abnormalities in Craniofacial Malformations in J. D. Kivlin [Ed.], Developmental Abnormalities of the Eye [International Ophthalmology Clinics, Spring 1984, Vol. 24, No. 1] Boston: Little, Brown, 1984).*

More recently Knoblock and Layer reviewed the association of clefting syndromes and retinal detachment [30]. Included were a variety of skeletal abnormalities in patients with hereditary vitreoretinal degeneration of various types, most of them being inherited in an irregular autosomal dominant manner.

In the Pierre Robin syndrome, consisting of cleft palate, mandibular micrognathia, and glossoptosis, nonspecific ophthalmopathy may be more frequent than has been generally appreciated. Smith and Stowe found nonspecific major lesions including esotropia, congenital cataract and glaucoma, microphthalmos, and retinal detachment [54].

In a survey of over 500 deaf children, Alexander noted 7 cases of Duane's syndrome [3]. Four other cases demonstrated restriction in horizontal movement of all four horizontal muscles, which may represent a rarer form of Duane's syndrome.

From the foregoing it would appear that, as a group, patients with facial clefts and deafness demonstrate a higher than usual frequency of ophthalmopathy and require critical surveillance by ophthalmologists. It should also be recognized that there is at least a fourfold increase in frequency of congenital anomalies in relatives of patients with facial clefts.

Hemifacial Microsomia

Hemifacial microsomia is known by many names, including otomandibular dysostosis, first and second branchial arch syndrome, and others. Gorlin and co-workers propose that Goldenhar's syndrome and oculoauriculo vertebral dysplasia, previously considered as separate entities, are variants of hemifacial microsomia [26]. Commonly associated eye findings include epibulbar dermoids; colobomas, generally of the upper lid; microphthalmos; and microcornea. While not a common finding, Duane's syndrome has been observed in a number of cases of hemifacial microsomia, especially the Goldenhar variant (Fig. 9-6).

In extreme cases the generally unilateral dysplasia includes the external ear, middle ear, cranial base, maxilla, mandible, facial nerve, muscles of mastication and facial expression, and absence of the parotid duct. Usually the other side is unaffected. When the facial asymmetry is severe the

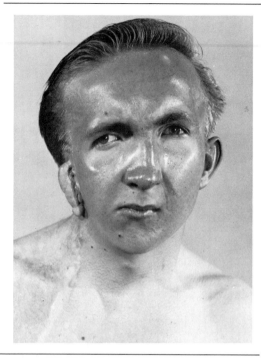

Fig. 9-7. *Hemifacial microsomia with partial reconstruction of right ear. Note asymmetry of face, the lower level of right orbit, and the exotropia.*

Fig. 9-8. *Terminal transverse defects with orofacial malformation (TTV-OFM) syndrome complex: ectrodactyly with orofacial malformation. Patient has unilateral facial nerve palsy, bilateral inability to abduct eyes, ectrodactyly, and tongue anomalies.*

(From M. T. Miller, Ocular Abnormalities in Craniofacial Malformations, in J. D. Kivlin [Ed.], Developmental Abnormalities of the Eye [International Ophthalmology Clinics, Spring 1984, Vol. 24, No. 1] Boston: Little, Brown, 1984.)

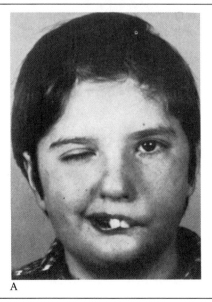

A

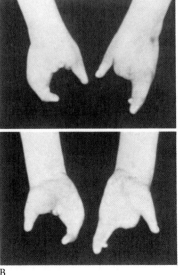

B

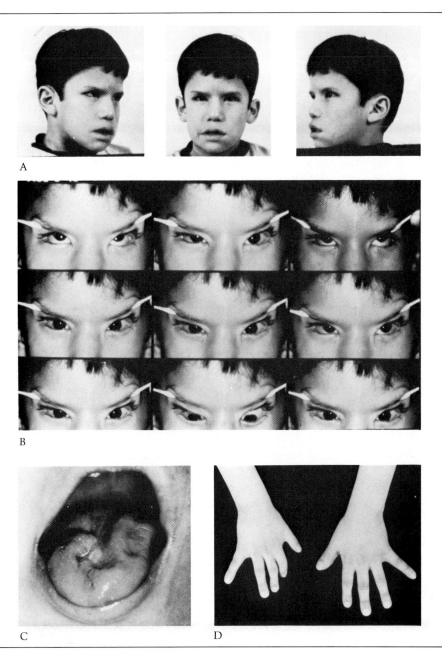

Fig. 9-9. *TTV-OFM syndrome complex: Möbius'
syndrome. Bilateral inability to abduct eye in patient
who also had bilateral facial nerve palsy, pectoralis
muscle defect and ipsilateral hand defect (Poland's
anomaly), and tongue anomaly. A. Masklike facies.
B. Typical motility. C. Tongue anomaly. D.
Clinodactyly of right hand.*

orbit in the affected side may be smaller and positioned lower than on the normal side (Fig. 9-7).

There is no clear inheritance pattern noted in this syndrome. Similarly, no evidence has been found for a hereditary pattern for oculovertebral dysplasia expressivity.

Möbius Type Syndromes—Terminal Transverse Defects with an Orofacial Malformation

The complex of terminal transverse defects with an orofacial malformation (TTV-OFM) includes a heterogeneous collection of syndromes with a wide variety of facial and limb anomalies [56]: the aglossia-adactyly syndrome, Hanhart's syndrome, ectrodactyly with orofacial malformations (Fig. 9-8), ankyloglossia syndrome, and Möbius' syndrome. A similar group of syndromes has been called oromandibular limb hypogenesis syndrome by Gorlin and associates [26].

The classic ocular feature noted in Möbius' syndrome is bilateral limitation of abduction associated with bilateral facial nerve palsy (Fig. 9-9). This form of strabismus also has been observed in Hanhart's syndrome, aglossia-adactyly, and other syndromes in this group. The apparent sixth and seventh nerve palsies may not be complete. The medial rectus muscles also often appear underactive in conjugate gaze, but convergence is frequently normal. Vertical eye movement may be normal in this group, but a few cases have shown vertical limitations that resemble restrictive syn-

Fig. 9-10. *Median facial cleft syndrome (frontonasal dysplasia) with hypertelorism, exotropia, nasal cleft, cleft of the left eyebrow, and widow's peak (forehead hair anomaly). Preoperative motility examination of patient demonstrates exotropia, V pattern of deviation, and overacting of inferior oblique muscles (mild). (From M. T. Miller and S. Pruzansky, Craniofacial Anomalies, in G. A. Peyman, D. Sanders, and M. F. Goldberg [Eds.] Principles and Practice of Ophthalmology [Vol. III], Philadelphia: Saunders, 1980.)*

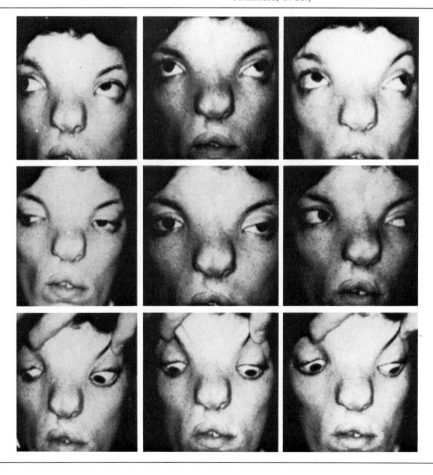

dromes more than the usual vertical palsies. An ocular motility disturbance resembling that of Duane's syndrome has been observed in a few patients in this syndrome complex [43].

Less frequent or characteristic ocular anomalies are epicanthal folds, abnormal slants to palpebral fissures, mild hypertelorism, microphthalmos, and nystagmus.

Ocular Hypertelorism

Ocular hypertelorism refers to a condition in which there is an increased separation between the bony orbits. It is an anatomic description rather than a diagnostic entity. Mild to moderate hypertelorism is found in a heterogeneous group of syndromes but occurs most prominently in the median facial cleft syndrome (frontonasal dysplasia) as a result of developmental arrest (Fig. 9-10). Characteristic findings of this syndrome are medial cleft nose, lip, and palate, a widow's peak, and cranium bifidum occultum. The most common ocular abnormality is a nonparetic form of exotropia. Infrequent findings are epibulbar der-

Fig. 9-11. *Postoperative motility examination of patient in Figure 9-10 shows significant decrease in exotropia but little change in versions. (From M. T. Miller and S. Pruzansky, Craniofacial Anomalies, in G. A. Peyman, D. Sanders, and M. F. Goldberg [Eds.], Principles and Practice of Ophthalmology [Vol. III], Philadelphia: Saunders, 1980.)*

moids, palpebral fissure changes, and optic atrophy, unless the hypertelorism is secondary to craniosynostosis.

In hypertelorism resulting from median facial cleft, the anterior part of the orbits are displaced laterally, but the separation is often within normal limits at the level of the optic canal. Exotropia is a very common finding in patients with moderate to severe degrees of hypertelorism and appears to result more from mechanical factors than from the structural abnormalities of the muscles noted in craniosynostosis patients. This conclusion results from the frequent observations that medial rotation of the orbits done at the time of surgery significantly decreases the exotropia and may produce esotropia in some patients (Fig. 9-11). There is rarely any associated limitation of lateral rectus function; therefore the esotropia must be the result of the anatomic change. Thus it is desirable, if possible, to defer surgery on the ocular muscles until the major reconstructive surgery is completed.

CONCLUSIONS

Craniofacial malformations are frequently associated with disease of the eye and its adnexa. While such syndromes have been recognized and studied for some time, the approach has generally been on a unidisciplinary basis. With the advent of in-

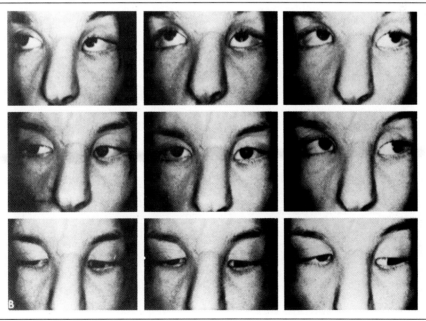

terdisciplinary programs for the study and care of the special patient with craniofacial birth defects, elucidation of the complex and interrelated dimensions of multiple organ malformations has led to a rational basis for comprehensive clinical management. As greater numbers of such syndromes come within the purview of ophthalmologists, previously undiscovered ophthalmopathy is encountered with increasing frequency.

With the advent of surgical techniques that permit reconstruction of orbital volume and shape and alteration in the angulation and distance between the orbits, a model system for the analysis of the interrelation of form and function has been created for ophthalmologic investigation.

REFERENCES

1. Abeles, M. Medullated optic nerve fibers accompanying oxycephaly and other cranial deformities. *Arch. Ophthalmol.* 16:188, 1936.
2. Aita, J. A. *Congenital Facial Anomalies with Neurologic Defects: A Clinical Atlas.* Springfield, Ill.: Thomas, 1969.
3. Alexander, J. Ocular abnormalities among congenitally deaf children. *Can. J. Ophthalmol.* 8:428, 1973.
4. Anderson, B., and Woodhall, B. Visual loss in primary skull deformities. *Trans. Am. Acad. Ophthalmol. Otolaryngol.* 57:497, 1953.
5. Archer, D. B., et al. Ophthalmic aspects of craniosynsotosis. *Trans. Ophthalmol. Soc.* 904:173, 1974.
6. Behr, C. Changes in the region of the bony canal in steeple skull. *Am. J. Ophthalmol.* 13:505, 1930.
7. Bertelsen, T. I. The premature synostosis of the cranial sutures. *Acta Ophthalmol.* [Suppl.] (*Copenh.*) 51, 1958.
8. Blodi, F. C. Development anomalies of the skull affecting the eye. *Arch. Ophthalmol.* 57:593, 1957.
9. Board, R. J., and Bunsic, J. R. The ocular effects of major reconstructive surgery in craniofacial disorders. Presented at the Association of Pediatric Ophthalmology and Strabismus meeting, Orlando, Florida, 1981.
10. Choy, A., Margolis, S., and Breinin, G. Ophthalmologic Complications of Craniofacial Surgery. In J. M. Converse, J. G. McCarthy, and D. Wood-Smith (Eds.), *Symposium and Diagnosis and Treatment of Craniofacial Anomalies.* St. Louis: Mosby, 1979. P. 519.
11. Choy, A. E., et al. Analysis of Preoperative and Postoperative Extraocular Muscle Function in Surgical Translocation of Bony Orbits: A Preliminary Report. In J. M. Converse, J. G. McCarthy, and D. Wood-Smith (Eds.), *Symposium on Diagnosis and Treatment of Craniofacial Anomalies.* St. Louis: Mosby, 1979. P. 128.
12. Converse, J. M. (Ed.) *Reconstructive Plastic Surgery: Principles and Procedures in Correction, Reconstruction and Transplantation.* Philadelphia: Saunders, 1964.
13. Cuttone, J., et al. Absence of the superior rectus in Apert's syndrome. *J. Pediatr. Ophthalmol. Strabismus* 16:349, 1979.
14. Cuttone, J., et al. The relationship between soft tissue anomalies around the orbit and globe and astigmatic refractive errors. *J. Pediatr. Ophthalmol. Strabismus* 17:29, 1980.
15. David, D., Poswillo, D., and Simpson, D. *The Craniosynostoses: Causes, National History and Management.* New York: Springer, 1982. P. 284.
16. Diamond, G. R., et al. Variations in extraocular muscle number and structure in craniofacial dysostosis. *Am. J. Ophthalmol.* 90:416, 1980.
17. Duke-Elder, S. *System of Ophthalmology,* Vol. 3: *Normal and Abnormal Development.* Part I. Embryology. St. Louis: Mosby, 1963.
18. Farnarier, G., et al. Les signes ophtalmologiques des craniosynostosis (à propos de 219 cas). *Bull. Soc. Ophtalmol. Fr.* 77:853, 1977.
19. Fogh-Anderson, P. *Inheritance of Harelip and Cleft Palate: Contribution to the Elucidation of the Etiology of the Congenital Clefts of the Face.* Copenhagen: Busck, 1942.
20. Franceschetti, A., and Klein, D. The mandibulofacial dysostosis: A new hereditary syndrome. *Acta Ophthalmol. Copenh.* 27:143, 1949.
21. Franceschetti, A., and Zwahlen, P. Un syndrome nouveau: Le dysostose mandibulofaciale. *Bull. Acad. Suisse Sci. Med.* 12:60, 1944.
22. Fraser, F. C. The genetics of cleft lip and cleft palate. *Am. J. Hum. Genet.* 22:336, 1970.
23. Friedenwald, H. An optic nerve atrophy associated with cranial deformity. *Arch. Ophthalmol.* 30:405, 1954.
24. Gobin, M. H. Sagittalization of the oblique muscles as a possible cause of the "A," "V," and "X" phenomena. *Br. J. Ophthalmol.* 13:52, 1968.
25. Gorlin, R. J., Cervenka, J., and Pruzansky, S. Facial clefting and its syndromes. *Birth Defects* 7(7):3, 1971.
26. Gorlin, R. J., Pindborg, J. J., and Cohen, M. M. *Syndromes of the Head and Neck* (2nd ed.). New York: McGraw-Hill, 1976.
27. Greaves, B., Walker, J., and Wybar, K. Disorders of ocular motility in craniofacial dysostosis. *J. R. Soc. Med..* 72:21, 1979.
28. Grüneberg, H. *The Pathology of Development: A Study of Inherited Skeletal Disorders in Animals.* New York: Wiley, 1963.
29. Ingraham, F. D., Alexander, E., Jr., and Matson, D. D. Clinical studies in craniosynostosis. *Surgery* 24:518, 1948.
30. Knoblock, W. H., and Layer, J. M. Clefting syndromes associated with retinal detachment. *Am. J. Ophthalmol.* 73:517, 1972.
31. Kreiborg, S., Pruzansky, S., and Pashayan, H. The Saethre-Chotzen syndrome. *Teratology* 6:287, 1972.

32. Laitinen, L., Miettinin, P., and Sulamaa, M. Ophthalmological observations in craniosynostosis. *Acta Ophthalmol.* [*Suppl.*] (*Copenh.*) 44–45:121, 1956.

33. Limon-Brown, E. (Ed.). *Proceedings of the 2nd International Strabismological Association.* Paris: Diffusion Generale de Librairie, 1974, p. 371.

34. Lindenberg, R., and Walsh, F. P. Vascular compressions involving intracranial visual pathways. *Trans. Am. Acad. Ophthalmol. Otolaryngol.* 68:677, 1964.

35. Lloyd, L. Craniofacial reconstruction: Ocular management of orbital hypertelorism. *Trans. Am. Ophthalmol. Soc.* 73:123, 1975.

36. Mafee, M., et al. High resolution computed tomography scanning in the evaluation of ocular motility. Presented at the Pediatric Ophthalmology and Strabismus Association meeting, Vancouver, Canada, 1983.

37. Marsh, J. Blepharo-canthal deformities in patients following craniofacial surgery. *Plast. Reconstr. Surg.* 61:842, 1978.

38. McLaurin, R. L., and Matson, D. D. Importance of early surgical treatment of craniosynostosis: Review of thirty-six cases treated during the first six months of life. *Pediatrics* 10:637, 1952.

39. Meskin, L. H., and Pruzanksy, S. Validity of the birth certificate in the epidemiologic assessment of facial clefts. *J. Dent. Res.* 46:1456, 1967.

40. Miller, M. Ocular motility patterns in craniosynostosis syndromes, abstracted. Presented at the meeting of the Association for Research in Vision and Ophthalmology, 1972.

41. Miller, M., and Folk, E. Strabismus associated with craniofacial anomalies. *Am. Orthoptic J.* 25:27, 1975.

42. Miller, M., and Pruzansky, S. Craniofacial Anomalies. In G. A. Peyman, D. R. Sanders, and M. F. Goldberg (Eds.), *Principles and Practice of Ophthalmology.* Philadelphia: Saunders, 1980. Vol. 3, p. 2354.

43. Miller, M. Personal observations, 1974.

44. Miller M., and Piest, K. Strabismus and refractive errors in mandibulofacial dysostosis. Unpublished data, 1984.

45. Morax, S., and Barraro, P. Signification du syndrome V avec double "upshoot." *J. Ophtalmol. Fr.* 1983.

46. Morax, S., and Beaumont, C. Relationship between motor defects of the eyes and cranio-orbital-facial malformations. Presented at the 4th International Symposium in Orbital Disorders, Amsterdam, 1981.

47. Mustardé, J. C. Congenital deformities in the orbital region. *Proc. R. Soc. Med.* 64:1121, 1971.

48. Ortiz-Monasterio, F., Fuente DelCampo, A., and Limon-Brown, E. Mechanism and Connection of V Syndrome in Craniofacial Dysostosis. In P. Tessier et al. (Eds.), *Symposium on Plastic Surgery in the Orbital Region.* St. Louis: Mosby, 1976. p. 246.

49. Parks, M. M., and Costenbader, F. D. Craniofacial

dysostosis (Crouzon's disease). *Am. J. Ophthalmol.* 33:782, 1959.

50. Piest, K. Miller, M., and Pruzanksy, S. Unpublished data, 1982.

51. Pruzansky, S., Miller, M., and Kammer, J. F. Ocular Defects in Craniofacial Syndromes. In M. F. Goldberg (Ed.), *Genetic and Metabolic Eye Disease* (1st ed.) Boston: Little, Brown, 1974. Pp. 487–498.

52. Robb, R. M. Objective measurement of interpupillary distance. *Pediatrics* 44:973, 1969.

53. Sherne, J. Dislocation of the eyeball as a complication of oxycephaly. *Br. Med. J.* 1:565, 1938.

54. Smith, J. L., and Stowe, F. R. The Pierre Robin syndrome (glossoptosis, micrognathia, cleft palate): A review of 39 cases with emphasis on associated ocular lesions. *Pediatrics* 27:128, 1961.

55. Stickler, G. B., et al. Hereditary progressive arthro-ophthalmopathy. *Mayo Clin. Proc.* 40:433, 1965.

56. Temtamy, S., and McKusick, V. A. Absence deformities as a part of syndrome. *Birth Defects* 14(3):73, 1973.

57. Tessier, P. Recent Improvements in Treatment of Facial and Cranial Deformities of Crouzon's Disease and Apert's Syndrome. In P. Tessier et al. (Eds.), *Symposium on Plastic Surgery in the Orbital Region.* St. Louis: Mosby, 1976. P. 271.

58. Tessier, P. Personal communication.

59. Urrets-Zavalía, A., Jr. Familial primary hypoplasia of the orbital margin. *Trans. Am. Acad. Ophthalmol. Otolaryngol.* 59:42, 1955.

60. Urrets-Zavalía, A., Jr., Solares-Zamora, J., and Olmos, H. R. Anthropological studies on the nature of cyclovertical squint. *Br. J. Ophthalmol.* 45:578, 1961.

61. Vignaud, J. Part III: Radiological Study of the Normal Skull in Premature and Newborn Infants. In F. Falkner (Ed.), *Human Development.* Philadelphia: Saunders, 1966.

62. Von Graefe, A. Ueber Neuroretinitis und gewisse Fallefulminirender Erblindung. *Albrecht von Graefes Arch. Klin. Exp. Ophthalmol.* 12:114, 1886.

63. Walker, J., and Wybar, K. Ocular Motility Problems in Craniofacial Dysostosis. In S. Moore, J. Mein, and L. Stockbridge (Eds.), *Orthoptics: Past, Present, Future.* New York: Grune & Stratton, 1976. P. 299.

64. Warkany, J. *Congenital Malformations: Notes and Comments.* Chicago: Year Book, 1971.

65. Weinstock, F. J., and Hardesty, H. H. Absence of superior recti in craniofacial dysostosis. *Arch. Ophthalmol.* 74:152, 1965.

66. Whitacker, L. A., et al. Combined report and complications in 793 craniofacial operations. *Plast. Reconstr. Surg.* 64:198, 1979.

67. Zaki, H. A. A., and Kenney, A. H. The bony orbital walls in horizontal strabismus. *Arch. Ophthalmol.* 57:418, 1957.

10

Strabismus

Marilyn T. Miller
Eugene R. Folk

DEFINITION OF STRABISMUS

For the purpose of this chapter, we define *strabismus* as any intermittent or constant abnormal ocular muscle imbalance that results in the object of regard not falling simultaneously on both maculae. The deviation may be present in one or all fields of gaze. We include microtropia herein but exclude phoria (unless associated with intermittent deviations). Because poor fusional amplitudes or other abnormal sensory states may be important factors in the causation of strabismus, they are discussed from that perspective but not as a form of strabismus. The rationale for this separation is that in most reports the incidence of strabismus in various populations is usually based on ocular misalignment (constant or intermittent).

Although some studies have not been designed to identify patients with microtropia, we have somewhat arbitrarily included this deviation under forms of strabismus. The cause of strabismus, the risk factors for the production of the ocular deviation, and the influence of genetic information on these characteristics are very complex and confusing. Although it would be desirable to omit the relationship of heterophoria to manifest deviations of any type, this is not possible as heterophoria is most often defined as a "latent strabismus," which implies that it is a risk factor for the development of strabismus. This, however, is not necessarily an accepted position, and whether the causes of heterophoria are genetic or environmental they could be different from those pro-

Supported in part by Grant EY-1792 from the National Eye Institute, Bethesda, Maryland.

ducing an intermittent or constant squint. On this controversial subject, we can only speculate that if families with a high frequency of manifest strabismus also have a high incidence of significant phorias, this would suggest that a tropia may often represent a "broken-down phoria." Waardenburg strongly suggests that esophoria and exophoria are inherited and that they may result in a manifest tropia if the degree of anomaly is severe or if there are secondary predisposing influences "which may be the product of accessory genes" [105]. He believes that the anomaly may be peripheral in nature but cannot exclude a central problem, although he rejects Worth's concept of primary disturbances of fusion [111].

In discussing the delicacy of coordinated ocular movement and "the non-obligatory, non-rigid and physiological nature of the system," Duke-Elder and Wybar noted that disturbances in ocular movement can result from a failure in the structural or functional development of the fixation reflexes [24]. Chavasse considers that obstructions of fixation reflexes fall into four main categories [62, 111]: (1) optical disease, which encompasses anisometropia, severe congenital ptosis, and intrinsic ocular abnormalities such as pathologic conditions of the cornea or ocular media or damage to the retina; (2) sensory obstructions that indicate failure of foveal development; (3) motor obstacles either static, such as anatomic factors, or kinetic, such as accommodation-convergence and neurogenic abnormalities; and (4) central obstructions. This last group is the most difficult to analyze as it often involves the concept of an anatomic fusion center. The work of Wiesel and Hubel has supplied some observable structural alteration to substantiate these theoretical considerations [109]. The role of genetic factors is fairly well documented in some of these groups of obstacles (e.g., various refractive errors, hereditary foveal developmental anomalies), while the hereditary influence of factors such as fusional deficiencies can only be inferred from statistics resulting from studies of family incidence. As in other types of genetic disease, the observed types of abnormalities may either be primary or secondary. For example, the abnormal shape or position of the bony orbit may modify the mechanical advantage of essentially normal ocular muscles, resulting in strabismus, amblyopia, and secondary changes in visual cortex. Possibly, some individuals with the same degree of structural deformity may not develop strabismus because of strong fusional reflexes or other central or refractive factors that are genetically influenced.

CATEGORIES OF STRABISMUS

To evaluate the genetic aspects of strabismus, we have decided somewhat arbitrarily to divide our discussion in this chapter into the following categories:

1. Concomitant strabismus with no known associated or myopathic disease in an otherwise "normal" child who has
   a. equal visual potential
   b. associated ocular abnormality or anisometropia
2. Strabismus associated with congenital systemic conditions or syndromes.
3. Congenital neurologic and restrictive motility abnormalities without other nonocular abnormalities.

Generalized myopathies with known hereditary patterns presenting at birth or early childhood have not been considered, although a few forms have familial patterns [107].

HISTORICAL CONSIDERATIONS

Role of Hereditary Factors

The importance of environmental influences or genetic factors on the causation of squint dates back to antiquity. Numerous legends offer explanations for misalignment of the eye, ranging from metaphysical or religious beliefs at one end of the spectrum (e.g., concepts of the "evil eye," various

displeasures of the gods) to environmental factors (such as malposition of the infant in the crib). Hippocrates noted that "children of parents having distorted eyes squint also for the most part" [44]. That strabismic parents beget strabismic offsprings is a well-accepted observation, but the incidence in families varies from 4 percent to a very high 52 percent in a report by Worth [111] and 65 percent in series by Pratt-Johnson and Lunn [82], Dufier and colleagues [23], and others [12, 24]. Such wide variations may relate to differences in sample size, definitions of strabismus, methods of ascertainment (i.e., history vs. examination), and the underlying incidence of squint in a target population. This last factor is most significant when using a multifactorial model.

In a large study of Greek strabismic children with affected first-degree relatives (brothers and sisters), Chimonidou and associates made some interesting observations [8]: (1) Of patients with early-onset strabismus, 42 percent had brothers or sisters with strabismus, compared to 54 percent with affected sibs in the later-onset squint patients. (2) Ninety-seven percent of sibs had the same type of strabismus as the proband. (3) About 50 percent of patients developed strabismus at about the same age as their sibs (within 1 year). These investigators examined one set of monozygotic twins who were raised in different environments. Both developed esotropia at age 3 years, which suggests a strong familial disposition for the development of strabismus.

Methods of Study

TWIN STUDIES

For the last 100 years research with twins has been a popular investigative approach in genetics for calculating the degree of genetic variability, the penetrance of a gene, and the significance of genetic and environmental factors in susceptibility to common disease. Comparison of the incidence of a trait, disease, or abnormality in monozygotic (MZ) twins is one of the most useful methods of arriving at these data. High degrees of concordance (both twins affected) do not necessarily imply high genetic susceptibility; significant differences between monozygotic and dizygotic (DZ) twin pairs also must be present to make this inference. For example, infectious disease shows a high concordance rate but does not imply significant genetic factors if it is equal in MZ and DZ twins. In 1875 Galton used the terms *nature* and *nurture* in his discussion of twin data [34], although he may not have understood all the implications of MZ and DZ twin evaluation.

The advantage of twin research is in the relative control of environmental (nongenetic) influences. Most differences in MZ pairs are assumed to be predominately due to environmental influences, although there also may be some random factors. These differences also occur in DZ pairs, but since DZ twins share only 50 percent of the genetic matter, they offer good control data. Numerous studies of genetic factors in strabismus have been based in part on data from twins [45, 57, 59, 86, 105, 107]. While this approach gives information on the degree of hereditary influence, it does not tell the mode of genetic transmission.

The "heritability" of a trait or disease is often used to imply the degree of genetic contribution to a specific phenotype and can be estimated from studies on twins using degrees of concordance. This method has significant limitations but is useful conceptually. Among the many formulas proposed to arrive at a numerical value [104], one simple formula proposed by Holzinger is as follows [47]:

$$H \text{ (heritability)} = C_{MZ} - C_{DZ}/100 - C_{DZ}.$$

C_{MZ} = percent concordance in monozygotic twins.

C_{DZ} = percent concordance in dizygotic twins.

The theoretical maximum is 1, and the minimum is 0. If the percentage of affected twins is the same in each group, implying an environmental cause, the value of H will be 0.

A heritability value allows the calculation of the approximate amount of phenotypic variation owing to genetic factors. Rubin and co-workers, using data from a survey of ophthalmologists of 50 countries, calculated heritability for a variety of ophthalmologic conditions and characteristics that might be considered obstructions to the development of fixation and fusion reflexes [86]. They concluded that the traits with high genetic influences ($H > 0.50$) are exotropia, hyperopia, and myopia; those with moderate genetic influences ($0.49 \geq H \geq 0.30$) include astigmatism, eccentric fixation, amblyopia, esotropia, and hyperopia.

Waardenburg reviewed the literature on various characteristics of strabismus in twins and noted the following concordance rates [105]:

	Monozygotic Twins (No.)	Dizygotic Twins (No.)
Esotropia	81% (56)	14% (7)

Waardenburg also observed that a number of amblyopic (MZ) twins were discordant or had a significant difference in degree of amblyopia; he concluded that ambylopia was not a primary defect, but occurred secondary to strabismus rather than being the precipitating factor. His data on exotropia were less extensive and somewhat inconclusive. One method (Table 10-1) he used to analyze this problem was to compare the number of amblyopic patients between two different populations [105].

The concordance rates in MZ twins in various studies have not always been consistent. Weekers and co-workers, who found three pairs of MZ twins concordant in seven pairs studied, but noted that the level of ametropia was similar in six pairs, concluded that the strabismus was secondary to the refractive errors [108].

DeVries and Houtman reported on 17 pairs of MZ twins in which at least one twin had strabismus [20]. They found concordance in only 8 of 17 pairs; no neonatal or extraneous factors explained the discordance. In the concordant group a number of pairs showed a large manifest deviation in one twin and a microstrabismus in the other twin. They concluded that these findings support the concept of a common pathogenic factor, influenced by heredity, that may result in a variety of sensory and motor disturbances of the oculomotor system. This is in agreement with the findings of Crone and Velzeboer, who investigated the frequency of different types of strabismus, clinical features, and hereditary history in a population with squint [13]. They felt that their data were best explained by a large pathogenic factor resulting in a variety of ocular motility disturbances, particularly the convergent types. They further suggested that the categories of convergent strabismus are artificial if they are meant to imply different causal mechanisms.

Kvapilíková studied the sensory status of 34 pairs each of MZ and DZ twins [59]. A high correlation coefficient of foveolar fusion was noted in the MZ twins (0.81), compared with the DZ twins (0.58), resulting in a high hereditability quotient of 0.59. They concluded that there was more than a 50 percent hereditary component in the variability of fusion.

Richter's study of strabismic families included 39 pairs of twins (27 DZ, 12 MZ) [83, 84]. She found concordance in amblyopia and retinal correspondence in about 44 percent of MZ twins but in only about 17 percent of DZ twins. For strabismus the concordance was about 92 percent for

Table 10-1. *Degree of Amblyopia in Various Twin Groups with Convergent Squint*

	Degree of amblyopia (%)
Average of whole population	67–75
Concordant squinting MZ twins	69–74
Concordant and discordant squinting MZ twins (same sexes)	74
Concordant and discordant squinting DZ twins (same and mixed sexes)	63
Pairs of sibs or other family members	68+

MZ = monozygotic; DZ = dizygotic.
Source: From P. J. Waardenburg [105].

Table 10-2. *Concordance of Concomitant Strabismus in 39 Pairs of Twins*

Twins	Concordant	Discordant	Total
MZ	11	1	12
DZ	7	20	27
Total	18	21	39

MZ = monozygotic; DZ = dizygotic.
Source: From S. Richter [84].

MZ pairs and about 26 percent for DZ pairs (Table 10-2). When concordance in MZ twins was four times higher than in DZ pairs, a multifactorial mode of inheritance was considered very probable.

It has been difficult to pool the data on twins or to arrive at a definite conclusion, because the methods of data collection and characteristics being evaluated are frequently different.

INCIDENCE OF STRABISMUS IN POPULATION AND FAMILIES

In analyzing any pathologic state in a population it is necessary to establish the criteria for those individuals considered affected, then determine by some unbiased, comprehensive method the frequency of the condition in the population of interest, and finally compare the incidence in various populations [1, 13, 49, 98, 105]. This is a very difficult and perhaps almost impossible task in strabismus. The affected individuals are usually young and not seriously ill and can be detected only by experienced examiners or sophisticated screening techniques. For example, the child with a microtropia cannot be identified by simple diagnostic screening. Similarly, it is misleading to compare prevalence of strabismus in two dissimilar populations without constant and controlled examination conditions. Therefore any figures of frequency from, for example, racially or culturally different groups, must be scrutinized closely as to how they were obtained before comparative conclusions can be proposed.

The accuracy of positive family history is often questionable. Obtaining data on frequency by questionnaire yields significant biases. The failure to recognize noncosmetic deviations that can be identified only through examination produces a high false-negative group, whereas epicanthal folds and facial anomalies producing pseudostrabismus give an inappropriately high number of affected individuals.

Kornder and colleagues studied the prevalence of strabismus in school-aged children in British Columbia identified by screening personnel with different training backgrounds compared with those identified by various batteries of screening examinations [58]. There was a significant difference in results between trained and untrained examiners and also between rates obtained from subjective methods only compared with objective plus subjective methods of evaluation. The "missed" group was primarily children with intermittent exotropia. The prevalence of strabismus obtained using a battery of tests was 4.5 percent. In this group 35 percent gave a positive response to one or more of three questions involving family members with eyes that turned in or out, poor vision in one eye from childhood, and wearing glasses before school age. In children with manifest squint, about 60 percent had a convergent squint and 38 percent a divergent squint.

Another important approach is to identify genetic and environmental differences by comparing the incidence of strabismus and refractive errors in an immigrant population of a given racial or cultural background to that of a native-born population. A comparison may also be made with the incidence in the immigrant population's country of birth. Eustace used this approach to study the prevalence of strabismus and refractive errors in second-generation West Indian children born in Birmingham, England, relating it to previous studies done on white children in the same hospital [28]. The prevalence of divergent squint was four times higher in the West Indian population than in the white group. Myopia was significantly more frequent in both types of squint, especially divergent, in the West Indian population. Amblyopia also was more common in that

Table 10-3. *Racial Distribution of Types of Esotropia in 500 Consecutive Children Referred to the Orthoptic Clinic, Honolulu*

| Race | Type of esotropia | | Total |
	Accommodative (or partly accommodative)	Nonaccommodative	
Caucasian	96 (79%)	26 (21%)	122
Oriental	33 (50%)	33 (50%)	66
Mixed	22 (51%)	21 (49%)	43
Total	151	80	231

Source: From M. R. Ing and S. W. Pang [49].

Table 10-4. *Population Frequency and Onset Time in Concomitant Squint (Swedish Children)*

Type of squint	Population frequency (%) (by 6 years)	Onset time
Constant esotropia	2.59 ± 0.205	45% in 1st year
Intermittent esotropia (corrected for loss)	0.93 ± 0.124	Developed equally each year
Constant exotropia	0.13 ± 0.047	Primarily 1st year
Intermittent exotropia	0.30 ± 0.071	40–50% 1st year
Vertical (not paretic)	0.05 ± 0.029	
Total (corrected)	4.0	—

Source: From W. Nördlow [79].

group, but perhaps the most significant finding was that anisometropia greater than 2 diopters existed in 65 percent of cases of amblyopia. Although information from a control population is necessary to make a final conclusion, these data suggest that anisometropia results in amblyopia, which may be the major factor contributing to the production of squint.

Racial differences in the distribution and incidence of concomitant strabismus have frequently been reported [46, 49, 63, 73, 75, 105–107]. Some studies have shown a lower rate of strabismus in the black population, with less accommodative esotropia than exotropia [49, 73, 75]. Ing and Pang showed a difference between accommodative and nonaccommodative esotropia in a Hawaiian population (Table 10-3) [49]. Nördlow examined 6,000 Swedish children to establish characteristics of concomitant convergent, divergent, and vertical squint (Table 10-4) [79].

RISK FACTORS FOR STRABISMUS

The concept of risk factors in strabismus implies either multifactorial inheritance or at least more than a monogenic mode of genetic transmission. These factors may be additive (and of near-equal value) or involve either accessory genes or environmental influences that modify the penetrance of a dominant gene. At this time these are theoretical and statistical considerations. What seems quite clear is that a variety of factors may contribute to the development of strabismus in a child.

An analysis of risk factors is more than an exercise to prove a multifactorial type of inheritance of ocular deviations. It offers the opportunity for better insight into the causation of strabismus and early identification of affected children, thus potentially affording an opportunity to intervene before a manifest deviation develops with ensuing sensory complications [50, 51]. If high hyperopia were a well-established risk factor in a family "predisposed" to the development of accommodative esotropia, early refraction and the prescription of a hyperopic correction in the very young child in this family would seem a rational approach. Unfortunately it would be difficult to prove the effectiveness of this preventive treatment in a prospective study, unless a large randomized clinical trial were initiated.

There have been many research efforts attempting to identify potential risk factors in strabismus [31]. One extensive study was undertaken at the University of Iowa in 1967 [39, 42, 43, 64–68, 78, 89, 91, 95–97]. A quantative methodologic approach was utilized to give information on the extent to which offspring resemble their parents for a large number of orthoptic and ophthalmologic measures, that is, to study the relative influence of genetic versus environmental factors on expression of a given trait. The relationship was expressed as the degree of heritability (h^2). To relate this information to the cause of strabismus, a second determination was undertaken associating these characteristics with the actual occurrence of strabismus. These investigators compared the phenotype and genetic variant, the mean, the heritability, and the relationship among the variables in families of children with concomitant strabismus with a control family population. Their work suggested that refractive error, convergence and divergence amplitudes, and accomodative convergence/ accomodation (AC/A) ratio were important variables; that convergence and divergence amplitudes were primary biologic differences in strabismic and nonstrabismic families with refractive errors; and that AC/A in some way interacted with these differences [96]. An interpretation of this type of information in the framework of the multifactorial model suggested that certain measurable characteristics that display a genetic predisposition alone do not cause or result in strabismus but that other factors (genetic or environmental) place the individual nearer the threshold for the development of strabismus.

Schlossman and Priestly in their study of 158 patients with strabismus in New York noted a positive family history in about 50 percent of those with esotropia and 37 percent of those with exotropia [87]. They reported that the direction of squint was almost always the same in affected family members, but that the subtype varied within the family. An interesting observation was that family members reacted similarly to surgical procedures. The authors felt that amblyopia and retinal correspondence were not inherited. They also suggested that there were at least two categories of causes of strabismus and each may have different modes of inheritance. The first category was defects in ectoderm involving nerve tissues; the second, defects in mesoderm causing abnormalities of structure or location of ocular muscles. Hyperopia was thought to be a risk factor in Schlossman and Priestly's study, but there was

not a direct correlation between the degree of hyperopia and the amount of squint [87]. Hyperopia may have played a significant role in the development of strabismus; once the squint occurred, however, the amount of deviation was not related to this degree of hyperopia in a dose-related manner. Amblyopia also appeared to be a secondary phenomenon and not genetically determined.

There is certainly no unanimity among studies concerning the relative importance of refractive error as a causal factor in strabismus, although many investigators believe that it is particularly important in accommodative esotropia [13, 69, 83, 84, 106, 108]. It is agreed, however, that refractive errors are strongly genetically determined. Sorsby and associates showed that the coefficient of correlation in studies on twins approaches the value expected for a quantative measure of inheritance from a number of additive genes contributing to the feature studied, that is, unity for MZ and 0.5 for DZ twins [93, 94]. Each component of refraction (e.g., corneal curvature) also shows independent normal distribution. Parent-sib and sib-sib studies also have supported this polygenic mode of inheritance in the refractive range between $+6$ and -4 diopters, although there is some evidence that the extreme ends of the refractive curves may have strong monogenic influence [93]. If refractive errors are a major contributor to some types of strabismus, then almost by definition there is a multifactorial inheritance, since refraction appears quite clearly to be due to multiple genes.

The risk factors and genetics of microtropia have been discussed by a number of authors who compared families of patients with microtropia to a control group [6, 60]. Cantolino and von Noorden found an increased incidence of primary micro-

Table 10-5. *Ocular Findings in Families* of Patients with Microtropia and Control Families*

Finding	Microtropic families	Control families
Strabismus	14/92 (15%)	3/77 (4%)
Sensory and motor anomalies	50/92 (54%)	20/77 (26%)
Refractive errors	28/92 (30%)	12/77 (16%)
Anisometropia	8/92 (9%)	1/77 (1%)
Microtropia	7/92 (8%)	0

*Parents and siblings.
Source: From S. J. Cantolino and G. K. von Noorden [6].

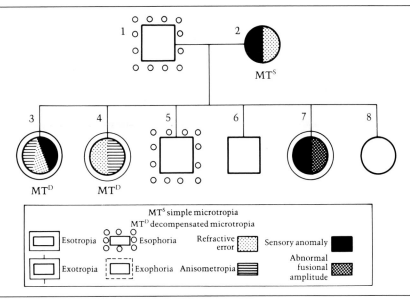

Fig. 10-1. *Pedigrees of microtropic propositi indicating associated refractive, sensory, and motor anomalies. (From S. J. Cantolino and G. K. von Noorden, Heridity in micoropia, Arch. Ophthalmol. 81: 753, 1969.)*

tropia in the families and also "decompensated microtropia," that is, microtropia occurring in other forms of esotropia after treatment [6]. They also noted a high level of sensory and motor anomalies in the microtropia group (54%) compared with control families (26%) (Table 10-5 and Fig. 10-1). There was more anisometropia (8.7% vs. 1.3%) in family members of children with strabismus than in the control families. These authors suggested that microtropia may be inherited in a multifactorial manner by the additive effect of many risk factors.

CONCOMITANT SQUINT

Possible Modes of Inheritance

Concomitant strabismus in patients without evidence of systemic abnormalities or an obvious medical or neurologic abnormality is the most common type of ocular motility disturbance. Authors have proposed both dominant and recessive types of autosomal mendelian transmission [17, 32, 87, 105]. More recently, a multifactorial mode of inheritance has been postulated as the best explanation of the familial tendency often observed in this large group of children [38, 52, 83, 84]. Because of the present popularity of this theory,

and the authors' personal bias, this mode will be considered in greater depth.

Multifactorial inheritance has been offered as the basis of many diseases. The more common types usually are neural tube defects and cleft palate. Many physical traits also appear to be controlled by multiple genes. Common examples of such traits are fingerprints, iris color and structure, refraction, height and weight, intelligence, and skin pigment [7, 39, 93, 94]. The hereditary component of certain forms of glaucoma also may be explained best by multifactorial transmission [33]. These entities show a familial aggregation; there is a higher incidence in families of the index case than in the population in general, but the inheritance pattern cannot be simply explained by a single-gene mode of transmission, environmental influences, or chromosomal aberrations [26, 27].

The conclusion that both genetic and environmental risk factors contribute to the development of strabismus is an attractive but at this point only a statistical concept not well proved or understood. The pattern of inheritance of many diseases believed to be on a multifactorial basis can often be explained by using one or two genes and varying the penetrance, frequency, and expressivity [10]. This is particularly true if combinations of dominant and recessive genes are used.

A few terms are frequently employed in the discussion of the theory and application of multifactorial inheritance. These expressions are not

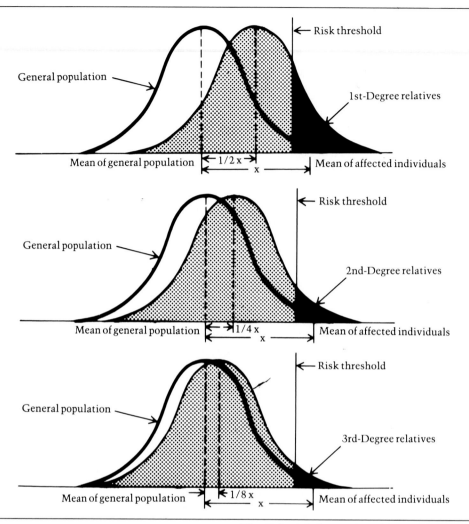

Fig. 10-2. *Multifactorial model patterns. "Normal" curves show size of risk group in relatives of differing consanguinity (dark areas) compared with that in general population (dotted areas). (From C. O. Carter, Multifactorial Genetic Disease, in V. McKusick and R. Clairborne [Eds.],* Medical Genetics, *New York: H. P. Publishing, 1973.).*

always uniformly defined, but the following are those most frequently used:

1. *Polygenic trait or disease*: a condition caused by the action of multiple genes, each having a small effect. A few conditions appear to result from many genes, with an additive effect and no environmental influences. While pure polygenic conditions are unlikely, they are integral to the understanding of multifactorial inheritance. There are, however, traits or diseases that may be influenced more by many genes than by the environment.
2. *Multifactorial trait or disease*: a condition resulting from the action of multiple genes (polygenic) plus environmental factors.

3. *Additive factors or genes*: genes or factors that display no dominance in the heterozygotes, exist at independent loci, and act cumulatively on the phenotype.
4. *Continuous distribution*: continuous gradation of a trait or attribute that can be measured on a scale (i.e., height, weight, finger whorls). The distribution is a normative curve; most individuals are near the mean or within one standard deviation of it.

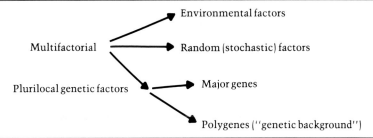

Fig. 10-3. *Vogel and Motulsky's modified conceptual model for causation of multifactorial disease. The importance of major genes is emphasized in the scheme. (From F. Vogel and A. G. Motulsky,* Human Genetics, *New York: Springer, 1979.)*

5. *Quasicontinuous distribution with "threshold effect"*: a model popularized by Falconer in which the genetic "liability" to a disease or a malformation is distributed continuously and is a result of many genes, acting usually in an additive fashion [29, 30]. The individual is not affected until a certain threshold is reached, that is, a certain critical number of factors, either genetic or environmental, are possessed (Fig. 10-2).

In its present form a multifactorial model implies a relatively numerous group of factors, environmental and genetic, that are essentially equal in value and demonstrate a normal distribution. The critics of this model point out that it is difficult to imagine a biologic system in which all factors contributing to a trait or risk for a disease state would be equal in importance and would have the same frequency in each population. This objection has resulted in modified multifactorial models in which "major gene" effects, dominance, and environmental effects have different degrees of importance (Fig. 10-3). However, if one increases the number of modifications, the new model cannot be differentiated statistically from two- and three-gene computerized models, especially when penetrance and recessiveness are considered in these theoretical systems.

The multifactorial mode of inheritance of disease with a threshold effect has the following characteristics and differences from either autosomal dominant (AD) or autosomal recessive (AR) modes of inheritance (Figs. 10-4 to 10-6): (1) The percentage of affected sibs is similar to the percentage of other affected first-degree relatives (not in AR). (2) There is a sharp decline in prevalence

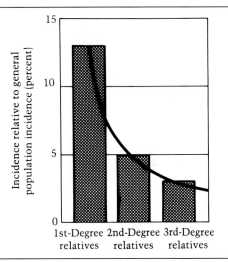

Fig. 10-4. *Theoretical curve derived from multifactorial model with threshold, as shown in Fig. 10-2. (From C. O. Carter,* Multifactorial Genetic Disease, *in V. McKusick and R. Claiborne [Eds.],* Medical Genetics, *New York: H. P. Publishing, 1973.)*

from first-degree to second-degree relatives (not AD). (3) The risk of recurrence varies from family to family (neither AR nor AD), with increased risk when there are greater numbers of affected near relatives, that is, when the family liability is higher. (4) If a difference in frequency exists between the sexes, there will be more affected relatives in the sex that exhibits the lowest population frequency (i.e., this group needs more liability factors to manifest the disease). A difference in frequency of strabismus in the two sexes has occasionally been noted [83, 84, 105]. (5) Consanguinity will increase the number of affected individuals (like AR). (6) The incidence in sibs is approximately equal to $\sqrt{p}$ (p = population incidence) [26, 27]. In one study from the Registry of Handicapped Children in Canada, $\sqrt{p}$ was 0.036 and the sib incidence was 0.035, which supports the polygenic model [90]. Risk of recurrence in a multifactorial model is based on the frequency of the

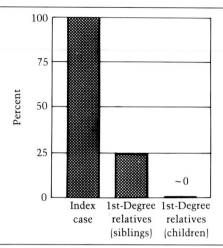

Fig. 10-5. *Single recessive gene model. This model fails to predict the observed incidence patterns in many common diseases thought to be inherited in a multifactorial manner, particularly the difference between first-degree sibs and first-degree children of affected individuals. (From C. O. Carter, Multifactorial Genetic Disease, in V. McKusick and R. Claiborne [Eds.], Medical Genetics, New York: H. P. Publishing, 1973.)*

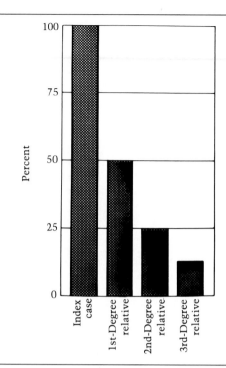

Fig. 10-6. *Single dominant gene model is equally nonpredictive. Here, in theory, the incidence should be directly proportional to the number of genes shared with the index case. (From C. O. Carter, Multifactorial Genetic Disease, in V. McKusick and R. Claiborne [Eds.], Medical Genetics, New York: H. P. Publishing, 1973.)*

disease in a population (*p*) and the number of presently affected family members [3, 15]. Curnow and Smith have devised one such set of calculations with various possible numbers of other affected parents, sibs, or both (Fig. 10-7) [15]. From their set of estimates, the recurrence risk of a disease with 4 percent frequency in the population for a third sib with two affected sibs would be approximately 30 percent (Fig. 10-7). It would be even higher if one or both parents were also affected.

The threshold concept is intellectually appealing to strabismologists because it would explain certain observed phenomenon, such as the development, in a few patients, of ocular deviations after minor interruptions in fusion that normally would not cause strabismus. For example, occasionally we observe a child who develops a squint that is not easily reversed after an eye has been patched for 1 day for a small corneal abrasion or comparably minor ocular problem. With the threshold concept of strabismus, one could postulate that the child's genetic liability had been just under the threshold, and that this minor environmental factor moved the degree of liability over the threshold, that is, from unaffected to affected.

In a study of a large population of families with strabismus, Dahlberg and Nördlow noted that their data would fit a recessive inheritance pattern with a population frequency of 2 to 3 percent and a penetrance of 30 to 35 percent [18]. However, their conclusion, based on general considerations and data in the literature, was that it probably was not a monohybrid type of hereditary pattern but, rather, that many genes and different types of inheritance were involved.

Dufier and colleagues studied 195 cases of idiopathic convergent concomitant squint and established three categories: alternating squint without amblyopia, squint with amblyopia, and accommodative squint [23]. After performing a complex segregation analysis, they concluded that if one assumes a monofactorial model (i.e., one gene locus) with genetic homogeneity and penetrance owing to chance and not genetic factors, the hypothesis of dominant autosomal inheritance with incomplete penetrance seems a more probable mode of inheritance than does recessive

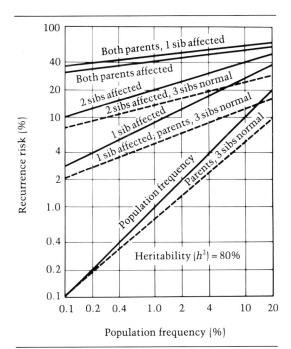

Fig. 10-7. *Recurrence risk for multifactorial inheritance in a variety of sibships with heritability of 80% Broken lines include normal relatives. (From R. N. Curnow and C. Smith, Multifactorial models for familial diseases in man, J. R. Stat. Soc. A 2: 131, 1975.)*

or multifactorial. However, this study did not permit the possibility of a few gene loci or mixed inheritance modes to be tested.

A study of French families with strabismus was conducted by Massin and Drouard [69]. They limited their study to families of strabismic children who had at least two affected siblings. They proposed that high hyperopia was dominantly inherited and suggested from their findings that the refractive error was genetically determined and the strabismus was a consequence. They also felt that essential convergent strabismus, that is, the type without significant hyperopia, showed a dominant mode of transmission. A few of the families had mixed types of convergent strabismus. Divergent strabismus also appeared to be dominantly inherited, with myopia noted in 50 percent of the patients. However, by including only families with two affected sibs of a strabismic child, they were analyzing only individuals at one tail of the multifactorial curve. Since the risk of recurrence of a multifactorially inherited disease is dependent on the frequency of the disease in the population and the number of already affected family members, in families that have a high "li-

ability" in a disease that has a significant population frequency (3–4%), a high ratio of affected parents and sibs will be present, and this may resemble a model of dominant inheritance with decreased penetrance (Fig. 10-7).

Rarely is the ophthalmologist asked by parents for a firm risk figure for the development of strabismus in future children, although they may inquire as to whether it "runs in the family." Genetic counseling requires that either a particular mode of inheritance is well established or that the approximate risks, based only on valid empirical data for the disease, are available. If a multifactorial type of inheritance is accepted for strabismus, then the recurrence risk will depend on the number of affected family members. Estimates then may be given using graphs or tables based on incidence of disease, heritability, and number of affected family members (Fig. 10-7) [3, 7, 14, 15, 54, 103].

Effect of Ocular Disease

Any impairment of vision can produce strabismus in many individuals, particularly if the involvement is asymmetric or unilateral. Children (or adults) with straight eyes and binocular vision frequently develop an ocular deviation within weeks after sustaining a serious injury. Older children and adults more frequently acquire exotropia than do very young children, in whom either esotropia or exotropia may result. In congenital cases, causal factors may range from easily visible disease such as cataract to a less obvious cause such as anisometropia.

Many genetically determined types of ophthalmic disease show an increased incidence of strabismus, either primary or secondary. A few examples would be Best's disease, Marfan's syndrome, certain hereditary cataracts, and nystagmus syndromes. Inheritance of the ocular defect follows well-recognized mendelian rules of inheritance, and the presence of strabismus relates to either the genetic background of the individual, the severity of the ocular pathology, or a combination of these [14]. However, not all patients with monocular or asymmetric pathology or anisometropia develop strabismus, which suggests that the individual's degree of genetic liability may affect whether strabismus ensues or the eyes remain straight. In the same way one could speculate that after the visual potential of the eye is improved, for example, by extracting a traumatic cataract, the success of restoring binocular vision and realigning the eyes may be partially influenced by genetic background of the individual.

STRABISMUS IN PATIENTS WITH ASSOCIATED NONOCULAR MALFORMATIONS

Apparent strabismus frequently is noted in children with genetic neurologic problems, metabolic diseases, chromosomal aberrations, and craniofacial malformations [36, 48, 71, 74, 92, 112]. Certain groups have a high incidence of associated ocular disease and secondary strabismus, in some craniofacial malformations the soft or bony craniofacial abnormalities result in pseudostrabismus, and in a few syndromes there may be a very characteristic form of strabismus (e.g., absence of abduction in Möbius' syndrome); however, in many conditions the strabismus is nonspecific but occurs at a high frequency. This nonspecific strabismus may be due to primary pathologic changes in the central nervous system adding another major liability factor for the development of strabismus in a susceptible individual. For example, in one series of patients with Waardenburg's syndrome, an autosomal dominant disease, 19 percent had convergent strabismus with no associated ocular pathology [19].

Exotropia in patients with hypertelorism is a very frequent finding, whether the hypertelorism is caused by median facial cleft, encephalocele, or craniosynostosis. A crucial question is whether the pattern results from the secondary, nonspecific, mechanical effect of an abnormally shaped bony orbit or from a primary defect of the central nervous or peripheral system or unusual muscle anomalies [74]. Possibly both explanations are correct for different syndrome types or even for different patients with the same syndrome.

The answer to this question becomes intriguing when considering the genetic implications of the strabismus. If it is only the degree of orbital separation that causes exotropia in most patients, then the anatomic deformity becomes the prime causal factor of the strabismus; however, it is possible that with only a moderate amount of hypertelorism the genetic background may be the determining factor as to whether a squint results. The strong influence of the anatomic malformation in hypertelorism is based on the observation that reconstructive surgery to reduce markedly the intraorbital distances frequently results in substantial improvement or cure of the exotropia [9].

Crouzon's and Apert's diseases are craniosynostosis syndromes with an autosomal dominant form of transmission. The orbits in the affected patients are markedly shallow and have other significant changes in shape. The most characteristic motility finding is a V pattern exotropia or esotropia with severely overacting inferior oblique muscles [71, 74]. Some patients also show underacting superior rectus muscles. While mechanical factors may be responsible for the motility disturbance, the anatomic finding at the time of ocular muscle surgery and on computed tomography scan indicates that the abnormal position and size of the ocular muscles play at least a contributory role [16, 21]. It could be speculated that the primary genetic influence causes changes in the normal development of the bony orbit in utero, and that the migration of the mesodermal tissue destined to be ocular muscles is secondarily affected, or, conversely, the genetic defect may directly disturb the normal development of some of the ocular muscles. It is very possible that superimposed mechanical factors modifying the action of the ocular muscles also may increase the characteristic V pattern noted in almost all even moderately affected patients.

Douglass attempted to identify complications of pregnancy and delivery that may be related to the development of strabismus in the infant [22]. In a study of children with early onset of squint he found a significantly high incidence of prematurity, spasticity, and mental retardation. A general increase in the incidence of other abnormalities (14.5%) suggested to him that many cases of early-onset strabismus are actually a type of congenital anomaly. He also noted strabismus in 50 percent of children and adults with cerebral palsy. The relationship of the development of squint to perinatal factors including prematurity was not established; there were variable types of data and a disagreement as to the degree and severity of the precipitating factors [13, 36, 79].

CONGENITAL INCOMITANT STRABISMUS

It seems desirable to separate the unusual category of incomitant strabismus into neurologic and restrictive syndromes, but in a number of clinical entities it is not completely established whether the restrictive motility is a secondary occurrence superimposed on a primary nuclear or peripheral cranial nerve palsy. Therefore both subgroups will be considered together, with emphasis on the clinical and genetic aspects.

Several unusual types of strabismus include limited ocular motility in some fields of gaze, no typical neurologic pattern, and restriction on forced duction testing. An example of this group is Duane's syndrome. Duane's retraction syndrome represents about 1 percent of all strabismus cases examined, making it an unusual but not rare form of ocular motor disturbance [55, 56]. While Duane's syndrome usually occurs as an isolated sporadic entity, familial patterns have been observed in 5 to 10 percent of cases [24, 81]. The most typical ocular motility findings are marked restriction on abduction, milder restriction on adduction, and retraction on adduction often accompanied by an upshoot or downshoot of the affected eye. Bilaterality is observed in about 20 percent of cases; females are more affected than males; the left eye is more frequently involved than the right. Further classifications of types of Duane's syndrome are dependent on deviations in primary position and relative limitations on horizontal gaze.

The hereditary tendency observed in Duane's syndrome is usually autosomal dominant transmission with incomplete penetrance and expressivity [25]. There are relatively few reports of affected twins, but concordance in MZ twins has been described [35, 70]. In one pair of twins there was a unilateral left eye involvement [35]; in another, a mirrorlike monocular situation existed [70]. Discordance in MZ twins also has been reported [85].

Many series in the literature indicate a variety of skeletal and hearing abnormalities in patients with Duane's syndrome [72, 80, 81]. The association is most frequently reported in two syndrome complexes—Wildervanck's syndrome and hemifacial microsomia, particularly the Goldenhar variant. From a pathologic perspective these syndrome complexes have hearing and ear abnormalities and cervical spine anomalies in common. Epibulbar dermoids are a frequent finding in the Goldenhar variant and also in a few cases of Wildervanck's syndrome [110]. The classic Wildervanck's syndrome (cervico-oculoacoustic) consists of the triad of Klippel-Feil anomalies of the spine, sensorineural deafness, and Duane's syndrome. Often patients manifest an incomplete syndrome. In contrast to those with hemifacial microsomia, patients with Wildervanck's syndrome frequently show a definite familial transmission with a predilection for females (50–70%). This has led some authors to suggest an X-linked dominant inheritance with lethality in males [110]. However, Kirkham postulates that the gene has incomplete penetrance with marked pleiotropic effects, and he believes that it is inherited in an autosomal dominant mode with factors modifying the expression in such a way that females are more at risk [55]. Hemifacial microsomia, on the other hand, usually occurs sporadically, although there is some evidence for a multifactorial mode of inheritance in some cases.

Another restrictive syndrome is congenital fibrosis syndrome. In its most extreme form a generalized fibrosis of almost all of the extraocular muscles results in a relatively immobile and fixed eye [5]. A much more common variant of the congenital fibrosis syndrome is characterized by bilateral ptosis and limitation of upward gaze with esotropia occurring when the patient attempts to look up. Exotropia may be present in downward gaze. The forced duction test is positive, and the muscles often appear fibrotic. The cause of the syndrome is unknown. It can be monocular as well as binocular, and there is often marked familial variation. We have one family in our clinic with two members who have a congenital fibrosis syndrome, each with a markedly different clinical appearance. One of the sibs has monocular involvement but all ocular muscles are affected, while the other sib has double levator palsy alone. Some families definitely exhibit an autosomal dominant inheritance pattern; however, autosomal recessive disease cannot be ruled out when only sibs manifest the disease [40].

Two interesting families with dominantly inherited congenital familial fibrosis, in which there was evidence of a nuclear or supranuclear causation, were reported by Cibis and co-workers [11]. This information supports a neurogenic cause with secondary fibrosis in these families.

Brown described a restrictive strabismus syndrome characterized by inability to elevate the eye in the adducted position, widening of palpebral fissures on adduction, and restriction in forced duction testing [4]. The congenital form is usually sporadic, but familial involvement has been described [37, 53].

Specific familial cranial nerve palsies have been reported not only of the sixth, third, and fourth nerves, but in also familial ptosis without associated ocular motility disturbances [41, 107]. In the TTV-OFM syndrome complex [100], which includes Möbius syndrome, a bilateral limitation of abduction has been reported in many. Most cases are sporadic but familial cases have been reported.

Chronic progressive external ophthalmoplegia is a slowly progressive paresis of the extraocular muscles and lid. It usually starts with ptosis and ultimately involves all of the muscles. The Urist version reflex test or other tests sensitive to small limitations of ocular movement frequently show the early manifestations of the weakening of the extraocular muscles in all cardinal positions of gaze [102]. Chronic progressive external ophthalmoplegia is a component of the Kearns-Sayre syndrome [2, 61, 77]. The most serious complication is a heart block that may occur in young people. Pigmentary degeneration of the retina is reported in some patients, in addition to various other anomalies. Both autosomal dominant and autosomal recessive pedigrees have been proposed in familial cases, although the disease more frequently occurs sporadically [88].

Blepharophimosis is a congenital disorder characterized by bilateral ptosis, a shortened palpebral fissure, epicanthus inversus, and a temporal displacement of the lower puncta. The patient may show pseudostrabismus, but at times there is an associated manifest deviation. Families demonstrating autosomal dominant transmission are well documented, but many authors have noted that the trait is transmitted more frequently through males than females. This finding has been explained by the association with primary amenorrhea in some affected females [101, 113]. It has been proposed that there are two different types of blepharophimosis based on the hormonal disturbance in the female [113].

CONCLUSIONS

Genetic factors in strabismus have been repeatedly investigated using many approaches: (1) the frequency of a positive family history obtained in children with strabismus; (2) the identification and relative importance of risk factors for development of common forms of ocular deviation; (3) the heritability of different types of squint and various ophthalmologic characteristics such as refraction and AC/A ratio; (4) the modes of inheritance that would be consistent with the experimental data; and (5) comparative studies of types of squint and risk factors as they relate to different cultural, geographic, or racial populations.

From these studies the one thing that appears irrefutable is that there is a significant hereditary component to the development of all types of concomitant squint, but that the familial incidence rates vary greatly, ranging from very low figures to 65 percent in some studies. One explanation of this difference is that true frequency differences do exist in populations because of different gene pools. Another important explanation is that the ascertainment of affected individuals is not constant from study to study.

One or more mendelian models of inheritance may adequately fit any one set of experimental results, especially if the postulated level of penetrance is low, but there is no model that is consistent with even the majority of studies on the inheritance of strabismus. There are many investigators who suggest that a multifactorial mode best explains the statistical data, although other complex two-gene mendelian models frequently also are statistically compatible. A more compelling argument for multifactorial inheritance is that a number of ophthalmologic measurements such as refraction and certain sensory characteristics show significant levels of heritability and also appear to be causal factors in the development of strabismus. Here, too, there is not a high level of agreement between the studies on the importance of any one factor as a major cause of a deviation.

A number of ophthalmologic or systemic syndromes have an associated high incidence of strabismus, which may be secondary to ocular malformations or a result of primary involvement of the oculomotor system centrally or peripherally. It is difficult to extract from these findings definite conclusions concerning strabismus in the normal child, although they may give some evidence that anatomic factors may play more of a role in the development of concomitant deviations than previously thought.

If it can be concluded from family studies that certain children are at significant risk for strabismus, some preventive actions might be possible. For these to be successful, the contributing factors for the development of squint must be identifiable in young children, and some practical intervention must be available. Such intervention would be very desirable, even if only for a small number of children, to prevent the abnormal, often irreversible, sensory adaptations that follow. At our present state of knowledge, however, this is only occasionally a practicable consideration.

REFERENCES

1. Adelstein, A. M., and Scully, J. Epidemiological aspects of squint. *Br. Med. J.* 3:334, 1967.
2. Bastiaensen, L., et al. Kearns syndrome: A heterogeneous group of disorders with CPEO, or a nosological entity? *Doc. Ophthalmol.* 52:207, 1982.
3. Bonaiti-Pellie, C., and Smith, C. Risk tables for ge-

netic counselling in some congenital malformations. *J. Med. Genet.* 11:374, 1974.

4. Brown, H. W. True and simulated superior oblique tendon sheath syndrome. *Doc. Ophthalmol.* 34:123, 1973.

5. Burian, H. M., and von Noorden, G. K. *Binocular Vision and Ocular Motility: Theory and Management of Strabismus.* St. Louis: Mosby, 1974. P. 388.

6. Cantolino, S. J., and von Noorden, G. K. Heredity in microtropia. *Arch. Ophthalmol.* 81:753, 1969.

7. Carter, C. O. Multifactorial Genetic Disease. In V. McKusick and R. Claiborne (Eds.), *Medical Genetics.* New York: H. P. Publishing, 1973. P. 199.

8. Chimonidou, E., et al. Family distribution of concomitant squint in Greece. *Br. J. Ophthalmol.* 61:27, 1977.

9. Choy, A. E., et al. Analysis of Preoperative and Postoperative Extraocular Muscle Function in Surgical Translocation of Bony Orbits: A Preliminary Report. In I. M. Converse, J. C. McCarthy, and D. Wood-Smith (Eds.). *Symposium on Diagnosis and Treatment of Craniofacial Anomalies.* St. Louis: Mosby, 1979. P. 128.

10. Chung, C. S., Ching, G. H. S., and Morton, N. E. A genetic study of cleft lip and palate in Hawaii: II. Complex segregation analysis and genetic risks. *Am. J. Hum. Genet.* 26:177, 1974.

11. Cibis, G. W., et al. Electromyography in Congenital Familial Ophthalmoplegia. In R. Reinedke (Ed.). *Strabismus II. Proceedings of the 4th Meeting of the International Strabismological Association, Asilomar, California, 1982.* New York: Grune & Stratton, 1984.

12. Cohn, H. Über vererbruny und Behandlung des Einwarts—Schieln. *Berl. Klin. Wochenschr.* 41:1047, 1904.

13. Crone, R. A., and Velzeboer, C. M. Statistics in strabismus in the Amsterdam youth. *Arch. Ophthalmol.* 55:455, 1956.

14. Cross, H. E. The heredity of strabismus. *Am. Orthoptic J.* 25:11–17, 1975.

15. Curnow, R. N., and Smith, C. Multifactorial models for familial diseases in man. *J. R. Stat. Soc. A* 2:131, 1975.

16. Cuttone, J., et al. Absence of the superior rectus in Apert's syndrome. *J. Pediatr. Ophthalmol. Strabismus* 16:349, 1979.

17. Czellitzer, A. Wie vererbt sich Schielen? *Klin. Monatsbl. Augenheilkd.* 79:519, 1922.

18. Dahlberg, G., and Nördlow, W. Genetics of convergent strabismus. *Acta Genet.* 2:1, 1951.

19. Dellemon, J. W., and Hageman, M. J. Ophthalmological findings in 34 patients with Waardenburg syndrome. *J. Pediatr. Ophthalmol. Strabismus* 15:341, 1978.

20. DeVries, B., and Houtman, W. A. Squint in monozygotic twins. *Doc. Ophthalmol.* 46:305, 1979.

21. Diamond, G. R., et al. Variations on extraocular muscle number and structure in craniofacial dysostosis. *Am. J. Ophthalmol.* 90:146, 1980.

22. Douglass, A. A. Nature and cause of squint of early onset. *Br. Orthoptic J.* 21:29, 1964.

23. Dufier, J. L., et al. Inheritance in the etiology of convergent squint. *Ophthalmologica* 179:225, 1979.

24. Duke-Elder, S., and Wybar, K. Ocular Motility and Strabismus. In S. Duke-Elder (Eds.), *System of Ophthalmology,* Vol. 6. St. Louis: Mosby, 1973.

25. Duke-Elder, S. *Textbook of Ophthalmology.* St Louis: Mosby, 1963. Vol. 3, Part 2, pp. 991–996.

26. Edwards, J. H. The simulation of Mendelism. *Acta Genet.* 10:63, 1960.

27. Edwards, J. H. Familial predisposition in man. *Br. Med. Bull.* 25:58, 1969.

28. Eustace, P. Myopia and divergent squint in West Indian children. *Br. J. Ophthalmol.* 56:559, 1972.

29. Falconer, D. S. Validity of the theory of genetic correlation. *J. Hered.* 45:42, 1954.

30. Falconer, D. S. The inheritance of liability to diseases with variable age of onset, with particular reference to diabetes mellitus. *Ann. Hum. Genet.* 31:1, 1967.

31. Franceschetti, A. T., and Burian, H. M. Gradient accommodative convergence/accommodative ratio in families with and without esotropia. *Am. J. Ophthalmol.* 70:558, 1970.

32. François, J.: *L'hérédité en Ophtalmologie.* Paris: Masson, 1958. Vol. 4, p. 291.

33. François, J. Genetic predisposition to glaucoma. *Dev. Ophthalmol.* 3:1, 1981.

34. Galton, F. The history of twins as a criterion of the relative powers of nature and nurture. *J. Anthropol. Inst.* 5:391, 1875.

35. Gedda, L., and Magistretti, S. Paracinesia adduttorio-enoftalmica gemello-familiane e albinismo oculare in altra famiglia. *Acta. Genet. Med. Gemellol (Roma)* 5:291, 1956.

36. Goldstein, H., et al. Perinatal factors associated with strabismus in Negro children. *Am. J. Public Health* 57:217, 1967.

37. Gowan, M., and Levy, J. Heredity in the superior oblique tendon sheath syndrome. *Br. Orthoptic J.* 25:91, 1968.

38. Griffin, J. R., et al. Heredity in congenital esotropia. *J. Am. Optom. Assoc.* 50:1237, 1979.

39. Grützner, P., Yazawa, K., and Spivey, B. E. Heredity and strabismus. *Surv. Ophthalmol.* 14:441, 1970.

40. Harley, R. D., Rodrigues, M. M., and Crawford, J. S. Congenital fibrosis of the extraocular muscles. *J. Pediatr. Ophthalmol.* 15:346, 1978.

41. Harris, D. J., Jr., et al. Familial congenital superior oblique palsy. Presented at the American Academy of Ophthalmology Meeting, November 1984, Atlanta, Georgia.

42. Hegmann, J. P., and DeFriess, J. C. Are genetic correlations and environmental correlations correlated? *Nature* 226:284, 1970.

43. Hegmann, J. P., Mash, A. J., and Spivey, B. E. Genetic analysis of human visual parameters in populations with varying incidences of strabismus. *Am. J. Hum. Genet.* 26:549, 1974.

44. Hippocrates. Air, water and places. In *The Genuine Works of Hippocrates*, transl. by F. Adams. New York: William Wood, 1886. P. 171.

45. Hofstetter, H. W. Accommodative convergence in identical twins. *Am. J. Optom. Arch. Am. Acad. Optom.* 25:480, 1948.

46. Holm, S. Le strabisme concomitant chez les pale-negrides au Gabon, Afrique Equatoriale Française: Contribution à la question de race et de strabisme. *Acta Ophthalmol.* 17:361, 1939.

47. Holzinger, K. J. The relative effect of nature and nuture influences on twin differences: I. *Educ. Psychol.* 20:241, 1929.

48. Howard, R. Chromosomal disease and strabismus. *Am. Orthoptic J.* 27:138, 1977.

49. Ing, M. R., and Pang, S. W. The Racial Distribution of Strabismus. In R. D. Reinecke (Ed.), *Strabismus: Proceedings of the 3rd Meeting of International Strabismological Association, May 1978, Japan.* New York: Grune & Stratton, 1978.

50. Ingram, R. M. The problem of screening children for visual defects. *Br. J. Ophthalmol.* 61:4, 1977.

51. Ingram, R. M. Refraction as a basis for screening children for squint and amblyopia. *Br. J. Ophthalmol.* 61:8, 1977.

52. Isenberg, S. Genetic Aspects of Strabismus. In A. Emery and D. Rimoin (Eds.), *Principles and Practice of Medical Genetics*, Vol. 1. Edinburgh: Churchill Livingstone, 1983.

53. Katz, N. N., Whitmore, P. U., and Beauchoup, G. R. Brown's syndrome in twins. *J. Pediatr. Ophthalmol. Strabismus* 18:32, 1981.

54. Keith, C. G. Genetics and counselling in ophthalmology. *Aust. J. Ophthalmol.* 9:74, 1981.

55. Kirkham, T. H. Genetics and Duane's syndrome. *Br. J. Ophthalmol.* 27:74, 1970.

56. Kirkham, T. H. Inheritance of Duane's syndrome. *Br. J. Ophthalmol.* 54:323, 1970.

57. Kondo, K., Mori, E., and Adachi, K. A study on squint in 21 cases of monozygotic twins. *Folia Ophthalmol. Jpn.* 26:166, 1975.

58. Kornder, L. D., et al. Detection of manifest strabismus in young children. *Am. J. Ophthalmol.* 77:211, 1974.

59. Kvapilíková, K. Heredity of the fusion capacity. *Cesk. Oftalmol.* 25:332, 1969.

60. Lang, J. Microtropia. *Int. Ophthalmol.* 6:33, 1983.

61. Leveille, A. S., and Newell, F. N. Autosomal dominant Kearns Sayre syndrome. *Ophthalmology (Rochester)* 87:99, 1980.

62. Lyle, T. K., and Bridgman, G. J. *Worth and Chavasse Squint.* London: Bailliere, Tindall & Cox, 1959.

63. Mann, I. *Culture, Race and Climate and Eye Disease: An Introduction to the Study of Geographical Ophthalmology.* Springfield, Ill.: Thomas, 1966.

64. Mash, A. J., and Spivey, B. E. Genetic aspects of strabismus. *Doc. Ophthalmol.* 34:285, 1973.

65. Mash, A. J., et al. Strabismus. In M. F. Goldberg (Eds.), *Genetic and Metabolic Eye Disease* (1st ed.). Boston: Little, Brown, 1974. P. 261.

66. Mash, A. J., Hegmann, J. P., and Spivey, B. E. Genetic analysis of indices of corneal power and corneal astigmatism in human populations with varying incidences of strabismus. *Invest. Ophthalmol.* 14:826, 1975.

67. Mash, A. J., Hegmann, J. P., and Spivey, B. E. Genetic analysis of vergence measures in populations with varying incidences of strabismus. *Am. J. Ophthalmol.* 79:978, 1975.

68. Mash, A. J., Hegmann, J. P., and Spivey, B. E. Genetic analysis of cover test measures and AC/A ratio in human populations with varying indices of strabismus. *Br. J. Ophthalmol.* 59:380, 1975.

69. Massin, M., and Drouard, E. Contribution à l'étude des strabismes concomitants familiaux. *Ann. Ocul. (Paris)* 198:323, 1965.

70. Mehdorn, E., and Kommerell, G. Inherited Duane's syndrome: Mirror-like localization of oculomotor disturbances in monozygotic twins. *J. Pediatr. Ophthalmol. Strabismus* 16:152, 1979.

71. Miller, M. Ocular motility problems in craniosynostosis syndromes (abstract). *Invest. Ophthalmol.* 2:1972.

72. Miller, M. T., and Pruzansky, S. Craniofacial Anomalies. In G. A. Peyman, D. R. Sanders, and M. F. Goldberg (Eds.), *Principles and Practice of Ophthalmology.* Philadelphia: Saunders, 1980. Vol. 3, pp. 2355–2455.

73. Miller, M. T. Unpublished data from study in Abak, Nigeria, 1982.

74. Miller, M. T., and Folk, E. R. Strabismus associated with craniofacial anomalies. *Am. Orthoptic J.* 25:27, 1975.

75. Miner, J. L. Some impressions of certain eye afflictions on the Negro as compared with the White race. *Trans. Am. Ophthalmol. Soc.* 12:460, 1910.

76. Molnár, L. Über die Vererbung des Schielens. *Klin. Monatsbl. Augenheilkd.* 150:557, 1967.

77. Nemet, P., Godel, V., and Lazar, M. Kearns-Sayre syndrome. *Birth Defects* 18(6):263, 1982.

78. Niederecker, O., Mash, A. J., and Spivey, B. E. Horizontal fusional amplitudes and versions. *Arch. Ophthalmol.* 87:283, 1972.

79. Nördlow, W. Squint: The frequency of onset at different ages and the incidence of some associated defects in a Swedish population. *Acta Ophthalmol. (Copenh.)* 42:1015, 1964.

80. O'Malley, E. R., Helvenston, E. M., and Ellis, F. D. Duane's retraction syndrome: Plus. Presented at the American Association of Pediatric Ophthalmology and Strabismus annual meeting, 1981.

81. Pfaffenbach, D. O., Cross, H. E., and Kearns, T. P. Congenital anomalies in Duane's retraction syndrome. *Arch. Ophthalmol.* 88:635, 1977.

82. Pratt-Johnson, J. A., and Lunn, C. T. Early case findings and the hereditary factor in strabismus. *Can. J. Ophthalmol.* 2:50, 1967.

83. Richter, S. *Untersuchungen über die Heredität des Strabismus Concomitans Abhandlungen aus dem*

Gebiete der Augenheilkunde (vol. 35). Leipzig: Thieme, 1967.

84. Richter, S. Zur Heredität des Strabismus concomitants. *Humangenetik* 3:235, 1967.

85. Rosenbaum, A. L., and Weiss, S. J. Monozygotic twins discordant for Duane's retraction syndrome. *J. Pediatr. Ophthalmol. Strabismus* 15:360, 1978.

86. Rubin, W., Helm, C., and McCormack, M. K. Ocular Motor Anomalies in Monozygotic and Dizygotic Twins. In R. Reinecke (Ed.), *Strabismus: Proceedings of the 3rd Meeting of the International Strabismological Association*, Asilomar, California, 1978. New York: Grune & Stratton, 1978. P. 89.

87. Schlossman, A., and Priestly, B. Role of heredity in etiology and treatment of strabismus. *Arch. Ophthalmol.* 47:1, 1952.

88. Schnitzler, E. R., and Robertson, W. C., Jr. Familial Kearns-Sayre syndrome. *Neurology (N.Y.)* 29:1172, 1979.

89. Scott, W. E., and Mash, A. J. Kappa angle measures of strabismus and nonstrabismus individuals. *Arch. Ophthalmol.* 89:18, 1973.

90. Simpson, N. E., and Alleslev, J. L. Association of children's diseases in families from record linkage data. *Can. J. Genet. Cytol.* 14:789, 1972.

91. Smith, D., et al. Selected ophthalmologic and orthoptic measurements of families. *Arch. Ophthalmol.* 87:278, 1972.

92. Smith, D. (Ed.). *Recognizable Patterns of Human Malformations.* Philadelphia: Saunders, 1976.

93. Sorsby, A. Biology of the Eye as an Optical System. In T. Duane (Ed.), *Clinical Ophthalmology.* Hagerstown, Md.: Harper & Row, 1979.

94. Sorsby, A., Leary, G. A., and Fraser, G. R. Family studies on ocular refraction and its components. *J. Med. Genet.* 3:269, 1966.

95. Spivey, B. E., and O'Neill, R. Computer input of patient examinations by means of optical scanning. *Arch. Ophthalmol.* 81:407, 1969.

96. Spivey, B. E. Strabismus: Factors in anticipating its occurrence. *Aust. J. Ophthalmol.* 8:5, 1980.

97. Spivey, B. E. Quantitative genetics and clinical medicine. *Trans. Am. Ophthalmol. Soc.* 54:661, 1976.

98. Spuhler, J. N. Empirical studies on quantative human genetics. In the use of vital and health statistics for genetic and radiation studies. United Nations Publication #61, XVII 8:241–252, 1962.

99. Starodubtseva, E. I. Heredity in ophthalmology. *Oftalmol. Zh.* 27:71, 1972.

100. Temtamy, S., and McKusick, V. A. Absence deformities as a part of a syndrome. *Birth Defects* 14(3):73, 1973.

101. Townes, P. L., and Meuchler, E. L. Blepharophimosis, ptosis, epicanthus inversus and primary amenorrhea. *Arch. Ophthalmol.* 97:1664, 1979.

102. Urist, M. Lateral version reflex test. *Am. J. Ophthalmol.* 63:808, 1967.

103. Vogel, F., and Kruger, J. Multifactorial Determination of Genetic Affections. In J. F. Crow and J. W. Neel (Eds.), *Proceedings of the 3rd International Congress on Human Genetics, Chicago, 1966.* Baltimore: Johns Hopkins Press, 1967, P. 436.

104. Vogel, F., and Motulsky, A. G. *Human Genetics.* New York: Springer, 1979. Appendix 4, 6; pp. 143–164.

105. Waardenburg, P. J. Squint and heredity. *Doc. Ophthalmol.* 7:422, 1954.

106. Waardenburg, P. J., Franceschetti, A., and Klein, D. *Genetics and Ophthlamology.* Assen, Netherlands: Royal Van Gorcum, 1961. Vol. 2, pp. 1009–1016.

107. Waardenburg, P. J. Anomalies of Persumably Peripheral Origin of the Extra-Ocular Muscles. In P. J. Waardenburg, A. Franceschetti, and D. Klein (Eds.), *Genetics and Ophthalmology.* Springfield, Ill.: Thomas, 1961. Vol 1, pp. 156–169; 415–439.

108. Weekers, R. P., et al. Contribution à l'étiologie du strabisme concomitant et de l'amblyopie par l'étude de jumeaux uni et bivitellins. *Bull. Soc. Belge Ophtalmol.* 112:146, 1956.

109. Wiesel, T. N., and Hubel, D. H. Single cell responses in striate cortex of kittens deprived of vision in one eye. *J. Neurophysiol.* 26:1003, 1963.

110. Wildervanck, I. S. Een cervico-oculo-acusticies syndrom. *Ned. Tijdschr. Geneeskd.* 104:260, 1960.

111. Worth, C. A. *Squint: Its Causes, Pathology and Treatment* (6th ed.). Philadelphia: Blakiston, 1903. Revised as *Worth's Squint, or the Binocular Reflexes and the Treatment of Squint* (7th ed.), edited by F. B. Chavasse. Philadelphia: Blakiston, 1939.

112. Wybar, K. Ocular motility disorders in pediatric disease. In R. Reinecke (Ed.), *Strabismus II: Proceedings of the 4th Meeting of the International Strabismological Association*, Asilomar, Calif., 1982. New York: Grune & Stratton, 1984. P. XXI.

113. Zlotogora, J., Sagi, M., and Cohen, T. The blepharophimosis, ptosis, and epicanthus inversus syndrome: Delineation of two types. *Am. J. Hum. Genet.* 35:1020, 1983.

11 Glaucoma

Robert B. Nixon
Charles D. Phelps

Primary open-angle glaucoma, primary angle-closure glaucoma, and primary congenital glaucoma are separate and distinct diseases. Each is inherited to some extent.

PRIMARY OPEN-ANGLE GLAUCOMA

The familial nature of primary open-angle glaucoma in adults is well documented in numerous pedigrees compiled during the past 130 years [83, 204]. In many instances the pedigrees appear to indicate simple autosomal dominant transmission: The disease appears in several successive generations, affecting females and males equally. In other pedigrees, however, affected individuals have unaffected parents, or the glaucoma skips generations, suggesting either autosomal recessive transmission or incomplete penetrance if the transmission is autosomal dominant.

Most of these pedigrees are from studies performed before gonioscopy came into routine use. It is often impossible to ascertain whether the family under study is afflicted by open-angle or closed-angle glaucoma. Furthermore, the diagnostic criteria for glaucoma vary from study to study and often are unspecified. As a result conclusions from these pedigrees about the mode of inheritance of primary open-angle glaucoma must be evaluated with skepticism.

A clinical epidemiologist studying the inheritance of primary open-angle glaucoma must de-

We are indebted to Steven M. Podos, M.D., a coauthor of this chapter in the first edition of this book, who made several helpful suggestions to the current authors.
This work was supported, in part, by Grants EY-03330 and RR-59 from the National Institutes of Health.

fine acceptable diagnostic criteria before attempting to answer questions regarding its mode of genetic transmission. For purposes of this review, primary open-angle glaucoma will be defined as a syndrome of high intraocular pressure, cupped optic disc, typical glaucomatous visual field abnormality, anterior chamber angle open by gonioscopy, and no underlying explanation for the high pressure. The partial syndromes of ocular hypertension and low-tension glaucoma will be included only when specifically stated. The syndrome of primary open-angle glaucoma is usually thought to be a single disease. However, we must not exclude the possibility that future investigation will show it to be a number of pathogenically distinct disorders with a similar clinical picture.

Genetic Transmission of Primary Open-Angle Glaucoma

Several surveys have estimated that between 13 and 47 percent of glaucoma is familial [2, 84]. Most of these surveys did not classify the variety of glaucoma by gonioscopy. However, ophthalmologists using adequate diagnostic criteria have identified many familial cases of primary open-angle glaucoma [48, 59, 69, 84, 86, 96, 99, 104]. Some surveys have found that up to 50 percent of patients with primary open-angle glaucoma have a relative who has also lost vision from the disease [86, 182]. Curiously, a family history is present on the maternal side of the family six to seven times more frequently than on the paternal side [144, 182].

Other investigators have looked at the preva-

Table 11-1. *Prevalence of Glaucoma in Relatives of Patients with Primary Open-Angle Glaucoma*

Author	Type of relative	Number	Percent
Leighton [122]	Siblings	2/38	5.3
	Children	3/74	4.0
Davies [71]	Siblings	2/29	6.9
	Children	0/61	0.0
Jay and Paterson [104]	Siblings	7/65	10.8
	Children	6/172	3.5
Miller and Paterson [141, 142, 143, 151, 153]	Siblings	8/50	16.0
	Children	9/75	12.0
	First-degree relatives	18/650	2.8
François [84]	Relatives	21/413	5.1
Kolker [116]	First-degree relatives	6/110	5.4
Perkins [154]	First-degree relatives	11/190	5.8

lence of glaucoma in individuals who have a relative with primary open-angle glaucoma [71, 84, 85, 104, 122, 141–143, 151, 153, 154]. This has ranged from 2.8 to 16 percent (Table 11-1); in contrast, only 0.47 to 1.43 percent of several large random populations surveyed in the United States, Great Britain, and Sweden have been found to have primary open-angle glaucoma [29, 58, 102, 110, 166].

Two features of primary open-angle glaucoma make its genetic study difficult. The first is the high prevalence of the incomplete syndromes of ocular hypertension and low-tension glaucoma. For example, a large proportion of glaucoma relatives do not have the full syndrome but have impaired aqueous outflow or high intraocular pressure [8, 25, 48, 71, 116, 141–143, 151]. It is difficult to classify these relatives in a pedigree analysis. The abnormalities of intraocular pressure undoubtedly forecast the eventual loss of visual field in some. However, no arbitrary level of intraocular pressure, outflow facility, or other currently available measurement will identify with reasonable certainty the eyes destined to lose visual field [22, 24]. Until our prognostic techniques improve, the diagnosis of glaucoma is best made on the basis of damaged visual function, even though the prevalence of glaucoma in relatives will, as a result, be underestimated.

The second feature is that the disease usually affects older people. Thus the occurrence of glaucoma in a family member can be ascertained only if serial examinations are performed over the individual's lifetime. The influence of age on the prevalence of open-angle glaucoma in family studies is particularly exemplified by the studies of Paterson and Miller [141, 143, 151, 153]. In an initial study of 125 siblings and children, they found 6 cases of glaucoma; in a follow-up study 9 years later, they found 11 more cases. The figures listed in Table 11-1 are misleading in two ways. Because they are prevalances of glaucoma at one point in time, they underestimate the risk of primary open-angle glaucoma's eventually developing in a relative of an afflicted individual. In addition, the seemingly higher prevalence of glaucoma in siblings than in children probably reflects only the greater average age of the siblings at the time of the studies.

Postulated Modes of Inheritance

The pattern of glaucoma inheritance remains controversial. Autosomal dominant transmission is favored by some [59, 75, 84, 86, 96, 99]. However, most recently acquired evidence supports either autosomal recessive transmission [33, 35, 39–41, 43, 44, 46] or polygenic, multifactorial inheritance [15, 22, 104].

In Becker's theory of *autosomal recessive transmission*, he proposes a genetic model in which a single allelic pair of genes determines the predisposition of an individual to develop primary open-angle glaucoma [33, 40, 44, 46]. Glaucoma occurs almost exclusively in individuals homozygous for the recessive "glaucoma" gene. However, time is required for development of glaucoma in such an individual, and penetrance of the gene's effect may be modified by other factors. Therefore not all homozygotes have glaucoma at the time of study or will develop glaucoma.

Becker further proposes that the response of an individual's intraocular pressure to prolonged topical application of corticosteriods may "unmask" his or her genetic predisposition to glaucoma. Some evidence (see Corticosteroid Responsiveness, below) suggests that the corticosteroid response is genetically determined with an autosomal intermediate recessive mode of inheritance: Homozygotes for the recessive gene mediating corticosteroid sensitivity respond with a marked elevation of intraocular pressure, homozygotes for the "nonresponder" gene have little or no change in pressure, and heterozygous individuals show a more modest elevation of pressure. Becker offers evidence that the gene determining corticosteroid responsiveness may be identical to his postulated recessive glaucoma gene [39, 40].

From the distribution in normal populations of intraocular pressure responses to topical corticosteroid application, the frequency of the recessive gene that determines corticosteroid sensitivity can be calculated to be between 20–25% [44]. Becker and Hahn suggest that forces governing natural selection allow such an unusually high frequency of a pathologic gene because the untoward effects of glaucoma occur after the reproductive age. Whether or not possession of the gene confers upon its bearer any survival advantage that may account for its high frequency has yet to be determined.

Becker and Hahn also point out that a characteristic feature in pedigrees of autosomal recessive traits with a high gene frequency is an impression of dominant inheritance produced by the reasonably frequent occurrence of matings of homozygotes with heterozygotes. Therefore what the authors of many published pedigrees interpreted to be dominance may actually have been quasidominance.

In his *polygenic, multifactorial theory* [15, 22], Armaly proposes that the inheritance of glaucoma is not specified by a single allelic pair of genes, but instead is the manifestation of the combined influences of many pairs of genes. Each of several measurable parameters of the glaucoma disease complex, including intraocular pressure [14, 25], outflow facility [25], and the horizontal cup-disc ratio [13], is inherited by polygenic transmission. Each shares some common genetic determinants with one or more of the others. The pair of genes governing the ocular hypertensive response to topical administration of corticosteroids is one of the multiple allelic pairs that influence these parameters. Armaly, measuring the corticosteroid response differently from Becker, agrees that it is inherited as a simple mendelian trait. However, he does not think a genetic susceptibility to a high corticosteroid response is always a prerequisite for inheritance of primary open-angle glaucoma.

Corticosteroid Responsiveness

The concept of monogenic inheritance of corticosteroid responsiveness is founded on (1) the demonstration within the total population of three subpopulations with respect to intraocular pressure responsiveness to topical corticosteroid administration, and (2) the demonstration in families that the responses of individuals can be predicted by the rules of mendelian segregation.

Becker and Armaly use different criteria for the measurement of corticosteroid responsiveness (Table 11-2). Becker measures the *absolute level* of intraocular pressure that is attained after 6 weeks

Table 11-2. *Measurement of Intraocular Pressure Response to Topical Application of Corticosteroids*

Criterion	Becker	Armaly
Corticosteroid preparation	Dexamethasone 0.1% (in early studies, betamethasone 0.1%)	Dexamethasone 0.1%
Dosage schedule	4 times daily	3 times daily
Duration	6 weeks	4 weeks
Parameter measured	Final applanation intraocular pressure (P_a)	Change in applanation intraocular pressure (ΔP_a)
Classification		
Low	nn: $P_a < 20$	$p^L p^L$: $\Delta P_a < 6$
Intermediate	ng: P_a 20–31	$p^L p^H$: ΔP_a 6–15
High	gg: $P_a > 31$	$p^H p^H$: $\Delta P_a > 15$

of topical dexamethasone 0.1% four times daily. (In earlier studies he used betamethasone 0.1% four times daily, and the response was similar.) Armaly measures the *change* in intraocular pressure after 4 weeks of topical dexamethasone 0.1% three times daily.

Both Becker and Armaly separated three levels of intraocular pressure responses to corticosteroid challenge by analyzing the distribution of the response in tested normal population samples. The frequency distribution curves were found to be skewed toward high responses. When the data were plotted as cumulative percent frequency curves, which for a single gaussian distribution should form a straight line, a statistically significant deviation from a straight line was noted by Becker for responses of 20 mm Hg or higher [33] and by Armaly for a pressure change of +6 mm Hg or more [15]. These deviations suggested the existence of more than one population: a normally distributed population of "nonresponders" and an uncharacterized population of "responders."

Using a pressure increase of 6 mm Hg or more to separate corticosteroid responders from nonresponders, Armaly replotted the cumulative percent frequency curve for the responders. Again the distribution was not gaussian, because of a small excess of individuals whose pressure rise exceeded 15 mm Hg. Becker, lacking a sufficient number of normal subjects to be certain of a third, higher-responding group, analyzed the corticosteroid responses of glaucoma subjects and relatives of those with glaucoma. A large proportion of these selected subjects were found to attain a final intraocular pressure of 20 mm Hg or higher. When their responses were plotted in a cumulative percent frequency curve, a deviation from a single gaussian distribution was again noted, this time at a final pressure of 32 mm Hg or higher. The mean and standard deviation of the final intraocular pressures of the lower-responding portion of this selected population (those with final pressures of less than 32 mm Hg) were almost identical to the mean and standard deviation of the final intraocular pressures of the higher-responding portion of the previously tested normal population, which suggested that the two groups composed one homogeneous subpopulation of intermediate responders.

Postulating a genetic determination of the corticosteroid response, Becker designated the genotypes of the low, intermediate, and high corticosteroid response groups as nn, ng, and gg respectively; Armaly used the designations P^LP^L,

Table 11-3. *Frequency of Corticosteroid Phenotypes** in Normal Subjects*

Observed			
Armaly [15]	P^LP^L	P^LP^H	P^HP^H
(n = 80)	66%	29%	5%
Becker [117]	nn	ng	gg
(n = 300)	58%	36%	6%
Predicted			
Gene frequency of 0.20	64%	32%	4%
Gene frequency of 0.25	56.25%	37.5%	6.25%

*See Table 11-2.

P^LP^H, and P^HP^H (Table 11-2). Becker's designation g for the high-response gene obviously refers to his hypothesis relating glaucoma and the corticosteroid response.

Table 11-3 lists the frequency of each level of response in random population samples. The table also shows the expected ratios of responses, should the response be controlled by a recessive gene with a frequency of 0.20 or 0.25. The observed frequencies of the different responses indicate a gene frequency in this range.

Analysis of the mean and standard deviation of responses in each of the three groups, classified by either method, reveals a slight overlap between low and intermediate groups and intermediate and high groups [15, 33]. The selected boundaries between the groups are admittedly arbitrary. The validity of the response classification can be criticized on theoretical grounds [174, 178]. Armaly and Becker defended both their classification criteria and their hypothesis of monogenic inheritance of corticosteroid responsiveness by demonstrating that the corticosteroid responses in family units are predictable from the laws of mendelian transmission.

Armaly studied 19 families with 75 children [10, 15]. Both parents and children were corticosteroid classified. Only one child had an unpredicted response. Furthermore, the ratios of low, intermediate, and high responses in the children of each type of family unit tested (P^LP^L × P^LP^L, P^LP^H × P^LP^H, and P^LP^H × P^HP^H) were exactly those predicted by classical mendelian assortment.

Becker and Kolker, in a similar study involving 100 offspring of patients with known corticosteroid phenotypes, found only one unexpected response [45]. Again, the proportion of low, intermediate, and high responses in the offspring of various parental combinations was almost exactly that predicted by the mendelian model.

Thus, much evidence supports the concept that corticosteroid responsiveness is determined by a single gene pair. However, evidence against the concept was found in a study of corticosteroid responses in twins by Schwartz and co-workers [177, 178]. They tested 37 monozygotic and 26 dizygotic twin pairs with topical dexamethasone. The frequency of similar responses was not significantly different in the two types of twins. Their disquieting conclusion was that environmental, not genetic, factors are the dominant determinants of the corticosteroid response.

A partial explanation for the discrepancy between the results of the twin study and the results of the earlier studies of Becker and Armaly is found in an analysis by Palmberg and co-workers of the reproducibility of the corticosteroid provocative test [150]. When a group of normal subjects were tested on several occasions, the proportion of low, intermediate, and high responders was the same on each occasion. However, the subjects in each response group differed from test to test. Considerable cross-over occurred between the low and intermediate response groups. Those who were high responders the first time tended to be high responders on subsequent testing. This suggested that only the high response "signal" consistently emerged above the "background noise" of the spontaneous variation of intraocular pressure. Because few of the twins were high responders, that study could not conclusively prove or disprove the genetic nature of the response.

In summary, the question of whether or not the corticosteroid response is inherited remains unresolved. Much of the literature that will be subsequently reviewed assumes a monogenic inheritance of the response.

Corticosteroid Responsiveness and Open-Angle Glaucoma

The relation of primary open-angle glaucoma to corticosteroid responsiveness may be investigated by corticosteroid provocative testing of patients with glaucoma and their relatives.

Becker found that 92 percent of patients with untreated primary open-angle glaucoma were high corticosteroid responders (gg) [33]. Armaly, testing primary open-angle glaucoma patients with high pressures, found the distribution of corticosteroid phenotypes to be $P^L P^L$, 6 percent; $P^L P^H$, 48 percent; and $P^H P^H$, 46 percent. Interestingly,

the distribution of responses in low-tension glaucoma was almost the same as in high-tension glaucoma [11]. Many other investigators [80, 114, 138, 146, 180, 181, 205] have confirmed an increased prevalence of corticosteroid responsiveness in glaucoma patients, although some have denied it [128, 147, 189].

One of the reasons Becker and Armaly disagreed on how frequently a high corticosteroid response occurs in primary open-angle glaucoma patients is the different yardsticks with which each measured the response. If the baseline intraocular pressure is 15 to 16 mm Hg, an individual's response to corticosteroid drops would be classified similarly by either method. At lower baseline intraocular pressures, Armaly's criteria tend to classify more individuals as high responders. On the other hand, at higher baseline pressures, Becker's criteria classify more individuals as high responders. Since most patients with glaucoma have high intraocular pressures, many more of them are classified as high responders by Becker's than by Armaly's criteria.

This raises the question whether the high frequency of gg responses observed by Becker in primary open-angle glaucoma patients is truly a genetic association or whether it merely reflects a high prevalance of elevated intraocular pressures in glaucoma patients. A related question is whether pathologic changes in the outflow passages of a glaucomatous eye may alter the phenotypic response of the eye to corticosteroid challenge. To answer these questions, offspring and siblings of patients with primary open-angle glaucoma have been tested with topical corticosteroids. If the high corticosteroid responses of glaucoma patients are indeed genetic in origin, their children and siblings, who for the most part do not have glaucoma or elevated intraocular pressures, should have increased prevalences of high and intermediate corticosteroid responses. Furthermore, the distribution of the three types of responses in glaucoma relatives will be predictable, given the frequency with which the "g" allele appears in the general population and the assumptions that the corticosteroid response is inherited in an intermediate recessive fashion.

Becker and co-workers found that high responses to corticosteroid testing do occur with increased frequency in children [41] and siblings [43] of glaucoma patients, and that the distribution of the responses in these relatives was very similar to that which would be predicted if the recessive genetic hypothesis were correct and if

Table 11-4. *Frequency of Corticosteroid Phenotypes* in Siblings and Children of Patients with Primary Open-Angle Glaucoma*

	Phenotype		
Relatives	nn	ng	gg
Siblings (n = 70)			
Observed [43]	19%	50%	31%
Predicted (gene frequency = 0.2)	20%	49%	31%
Children (n = 100)			
Observed [41]	1%	82%	17%
Predicted (gene frequency = 0.2)	0%	80%	20%

*See Table 11-2.

the gene frequency were 0.2 (Table 11-4). This evidence strongly supports Becker's hypothesis that an individual's corticosteroid response, measured by the final pressure attained, does reveal his or her glaucoma genotype, and that primary open-angle glaucoma is, indeed, recessively inherited.

Armaly also found that the corticosteroid responsiveness of glaucoma offspring was consistent with a genetic origin for the high responses in primary open-angle glaucoma patients. He studied 14 families in which one of the two parents had glaucoma [11]. Both parents and children were corticosteroid classified. The agreement of the observed responses with the predicted ratios of responses was good. Although 6 of the 58 offspring had responses that were not predictable from their parents', 5 of the 6 unpredicted responses were just 1 mm Hg over the limit of those predicted.

An increased frequency of corticosteroid responsiveness in relatives of those with glaucoma has been confirmed by Paterson [152] and François and colleagues [87], although the latter did not find the frequency of responsiveness in parents and children of glaucoma patients to be as high as would be predicted from Becker's model.

What is the prognosis of a nonglaucomatous individual with a high corticosteroid response? In a study by Kitazawa and Horie, 35 subjects who were high responders by Armaly's criteria were followed for an average of 12.2 years and a minimum of 10 years [106]. Of 22 patients who originally had pressures less than 22 mm Hg on three successive visits, 5 eventually developed ocular hypertension and 2 of these showed glaucomatous defects. Even more striking was the development of visual field defects in 7 of 13 subjects who were originally classified as ocular hypertensives (in-

traocular pressure greater than 21 mm Hg on at least three successive visits).

Inheritance of Intraocular Pressure and Outflow Facility

Intraocular pressure and outflow facility are *quantitative traits;* that is, they are measurable characteristics that have a continuous frequency distribution curve. Other classic examples of quantitative traits include body stature, intelligence, blood pressure, and the refraction of the eye. Quantitative traits are often designated as multifactorial or polygenic, because they are determined by many factors, some environmental and some genetic.

As with other multifactorial traits, individuals tend to resemble their siblings and parents with regard to intraocular pressure and outflow facility [14, 25, 129]. As with other multifactorial traits this resemblance may not be purely genetic. Although one study by Armaly demonstrated no significant correlation between the intraocular pressure in husband and wife pairs [9], Bengtsson has presented evidence to the contrary [57]. He found the correlation between the husband and wife pairs for intraocular pressure to be highly significant and of the same order of magnitude as that in relatives sharing a common genetic background.

A family history of glaucoma is one factor that influences the level of intraocular pressure and outflow facility. Intraocular pressure on the average is higher and the average outflow facility is lower in individuals with a family history of glaucoma than in those lacking such a family history (Table 11-5) [8, 48, 116, 142]. In one study, an intraocular pressure exceeding 20 mm Hg was found in 35 percent of eyes if there was a family history of glaucoma, but in only 18 percent of eyes if such a family history was lacking [8].

Becker and co-workers, studying families in which at least two persons have glaucoma, found an intraocular pressure of 30 mm Hg or more in 5.5 percent of the unaffected relatives; the prevalence in relatives over the age of 40 years rose to 9.7 percent (Table 11-5) [48]. Low outflow facilities and P_0/C ratios (P_0 = pressure; C = outflow facility) exceeding 100 also are more frequent in the eyes of glaucoma relatives [25, 48, 71, 141, 143, 151].

Another important factor in determination of an individual's intraocular pressure and outflow facility is his or her predisposition to corticosteroid-induced intraocular pressure elevations

Table 11-5. *Introcular Pressure in Relatives of Those with Glaucoma*

Author	Intraocular pressure (mm Hg)	First-degree relatives All ages	First-degree relatives Over 40 years
Becker and co-workers [48]	>30	5%	10%
Armaly [8]	>20	35%	—
Miller [142]	>21	10%	15%
Kolker [116]	>21	12%	—

(Table 11-6) [16, 25, 37]. High corticosteroid responders have significantly higher mean intraocular pressure and lower mean outflow facility than do nonresponders.

Cupping of the Optic Nerve

Cupping of the optic nerve may be acquired, as in glaucoma, or it may be congenital. Although some studies show a slight increase in cup size with aging, this effect is not great in normal eyes [179].

One way to measure the size of the optic cup is to estimate the ratio of the horizontal diameter of the cup to the horizontal diameter of the disc; that is, the horizontal C/D ratio. The distribution of horizontal C/D ratios in the normal population is markedly skewed toward low values; the horizontal C/D ratio was less than 0.4 in 85 percent of one population of normal subjects [13]. Nevertheless, a small but significant number of otherwise healthy eyes have congenitally large cups, which may be confused with glaucomatous cupping.

Armaly demonstrated that the horizontal C/D ratio of an individual resembled that of his or her parents and siblings, but not that of his or her spouse [9, 13]. In a few families in which the two parents had markedly dissimilar horizontal C/D ratios, the ratio of the offspring tended to resemble the averages of the parents' ratios, rather than resembling one parent more than the other. These observations are consistent with multifactorial inheritance of cup size. Further corroboration of the heritability of size of the optic cup has been pointed out by Schwartz and colleagues, who compared the intrapair differences in 37 pairs of monozygotic and 26 pairs of dizygotic twins [176]. Intrapair variance for monozygotic twins was significantly less.

Eyes with a horizontal C/D ratio exceeding 0.3 are more likely than those with a lower ratio to have an intraocular pressure of 20 mm Hg or higher, an outflow facility of 0.14 μl/min/mm Hg or lower, or both [19, 26]. This may result from the three parameters' (cup size, intraocular pressure, and outflow facility) sharing in common at least one genetic determinant, the allelic pair of genes governing corticosteroid responsiveness. Armaly finds the frequency of horizontal C/D ratios exceeding 0.3 to be 15 percent in nn individuals, 20 percent in ng individuals, and 52 percent in gg individuals [14].

The prevalence of large cups (horizontal C/D ratio exceeding 0.3) in normal eyes is similar in

Table 11-6. *Relationship of Intraocular Pressure and Outflow Facility to Corticosteroid Phenotype**

Phenotype	Number	Applanation pressure (mm Hg)	Outflow facility (μl/min/mm Hg)
Armaly [16] (mean ± S.D.)			
$p^L p^L$	169	15.0 ± 3.0	0.29 ± 0.10
$p^H p^H$	44	16.8 ± 2.0	0.22 ± 0.07
Becker [37] (mean ± S.D.)			
nn	100	14.5 ± 2.2	0.30 ± 0.05
ng	200	16.0 ± 2.5	0.26 ± 0.05
gg	250	19.2 ± 3.3	0.18 ± 0.06

*See Table 11-2.

Table 11-7. *Racial Influences on Horizontal Cup-Disc Ratio*

Classification	Cup-disc ratio greater than 0.3		
	Blacks	Whites	All
nn*	4/24 (16.7%)	26/176 (14.8%)	30/200 (15%)
ng*	6/34 (17.6%)	34/166 (20.5%)	40/200 (20%)
gg*	41/68 (60.3%)	89/182 (48.9%)	130/250 (52%)
Primary open-angle glaucoma	61/66 (92.4%)	184/234 (78.6%)	245/300 (82%)
Opposite eye, unilateral primary open-angle glaucoma	—	—	48/80 (60%)

*See Corticosteroid Responsiveness in text for explanation.
Source: Unpublished data provided by S. M. Podos and B. Becker.

black and white populations. However, large cups in glaucomatous eyes are more prevalent among blacks than among whites (Table 11-7) [161]. The pathogenesis of glaucomatous optic atrophy may differ in the two races, socioeconomic factors may impede early glaucoma diagnosis in black populations, or response to treatment differ [68, 125].

Documented enlargement of the cup or an asymmetry of the cupping (in which the horizontal C/D ratio of one eye exceeds that of its fellow by more than 0.2) strongly indicates acquired nerve damage [18, 82, 207]. An inequality of horizontal C/D ratios in the two eyes exceeding 0.2 is seen in less than 1 percent of a randomly selected population [13].

The frequency of horizontal C/D ratios exceeding 0.3 in the unaffected eye of patients with unilateral glaucoma is 56 to 60 percent [21, 37]. There is some evidence suggesting that eyes with genetically determined large cups are more susceptible to glaucomatous damage than are eyes with small cups [17, 21, 37, 211], but this may merely be a sign of early damage in the fellow eye that precedes any visual field changes. The high frequency of large cups in the fellow eyes of patients with unilateral glaucoma resembles that in high corticosteroid responders (52%) [37] but is much greater than the frequency (27%) in a population of eyes with ocular hypertension (selected for intraocular pressures greater than 19 mm Hg and normal visual fields in both eyes of the patient) [21].

Association of Systemic Markers with Primary Open-Angle Glaucoma

Patients with primary open-angle glaucoma are found to differ from the normal population when examined for abnormalities of glucose metabo-

lism, phenylthiocarbamide tasting, and plasma cortisol suppression after systemic administration of corticosteroids [36]. High responders to topical corticosteroids (gg individuals) resemble glaucoma patients and differ from the remaining nonglaucomatous population when tested for the first two of these systemic characteristics. There also appears to be an increased prevalence of migraine headache in patients with low-tension glaucoma [160].

GLUCOSE METABOLISM

Abnormalities of glucose metabolism are common in patients with primary open-angle glaucoma, and 6 to 13 percent of glaucoma patients have known diabetes mellitus [22, 27, 38, 98, 130, 137, 168]. Those glaucoma patients who are not clinically diabetic frequently have positive glucose tolerance test results [38, 49, 168, 173]. Abnormal glucose tolerance test results occur with similar frequency in high corticosteroid responders (Table 11-8) [12, 38, 49]. Interestingly, positive results on glucose tolerance tests occur more frequently in those gg individuals who have large horizontal C/D ratios than in those with small horizontal C/D ratios [38].

Conversely, primary open-angle glaucoma occurs in 4 to 11 percent of diabetic patients [27, 64, 167]; these prevalences are several times those of nondiabetic control populations. Increased prevalences of intermediate and high corticosteroid responders have also been found among diabetic patients, both juvenile and adult [34, 38].

Armaly, however, reports an increased prevalence of corticosteroid responders only among juvenile diabetic patients, not among diabetic adults. Furthermore, when he tested seven par-

Table 11-8. *Glucose Tolerance Test Results in Patients Over 40 Without Overt Diabetes*

Classification	Number	Glucose tolerance abnormal*
nn†	50	2%
ng†	70	4%
gg†	100	17%
Primary open-angle glaucoma	120	22%

*Sum of plasma glucose at 0, 1, 2, and 3 hr ≥ 600 mg/100 ml.
†See Corticosteroid Responsiveness in text for explanation.
Source: Modified from B. Becker [38].

Table 11-9. *Intraocular Pressure in Diabetic Patients*

Classification	Intraocular pressure >20 mm Hg	Intraocular pressure >23 mm Hg
Adult diabetics	18–21%	5–12%
Nondiabetics (over age 40)	9.6%	1.8%
Juvenile diabetics	21–30%	6–15%

Source: Modified from B. Becker [34, 38].

ents of four diabetic children who were corticosteroid responders, none of the parents responded [15]. This indicates that diabetes may modify the phenotypic response to corticosteroid testing and that the gene governing corticosteroid responsiveness may not necessarily be more prevalent among diabetics.

The relationship between intraocular pressure and diabetes mellitus is not universally agreed on. Some series of diabetic patients are reported to have a higher mean intraocular pressure than normal control subjects, particularly if patients of all ages are pooled [28, 66, 103, 130] or if only children are examined [172, 200]. In one series older diabetic individuals actually had a lower mean intraocular pressure than comparable unselected control subjects, and a tendency toward a higher mean intraocular pressure could be detected only in younger diabetic patients [23].

Adult diabetic patients have a greater prevalence of intraocular pressure exceeding 20 and 23 mm Hg than do comparable nondiabetic control subjects (Table 11-9) [34, 38]. The same is probably true for juvenile diabetic patients, although control measurements for nondiabetic children are not available.

In the Framingham eye study the prevalence of diabetes was two to three times higher in persons with pressures greater than 21 mm Hg than in persons with lower pressures [110]. (Interestingly, in this study there was no relationship between glaucoma and diabetes.)

A fascinating relationship between the stages of diabetic retinopathy and the level of the intraocular pressure is discussed by Becker in his Edward Jackson Memorial Lecture [38]. Diabetic pa-

tients whose retinopathy is proliferative have lower intraocular pressures than do diabetic patients without proliferative retinopathy [38, 42, 66]. Furthermore, topical corticosteroid testing in diabetic adults reveals a significantly greater prevalence of high responders among diabetic patients without proliferative retinopathy than among nondiabetics or diabetics with proliferative retinopathy [38, 42]. In fact, the distribution of responses in diabetic patients with proliferative retinopathy resembles that of the normal population. These findings have prompted a suggestion that corticosteroid provocative testing may be of value in determining the prognosis of diabetic retinopathy [38].

A final observation about the relationship of diabetes to glaucoma is that diabetes may weaken the resistance of the optic nerve to glaucomatous damage. Becker found that glaucomatous patients with positive results on glucose tolerance tests lose visual field at lower levels of intraocular pressure than do those with negative results [38]. Armaly, in a 10-year study of nearly 4,000 subjects with initially normal visual fields, found only 4 individuals in whom glaucomatous visual field defects subsequently developed [20]. Three of these were overtly diabetic, and the fourth had a positive glucose tolerance test result. It should be noted, however, that two multivariate analyses of glaucomatous risk factors have found diabetes to be of only slight importance as a predictor of future visual field loss [78, 79, 97].

PHENYLTHIOCARBAMIDE TASTING

Sensitivity to the bitter taste of phenylthiocarbamide (PTC) is distributed bimodally in the general population. Thirty percent of whites are relatively insensitive and are classified nontasters; nontasting is much less frequent in black populations. PTC nontasting is inherited as a simple mendelian recessive trait.

There is disagreement regarding the prevalence of PTC nontasters among open-angle glaucoma patients. While Kalmus and Lewkonia could find no difference in the prevalence of nontasting among control subjects, primary open-angle glaucoma patients, and ocular hypertensive patients [106], Becker and Morton found a 55 percent prevalence of PTC nontasters in open-angle glaucoma patients [50]. Becker and Kolker found a similar high prevalence (53 percent) in individuals with a gg phenotype [46]. In contrast, the prevalance of nontasting in the ng and nn phenotypes was 32 percent and 25 percent, respectively. These figures apply only to white populations.

THYROID FUNCTION

The prevalence of a low serum protein-bound iodine (PBI) has been found to be higher in gg corticosteroid responsive and glaucomatous individuals than in corticosteroid nonresponders [46, 47]. However, later studies have shown no significant differences between nn, ng, gg, or primary open-angle glaucoma individuals in the more specific tests of thyroid function: thyroxine (T_4), triiodothyronine (T_3) resin uptake, or thyroid-stimulating hormone (TSH) [118].

PLASMA CORTISOL

The production of endogenous cortisol by the cells of the adrenal cortex is regulated by a hypothalamic-pituitary feedback system that is closely attuned to the level of circulating glucocorticoids. Administration of an exogenous corticosteroid, such as dexamethasone, inhibits production of adrenocorticotropic hormone (ACTH) by the pituitary gland. Lacking the stimulus of ACTH, the adrenal cortex decreases its production of cortisol.

The suppressibility of endogenous cortisol production by exogenous dexamethasone is tested by administering an oral dose of dexamethasone at 11 P.M. and measuring the plasma cortisol at 8 A.M. the following morning. This measurement is compared with a control measurement obtained at 8 A.M. the preceding morning.

A dose-dependent response is noted (Table 11-10) [54]. After 1 mg of dexamethasone, plasma cortisol in both nn and ng populations and glaucoma populations decreases as expected [52, 54]. If a 0.25-mg dose of dexamethasone is used, plasma cortisol is suppressed in only 27 percent of the nn and ng populations. In contrast, suppression is still seen in 83 percent of the glaucoma population [162]. Thus, glaucoma patients are more sensitive than nn and ng populations to plasma cortisol suppression by exogenously administered glucocorticoids, as well as being more sensitive to the ocular hypertensive effect of topically administered corticosteroids.

Dexamethasone suppression testing in gg individuals separates three groups: one group with "normal" sensitivity (i.e., resembling that of the nn and ng populations), a second group with increased sensitivity (i.e., resembling that of the glaucoma population), and a third group that is insensitive to the effect of exogenous dexamethasone [54, 162]. This third group includes 29 percent of the gg population. The significance of the relative insensitivity to dexamethasone suppression in this group of gg subjects is unclear. The demonstration of a difference between some high corticosteroid responders and glaucoma patients in this characteristic, in contrast to the similarities found in topical corticosteroid testing, PTC tasting, glucose tolerance testing, aqueous humor dynamics, and horizontal C/D ratios, may be a significant clue in the search for indicators of susceptibility to visual field loss [119].

Levene and Schwartz, measuring plasma cor-

Table 11-10. *Dexamethasone Suppression of Plasma Cortisol*

| Classification | Number | Frequency (%) of suppression* after dexamethasone | | |
		1.0 mg	0.5 mg	0.25 mg
nn, ng[†]	37	100	62	27
Primary open-angle glaucoma	35	100	100	83

*Ratio 8 A.M.$_1$/8 A.M.$_0$ ≤ 0.75.
†See Corticosteroid Responsiveness in text for explanation.
Source: Modified from B. Becker et al. [52] and B. Becker and C. K. Ramsey [54].

tisol levels before and *24 hours* after oral administration of 0.75 mg of dexamethasone have observed relatively poor plasma cortisol suppression in high intraocular pressure responders to topical corticosteroids [126]. Their data are obviously in disagreement with Becker's data on the hypersensitivity of most glaucoma patients and many high corticosteroid responders to dexamethasone suppression testing, although they may fit with the 29 percent of Becker's high responders who are relatively insensitive. The discrepancies between the results of the two studies indicate that the time at which plasma cortisol is measured after dexamethasone administration is a critical variable.

Schwartz and Levene [175], in contradistinction to Krupin and co-workers [119], found that baseline plasma cortisol levels tend to be higher in open-angle glaucoma patients with field loss than in age-matched normal subjects or ocular hypertensive patients with no field loss. They speculated that higher plasma cortisol levels in glaucoma patients may represent a basic metabolic difference that predisposes them to visual field loss or may merely reflect a stimulus to cortisol production by the diminished light input or the psychological stresses that accompany glaucomatous blindness.

Levene and associates, in a study of families, were unable to demonstrate inheritance of plasma cortisol levels [127]. A significant correlation of cortisol levels was found between husbands and wives, as well as among first-degree relatives, which suggests a strong environmental influence.

The search for the underlying mechanism of corticosteroid sensitivity at the cellular level has led to contradictory results. While early studies showed an increased sensitivity of lymphocytes from glaucoma patients to the inhibiting effect of corticosteroids on their transformation when stimulated by phytohemagglutinin [149], others have been unable to demonstrate any significant difference between lymphocytes from normal subjects and those from patients with open-angle glaucoma [55, 139, 188]. It now seems likely that the initial results were due not to difference in disease status but instead to a stress reaction of the glaucoma patients who were hospitalized.

Although there may be no difference in cortisol metabolism of lymphocytes between corticosteroid-responsive individuals and nonresponders, Southren and co-workers have shown that cells cultured from the trabecular meshwork of people with primary open-angle glaucoma do differ in the metabolism of cortisol from normal controls [187]. Two alterations were found: a marked increase (more than 100 times) in Δ^4-reductase activity and a decrease (fourfold) in 3-oxidoreductase activity. The changes persisted through many generations of tissue cultures. The prevalance and heritability of these metabolic alterations remain to be determined.

MIGRAINE AND LOW-TENSION GLAUCOMA

Recent evidence suggests a link between low-tension glaucoma and migraine headache [160]. One of us (C.D.P) and Corbett found a significantly higher prevalence of headache with migrainous features (unilaterality, nausea and vomiting, and visual prodromata) in these patients compared to those with primary open-angle glaucoma, ocular hypertension, or normal subjects. Up to 29.6 percent of those with low-tension glaucoma had migrainous symptoms, compared to 19.5 percent of normal subjects. This suggests that the vasospasm associated with migraine may produce not only intermittent symptoms of cerebral ischemia but also chronic intermittent ischemia of the optic nerve. Treatment using systemic β-adrenergic blocking drugs may be of benefit in these patients.

Inherited Ocular Abnormalities Often Associated with Primary Open-Angle Glaucoma

MYOPIA

Myopia is, at least in part, inherited, although the pattern of transmission and the effect of environmental factors are controversial [7, 30, 31, 77, 81, 107]. A possible association between myopia and primary open-angle glaucoma is suggested by several observations. Myopia of more than 1 diopter is strikingly prevalent in primary open-angle glaucoma patients. It is found in 27 to 32 percent of glaucoma patients, compared to 18 to 20 percent of age-matched persons in the general population [73, 155, 157, 171]. There is a weak correlation between myopia and ocular hypertension [56, 62], but this is not enough to account for the association with open-angle glaucoma. The explanation, instead, seems to be that myopes with ocular hypertension are at a much higher risk of developing a glaucomatous field defect than are emmetropes or hyperopes [131, 157].

Curtin has shown a positive correlation be-

Table 11-11. *Corticosteroid Phenotypes* in Patients with High Myopia and Krukenberg's Spindles*

		Phenotype		
Classification	Number	nn	ng	gg
Nonmyopic	200	60%	35%	5%
Myopia >5 D	30	15%	50%	37%
Krukenberg's spindles	15	27%	60%	13%
Primary open-angle glaucoma siblings	70	19%	50%	31%

*See Corticosteroid Responsiveness in text for explanation.
Source: Adapted from Kolker and Hetherington [117].

tween axial eye length and primary open-angle glaucoma: The incidence of primary open-angle glaucoma rises from 3 percent in myopes with an axial length below 26.5 mm to 28 percent in those with an axial length greater than 33.5 mm [70].

Eyes with myopia of greater than 5 diopters, when tested with topical corticosteroids, respond with large increases in intraocular pressure more frequently than do eyes of the general population (Table 11-11) [117, 163]. The distribution of corticosteroid phenotypes in persons with high myopia also resembles that of close relatives of patients with primary open-angle glaucoma.

Although myopia appears to be a risk factor in the development of glaucoma, it may in fact have a salutary effect in improving the long-term prognosis of a glaucoma patient once the intraocular pressure is controlled by treatment. This is true irrespective of patient age, type of treatment, or initial appearance of the optic disc [158].

Multifactorial Inheritance of Primary Open-Angle Glaucoma

The inheritance of primary open-angle glaucoma is closely related to the inheritance of susceptibility to corticosteroid-induced intraocular pressure elevations. The allelic pair of genes governing the corticosteroid response, if this response is indeed inherited, may be the primary genetic determinant of glaucoma, or it may be only one of several allelic pairs involved in the inheritance of glaucoma. Whether one subscribes to a theory of monogenic recessive or polygenic transmission of glaucoma depends in large part on the correlation one finds between glaucoma and corticosteroid responsiveness. This correlation in turn depends on how one measures the corticosteroid response.

Proponents of the recessive theory must invoke other modifiers, such as endocrinous, cardiovascular, environmental, or additional genetic factors, to explain why glaucoma does not occur in all individuals with the gg corticosteroid phenotype, and why, when it does occur, it appears at various ages and with different degrees of severity. Thus the hypothesized recessive transmission is also multifactorial. Disagreement between the two theories rests solely on whether a homozygous pair of genes for high corticosteroid sensitivity is a requisite for the development of glaucoma. It is neither possible nor necessary for the clinician, with currently available information, to decide which view is "correct"; practical implications are the same.

Knowledge that primary open-angle glaucoma is inherited and is frequently associated with other conditions or measurable features makes the problems of screening and detection more manageable. Alerting signals that should initiate an investigation for primary open-angle glaucoma include the following:

1. A family history of glaucoma
2. High intraocular pressure or low outflow facility
3. High intraocular pressure after topical use of corticosteroids
4. Large, unequal, or vertically elongated cupping of the optic nerves
5. Optic disc hemorrhage
6. Myopia
7. Central retinal vein occlusion

The clinician has an obligation to urge that relatives of glaucoma patients be screened for glaucoma, with periodic reexaminations when the initial check is negative. The clinician should also investigate all of his or her patients with glaucoma or elevated intraocular pressures for diabetes mellitus.

SECONDARY GLAUCOMAS

Genetic factors have little influence on the occurrence of most varieties of secondary glaucoma. A few exceptions exist, the most obvious being the severe glaucoma that follows prolonged and unsupervised application of corticosteroid-containing collyria or ointments to a genetically susceptible eye.

Angle-Recession Glaucoma

A less obvious exception is the chronic glaucoma that develops months to years after blunt trauma of sufficient force to produce a recession of the anterior chamber angle. Armaly, intending to use this obviously secondary glaucoma as a control for his study of primary open-angle glaucoma and the corticosteroid response, applied topical corticosteroids to the uninvolved eyes of 11 patients with contusion angle glaucoma [11]. He was surprised to find that 5 of the patients possessed a $P^H P^H$ phenotype and the remaining 6 were $P^L P^H$. There were no nonresponders. In contrast, 3 of 4 patients with unilateral post-traumatic angle recession but no secondary glaucoma tested $P^L P^L$; the remaining patient tested $P^L P^H$. These findings suggest that a blunt blow to the eye of sufficient force to produce a tear into the ciliary body will cause glaucoma only in eyes genetically predisposed.

Spaeth compared the corticosteroid response of 15 patients with angle recession and 9 patients without angle recession, all of whom had had a hyphema secondary to blunt trauma 2 years previously [190]. A greater prevalence of corticosteroid responsiveness was found in the uninvolved fellow eyes of the patients in whom trauma had produced an angle recession (4 high, 5 intermediate, and 6 low responders) than in the patients in whom no angle recession was visible (5 intermediate and 4 low responders). A possible interpretation of these results is that blunt ocular trauma will produce an angle-recession injury more frequently in patients who are high responders to corticosteroids.

Central Retinal Vein Occlusion

Central retinal vein occlusion is associated with two types of glaucoma. The first is a devastating hemorrhagic glaucoma that follows the vein occlusion after a latent period of several weeks or months and is produced by synechial closure of the anterior chamber angle in association with neovascularization on the anterior surface of the iris. Less dramatic, but perhaps more important for the patient's ultimate visual prognosis, is the association of central retinal vein occlusion with preexisting primary open-angle glaucoma. Not only does retinal vein occlusion occasionally complicate known glaucoma [53, 74, 117, 186], but the fellow eyes of patients with unilateral central vein occlusion often harbor unsuspected primary open-angle glaucoma [201]. The vein occlusion may be asymptomatic, and after its resolution the only evidence may be the presence on the disc of venous loops or collateral vessels [101].

The prevalence of primary open-angle glaucoma or of abnormal water-provocative tonograms in the fellow eyes of patients with unilateral central retinal vein occlusion is about 35 percent [169, 201]. This prevalence increases to between 62 and 82 percent of the fellow eyes of patients with a unilateral central retinal vein occlusion that has been complicated by a secondary neovascular glaucoma [117, 169, 197, 201]. Furthermore, in the group with secondary neovascular glaucoma, an intraocular pressure elevation after topical application of corticosteroids occurs in 50 percent of the fellow eyes that have normal water-provocative tonograms [197]. Therefore, not only does primary open-angle glaucoma predispose to central retinal vein occlusion, but preexisting glaucoma, abnormalities of aqueous outflow, or corticosteroid sensitivity may increase the susceptibility of an eye with a central retinal vein occlusion to the subsequent development of rubeosis iridis and neovascular glaucoma.

Glaucomatocyclitic Crisis

In a series of 5 patients with unilateral glaucomatocyclitic crisis, the corticosteroid phenotypic classifications of the opposite eye were gg in 4 and nn in 1, which suggests a possible relation between this rare syndrome and primary open-angle glaucoma [108]. However, in another series of 15 patients with glaucomatocyclitic crisis, corticosteroid testing did not reveal an unusually high number of responders [170]. Lending support to a thesis that glaucomatocyclitic crisis and primary open-angle glaucoma may be related, Kass and coworkers reported a series of 11 patients, 5 of whom had glaucomatous visual field defects in the affected eye as well as the opposite eye [108]. Interestingly, 4 of 7 patients tested either had overt diabetes or had positive glucose tolerance test results.

Exfoliative Glaucoma

The results of corticosteroid testing in exfoliative glaucoma, the glaucoma associated with pseudoexfoliation of the lens capsule, are especially interesting, for this condition in many other respects is similar to primary open-angle glaucoma. However, the distribution of corticosteroid responses in patients with exfoliative glaucoma resembles that of the normal population [92, 165], and in those with pseudoexfoliation but no glaucoma the prevalence of steroid-induced intraocular pressure elevation is even less than that in a random population [196]. These findings suggest that exfoliative glaucoma is not the same as primary open-angle glaucoma and, instead, is secondary to plugging of the trabecular meshwork by exfoliative material. Genetic factors may still play a role, because pseudoexfoliation, with or without glaucoma, often appears in several members of a family [1, 115, 165, 195]. Whether this familial occurrence depends on environmental or genetic factors is not well worked out.

Pigmentary Glaucoma

Pigmentary glaucoma, typically an open-angle glaucoma in young myopic males, is characterized by Krunkenberg's spindles, pigment deposition in the trabecular meshwork, and concentric peripheral atrophy of the iris pigment epithelium. It was described by Sugar and Barbour as an entity distinct from primary open-angle glaucoma [194]. However, eyes with primary open-angle glaucoma also may have trabecular pigmentation [196], although usually they lack the other features of the pigment dispersion syndrome. Furthermore, patients with classical pigmentary glaucoma may have relatives with open-angle glaucoma or abnormal water-provocative test results but no evidence of pigment dispersion [51]. Finally, topical corticosteroid testing in persons with Krukenberg's spindles but with neither glaucoma nor a family history of glaucoma reveals an increased prevalence of high and intermediate responders (Table 11-11) [51, 210]. It is possible that pigmentary glaucoma occurs in eyes with pigment dispersion whose trabecular meshworks are unable to handle the pigment load because of genetic predisposition. The pigment dispersion itself may arise because of a deep anterior chamber and peripheral concavity of the iris [65], anatomic features that are also genetically determined.

Other Secondary Glaucomas

In other forms of secondary glaucoma, such as aphakic glaucoma with peripheral anterior synechiae and chronic angle-closure glaucoma unresponsive to iridectomy, the prevalences of the various corticosteroid phenotypes do not differ from those of the random population [32].

PRIMARY ANGLE-CLOSURE GLAUCOMA

Primary angle-closure glaucoma occurs when the peripheral portion of the iris bows forward against the trabecular meshwork, blocking outflow of aqueous humor from the eye. The diagnosis of primary angle-closure glaucoma is made when gonioscopy reveals a closed angle of the anterior chamber and no underlying cause such as inflammatory synechiae, rubeosis iridis, intraocular tumor, lens dislocation, or a leaking anterior chamber wound can be found. Angle closure may be intermittent, with acute elevations of the intraocular pressure and associated symptoms of pain, congestion, blurred vision, and halos; or it may be insidious, in all other respects mimicking primary open-angle glaucoma. The mechanism of angle closure is thought to be a relative pupillary block; in a susceptible eye, apposition of the pupillary region of the iris to the lens causes resistance to flow of aqueous humor from the posterior chamber into the anterior chamber. To maintain aqueous flow across this resistance, aqueous pressure in the posterior chamber must exceed that in the anterior chamber. The pressure differential between the two chambers pushes the flaccid peripheral iris forward against the cornea, closing the angle.

Since the time of von Graefe [203] and Priestly Smith [183], it has been noted that in certain primary glaucomas, especially of the acute congestive variety, the eyes have shallow anterior chambers. It has also long been observed that intraocular pressure elevations following mydriasis occur more frequently in shallow-chambered eyes [184, 193]. The depth of the anterior chamber follows a normal distribution curve in the general population [199]. The more shallow the anterior chamber, the greater is the likelihood of glaucoma. Up to 85 percent of eyes with a depth of less than 1.5 mm will develop angle-closure glaucoma [6]. The anterior chamber depth is also normally distributed in patients with angle-closure glaucoma, with a mean depth of about 1.8 mm and a calculated threshold for risk of angle-closure glaucoma of less than 2.5 mm [135]. Soon after gonioscopic classification of the glaucomas was introduced by Barkan, closed or narrow anterior chamber angles were associated with shallow anterior chambers [93]. Hypermetropia, often associated with shallow anterior chambers, was found to be prevalent in angle-closure glaucoma [192]. Eyes afflicted with angle-closure glaucoma also have smaller corneas [5, 93, 121, 185].

The common denominator of all these concurring factors, that is, angle closure, hypermetropia, shallow anterior chambers, small corneas, and small eyes, may be a disproportion between the size of the lens and the size of the eyeball [133, 134]. Lowe finds that in eyes with angle-closure glaucoma the lenses are thicker and more anteriorly situated, and the axial lengths are shorter than in normal eyes [133]. This disproportion produces a shallow anterior chamber with a forward position of the anterior lens surface, increasing the possibility of relative pupillary block and angle closure. Lens size, lens position, axial eyeball length, and anterior chamber depth are quantitative characteristics that probably are inherited in a multifactorial fashion. Tomlinson and Leighton have supported the concept that angle-closure glaucoma has a multifactorial causation by studying a group of angle-closure glaucoma patients, their siblings, and their offspring, comparing them to control subjects matched for age, sex, and refractive error [198]. As Clarke has pointed out, in diseases of multifactorial causation, first-degree relatives, that is, siblings and offspring, will be midway between resembling their affected relative and a matched control subject because they have inherited half of the "pathologic" genes from their parents [67]. Therefore, if the first-degree relative has ocular dimensions important in the development of angle-closure glaucoma that partially resemble those of the affected sibling or parent, it supports a multifactorial causation of angle-closure glaucoma. Tomlinson and Leighton found this to be true for corneal diameter, anterior chamber depth, lens thickness, and axial eye length.

Primary angle-closure glaucoma occasionally occurs in more than one member of a family [4, 132]. The reported prevalence of angle-closure glaucoma in relatives of affected patients varies from less than 1 percent to 12 percent [4, 123,

135, 151, 154]. Prevalance tends to be higher in siblings than in children, which supports a multifactorial cause of angle-closure glaucoma [4, 123]. Narrow angles are found in 20 to 32 percent of relatives of patients with angle-closure glaucoma [151, 191]. Before gonioscopy some family studies of primary open-angle glaucoma appeared to show autosomal dominant inheritance. Now it seems more likely that an anatomic predisposition to angle-closure glaucoma is inherited in a polygenic manner.

Patients with primary angle-closure glaucoma do not differ from the normal population in distribution of corticosteroid responsiveness [45, 111, 138]. However, when white patients with angle-closure glaucoma were tested for sensitivity to the taste of PTC, another inherited marker, only 17 percent were nontasters, compared with 28 percent of a normal population and 53 percent of a primary open-angle glaucoma population [50].

Racial differences in presentation and incidence of primary closed-angle glaucoma may be of genetic origin. In blacks primary angle-closure glaucoma is usually chronic and insidious, and the classic acute congestive variety is rare [2, 202]. In Japan and Southeast Asia primary angle-closure glaucoma is more common than primary open-angle glaucoma [112, 136]. Eskimos have the highest prevalance of primary angle-closure glaucoma of any population group studied [3, 76]. More than 2 percent of Eskimos over the age of 40 in both Greenland and Canada have primary angle-closure glaucoma, and over 10 percent of Eskimo women over 60 years old are affected. This compares to the 0.07 percent prevalence in a Welsh community surveyed by Hollows and Graham [102].

CONGENITAL GLAUCOMA

Primary Congenital Glaucoma

Primary congenital glaucoma is a rare disease in which anomalous development of structures in the anterior chamber angle produces abnormal resistance to outflow of aqueous humor from the eye. It is termed *congenital* because the outflow blockade is present at birth, but clinical features of photophobia, corneal enlargement and edema, and glaucomatous optic atrophy may not become evident until the child is several weeks or months old. Primary congenital glaucoma is unassociated with other major ocular abnormalities or systemic syndromes.

Most studies find that approximately 1 of every 8 or 10 cases of primary congenital glaucoma is familial [83, 204], and some authors report a 20 to 40 percent prevalence of familial cases [72, 85, 145]. Familial occurrence, by itself, does not indicate a genetic origin. However, a few reported instances of primary congenital glaucoma in twins provide striking evidence for a hereditary basis. At least 13 pairs of monozygotic twins with the defect have been described; in all of these except one [88] both children had glaucoma. In contrast, in all but one pair of dizygotic twins, only one child was affected [140, 209].

The genetic transmission of congenital glaucoma is controversial, and there may be several modes of inheritance. Until recently most authors have favored an autosomal recessive heredity. There are several points favoring this pattern. When familial, the disease frequently affects two or more offspring of healthy parents; other offspring are unaffected [63, 72, 204]. Genčík and colleagues reported that 41 percent of 118 patients with primary congenital glaucoma had consanguineous parents [89]; other authors have reported consanguinity rates of 4 to 8 percent [63, 140, 204].

The relative infrequency (10.7–14%) of familial primary congenital glaucoma [63, 83, 204] should not be misleading; many of the sporadic cases are probably also genetic. A recessively transmitted disease will afflict (assuming 100% penetrance) only 25 percent of the offspring of two heterozygotic "carrier" parents. Thus it is relatively unlikely that more than one child in a small family will be affected. Furthermore, in some siblings who are homozygous for the recessive genes glaucoma may fail to develop because of incomplete penetrance. Penetrance varies from nearly 100 percent in some pedigrees [83, 204] to 40 percent in the primary congenital glaucoma families of Copenhagen [208]. One factor affecting penetrance may be the child's sex; 3 of 5 patients with primary congenital glaucoma are males. It is significant that this ratio is the same in familial and nonfamilial cases. (In contrast, 63 percent of 47 reported Japanese patients have been female, which suggests that race may also influence penetrance [204].) Finally, new mutations and phenocopies (for example, congenital glaucoma produced by intrauterine rubella infection) may account for some nonfamilial cases.

A few families are reported in which two successive generations are afflicted [63, 83, 105, 140, 204]. These families may have a dominant form of congenital glaucoma (clinically identical to the recessive form) or may represent quasidominance, as in the marriage of a homozygote to a hetero-

Table 11-12. *Congenital Glaucoma Associated with Other Inherited Entities*

Primary disease	Mode of inheritance	Mechanism(s) of glaucoma
Aniridia	Autosomal dominant	Developmental anomaly of anterior chamber angle
Rieger's and Axenfeld's anomalies	Autosomal dominant	Developmental anomaly of anterior chamber angle
Peters' anomaly	Autosomal recessive	Developmental anomaly of anterior chamber angle
Lowe's oculocerebrorenal syndrome	X-linked recessive	Developmental anomaly of anterior chamber angle
Neurofibromatosis	Autosomal dominant	Developmental anomaly of anterior chamber angle, or tumor in meshwork
Marfan's syndrome	Autosomal dominant	Developmental anomaly of anterior chamber angle, or pupillary block by dislocated lens
Homocystinuria	Autosomal dominant	Pupillary block by dislocated lens
Marchesani's syndrome	Autosomal dominant or recessive (?)	Pupillary block by spherophakic lens
Microcornea or microphthalmos	Autosomal dominant or recessive	Angle-closure glaucoma
Retinoblastoma	Autosomal dominant	Angle closure secondary to forward displacement of the lens-iris diaphragm, rubeosis iridis with peripheral anterior synechiae, or inflammation

zygote. Westerlund estimates that 2.8 percent of the population of Copenhagen are heterozygotic carriers of congenital glaucoma [208]. Thus the possibility of a homozygote marrying a heterozygote is 1 in 35, with the odds increasing in consanguineous marriages.

Several studies have supported multifactorial inheritance [63, 72, 90, 91, 140]. Some factors favoring this mode of inheritance include a low number of affected siblings compared to expected numbers, a substantially decreased incidence in second-degree relatives compared to first-degree relatives, similarity in phenotypes between siblings, a parental prevalence of 2.7 to 4.4 percent, a nearly 30 percent incidence of unilaterality, and variable expressivity between families [36, 63].

Rarely, congenital glaucoma is found in some members of a family and primary open-angle glaucoma in others. Such concurrence may be the chance coincidence of two different diseases in one family. An alternate possibility is that the onset of primary congenital glaucoma in some children may be insidious, and mild cases may not become clinically manifest until later in life. Inherited susceptibility to corticosteroid-induced elevations of intraocular pressure occurs no more frequently among parents of primary congenital glaucoma patients than among the normal population [45, 109, 124].

Congenital Glaucoma Associated with Other Inherited Conditions of Children

Congenital glaucoma may be associated with other inherited conditions, ocular or systemic, that include among their manifestations a congenital anterior chamber angle anomaly. This anomaly may or may not resemble that seen in primary congenital glaucoma. Angle-closure glaucoma secondary to inherited abnormalities of the eye also may occur in infants and children. These various forms of glaucoma are listed, together with their modes of inheritance, in Table 11-12. This list, which includes only those forms of congenital and angle-closure glaucoma associated with inherited conditions, does not include the Sturge-Weber syndrome, which probably is not inherited. Several other inherited disorders, including Turner's syndrome, trisomy 13, trisomy 18, the systemic mucopolysaccharidoses, and the oculodentodigital syndrome, in which congenital glaucoma is only rarely manifested, are also not included in the list.

REFERENCES

1. Aasved, H. Study of relatives of persons with fibrillopathia epitheliocapsularis (pseudoexfoliation of the lens capsule). *Acta Ophthalmol. (Copenh.)* 53:879, 1975.

2. Alper, M. G., and Laubach, J. L. Primary angle-closure glaucoma in the American Negro. *Arch. Ophthalmol.* 79:663, 1968.

3. Alsbirk, P. H. Angle-closure glaucoma surveys in Greenland Eskimos. A preliminary report. *Can. J. Ophthalmol.* 8:260, 1973.

4. Alsbirk, P. H. Anterior chamber depth and primary angle-closure glaucoma: II. A genetic study. *Acta Ophthalmol. (Copenh.)* 53:436, 1975.

5. Alsbirk, P. H. Corneal diameter in Greenland Eskimos: Anthropometric and genetic studies with special reference to primary angle-closure glaucoma. *Acta Ophthalmol. (Copenh.)* 53:635, 1975.

6. Alsbirk, P. H. Primary angle-closure glaucoma: Oculometry, epidemiology, and genetics in a high risk population. *Acta Ophthalmol. [Suppl.] (Copenh.)* 127:5, 1976.

7. Angle, J., and Wissmann, D. A. The epidemiology of myopia. *Am. J. Epidemiol.* 111:220, 1980.

8. Armaly, M. F. On the distribution of applanation pressure: I. Statistical features and the effect of age, sex, and family history of glaucoma. *Arch. Ophthalmol.* 73:11, 1965.

9. Armaly, M. F. Applanation pressures in husband-wife pairs. *Am. J. Ophthalmol.* 62:635, 1966.

10. Armaly, M. F. The heritable nature of dexamethasone-induced ocular hypertension. *Arch. Ophthalmol.* 75:32, 1966.

11. Armaly, M. F. Inheritance of dexamethasone hypertension and glaucoma. *Arch. Ophthalmol.* 77:747, 1967.

12. Armaly, M. F. Dexamethasone ocular hypertension and eosinopenia, and glucose tolerance test. *Arch. Ophthalmol.* 78:193, 1967.

13. Armaly, M. F. Genetic determination and cup/disc ratio of the optic nerve. *Arch. Ophthalmol.* 78:35, 1967.

14. Armaly, M. F. The genetic determination of ocular pressure in the normal eye. *Arch. Ophthalmol.* 78:187, 1967.

15. Armaly, M. F. Topical Dexamethasone and Intraocular Pressure. In W. Leydhecker (Ed.), *International Symposium on Glaucoma*, Tutzing, 1966. Basel: Karger, 1967. P. 73.

16. Armaly, M. F. Genetic factors related to glaucoma. *Ann. N.Y. Acad. Sci.* 151:861, 1968.

17. Armaly, M. F. Cup/disk ratio in early open-angle glaucoma. *Doc. Ophthalmol.* 26:526, 1969.

18. Armaly, M. F. The correlation between appearance of the optic cup and visual function. *Trans. Am. Acad. Ophthalmol. Otolaryngol.* 73:898, 1969.

19. Armaly, M. F. The optic cup in the normal eye: I.

Cup width, depth, vessel displacement, ocular tension, and outflow facility. *Am. J. Ophthalmol.* 68:401, 1969.

20. Armaly, M. F. The visual field defect and ocular pressure level in open-angle glaucoma. *Invest. Ophthalmol.* 8:105, 1969.

21. Armaly, M. F. Optic cup in normal and glaucomatous eyes. *Invest. Ophthalmol.* 9:425, 1970.

22. Armaly, M. F. The Genetic Problem of Chronic Simple Glaucoma. In M. P. Solanes (Ed.), *International Congress of Ophthalmology: Proceedings of the XXI Congress, Mexico, 1970.* Amsterdam: Excerpta Medica, 1971. P. 278.

23. Armaly, M. F., and Baloglou, P. J. Diabetes mellitus and the eye: II. Intraocular pressure and aqueous outflow facility. *Arch. Ophthalmol.* 77:493, 1967.

24. Armaly, M. F., et al. Biostatistical analysis of the collaborative glaucoma study: I. Summary report of the risk factors for glaucomatous visual field defects. *Arch. Ophthalmol.* 98:2163, 1980.

25. Armaly, M. F., Monstavicius, B. F., and Sayegh, R. E. Ocular pressure and aqueous outflow facility in siblings. *Arch. Ophthalmol.* 80:354, 1968.

26. Armaly, M. F., and Sayegh, R. E. The cup/disc ratio: The findings of tonometry and tonography in the normal eye. *Arch. Ophthalmol.* 82:191, 1969.

27. Armstrong, J. R., et al. The incidence of glaucoma in diabetes mellitus: A comparison with the incidence of glaucoma in the general population. *Am. J. Ophthalmol.* 50:55, 1960.

28. Bankes, J. L. K. Ocular tension and diabetes mellitus. *Br. J. Ophthalmol.* 51:557, 1967.

29. Bankes, J. L. K., et al. Bedford glaucoma survey. *Br. Med. J.* 1:791, 1968.

30. Basu, S. K., and Jindal, A. Genetic aspects of myopia among Dawoodi Bohras. *Hum. Hered.* 33:163, 1983.

31. Bear, J. C., and Richler, A. Environmental influences on ocular refraction. *Am. J. Epidemiol.* 115:138, 1982. Taylor, H. R. Reply to above letter. *Am. J. Epidemiol.* 115:139, 1982.

32. Becker, B. The effect of topical corticosteroids in secondary glaucomas. *Arch. Ophthalmol.* 72:769, 1964.

33. Becker, B. Intraocular pressure response to topical corticosteroids. *Invest. Ophthalmol.* 4:198, 1965.

34. Becker, B. Diabetes and Glaucoma. In S. J. Kimura and W. M. Caygill, *Vascular Complications of Diabetes Mellitus.* St. Louis: Mosby, 1967. P. 43.

35. Becker, B. Topical Corticosteroids and Intraocular Pressure. In B. Becker and R. C. Drews (Eds.), *Current Concepts in Ophthalmology.* St. Louis: Mosby, 1967. P. 132.

36. Becker, B. Glaucoma: Recent endocrine studies. *Acta Soc. Ophthalmol. Jpn.* 73:2614, 1969.

37. Becker, B. Cup/disk ratio and topical corticosteroid testing. *Am. J. Ophthalmol.* 70:681, 1970.

38. Becker, B. Diabetes mellitus and primary open-angle glaucoma. *Am. J. Ophthalmol.* 71:1, 1971.

39. Becker, B. The genetic problem of chronic simple glaucoma. *Ann. Ophthalmol.* 3:351, 1971.

40. Becker, B. The Genetic Problem of Chronic Simple Glaucoma. In M. P. Solanes (Ed.), *International Congress of Ophthalmology. Proceedings of the XXI Congress, Mexico, 1970.* Amsterdam: Excerpta Medica, 1971. P. 286.

41. Becker, B., and Ballin, N. Glaucoma and corticosteroid provocative testing. *Arch. Ophthalmol.* 74:621, 1965.

42. Becker, B., et al. Intraocular pressure and its response to topical corticosteroids in diabetes. *Arch. Ophthalmol.* 76:477, 1966.

43. Becker, B., and Chevrette, L. Topical corticosteroid testing in glaucoma siblings. *Arch. Ophthalmol.* 76:484, 1966.

44. Becker, B., and Hahn, K. A. Topical corticosteroids and heredity in primary open-angle glaucoma. *Am. J. Ophthalmol.* 57:543, 1964.

45. Becker, B., and Kolker, A. E. Topical corticosteroid testing in conditions related to glaucoma. *Int. Ophthalmol. Clin.* 6:1005, 1966.

46. Becker, B., and Kolker, A. E. The corticosteroid intraocular pressure response: Thyroid function and phenylthiourea taste test. *Doc. Ophthalmol.* 26:313, 1969.

47. Becker, B., Kolker, A. E., and Ballin, N. Thyroid function and glaucoma. *Am. J. Ophthalmol.* 61:997, 1966.

48. Becker, B., Kolker, A. E., and Roth, F. D. Glaucoma family study. *Am. J. Ophthalmol.* 50:557, 1960.

49. Becker, B., and LeBlanc, R. P. The glucose tolerance test and the response of intraocular pressure to topical corticosteroids. *Diabetes* 19:715, 1970.

50. Becker, B., and Morton, W. R. Phenylthiourea taste testing and glaucoma. *Arch. Ophthalmol.* 72:323, 1964.

51. Becker, B., and Podos, S. M. Krukenberg's spindles and primary open-angle glaucoma. *Arch. Ophthalmol.* 76:635, 1966.

52. Becker, B., et al. Plasma cortisol suppression in glaucoma. *Am. J. Ophthalmol.* 75:73, 1973.

53. Becker, B., and Post, L. T. Retinal vein occlusion: Clinical and experimental observations. *Am. J. Ophthalmol.* 34:677, 1951.

54. Becker, B., and Ramsey, C. K. Plasma cortisol and the intraocular pressure response to topical corticosteroids. *Am. J. Ophthalmol.* 69:999, 1970.

55. Ben-Ezra, D., Ticho, U., and Sacks, U. Lymphocyte sensitivity to glucocorticoids. *Am. J. Ophthalmol.* 83:866, 1976.

56. Bengtsson, B. Some factors affecting the distribution of intraocular pressures in a population. *Acta Ophthalmol. (Copenh.)* 50:33, 1972.

57. Bengtsson, B. Resemblance between tonometer readings on relatives and spouses. *Acta Ophthalmol. (Copenh.)* 54:27, 1976.

58. Bengtsson, B. The prevalence of glaucoma. *Br. J. Ophthalmol.* 65:46, 1981.

59. Bessiére, D., and Le Goff, J. L. À propos de quelques cas familiaux de glaucome chronique simple. *Bull. Soc. Ophtalmol. Fr.* 63:789, 1963.

60. Bigger, J. F., Palmberg, P. F., and Becker, B. Increased cellular sensitivity to glucocorticoids in primary open-angle glaucoma. *Invest. Ophthalmol.* 11:832, 1972.

61. Bigger, J. F., Palmberg, P. F., and Zink, H. A. In vitro corticosteroid: Correlation response with primary open-angle glaucoma and ocular corticosteroid sensitivity. *Am. J. Ophthalmol.* 79:92, 1975.

62. Bonomi, L., Mecca, E., and Massa, F. Intraocular pressure in myopic anisometropia. *Int. Ophthalmol.* 5:145, 1982.

63. Briard, M. L., et al. The genetics of congenital glaucoma: A study of 231 cases. *J. Genet. Hum.* (Suppl. 24):107, 1976.

64. Brooser, G. Diabetes gondozas soran vegzett glaukoma szures adatal elozetes kozles. *Szemeszet* 105:283, 1968. (Abstract in *Excerpta Medica XII* 23:259, 1969.)

65. Campbell, D. G. Pigmentary dispersion and glaucoma: A new theory. *Arch. Ophthalmol.* 97:1667, 1979.

66. Christiansson, J. Intraocular pressure in diabetes mellitus. *Acta Ophthalmol.* (*Copenh*) 39:155, 1961.

67. Clarke, C. A. Genetic counselling. *Br. Med. J.* 1:606, 1972.

68. Coulehan, J. L., Helzlsower, K. J., and Rogers, K. D. Racial differences in intraocular tension and glaucoma surgery. *Am. J. Epidemiol.* 111:759, 1980.

69. Crombie, A. L., and Cullen, J. F. Hereditary glaucoma: Occurrence in five generations of an Edinburgh family. *Br. J. Ophthalmol.* 48:143, 1964.

70. Curtin, B. J. Myopia: A review of its aetiology, pathogenesis, and treatment. *Surv. Ophthalmol.* 1:1, 1970.

71. Davies, T. G. Tonographic survey of the close relatives of patients with chronic simple glaucoma. *Br. J. Ophthalmol.* 52:32, 1968.

72. Demenais, F., et al. Congenital glaucoma: Genetic models. *Hum. Genet.* 46:305, 1979.

73. Diaz-Dominguez, D. Sur les rapports de la grande myopie et de l'hypertension oculaire. *Ann. Ocul.* (*Paris*) 194:597, 1961.

74. Dobree, J. H. Venous obstruction and neovascularization at the disc in chronic glaucoma. *Trans. Ophthalmol. Soc. U.K.* 72:229, 1957.

75. Dodinval, P., Prijot, E., and Weekers, R. L'hérédité du glaucoma à angle ouvert. *J. Med. Genet.* 7:244, 1970.

76. Drance, S. M. Angle-closure glaucoma among Canadian Eskimos. *Can. J. Ophthalmol.* 8:252, 1973.

77. Drance, S. M. Myopia: Genes or environment? *Can. Med. Assoc. J.* 112:552, 1975.

78. Drance, S. M., et al. Use of discriminant analysis: II. Identification of persons with glaucomatous visual field defects. *Arch. Ophthalmol.* 96:1571, 1978.

79. Drance, S. M., et al. Multivariate analysis in glaucoma: Use of discriminant analysis in predicting glaucomatous visual field damage. *Arch. Ophthalmol.* 99:1019, 1981.

80. Drance, S. M., and Scott, S. A comparison of action of dexamethasone and medrysone on human intraocular pressure. *Can. J. Ophthalmol.* 3:159, 1968.

81. Duke-Elder, S. *System of Ophthalmology, Vol. 5: Ophthalmic Optics and Refraction.* St. Louis: Mosby, 1970. P. 268.

82. Fishman, R. S. Optic disc asymmetry: A sign of ocular hypertension. *Arch. Ophthalmol.* 84:590, 1970.

83. François, J. *Heredity in Ophthalmology.* St. Louis: Mosby, 1961.

84. François, J. Genetics and primary open-angle glaucoma. *Am. J. Ophthalmol.* 61:652, 1966.

85. François, J. Genetic Predisposition to Glaucoma. In W. Straub (Ed.) *Developments in Ophthalmology,* Vol. 3. New York: Karger, 1981. P. 1.

86. François, J., and Heintz-De Bree, C. Personal research on the heredity of chronic simple (open-angle) glaucoma. *Am. J. Ophthalmol.* 62:1067, 1966.

87. François, J., Heintz-De Bree, C., and Tripathi, R. C. The cortisone test and the heredity of primary open-angle glaucoma. *Am. J. Ophthalmol.* 62:844, 1966.

88. Fried, K., Sach, R., and Krakowsky, D. Congenital glaucoma in only one of identical twins. *Ophthalmologica* 174:185, 1977.

89. Genčík, A., Genčíková, A., and Gerinec, A. Genetic heterogeneity of congenital glaucoma. *Clin. Genet.* 17:241, 1980.

90. Genčík, A., et al. Notes on the genetics of congenital glaucoma. *Ophthalmologica* 179:209, 1979.

91. Genčíková, A., and Genčík, A. Congenital glaucoma in Gypsies from Slovakia. *Hum. Hered.* 32:270, 1982.

92. Gillies, W. E. Corticosteroid-induced ocular hypertension in pseudoexfoliation of lens capsule. *Am. J. Ophthalmol.* 70:90, 1970.

93. Gradle, H. S., and Sugar, H. S. Concerning the chamber angle: III. A clinical method of goniometry. *Am. J. Ophthalmol.* 23:1135, 1940.

94. Greve, E. L., and Furono, F. Myopia and glaucoma. *Albrecht von Graefe Arch Klin. Exp. Ophthalmol.* 213:33, 1980.

95. Haag, C. Das Glaukom der Jugendlichen. *Klin. Monatsbl. Augenheilkd.* 54:133, 1915.

96. Harris, D. The inheritance of glaucoma: A pedigree of familial glaucoma. *Am. J. Ophthalmol.* 60:91, 1965.

97. Hart, W. M., Jr., et al. Multivariate analysis of the risk of glaucomatous visual field loss. *Arch. Ophthalmol.* 97:1455, 1979.

98. Hauff, D. Glaukom und Diabetes. *Ophthalmologica* 160:391, 1970.

99. Havener, W. H. Chronic simple glaucoma: Hereditary aspects. *Am. J. Ophthalmol.* 40:828, 1955.

100. Hiller, R., Sperduto, R. D., and Krueger, D. E. Race,

iris pigmentation, and intraocular pressure. *Am. J. Epidemiol.* 115:674, 1982.

101. Hitchings, R. A., and Spaeth, G. L. Chronic retinal vein occlusion in glaucoma. *Br. J. Ophthalmol.* 60:694, 1976.

102. Hollows, F. C., and Graham, P. A. Intraocular pressure, glaucoma, and glaucoma suspects in a defined population. *Br. J. Ophthalmol.* 50:570, 1966.

103. Jain, I. S., and Luthra, C. L. Diabetic retinopathy: Its relationship with intraocular pressure. *Arch. Ophthalmol.* 78:198, 1967.

104. Jay, B., and Paterson, G. The genetics of simple glaucoma. *Trans. Ophthalmol. Soc. U.K.* 90:161, 1970.

105. Jerndal, T. Familial congenital glaucoma with dominant heredity. *Acta Ophthalmol. (Copenh.)* 46:459, 1968.

106. Kalmus, H., and Lewkonia, I. Relation between some forms of glaucoma and phenylthiocarbamide tasting. *Br. J. Ophthalmol.* 57:593, 1973.

107. Karlsson, J. L. Evidence for recessive inheritance of myopia. *Clin. Genet.* 7:197, 1975.

108. Kass, M. A., Becker, B., and Kolker, A. E. Glaucomatocyclitic crisis and primary open-angle glaucoma. *Am. J. Ophthalmol.* 75:668, 1973.

109. Kaufman, P. L., and Kolker, A. E. Ocular findings and corticosteroid responsiveness in parents of children with primary infantile glaucoma. *Invest. Ophthalmol.* 14:46, 1975.

110. Kini, M. M., et al. The Framingham Eye Study: The prevalence of senile cateract, diabetic retinopathy, senile macular degeneration, and open angle glaucoma. *Am. J. Ophthalmol.* 85:28, 1978.

111. Kitazawa, Y. Primary angle-closure glaucoma: Corticosteroid responsiveness. *Arch. Ophthalmol.* 84:724, 1970.

112. Kitazawa, Y. Personal communication, 1971.

113. Kitazawa, Y., and Horie, T. The prognosis of corticosteroid-responsive individuals. *Arch. Ophthalmol.* 99:819, 1981.

114. Kitazawa, Y., and Takeuchi, T. The effects of betamethasone in normal and glaucomatous eyes. *Acta Soc. Ophthalmol. Jpn.* 69:2031, 1965.

115. Knape, B., and Raitta, C. Familiares Vorkommen von Pseudoexfoliation und Glaukom. *Acta Ophthalmol. (Copenh.)* 48:434, 1970.

116. Kolker, A. E. Glaucoma family study: Ten-year follow-up (preliminary report). *Isr. J. Med. Sci.* 8:1357, 1972.

117. Kolker, A. E., and Hetherington, J., Jr. *Becker-Shaffer's Diagnosis and Therapy of the Glaucomas* (3rd ed.). St. Louis: Mosby, 1970.

118. Krupin, T., et al. Thyroid function and the intraocular pressure response to topical corticosteroids. *Am. J. Ophthalmol.* 83:643, 1977.

119. Krupin, T., Podos, S. M., and Becker, B. Effect of diphenylhydantoin on dexamethasone suppression of plasma cortisol in primary open-angle glaucoma. *Am. J. Ophthalmol.* 71:997, 1971.

120. Lacroix, A. La tension oculaire dans la myopia élevée progressive chez l'adulte. *Ann. Ocul. (Paris)* 159:730, 1922.

121. Lee, D. A., Brubaker, R. F., and Ilstrup, D. M. Anterior chamber dimensions in patients with narrow angles and angle-closure glaucoma. *Arch. Ophthalmol.* 102:46, 1984.

122. Leighton, D. A. Studies on relatives of glaucoma patients. *Proc. R. Soc. Med.* 61:542, 1968.

123. Leighton, D. A. Survey of the first-degree relatives of glaucoma patients. *Trans. Ophthalmol. Soc. U.K.* 96:28, 1976.

124. Leighton, D. A., and Phillips, C. I. Infantile glaucoma: Steroid testing in parents of affected children. *Br. J. Ophthalmol.* 54:27, 1970.

125. Leske, M. C. The epidemiology of open-angle glaucoma: A review. *Am. J. Epidemiol.* 118:166, 1983.

126. Levene, R. Z., and Schwartz, B. Depression of plasma cortisol and the steroid ocular pressure response. *Arch. Ophthalmol.* 80:461, 1968.

127. Levene, R. Z., Schwartz, B., and Workman, P. L. Heritability of plasma cortisol. *Arch. Ophthalmol.* 87:389, 1972.

128. Levene, R., et al. Topical corticosteroid in normal patients and glaucoma suspects. *Arch. Ophthalmol.* 77:593, 1967.

129. Levene, R. Z., et al. Heritability of ocular pressure in normal and suspect ranges. *Arch. Ophthalmol.* 84:730, 1970.

130. Lieb, W. A., et al. Diabetes mellitus and Glaukom. *Acta Ophthalmol. [Suppl.] (Copenh.)* 94:1, 1967.

131. Linnér, E. The association of ocular hypertension with the exfoliation syndrome, the pigmentary dispersion syndrome, and myopia. *Surv. Ophthalmol.* 25:1477, 1980.

132. Lowe, R. F. Primary angle-closure glaucoma: Family histories and anterior chamber depths. *Br. J. Ophthalmol.* 48:191, 1964.

133. Lowe, R. F. Causes of shallow anterior chamber in primary angle-closure glaucoma: Ultrasonic biometry of normal and angle-closure glaucoma eyes. *Am. J. Ophthalmol.* 67:87, 1969.

134. Lowe, R. F. Aetiology of the anatomical basis for primary angle-closure glaucoma: Biometrical comparisons between normal eyes and eyes with primary angle-closure glaucoma. *Br. J. Ophthalmol.* 54:161, 1970.

135. Lowe, R. F. Primary angle-closure glaucoma: Inheritance and environment. *Br. J. Ophthalmol.* 56:13, 1972.

136. Mann, I. *Culture, Race, Climate and Eye Disease: An Introduction to the Study of Geographical Ophthalmology.* Springfield, Ill.: Thomas, 1966.

137. Marré, E., and Marré, M. Ein Beitrage zum Glaukom bei Diabetes mellitus. *Klin. Monatsbl. Augenheilkd.* 153:396, 1968.

138. Masuda, H. The steroid ocular pressure response in the glaucomatous eye. *Acta Soc. Ophthalmol. Jpn.* 73:2060, 1969.

139. McCarty, G., Schwartz, B., and Miller, K. Absence of lymphocyte glucocorticoid hypersensitivity in primary open-angle glaucoma. *Arch. Ophthalmol.* 99:1258, 1981.

140. Merin, S., and Morin, D. Heredity of congenital glaucoma. *Br. J. Ophthalmol.* 56:414, 1972.

141. Miller, S. Outflow value in immediate descendants of parents with glaucoma simplex. *Trans. Ophthalmol. Soc. U.K.* 81:577, 1961.

142. Miller, S. J. Genetics of glaucoma and family studies. *Trans. Ophthalmol. Soc. U.K.* 98:290, 1978.

143. Miller, S. J. H., and Paterson, G. D. Studies on glaucoma relatives. *Br. J. Ophthalmol.* 46:513, 1962.

144. Morgan, R. W., and Drance, S. M. Chronic open-angle glaucoma and ocular hypertension: An epidemiological study. *Br. J. Ophthalmol.* 59:211, 1975.

145. Nakajima, A., Fujiki, K., and Tanake, U. Genetics of buphthalmos. Presented at the 7th Congress of the Asia-Pacific Academy of Ophthalmology, Karachi, Japan, 1979.

146. Nicholas, J. P. Topical corticosteroids and aqueous humor dynamics. *Arch. Ophthalmol.* 72:189, 1964.

147. Nordmann, J., et al. Le test à la cortisone dans le glaucome simple à champ visuel normal. *Ophthalmologica* 150:46, 1965.

148. Packer, H., Deutsch, A. R., and Deweese, M. K. Frequency of glaucoma in three population groups. *J.A.M.A.* 188:123, 1964.

149. Palmberg, P. F., and Bigger, J. F. Corticosteroid inhibition of titrated thymidine uptake by phytohemagglutinin stimulated human lymphocytes: Correlations of in vitro responses to ocular steroid response phenotypes. Presented at the meeting of the Association for Research in Vision and Ophthalmology, Sarasota, Florida, Apr., 1972.

150. Palmberg, P. F., et al. The reproducibility of the intraocular pressure response to dexamethasone. *Am. J. Ophthalmol.* 80:844, 1975.

151. Paterson, G. Studies on siblings of patients with both angle-closure and chronic simple glaucoma. *Trans. Ophthalmol. Soc. U.K.* 81:561, 1961.

152. Paterson, G. Studies of the response to topical dexamethasone of glaucoma relatives. *Trans. Ophthalmol. Soc. U.K.* 85:295, 1965.

153. Paterson, G. A nine-year follow-up of studies of first-degree relatives of patients with glaucoma simple. *Trans. Ophthalmol. Soc. U.K.* 90:515, 1970.

154. Perkins, E. S. Family studies in glaucoma. *Br. J. Ophthalmol.* 58:529, 1974.

155. Perkins, E. S. Morbidity from myopia. *Sight Sav. Rev.* 1979. P. 11.

156. Perkins, E. S., and Jay, B. S. Pigmentary glaucoma. *Trans. Ophthalmol. Soc. U.K.* 80:153, 1960.

157. Perkins, E. S., and Phelps, C. D. Open-angle glaucoma, ocular hypertension, low-tension glaucoma, and refraction. *Arch. Ophthalmol.* 100:1464, 1982.

158. Phelps, C. D. Effect of myopia on prognosis in treated primary open-angle glaucoma. *Am. J. Ophthalmol.* 93:622, 1982.

159. Phelps, C. D., et al. Blood reflux into Schlemm's canal. *Arch. Ophthalmol.* 88:625, 1972.

160. Phelps, C. D., and Corbett, J. J. Migraine and low-tension glaucoma. *Invest. Ophthalmol.* 26:1105, 1985.

161. Podos, S. M., and Becker, B. Unpublished data.

162. Podos, S. M., et al. Diphenylhydantoin and cortisol metabolism in glaucoma. *Am. J. Ophthalmol.* 74:498, 1972.

163. Podos, S. M., Becker, B., and Morton, W. R. High myopia and primary open-angle glaucoma. *Am. J. Ophthalmol.* 62:1039, 1966.

164. Pohjanpelta, P., and Hurskainen, L. Studies on relatives of patients with glaucoma simplex and patients with pseudoexfoliation of the lens capsule. *Acta Ophthalmol. (Copenh.)* 50:255, 1972.

165. Pohjola, S., and Horsmanheimo, A. Topically applied corticosteroids in glaucoma capsulare. *Arch. Ophthalmol.* 85:150, 1971.

166. Popovic, V. The glaucoma population in Gothenburg. *Acta Ophthalmol. (Copenh.)* 60:745, 1982.

167. Pur, S. Diabetes mellitus a glaukom. *Cesk. Oftalmol.* 22:427, 1966. (Abstract in *Excerpta Medica XII* 21:172, 1967.)

168. Radian, A. B., et al. Glaucom si diabet. *Oftalmologica* (Bucharest) 12:219, 1968. (Abstract in *Excerpta Medica XII* 23:162, 1969.)

169. Raitta, C. Der Zentralvenen- und Netzhautvenenverschluss. *Acta Ophthalmol. [Suppl.] (Copenh.)* 83:1, 1965.

170. Raitta, C., and Klemetti, A. Steroidbelastung bei Posner-Schlossmanschem Syndrom. *Albrect von Graefes Arch. Klin. Exp. Ophthalmol.* 174:66, 1967.

171. Roberts, J., and Rowland, M. Refraction status and motility defects of persons 4–74 years, U.S., 1971–1972. Vital and Health Statistics series 11, National Health Survey 206, U.S. Department of Health, Education, and Welfare Publication (PHS) 78-1651, 1978.

172. Safir, A., et al. Ocular abnormalities in juvenile diabetes: Frequent occurrence of abnormally high tensions. *Arch. Ophthalmol.* 76:557, 1966.

173. Schlote, H. W., and Marré, E. Latente diabetische Stoffwechsellage und Glaucoma simplex. *Klin. Monatsbl. Augenheilkd.* 156:67, 1970.

174. Schwartz, B. The response of ocular pressure to corticosteroids. *Int. Ophthalmol. Clin.* 6:929, 1966.

175. Schwartz, B., and Levene, R. Z. Plasma cortisol differences between normal and glaucomatous patients: Before and after dexamethasone suppression. *Arch. Ophthalmol.* 87:369, 1972.

176. Schwartz, J. T., Reuling, F. H., and Feinleib, M. Size of the physiologic cup of the optic nerve head: Hereditary and environmental factors. *Arch. Ophthalmol.* 93:776, 1975.

177. Schwartz, J. T., et al. Twin heritability study of the corticosteroid response. *Trans. Am. Acad. Ophthalmol. Otolaryngol.* 77:126, 1973.

178. Schwartz, J. T., et al. Twin study on ocular pressure after topical dexamethasone: I. Frequency distribution of pressure response. *Am. J. Ophthalmol.* 76:126, 1973.

179. Schwartz, J. T., Reuling, F. H., and Garrison, R. J. Acquired cupping of the optic nerve head in normotensive eyes. *Br. J. Ophthalmol.* 59:216, 1975.

180. Segal, P., and Skwierczynska, J. Badania nad wplywem miejscowego podawania ultrakortenolu na cisnienie srodoczne. *Klin. Oczna* 37:503, 1967. (Abstract in *Excerpta Medica XII* 22:28, 1968.)

181. Shikunova, R. P. Corticosteroid test and heredity in primary glaucoma. *Vestn. Oftalmol.* 3:43, 1970. (Abstract in *Excerpta Medica XII* 25:171, 1971.)

182. Shin, D. H., Becker, B., and Kolker, A. E. Family history in primary open-angle glaucoma. *Arch. Ophthalmol.* 95:598, 1977.

183. Smith, P. On the shallow anterior chamber of primary glaucoma. *Ophthalmol. Rev.* 6:191, 1887.

184. Smith, P. Glaucoma problems. *Ophthalmol. Rev.* 30:161, 1911.

185. Smith, P. Glaucoma problems. *Ophthalmol. Rev.* 31:193, 1912.

186. Smith, R. Concerning glaucoma and retinal venous occlusion. *Trans. Ophthalmol. Soc. U.K.* 75:265, 1955.

187. Southren, A. L., et al. Altered cortisol metabolism in cells cultured from trabecular meshwork specimens obtained from patients with primary open-angle glaucoma. *Invest. Ophthalmol. Vis. Sci.* 24:1413, 1983.

188. Sowell, J. G., et al. Primary open-angle glaucoma and sensitivity to corticosteroids in vitro. *Am. J. Ophthalmol.* 84:715, 1977.

189. Spaeth, G. L. Effects of topical dexamethasone on intraocular pressure and the water drinking test. *Arch. Ophthalmol.* 76:772, 1966.

190. Spaeth, G. L. Traumatic hyphema, angle recession, dexamethasone hypertension, and glaucoma. *Arch. Ophthalmol.* 78:714, 1967.

191. Spaeth, G. L. Gonioscopy: Uses old and new. The inheritance of occludable angles. *Ophthalmology (Rochester)* 85:222, 1978.

192. Sugar, H. S. The mechanical factors in the etiology of acute glaucoma. *Am. J. Ophthalmol.* 24:851, 1941.

193. Sugar, H. S. Anatomic factors that influence the depth of the anterior chamber: Their significance. *Am. J. Ophthalmol.* 25:1341, 1942.

194. Sugar, H. S., and Barbour, F. A. Pigmentary glaucoma: A rare clinical entity. *Am. J. Ophthalmol.* 32:90, 1949.

195. Tarkkanen, A. Pseudoexfoliation of the lens capsule. *Acta Ophthalmol. [Suppl.] (Copenh.)* 71:1, 1962.

196. Tarkkanen, A., and Horsmanheimo, A. Topical corticosteroids and nonglaucomatous pseudoexfoliation. *Acta Ophthalmol. (Copenh.)* 44:323, 1966.

197. Tarkkanen, A., Raitta, C., and Vannas, S. Corticosteroide und hamorrhagisches Glaukom nach Zentralvenenverschluss. *Albrecht von Graefes Arch. Klin. Exp. Ophthalmol.* 171:307, 1967.

198. Tomlinson, A., and Leighton, D. A. Ocular dimensions in the heredity of angle-closure glaucoma. *Br. J. Ophthalmol.* 57:475, 1973.

199. Törnquist, R. Shallow anterior chamber in acute glaucoma: A clinical and genetic study. *Acta Ophthalmol. (Suppl.) (Copenh.)* 39:1, 1953.

200. Traisman, H. S., et al. Intraocular pressure in juvenile diabetics. *Am. J. Ophthalmol.* 64:1149, 1967.

201. Vannas, S., and Tarkkanen, A. Retinal vein occlusion and glaucoma: Tonographic study of the incidence of glaucoma and of its prognostic significance. *Br. J. Ophthalmol.* 44:583, 1960.

202. Venable, H. P. Glaucoma in the Negro. *J. Natl. Med. Assoc.* 44:7, 1952.

203. von Graefe, A. Über die Iridectomie bei Glaucom und über den glaucomatösen Process. *Albrecht von Graefes Arch. Ophthalmol.* 3:456, 1857.

204. Waardenburg, P. J., Franceschetti, A., and Klein, D. *Genetics and Ophthalmology*, Vol. 1. Springfield, Ill.: Thomas, 1961.

205. Weekers, R., Grieten, J., and Collignon-Brach, J. Contribution à l'étude de l'hypertension oculaire provoquée par la dexamethasone dans le glaucome à angle ouvert. *Opthalmologica* 152:81, 1966.

206. Weekers, R., Lavergne, G., and Prijot, E. La correction des mesures tonometriques chez les sujets à rigidité oculaire basse ou haute. *Ann. Ocul. (Paris)* 191:26, 1958.

207. Weisman, R. L., et al. Vertical elongation of the optic cup in glaucoma. *Trans. Am. Acad. Ophthalmol. Otolaryngol.* 77:157, 1973.

208. Westerlund, K. E. *Clinical and Genetic Studies on the Primary Glaucoma Diseases.* Copenhagen: Busck, 1947.

209. Widstrom, G., and Henschen, A. The relation between P.T.C. taste response and protein bound iodine in serum. *Scand. J. Clin. Lab. Invest. (Suppl.)* 69:257, 1963.

210. Wilensky, J. T., Buerck, K. M., and Podos, S. M. Krukenberg's spindles. *Am. J. Ophthalmol.* 79:220, 1975.

211. Yablonski, M. E., et al. Prognostic significance of optic disk cupping in ocular hypertensive patients. *Am. J. Ophthalmol.* 89:585, 1980.

12

Corneal Diseases

Corey A. Miller
Jay H. Krachmer

In this chapter, two categories of corneal disorders will be described: corneal dystrophies and corneal disorders associated with inherited systemic disease.

The corneal dystrophies are primary, bilateral, inherited disorders of the cornea that occur unaccompanied by systemic disease [94]. The age at onset, symptoms, mode of progression, and clinical features of an individual dystrophy vary but tend to remain the same within a given pedigree [121]. Most dystrophies are inherited in an autosomal dominant fashion with varying degrees of penetrance and expressivity. Clinical manifestations usually occur in the first few decades of life and are stationary or slowly progressive. Inflammation and vascularization may be secondary changes [410].

Most of the corneal dystrophies may be identified by their morphologic characteristics (Fig. 12-1) and typical history of onset and progression. The family history and examination of family members may be of great benefit in the diagnosis of unusual cases. The histopathology, especially ultrastructural pathology, is well documented for most of the dystrophies, yet relatively little is known concerning their pathogenesis [218, 301]. Histochemical methods have provided identification of some of the deposited or altered substances in these disorders. Further insight will be provided by tissue culture techniques that allow study in a dynamic state.

Certain corneal changes, often resembling the corneal dystrophies, are found in a variety of inherited skin and metabolic disorders [115, 119]. In some of these genetic conditions, the corneal alterations may be so characteristic as to be pathognomonic of the disease; in others they are nonspecific and often secondary to adnexal involvement.

The clinical, genetic, and histochemical aspects of these two groups of disorders will be presented in this chapter. A modified topographic classification, based on the level of origin of the early corneal changes, will be used for the corneal dystrophies (Table 12-1) [112, 121, 259, 410, 411]. The other disorders will be divided into those with primary dermatologic changes and those associated with known metabolic defects.

CORNEAL DYSTROPHIES

Dystrophies of the Epithelium and Bowman's Membrane

MEESMANN'S DYSTROPHY

Juvenile hereditary epithelial dystrophy was first described by Pameijer [288] and was more comprehensively detailed by Meesmann and Wilke [271, 272]. It is a rare, bilaterally symmetrical, autosomal dominant disorder that may present in the first year of life as epithelial cysts [47, 360]. Symptoms are rare until middle age when the cysts begin to rupture onto the ocular surface causing intermittent tearing, pain, and photophobia. Vision may be slightly diminished because of an irregular corneal surface or moderately decreased if there is subepithelial scarring. Diminished corneal sensation is a late finding in some cases. Treatment is rarely required and usually involves only symptomatic management of the surface problems.

Myriads of fine, round vacuoles are present in the epithelium, most prominently in the intrapalpebral zone, although they involve the entire

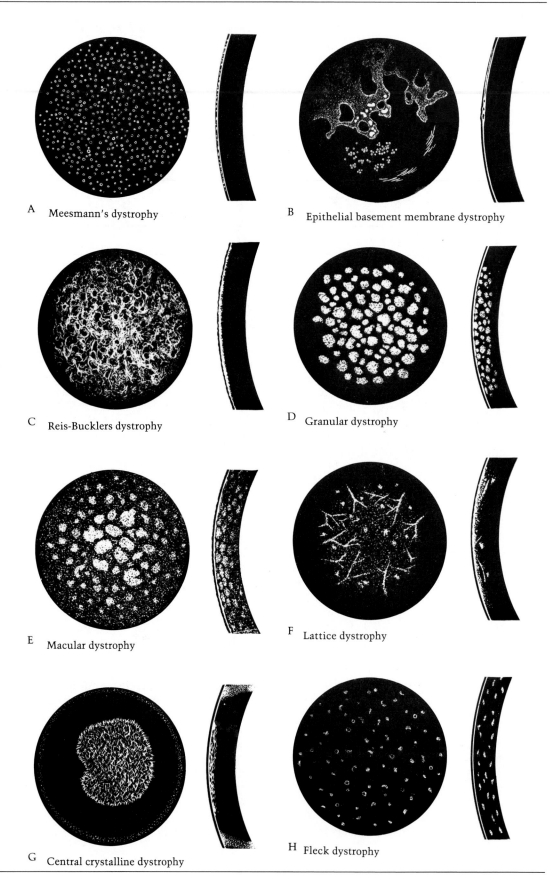

A   Meesmann's dystrophy

B   Epithelial basement membrane dystrophy

C   Reis-Bucklers dystrophy

D   Granular dystrophy

E   Macular dystrophy

F   Lattice dystrophy

G   Central crystalline dystrophy

H   Fleck dystrophy

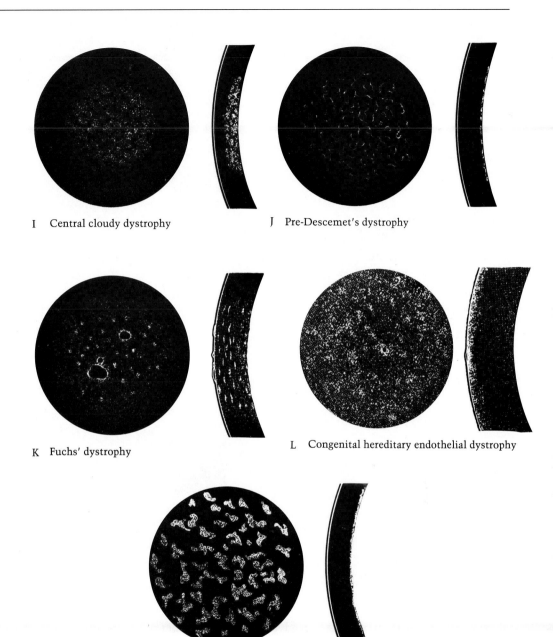

I   Central cloudy dystrophy

J   Pre-Descemet's dystrophy

K   Fuchs' dystrophy

L   Congenital hereditary endothelial dystrophy

M   Posterior polymorphous dystrophy

Fig. 12-1. *Representative clinical appearance of various types of corneal dystrophy. (Figs. B and J from G. O. Waring, M. M. Rodrigues, and P. R. Laibson [410].)*

Table 12-1. *Classification of the Corneal Dystrophies Described in This Chapter*

Epithelium and Bowman's membrane
   Meesmann's dystrophy (juvenile hereditary
     epithelial dystrophy)
   Epithelial basement membrane dystrophy (map-dot-
     fingerprint dystrophy)
   Dystrophic recurrent erosion
   Reis-Bücklers dystrophy
   Anterior membrane dystrophy (Grayson-Wilbrandt)
   Honeycomb dystrophy (Thiel and Behnke)
   Inherited band-shaped keratopathy
   Anterior mosaic dystrophy
Stroma
   Granular dystrophy (Groenouw's type I)
   Macular dystrophy (Groenouw's type II)
   Lattice dystrophy (Biber-Haab-Dimmer)
   Gelatinous-drop-like dystrophy
   Central crystalline dystrophy (Schnyder)
   Fleck dystrophy (speckled dystrophy)
   Central cloudy dystrophy (François)
   Posterior amorphous corneal dystrophy
   Congenital hereditary stromal dystrophy
   Pre-Descemet's dystrophy
Endothelium and Descemet's membrane
   Cornea guttata
   Fuchs' dystrophy
   Congenital hereditary endothelial dystrophy
     (Maumenee)
   Posterior polymorphous dystrophy (Koeppe)
Ectatic dystrophies
   Keratoconus

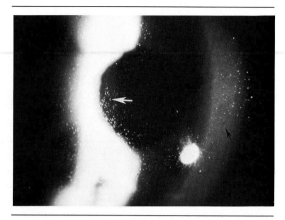

Fig. 12-2. *The cysts in Meesmann's dystrophy appear as gray dots on focal illumination (black arrow) and refractive vesicles on indirect illumination (white arrow).*

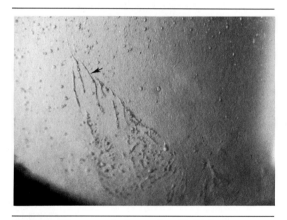

Fig. 12-3. *Meesmann's dystrophy. Multiple fine vesicles stand out in retroillumination. Coalescence of these droplets may form clusters or refractile lines (arrow).*

cornea (Fig. 12-2). In retroillumination they appear as cysts or vacuoles (Fig. 12-3). With direct focal illumination the appearance is that of discrete gray dots. Ruptured cysts on the surface stain with fluorescein; however, the intraepithelial cysts do not fluoresce. Whorl, crescentic, wedge, and cluster distributions of the vesicles have been noted [272]. The intervening cornea is usually clear. Serpiginous gray lines and small amorphous subepithelial opacities, in addition to the characteristic fine whitish dots, were found in the patients described by Stocker and Holt [370]. Histologic study in this family showed a separation of basement membrane from Bowman's membrane by an amorphous layer with a nodular distribution that stained with periodic acid–Schiff (PAS).

In Meesmann's dystrophy light microscopy demonstrates an epithelial layer that is variably thickened or thinned with cytoplasmic vacuolation and diffuse disorganization [47, 109, 235]. The deeper and more superficial mature epithelial cells

appear morphologically similar, lacking the normal transition. Intraepithelial cysts occasionally open onto the surface, distorting the surface regularity. Basal layer mitoses are often seen, and variable increased amounts of glycogen have been reported in the more superficial epithelial layers. Small, usually round, debris-filled intraepithelial cysts ranging from 10 to 100 μm are found throughout the epithelial layers, most characteristically in the anterior third. The intracystic debris stains for glycosaminoglycans with alcian blue and colloidal iron stains and probably represents degenerated cellular products [62]. An abnormally thickened, often multilaminar epithelial basement membrane is present with pedunculated excrescences extending into the epithelium. The anterior portion of this membrane, like the intracystic debris, stains for glycosaminoglycans.

Electron microscopy shows a material described as "peculiar substance" within the epithelial cells, most prominently in the basal layers [104, 235, 289]. These regular aggregates are in close proximity to the tonofilaments and desmosomes in the cytoplasm. The cysts are lined with membranes of the adjacent epithelial cells forming a corrugated microvillous wall. Cysts contain a spectrum of degenerated cell products from recognizable cell organelles to a vacuolated homogeneous substance. Little peculiar substance is found within these cysts. Other investigators have found electron-dense bodies similar to lysosomes in Meesmann's dystrophy [283]. The thickened basement membrane is formed by a homogeneous posterior layer and an anterior, more atypical, accumulation of basement membrane material. The rest of the cornea is normal without apparent modification of Bowman's membrane or deeper stroma.

The cause and the specific biochemistry of the peculiar substance are unknown. The dystrophy appears to be a primary result of the accumulation of this material within the cells. The increased cell turnover, thickened basement membrane, and cell degeneration are probably secondary changes.

Most affected individuals retain normal vision and are only intermittently symptomatic. However, sometimes subepithelial scarring and surface irregularity lead to moderately reduced vision. Epithelial debridement is followed by a recurrence of the cysts, which, however, may be slow to form and not always as severe as the original involvement. Superficial keratectomy has been reported with normal re-epithelialization [62], but recurrent epithelial involvement has occurred after lamellar and penetrating keratoplasty [370].

EPITHELIAL BASEMENT MEMBRANE DYSTROPHY
(MAP-DOT-FINGERPRINT DYSTROPHY)

The term *epithelial basement membrane dystrophy* has been used to describe a variety of anterior corneal disorders including Cogan's microcystic epithelial dystrophy, fingerprint dystrophy, map-dot-fingerprint dystrophy, anterior membrane dystrophy, nontraumatic recurrent erosion, and net and bleb dystrophies.

Cogan and associates noted bilateral grayish white spheres, usually 0.1 to 0.5 mm in diameter, in the superficial cornea of 5 unrelated adult female patients [61]. These centrally located, irreg-

ular or comma-shaped opacities did not significantly decrease visual acuity and remained asymptomatic in 3 of the patients. The "microcystic dystrophy of the corneal epithelium" did not progress, but individual lesions did appear and disappear over short intervals. Histopathologic specimens from 2 patients showed intraepithelial cysts containing pyknotic nuclei and cytoplasmic debris. An anomalous basement membrane was also found within the epithelial layer.

Guerry described 9 additional patients with subtle, faint, geographic configurations at times in conjunction with "putty grey dots" [165]. These map figures were noted to change location, contour, and size with observation. "Maplike epithelial dystrophy of the cornea" was usually asymptomatic and nonprogressive. Fingerprint lines in the cornea were elucidated by Guerry in a 1950 report [164], but similar, although more coarse, changes had been described by Vogt [402]. These fine wavy lines had a whorl-like contour, and family members were unaffected. Histologic study of fingerprint lines demonstrated folding and reduplication of the basement membrane. Subsequent studies have demonstrated the concomitant appearance of map, dot, and fingerprint changes of the cornea [236, 392, 428]. Related bleb and netlike patterns with distinctive histopathology have also been reported [78]. A high percentage of patients with these latter findings had recurrent erosions. No hereditary pattern was established.

Recently the terms *map-dot-fingerprint dystrophy* and *epithelial basement membrane dystrophy* have been used to refer to this group of often coexistent disorders. An autosomal dominant pattern of inheritance was suggested by a study in which the proband displayed moderately large intraepithelial putty-colored microcysts of Cogan or moderately pronounced gray sheets of intraepithelial basement membrane material with maplike borders [237]. Subsequent studies have shown similar, but milder, clinical findings to be present in a large percentage of the asymptomatic general population [417]. This has raised the question of whether this process is truly a dystrophy.

The most prevalent and probably the earliest clinical change is the maplike area. Slit-lamp examination methods that are helpful in visualizing the maps are a broad oblique beam with an undilated pupil, red reflex through a dilated pupil, and fluorescein, which stains negatively over the heaped-up epithelium. Maps are diffusely circumscribed areas with a central ground-glass appearance and oval clear lacunae (Fig. 12-4). The mar-

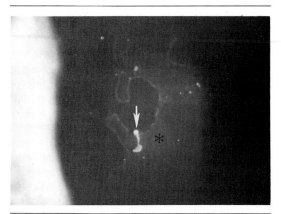

Fig. 12-4. *Slit-lamp photograph of cornea in epithelial basement membrane dystrophy. Map (asterisk) with diffuse ground-glass appearance on oblique illumination. The well-circumscribed dots are seen underneath the map. A larger microcyst (arrow) can be seen to extend from underneath the intraepithelial layer into a clear zone.*

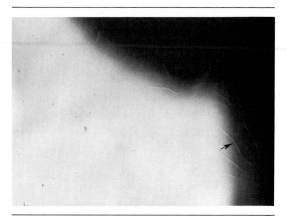

Fig. 12-5. *Fingerprint lines (arrow) in epithelial basement membrane dystrophy appear refractile by indirect illumination from the iris.*

gins are sharply demarcated from the surrounding clear cornea and are elevated. These typical patches range in size from several hundred microns to areas covering several square millimeters or more.

Dots are fine gray-white round, oblong, or comma-shaped opacities seen in the central cornea, usually underneath the maplike changes (Fig. 12-4). They may become confluent with lobulated smooth margins and may stain if they open onto the ocular surface. Blebs are clustered, fine, clear bubbles seen only with indirect illumination from the iris or in red reflex. Clusters of the blebs may form a refractile sheet with a lobulated margin. The individual blebs are much smaller than the dotlike changes. Nets are composed of rows of blebs that seem to follow the normal corneal mosaic.

Fingerprint lines require diligent examination for detection and consist of concentric, often curvilinear, parallel lines clustered in the central or midperipheral cornea (Fig. 12-5). They appear as cylindrical processes, which may branch or may be club shaped at their termination. Fingerprints are best seen by indirect illumination of the iris or in red reflex from the fundus. Fluorescein may highlight their presence. They are the least frequently encountered of the principal triad of findings in epithelial basement membrane dystrophy. Similar changes are found in a variety of other conditions [39]. *Fibrillary lines* are often seen in normal corneas, and *shift lines* can be present in Fuchs' dystrophy [37]. Mares' tails and tram lines are also variants of fingerprints.

Symptoms vary in epithelial basement membrane dystrophy depending on the population selection. Most patients remain asymptomatic. In others the disorder may become manifest after the third decade of life as recurrent epithelial erosion or transient episodes of decreased visual acuity. The erosions characteristically occur over a period of up to a few years, with spontaneous improvement [410]. Approximately 50 percent of individuals with recurrent erosion syndrome manifest some of the clinical features of epithelial basement membrane dystrophy [42].

Treatment of the acute erosions includes use of 5% sodium chloride drops during the day and a similar ointment at night. Topical osmotic colloidal solutions at bedtime have also been successful [111]. Patching and cycloplegia may be necessary. Recalcitrant cases may require a therapeutic soft contact lens for an extended period with the concomitant use of sodium chloride. Superficial epithelial keratectomy, in addition to the above measures, has also proven beneficial in selected cases [49].

Histopathologically, the maplike changes are formed by aberrant multilaminar projections of a thickened basement membrane into the overlying epithelium. These 2- to 6-μm-thick layers are composed of a fine fibrillogranular material and may be fragmented or discontinuous with rolled or club-shaped terminations. They separate the epithelium into anterior and posterior lamellae. The epithelial cells in the anterior lamella show normal intercellular junctions but do not develop good hemidesmosomal connections to the underlying aberrant basement membrane [62, 79, 326].

Dots are actually pseudocysts that contain nuclear and cytoplasmic debris. In most studies, these

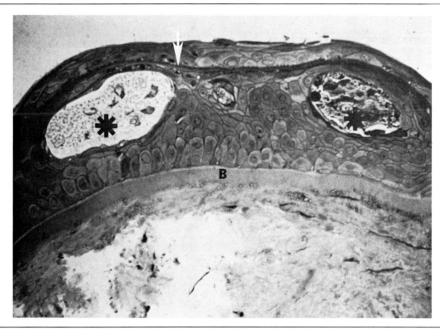

Fig. 12-6. *Light micrograph of cornea in epithelial basement membrane dystrophy showing abnormal intraepithelial membrane (arrow) and two large microcysts (asterisks) abutting against its posterior surface. Bowman's membrane (B) is intact.*

(Paraphenylenediamine, ×165 before 30% reduction.) (From M. M. Rodrigues et al., Arch. Ophthalmol. *92:475, 1974. Copyright 1974, American Medical Association.)*

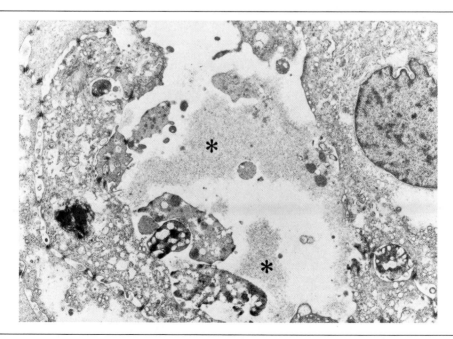

Fig. 12-7. *Transmission electron micrograph of a developing intraepithelial pseudocyst in epithelial basement membrane dystrophy. Fine granular debris (asterisks) as well as other cell products are seen within the pseudocyst. (×8,000 before reduction.)*

(From J. A. Fogle et al. Published with permission from the American Journal of Ophthalmology *79:925–940, 1974. Copyright by the Ophthalmic Publishing Company.)*

were located immediately posterior to the basement membrane projections (Fig. 12-6). They are occasionally surrounded by multinucleated cells. Villous processes of the surrounding cells may give a corrugated appearance to the borders of the pseudocysts (Fig. 12-7). Similar, although usually smaller, pseudocysts occur unassociated with the map changes and occasionally are seen opening onto the anterior epithelial surface [62, 79, 326, 428].

The fingerprint lines also are formed by insinuation of a basement-membrane-enclosed material into the overlying epithelium (Fig. 12-8). The core of these projections consists of closely packed granules approximately 80 Å in diameter with larger fibrils (125–170 Å in diameter) located near the free ends of the structures [35]. A similar fibrillogranular substance may be found to comprise the thickened basement membrane layer. Subepithelial plaques, sometimes with mushroom-shaped configurations, have also been noted in some cases. Bowman's layer and the stroma are usually uninvolved (Fig. 12-8) [79, 326].

Blebs are formed by deposition of a somewhat similar fibrillogranular protein between Bowman's layer and epithelial basement membrane in a mound configuration. These mounds are the clinically visible blebs. The overlying epithelium is usually normal [78].

The pathogenesis of epithelial basement membrane dystrophy probably involves the primary synthesis of an abnormal basement membrane with intraepithelial extension. This material then blocks the normal epithelial maturation, resulting in aberrant cells and focal collections of cellular debris [62, 326]. Another theory is that an abrasion or epithelial looseness allows two layers of basal cells to come together or one to override the other creating the midepithelial layer. Other investigators have suggested a primary epithelial fibrillopathy or altered epithelial metabolism in the production of this disorder [79, 326].

DYSTROPHIC RECURRENT EROSION

Clinical recurrent corneal erosion is a relatively common disorder usually precipitated by injury from paper products or fingernails but often occurring without a history of trauma [54]. Some of these spontaneous erosions are inherited, and even those occuring after trauma may show a genetically determined predisposition [42].

Fig. 12-8. *Phase-contrast micrograph of fingerprint lines demonstrates projections of abnormal basement membrane (arrows) into the overlying epithelium (Ep). Bowman's layer (B) and stroma (S) are normal in appearance. (Paraphenylenediamine, × 800 before 24% reduction.) (Courtesy of Kenneth R. Kenyon.)*

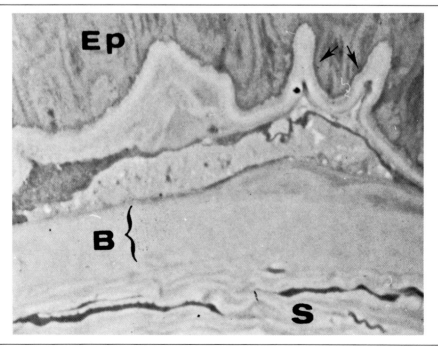

Pedigrees with a dominant history of recurrent erosions spanning several generations have been reported since the initial report of a family by Franceschetti [114]. In most of these families the onset of symptoms was in the first decade of life, and erosions were frequently bilateral [405]. Recurrences were noted to occur over multiple sites in the cornea, in contrast to the typical course of acquired post-traumatic erosion. Epithelial slippage, microcyst formation, epithelial edema, bullae, filaments, or frank epithelial loss may be apparent during the acute erosive episode, which characteristically has its onset in the early morning hours. Increased nocturnal epithelial hydration with lid-corneal adhesion may worsen disruption of the epithelium in predisposed individuals. Pain, photophobia, tearing, and blepharospasm are immediate symptoms. Vision may be reduced during this acute episode, but recovery is usually complete. With increasing age, the severity and frequency of erosive episodes diminishes.

Subtle corneal changes, including epithelial irregularity and edema, intraepithelial microcysts, and mild subepithelial haze, may persist between erosive episodes. These findings are best appreciated with retroillumination or when viewed against a dilated pupil. Topical fluorescein may accentuate surface irregularities and occasionally is taken up by intraepithelial cysts. Significant subepithelial scarring is unusual in the absence of secondary complications and may suggest the presence of other underlying disorders or dystrophies.

Histopathology in a case of spontaneous erosion demonstrated intraepithelial cysts with cellular debris, epithelial edema with degenerative changes in some of the basal epithelial cells, and a deficiency or lack of hemidesmosomes [120]. Focal absence of the basement membrane and associated hemidesmosomes has been shown in recurrent erosion after trauma [153]. Although no specific pathology has been reported in known inherited recurrent erosions, similar alterations in the epithelial basement membrane and associated basement membrane complexes may be involved.

Recurrent erosion is part of the natural history of some corneal dystrophies [107]. It occurs most frequently in epithelial basement membrane dystrophy, which shares many of the characteristics of dystrophic recurrent erosion. Reis-Bücklers, macular, and lattice dystrophies may also present with freqeunt and prominent recurrent corneal erosions at certain stages. Meesmann's dystrophy and the variant forms of Reis-Bücklers dystrophy including honeycomb and anterior membrane dystrophies are less likely to produce recurrent erosions. Ultrastructural examination in some of the other dystrophies with frequent erosions has demonstrated abnormal basement membrane complexes with loss of hemidesmosomes and anchoring fibrils [107]. Fuchs' dystrophy may also produce epithelial breakdown on the basis of increasing epithelial edema. Congenital hereditary endothelial dystrophy, although associated with marked corneal edema, usually does not produce corneal erosion.

REIS-BÜCKLERS DYSTROPHY

Reis-Bücklers dystrophy was first clearly documented by Reis, who described siblings with an annular corneal disorder [319]. Recurrent attacks of photophobia and irritation occurred in childhood with progressive visual loss caused by anterior corneal opacities. Four generations of the same family were later detailed by Bücklers, who documented the dominant inheritance and strong penetrance [45].

This dystrophy usually presents in childhood with recurrent episodes of unilateral painful erosions eventually involving both eyes and occurring as frequently as two or three times per month. The earliest slit-lamp findings include a reticular superficial corneal opacification at the level of Bowman's membrane. Some patients have rapid progression and a succession of painful erosions, while others have a delayed onset of symptoms until the second or third decade [169].

The clinical course usually involves progressive corneal opacification and relatively fewer acute erosive episodes with time. Corneal sensation is often markedly diminished. The dystrophy is most often subjectively quiescent in the third and fourth decades except for residual decreased vision secondary to surface irregularity and opacification. The visual result may be variable even within the same pedigree.

Examination reveals an irregular corneal surface with varying thickness of the epithelial layer. Gray-white opacities in the subepithelial area take on a variety of forms: linear, geographic, ringlike, honeycomb, fishnet, or alveolar (Fig. 12-9). Sometimes there is a more mottled presentation with mounds, dots, and plaques. Occasionally the intervening areas are clear, but usually there is a diffuse ground-glass appearance. Ridges or mounds

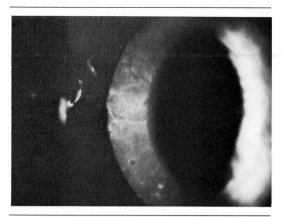

Fig. 12-9. *Slit-lamp photograph of cornea in Reis-Bücklers dystrophy demonstrates diffuse haziness with superimposed localized opacities of various morphologies that are best seen with oblique illumination.*

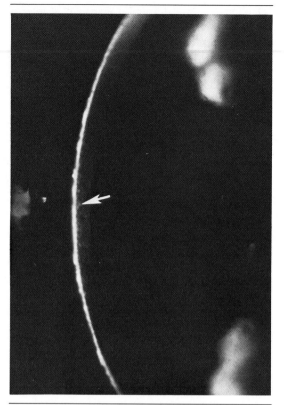

Fig. 12-10. *The narrow slit-lamp beam shows the anterior location of the opacities and overlying surface irregularity in Reis-Bücklers dystrophy. Smaller, punctate opacities are also present in the midstroma to superficial stroma (arrow).*

project forward from the level of Bowman's membrane into the epithelium (Fig. 12-10). The opacities are most dense in the central or midperipheral cornea, often creating an annular appearance, but on close examination they can be seen to involve the entire cornea. The underlying anterior stroma may contain discrete refractile opacities or have a diffuse ground-glass appearance. Hudson-Stähli lines and prominent corneal nerves are often present [195]. Irregular astigmatism and distorted keratoscopic mires owing to surface irregularity may be found in all stages.

Light microscopy confirms the varying thickness of the epithelial layer [160, 180, 295]. Degenerative findings include intracellular and intercellular edema, subepithelial fluid pockets containing glycogen, darkly staining cells, and intercellular vacuoles. Bowman's membrane is nearly totally replaced by an eosinophilic, PAS-positive material that appears stratified and mildly cellular and may project into the epithelium. Similar material is sometimes seen in the anterior stroma. Inflammatory changes are conspicuously absent.

Ultrastructural examination of Bowman's layer shows closely packed collagen fibers with a diameter of 300 to 400 Å with normal periodicity interspersed with clumps and sheets of short, dense, half-moon–shaped tubular microfibrils with a diameter of approximately 100 Å [2, 160, 180, 295]. Cross-striations are apparent in these smaller microfibrils. Fibroblasts are present in the anterior stroma. Disordered basement membrane complexes are present overlying these areas and where the basement membrane is absent. An accumulation of collagen and microfribils may also be seen between Bowman's layer and the overlying epithelium (Fig. 12-11). The posterior stroma, Descemet's membrane, and endothelium are usually normal.

The cause and the specific nature of the characteristic fibrils in this dystrophy remain unclear. Some investigators believe the disorder primarily relates to a degeneration of Bowman's membrane that results in the basement membrane and epithelial changes [160, 180]. Later, Bowman's membrane is replaced with collagen and microfibrils probably produced by fibroblast-like cells in the anterior stroma. Other theories include primary epithelial, epithelial basement membrane, and neurotrophic causes [432].

Treatment involves the medical management of erosions. The superficial opacification may be treated by curettage and superficial keratectomy

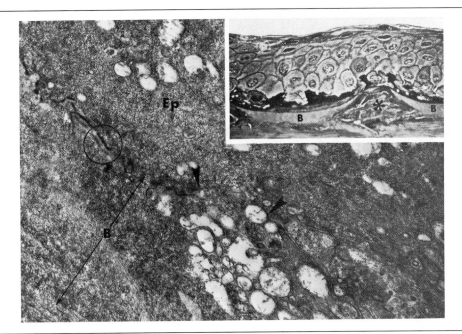

Fig. 12-11. *Histopathology of Reis-Bücklers dystrophy. Transmission electron microscopy demonstrates thin remnants of Bowman's layer (B) and masses of smaller-diameter fibrils. Hemidesmosomes (circle) are discontinuous, and there is apparent continuity (arrowheads) between the basal cell cytoplasm (Ep) and underlying cellular debris. (× 30,000 before 30% reduction.) Inset, Phase-contrast microscopy* demonstrates disruption of Bowman's membrane (B) by a fibrous-appearing material (asterisk). (Paraphenylenediamine, × 800 before 30% reduction.) (From J. A. Fogle et al. Published with permission from the American Journal of Ophthalmology 79:925–940, 1974. Copyright by the Ophthalmic Publishing Company.)

[430]. More advanced cases have been treated with lamellar and penetrating keratoplasties. Recurrence of this dystrophy in grafts is well recognized (Fig. 12-12) [432].

Fig. 12-12. *Recurrence of Reis-Bücklers dystrophy in a corneal graft. A fine granular appearance is present in the central graft, and more typical superficial opacities are seen in the periphery.*

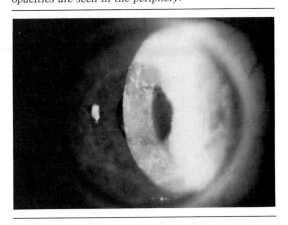

ANTERIOR MEMBRANE DYSTROPHY (GRAYSON-WILBRANDT)

A condition with a clinical appearance similar to that of Reis-Bücklers dystrophy was described by Grayson and Wilbrandt in two generations of a single pedigree [158]. This disorder did not become clinically apparent until 10 years of age. Episodes of pain and injection of the eye were unusual. Corneal sensitivity was normal, and the corneal nerves were usually prominent. Vision was variably affected, ranging from 20/20 in the first generation to 20/200 in the proband.

Slit-lamp examination showed amorphous gray-white opacities of various sizes over the entire cornea that did not stain with fluorescein. These seem to consist of mounds extending into the epithelium from a thickened Bowman's membrane. The intervening anterior cornea was relatively clear (Fig. 12-13). Small refractile bodies were present in the corneal stroma, but Descemet's membrane and the endothelium appeared normal. Light microscopy performed on a lamellar specimen taken from the proband showed the varying thickness of the epithelial layer with epithelial cells of different sizes and shapes, some with pyknotic nuclei. A PAS-positive material accumulated beneath the epithelium, at times replacing Bowman's membrane, and invaded the basal epithelial layers. No stromal changes were found to account for the clinically detected refractile figures [166].

Similar histopathologic changes were found post mortem in an elderly black woman whose ocular condition was never clinically demonstrated [106]. Light microscopy showed a PAS-positive subepithelial layer of varying thickness with some embedded cells. Ultrastructural study of this layer showed a fibrillogranular substance with occasional random collagen fibrils and embedded fibrocytes. Thickening or focal loss of the epithelial basement membrane and a lack of hemidesmosomes were demonstrated. Bowman's layer was relatively intact as were the deeper corneal layers.

A case with a similar age of onset and mild clinical findings accompanied by slightly more prominent erosions has been included by some investigators in this group of disorders [160]. However, histopathology of a superficial keratectomy specimen demonstrated a dense, nonfibrillar material replacing Bowman's layer with overlying lack of normal basal epithelial structures.

Fig. 12-13. *Slit-lamp photographs of cornea in anterior membrane dystrophy. A. Dense opacities in the central cornea. B. Relatively clear intervening stroma in an area of the cornea with fewer opacities.*

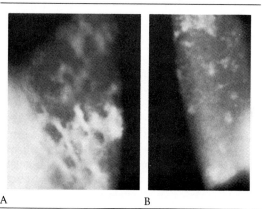

A   B

This disorder, like anterior membrane dystrophy, may be part of a spectrum of anterior corneal dystrophies that represent either different expressions of a similar genetic defect or morphologically similar changes occurring with different genetic input.

HONEYCOMB DYSTROPHY (THIEL AND BEHNKE)

Thiel and Behnke described a subepithelial dystrophy with an unusual clinical appearance that was transmitted as an autosomal trait in a family over 11 generations [383]. Of 234 members in this pedigree, 74 patients were examined, and 26 were found to be affected. The dystrophy presented in childhood with recurrent erosions and progressive visual loss. A bilateral, characteristic, honeycomb-like opacity was seen in the axial subepithelial region in affected individuals, usually by the second decade of life. The septa seemed to project into the overlying epithelium; however, the corneal surface was described as smooth and mirrorlike. The peripheral 1 to 2 mm of the cornea was uninvolved. Corneal sensation was not significantly decreased. Vision varied from 20/25 in younger family members to the 20/100 range in older individuals. Erosive symptoms occurred once or twice yearly in adult patients, usually becoming quiescent by the fourth to sixth decade of life. This disorder differs from Reis-Bücklers dystrophy by showing less severe visual involvement, a later onset, normal corneal sensation, typical honeycomb morphology, and a smooth corneal surface. A honeycomb-like pattern, however, can be a finding in patients with Reis-Bücklers dystrophy [295].

Histopathologic findings have been reported in 1 case of a clinical honeycomb pattern in a 61-year-old man who had poor vision since childhood and a family history of Reis-Bücklers corneal dystrophy [431]. Light microscopy demonstrated an irregular epithelial layer with dark cells having processes extending through a PAS-positive subepithelial layer. The epithelial basement membrane was irregularly thickened, split, duplicated, or fragmented, but Bowman's membrane was intact. Ultrastructural study showed a dense material with banded structure in the basement membrane layer. There were nodular protrusions of this layer into the overlying epithelium. The fine structure of Bowman's layer showed occasional degenerative changes, but no curly fibrils characteristic of Reis-Bücklers dystrophy were encountered. These pathologic findings were contrasted to those in a 27-year-old niece of the above patient who demonstrated the typical findings of Reis-Bücklers dystrophy [431].

Epithelial basement membrane changes, especially thickening of this membrane, are present in most of the anterior dystrophies and may also be found in chronic corneal edema. Thickening of the epithelial basement membrane is a prominent feature of both honeycomb dystrophy and anterior membrane dystrophy but is not typically a feature of Reis-Bücklers dystrophy. There is little involvement of Bowman's membrane in honeycomb dystrophy, in contrast to Reis-Bücklers dystrophy, in which the layer is invariably affected. Despite these differences in histopathologic findings, the wide spectrum of appearance of patients with Reis-Bücklers dystrophy and the concurrent appearance of the dystrophy described by Thiel and Behnke in a single pedigree favor the classification of honeycomb dystrophy, along with anterior membrane dystrophy (Grayson-Wilbrandt), as variants of Reis-Bücklers corneal dystrophy [295, 431].

INHERITED BAND-SHAPED KERATOPATHY

Calcific band keratopathy results from deposition of calcium salts in the epithelium and Bowman's layer and between anterior stromal lamellae in an interpalpebral distribution [304]. It is usually the result of ocular or systemic disorders, trauma, or the use of certain drugs [240]. The most common ocular causes are chronic glaucoma, uveitis, keratitis, and phthisis bulbi. Systemic causes include a variety of disorders resulting in hypercalcemia or uremia. Similar changes have been reported in elastotic degeneration; however, light microscopic staining and characteristic ultrastructural findings help to differentiate this disorder from typical calcific band keratopathy [75]. The early stages of gelatinous-drop-like corneal dystrophy, which is a disorder of amyloid deposition, may also have a similar clinical presentation [200]. Band keratopathy occurs as a secondary manifestation in certain hereditary diseases such as the X-linked recessive disorder termed Norrie's disease [267], which is probably the same disorder as the condition known as Episkopi blindness [380].

The clinical appearance of band keratopathy is extremely characteristic. Early lesions consist of a slight haze at the level of Bowman's membrane in an interpalpebral distribution in the peripheral cornea, being separated from the limbus by a clear zone. Sparse, clear, round areas of Bowman's

membrane remain clinically uninvolved and may correspond to areas of passage of corneal nerves. The clear areas give a fenestrated appearance to the total band (Fig. 12-14). Progression is usually from the involved peripheral area centrally, but some cases show central involvement that occasionally takes on a mosaic appearance similar to that of anterior crocodile shagreen. Eventually, the entire palpebral zone is involved, and epithelial erosion and ulceration may occur. Until this stage, however, corneal sensation usually remains intact. The peripheral corneal changes are more apparent in band keratopathy associated with systemic hypercalcemia, and changes may also be apparent in the bulbar conjunctiva in a palpebral distribution.

A separate etiologic category has been described with a clinical appearance similar to typical secondary calcific band keratopathy. This hereditary primary type has been described in both childhood and senile forms [94]. The senile form was documented in a report of two brothers, aged 66

Fig. 12-14. *Slit-lamp appearance of band keratopathy. Clear areas* (arrows) *within the band give a fenestrated appearance.*

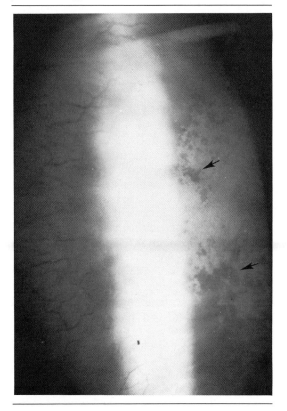

and 71 years, who demonstrated band keratopathy [399]. The childhood variety was seen in an 11-year-old boy and his 16-year-old sister [134]. This form was also observed in three of nine children in a consanguineous pedigree in which the maternal grandparents were first cousins [376]. The band-shaped opacity developed at puberty in two of these involved children but was congenital in the third sibling. Clinically, the opacity was denser centrally and consisted of small gray opacities having the appearance of tapioca grains [376].

Vertical transmission through a pedigree was described by Glees, who reported band-shaped keratopathy appearing in a father and son [146]. Bilateral band-shaped corneal dystrophy was reported in an 18-year-old patient by Lisch [251]. Similar clinical changes were present in the maternal grandmother of the propositus but involved only one eye, which also had keratoconus. Band-shaped dystrophy was felt to be inherited in an autosomal dominant fashion, but further documentation of this supposition awaits further family studies.

ANTERIOR MOSAIC DYSTROPHY

Gray-white polygonal opacities at the level of Bowman's membrane separated by clear spaces occur in anterior mosaic dystrophy, a rare, bilaterally symmetrical dystrophy [305]. Familial juvenile- and adult-onset forms of the dystrophy have been reported. Corneal sensation is intact in milder cases, and vascularization does not occur. Dominant inheritance was documented in two generations of one family [298]. In this pedigree the corneal changes were manifest later in life with no significant effect on visual acuity.

A similar axial pattern (anterior crocodile shagreen) usually is seen as a sporadic senile change unassociated with other ocular or systemic disorders. Early band keratopathy may show a similar pattern. The anterior mosaic pattern should also be differentiated from posterior crocodile shagreen, which is a senile change at the level of Descemet's membrane. A family was described in which the father had band keratopathy and his son had anterior crocodile shagreen [397]. The anterior mosaic pattern has also been seen in association with X-linked recessive megalocornea [24, 260]. Secondary forms have appeared after trauma and in phthisical globes [390]. Histopathology of secondary forms has been done, but the primary form has not been studied pathologically.

The dystrophy takes its morphology from the anterior corneal mosaic, which can be demonstrated in the normal cornea by flattening the corneal surface [36]. This is most commonly seen in the fluorescein pattern during applanation tonometry.

Stromal Dystophies

In 1890 Groenouw described an entity termed *noduli corneae* [161]. Later documentation traced the disease through four generations of the same family. In 1938 Bücklers divided these cases into two different dystrophies [44]. The nodular type (Groenouw's type I), now more commonly termed *granular dystrophy*, is dominantly inherited. Groenouw's type II is the recessive disorder *macular dystrophy*.

In 1890 Biber [19] described a reticular dystrophy that was shown in 1899 by both Haab [166] and Dimmer [89] to have a dominant mode of transmission. *Lattice dystrophy* completes the triad of the classic stromal dystrophies (Table 12-2).

Other dystrophic conditions of the stroma have been documented. This chapter will cover gelatinous-drop-like dystrophy, central crystalline dystrophy of Schnyder, fleck dystrophy, central cloudy corneal dystrophy of François, posterior amorphous corneal dystrophy, congenital hereditary stromal dystrophy, and pre-Descemet's dystrophy. Polymorphic stromal "dystrophy" will also be discussed, although it is probably a degeneration.

GRANULAR DYSTROPHY

Granular dystrophy (Groenouw's type I) is an autosomal dominant condition that usually produces clinical findings in the first or second decade of life [29, 349]. Discrete, gray-white opacities are seen in the anterior axial stroma (Fig. 12-15). The opacities are of different sizes and shapes and have the appearance of bread crumbs [94]. The intervening stroma is clear, and vision is usually not affected early in the disease. Gradually the opacities enlarge, coalesce, multiply, and often spread to involve the deeper and more peripheral stroma. However, the peripheral 2 to 3 mm of the stroma is not clinically involved. The lesions may destroy or elevate Bowman's membrane, resulting in surface irregularity, but epithelial erosions occur less frequently than with lattice dystrophy.

Table 12-2. *Classic Stromal Dystrophies*

Feature	Granular	Macular	Lattice
Inheritance	Autosomal dominant	Autosomal recessive	Autosomal dominant
Onset	First or second decade	First decade	First decade
Erosions	Rare	Occasional	Frequent
Vision	Diminished by fourth or fifth decade	Diminished by second decade	Diminished by second or third decade
Opacities	Discrete with sharp borders; do not extend to limbus; intervening stroma clear early but becomes hazy	Indistinct margins; hazy intervening stroma early; opacities extend to limbus; endothelium affected; central lesions more anterior, peripheral lesions more posterior	Branching lines, dots, and axial haze; intervening stroma relatively clear; limbal extension only in severe cases
Corneal thickness	Normal	Thinned	Normal
Characteristic histochemical stains	Masson trichrome, Luxol fast blue, antibodies to microfibrillar protein	Periodic acid–Schiff, colloidal iron, alcian blue, metachromatic dyes	Periodic acid–Schiff, Congo red, thioflavine-T (fluorescence), crystal violet (metachromasia); positive birefringence and dichroism
Material accumulated	Hyalin	Glycoprotein	Amyloid
Electron microscopic findings	Electron-dense rod-shaped structures surrounded by 8- to 10-nm microfibrils	Membrane-limited vacuoles filled with fibrillogranular material or lamellar bodies; similar vacuoles in endothelium	Characteristic 8- to 10-nm electron-dense nonbranching amyloid fibrils

Vision deteriorates slowly in most families, although pedigrees with a more rapid course have been reported [94, 167]. Visual impairment is rarely severe until after the fifth decade of life. Corneal sensitivity is variably affected. Isolated cases have been reported although familial occurrence with a dominant mode of inheritance has been well documented [94]. The clinical features of the dystrophic process tend to be uniform within pedigrees.

Slit-lamp examination may show fine dots and radial lines in the superficial stroma in the first decade of life. Later, focal white opacities in the anterior stroma take on a variety of shapes including those of doughnuts, stars, and snowflakes (Fig. 12-16). They are opaque using focal illumination and are partially translucent on retroillumination. There may be any number of these opacities. Aggregates of the individual lesions take many forms including chains, rings, or branching patterns. Initially the intervening cornea is clear, but with time a diffuse ground-glass appearance develops. Occasionally, the white dots are so numerous that the entire central cornea appears hazy.

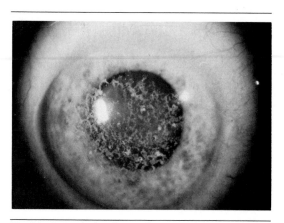

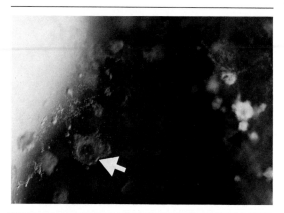

Fig. 12-15. *Granular dystrophy. Note discrete stromal opacities that spare the corneal periphery.*

Fig. 12-16. *Higher-magnification slit-lamp photograph of the lesions in granular dystrophy. In focal illumination the lesions are opaque* (black arrow); *in retroillumination they appear partially translucent and refractile. Individual lesions show irregular margins and may have clear centers* (white arrow).

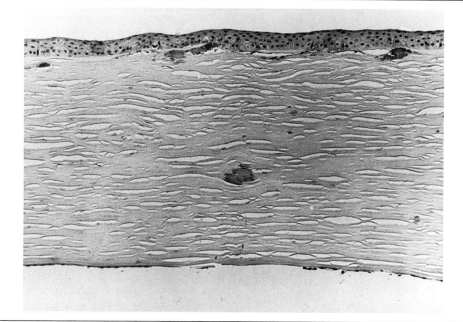

Fig. 12-17. *Light microscopy in granular dystrophy shows discrete staining deposits at various stromal levels and in the subepithelial region. (PAS, ×125 before 30% reduction.)*

There may be mild irregularity of the corneal surface with variable fluorescein staining and tear film breakup [94].

Light microscopy demonstrates deeply staining, eosinophilic, rod- or trapezoid-shaped deposits in the stroma and subepithelial areas (Fig. 12-17). These hyaline deposits stain bright red with Masson trichrome stain and may be PAS-positive [196]. The peripheral portion of the deposits may stain with Congo red [187]. There is a positive reaction in the deposits with antibodies to microfibrillar protein [329].

Typical ovoid or angular deposits may also be found within the epithelium in primary cases and are very typical of recurrent dystrophy [193, 361, 426]. The basement membrane is focally absent. Irregular, electron-dense, rod-shaped structures 100 to 500 μm wide are present in the extracellular spaces on ultrastructural examination (Fig. 12-18). Keratocytes may show degeneration or be normal in appearance [361]. The elongated discrete deposits may take on various morphologies including filamentous, "moth-eaten," or homogeneous

on higher resolution. There may be 8- to 10-nm tubular microfibrils surrounding these lesions (Fig. 12-19) [329].

The chemical composition of the larger deposits in granular dystrophy is not completely understood. *Hyaline* is a descriptive term in light microscopy that does not indicate the chemical nature of the deposits. The deposits are probably noncollagenous protein containing tyrosine, tryptophan, and sulfur-containing amino acids. Microfibrillar proteins and phospholipids have recently been demonstrated [329]. The dystrophy may be due to abnormal synthesis or handling of protein or phospholipids, which are the principal components of biologic cell membranes. The epithelial findings in recurrent granular dystrophy and its early superficial course favor an epithelial genesis of this disorder. Other investigators feel the stromal keratocyte is the primary source of the deposits in granular dystrophy [3, 193, 221].

Penetrating keratoplasty is indicated in cases of significantly diminished vision. Recurrences may appear early after keratoplasty with typical superficial findings on histology [426]. Treatment of superficial recurrence by debridement or superficial keratectomy with good results has been reported [241].

Apparent variants of granular dystrophy with an earlier onset of painful erosive episodes simulating the course of Reis-Bücklers dystrophy have

Fig. 12-18. *Transmission electron micrograph of cornea in granular dystrophy. Focal electron-dense deposits (asterisk) are seen in the superficial stroma. Similar-appearing smaller deposits (arrows) are found in the basal epithelial cells (E). ($\times$ 12,900 before 30% reduction.) (From M. M. Rodrigues et al.,* Arch. Ophthalmol. *101:802, 1983.)*

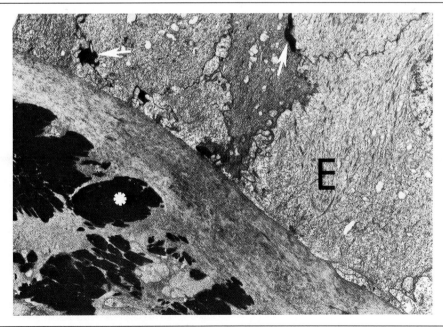

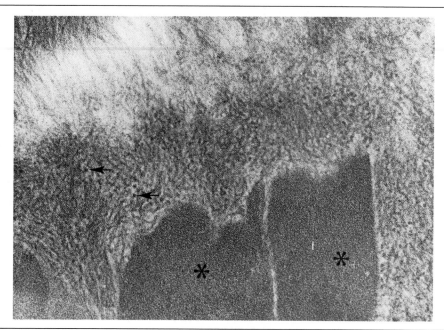

Fig. 12-19. *High-magnification transmission electron micrograph of cornea in granular dystrophy. The rod-shaped deposits (asterisks) in this case have a fine filamentous pattern. Surrounding these lesions are 8- to 10-nm microfibrils (arrows). (×165,000 before 30% reduction.) (From M. M. Rodrigues et al., Arch. Ophthalmol. 101:802, 1983.)*

been described. The intervening stroma is hazy, and the granular lesions may extend to the limbus. Vascularization and scarring are more prominent [167, 404].

MACULAR DYSTROPHY

Macular dystrophy is the least common of the classic stromal dystrophies (granular, macular, lattice) and like other recessive disorders is more severe and occurs often in pedigrees with consanguineous marriage [94]. This bilateral and usually symmetrical disorder begins in the first decade of life as a fine superficial axial corneal haze. Eventually the entire corneal stroma becomes involved, and deep peripheral involvement may form projections into the anterior chamber [121]. A diffuse opacity consisting of multiple irregular gray-white nodules develops (Fig. 12-20). Surface irregularity occurs with accompanying decreased corneal sensation. However, recurrent erosion is much less frequent than with lattice dystrophy. Photophobia is a prominent feature of macular dystrophy and often seems out of proportion to the clinical involvement. Usually by the age of 20 to 30 the patient has lost useful vision and requires penetrating keratoplasty.

Clinical examination in early stages shows a central, faint, ground-glass haze in the superficial cornea. Developing within this matrix are mul-

Fig. 12-20. *Diffuse slit-lamp photograph of cornea in macular dystrophy showing mottled central involvement and more discrete peripheral opacities.*

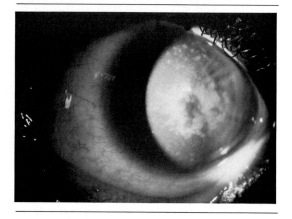

tiple small, gray-white opacities with irregular configurations and borders. These opacities are more prominent and superficial in the axial cornea and deeper and more discrete in the peripheral stroma (Fig. 12-21). Corneal guttae appear, and Descemet's membrane takes on a slate gray appearance. In the later stages surface irregularity owing to the elevated nodules occurs, and the stroma is diffusely involved with opaque nodules. However, unlike other stromal dystrophies in which corneal thickness is normal, pachymetry demonstrates significantly reduced corneal thickness in macular dystrophy [97]. If the endothelium is sufficiently affected, decompensation resulting in stromal and epithelial edema occurs. In such cases the corneal thickness will increase to what would be normal or even thickened for a nondystrophic cornea.

The clinical distinction between early macular and granular dystrophies may be difficult [44]. Fo-

Fig. 12-21. *Slit-lamp appearance in macular dystrophy demonstrates the anterior stromal location and diffuse nature of the central corneal involvement. The peripheral focal opacities are located in the posterior stroma* (arrow).

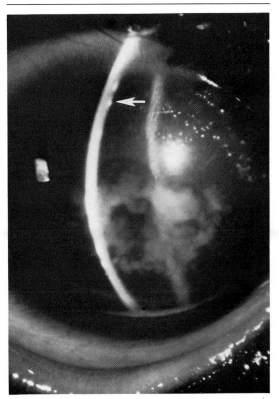

cal, rather discrete opacities in the superficial stroma appear early in both conditions. However, the early intervening stromal haze, involvement of the peripheral and deep stroma, decreased corneal thickness, and recessive family history help to distinguish macular dystrophy.

Light microscopy demonstrates nonspecific epithelial changes with degeneration, especially of the basal cells. Mononuclear cells and collections of carbohydrate-rich material have been noted in the subepithelial area. Bowman's membrane is irregular and either partially or totally absent. Portions of the membrane may be replaced by a basement-membrane-like material or a hyaline membrane often with embedded histiocytes [358].

Special stains show accumulation of glycosaminoglycan-like substance within stromal keratocytes as well as in the subepithelial and Bowman's histiocytes, surrounding stroma, Descemet's membrane, and endothelium [196, 358]. Colloidal iron and alcian blue stains are particularly useful in demonstrating the deposits within and surrounding the keratocytes. The most involved keratocytes are usually located in the more superficial or deeper layers of the stroma (Fig. 12-22) [226].

Electron microscopy demonstrates abundant endoplasmic reticulum and prominent Golgi systems in the epithelial cells [358]. The keratocytes contain membrane-limited intracytoplasmic vacuoles of various sizes usually found in conjunction with the rough endoplasmic reticulum [127]. These vacuoles are clear or contain a granular or fibrillar material of moderate electron density or lamellar bodies. Large vacuoles may distend the keratocyte up to three times the normal size (Fig. 12-23) [127, 226, 388]. Also present in the distended cells are various types of cytoplasmic lysosomes [130].

The surrounding normal stromal structure is interrupted by many membrane-limited vesicles often containing osmiophilic granular deposits (Fig. 12-24). Degenerated keratocyte components and patches of fibrillogranular substance may also be found [127]. Both the intracellular and the extracellular glycosaminoglycan-like accumulations can be localized using silver stains in conjunction with electron microscopy [218].

The anterior banded portion of Descemet's membrane is normal [127, 358]. However, the posterior portion is usually filled with small, electron-lucent vacuoles and osmiophilic membrane-like structures creating a honeycomb pattern [127, 141]. Multiple guttate excrescences are present

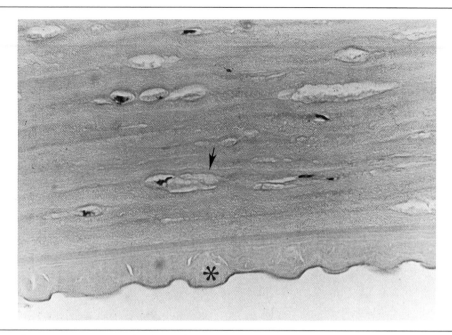

Fig. 12-22. *Light microscopy in macular dystrophy demonstrates accumulation of material in the keratocytes (arrow). Guttate excrescences (asterisk) are also present. (×125 before 30% reduction.)*

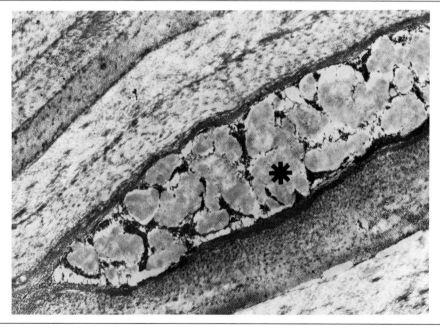

Fig. 12-23. *Macular dystrophy. A stromal keratocyte is distended by membrane-limited cytoplasmic vacuoles containing a fine granular material (asterisk). (×21,000.) (Courtesy of Merlyn M. Rodrigues.)*

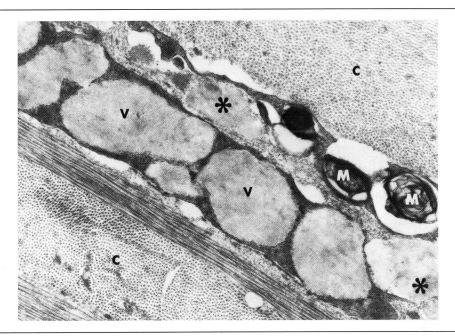

Fig. 12-24. *Micrograph of cornea in macular dystrophy. Vacuoles (V) filled with a fibrillogranular material are present in a stromal keratocyte. Similar material (asterisk) and membranous osmiophilic whorls (M) are seen adjacent in the keratocyte in the extracellular space. Stromal collagen fibrils (C) appear normal. (×22,700 before 30% reduction.) (From R. C. Snip, K. R. Kenyon, and W. R. Green, Macular corneal dystrophy: Ultrastructural pathology of corneal endothelium and Descemet's membrane. Invest. Ophthalmol. 12:88, 1973.)*

that contain irregular deposits of a fibrillogranular material similar to the stromal deposits [127]. The endothelium has also been reported to contain small vesicles filled with a fibrillogranular substance similar to those found in the keratocytes [127, 252].

Autosomal recessive disorders classically result from a single enzyme defect. Many families with macular dystrophy have been linked together by extensive genealogical investigations [218]. Expression of this mutant gene has been amplified in some pedigrees by the high number of consanguineous marriages. Although most investigators agree that the primary defect lies within the keratocyte, the exact enzyme defect remains unknown [138, 219].

In normal corneas the extracellular matrix consists of mainly type I collagen and two proteoglycans, keratan sulfate and chondroitin sulfate. Organ culture studies show that little or no keratan sulfate is synthesized by corneas with macular dystrophy [225]. Instead, a glycoprotein that is immunologically identical to the protein core of keratan sulfate is synthesized and accumulates both within the keratocytes and in the extracellular matrix [173, 174]. Macular dystrophy seems to result from a defect in the conversion of a glycoprotein precursor into a proteoglycan by the addition of keratan sulfate side chains, but, as stated above, the specific enzymatic defect remains undetermined.

Macular dystrophy can be distinguished from the systemic mucopolysaccharidoses [310]. In the latter disorders there is a deficiency in the breakdown of the glycosaminoglycan portion of different proteoglycans resulting in their accumulation and deposition in a variety of tissues. In the cornea this material initially accumulates within intracellular Golgi-derived lysosomes. Epithelial involvement is prominent, and Descemet's membrane is normal in the systemic mucopolysaccharidoses, in contrast to the findings in macular dystrophy. Extracorneal tissue and urine study results are normal in macular corneal dystrophy, although conjunctival changes have been demonstrated in the near limbal conjunctiva [253, 310].

Treatment of macular dystrophy involves tinted lenses to reduce the prominent photophobia, medical management of occasional erosions, and, ultimately, penetrating keratoplasty, which has a very favorable prognosis. The dystrophy rarely may recur in the donor tissue in both lamellar [224, 324] and penetrating grafts [224]. Recent work, however, has shown that donor keratocytes may survive for prolonged periods and that recurrence probably is the result of excessive glycoprotein production by affected host keratocytes [224, 284].

LATTICE DYSTROPHY

Lattice dystrophy usually presents in the first decade of life with symptoms of recurrent erosion or visual disturbance [368]. Younger asymptomatic patients may show characteristic early findings of the dystrophy including anterior refractile stromal dots (Fig. 12-25) and filamentous lines, subepithelial white spots (Fig. 12-26), and axial stromal haze (Fig. 12-27) [92]. Unusual pedigrees have shown a clinical and symptomatic onset in the fourth decade or later [80, 313].

With time the fine refractile lines become thicker and more radially oriented, involving deeper layers of the stroma. Recurrent erosions begin that cause irregularity of the epithelial surface and resultant diminished visual acuity. Individuals with typical stromal involvement without erosion may be asymptomatic and retain good vision. Other relatives of patients with lattice dystrophy may have recurrent epithelial erosions without characteristic stromal involvement [80].

Progressive clouding of the intervening stroma and scarring from recurrent erosions occur. The resultant dense, subepithelial opacities may obscure the lattice pattern. Concomitant decreased central corneal sensation usually occurs, and the patients may become symptomatically stable. Vascularization occurs secondarily in cases with extensive erosions. Unilateral and sector involvement of this dystrophy have been reported [240, 273, 311]. These unusual presentations tend to

Fig. 12-25. *Lattice dystrophy. Retroillumination shows refractile stromal dots* (arrow) *without lattice lines in a 13-year-old patient.*

Fig. 12-26. *Slit-lamp photograph of cornea of 10-year-old patient with early findings of lattice dystrophy. Subepithelial opacities* (arrow) *are present in the central cornea.*

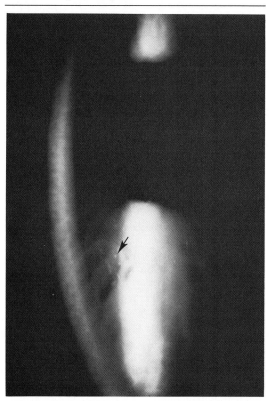

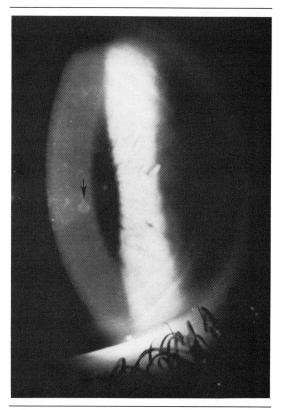

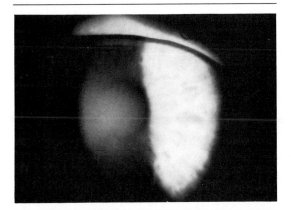

Fig. 12-27. *Diffuse anterior stromal haze in a young asymptomatic patient with lattice dystrophy demonstrated with broad oblique slit-lamp illumination.*

have a later onset and more benign clinical course than typical lattice dystrophy.

Slit-lamp examination shows refractile filamentous lines, refractile and nonrefractile dots, and, less frequently, a diffuse whitish stromal haze. The lattice filaments may be fine and delicate or broad and coarse with nodular dilatations. Typically they are radially oriented with dichotomous branching near their central terminations and are found to overlap each other in various stromal levels. The far peripheral cornea remains uninvolved except in the most severe cases. Indirect or retroillumination shows the rodlike nature and double contour of these lines with an optically clear center (Fig. 12-28). In focal illumination the filaments are opaque with finely irregular margins. Advanced cases can show fluorescence when illuminated with the blue slit-lamp light. Subepithelial or epithelial involvement with surface irregularity and irregular astigmatism is usually present.

Refractile, glassy, homogeneous, discrete dots or opaque, more irregular opacities occur with the filaments or in a linear fashion creating pseudo-filaments. These minute gray nebulae are similar to the early findings in granular and macular dystrophies.

A fine anterior, axial, stromal haze may be present and is seen best with a broad oblique beam. As the dystrophy advances, the dot opacities coalesce, the lattice lines become thicker and more opaque, and the intervening stroma becomes opaque in a fine granular pattern. A central disc-shaped opacity in the subepithelial and anterior

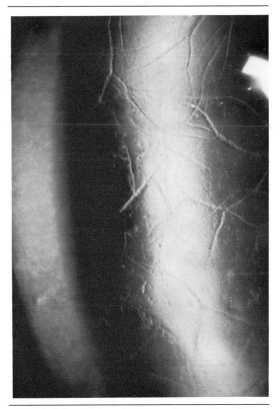

Fig. 12-28. *High-power slit-lamp photograph in lattice dystrophy. Delicate, branching, refractile filaments and smaller refractile dots are seen in retroillumination.*

stromal layers may obscure the central, typical lattice figures. Yellow or amber refractile material may accumulate in the subepithelial area and has been identified as elastotic degeneration [80, 93].

Histopathology reveals an irregular epithelium. The basal cells may be swollen, vacuolated, or pyknotic [196, 433]. The epithelial basement membrane is usually thickened and in places lacks normal hemidesmosomal structure [107, 433]. Bowman's membrane is thicker or thinner than normal and may be fragmented, especially in its periphery. A variably thick eosinophilic layer separating epithelial basement membrane from Bowman's layer may be present; it is composed of amyloid and collagen (Fig. 12-29) [123]. The corneal stroma contains a myriad of large, irregular, eosinophilic deposits that distort the normal corneal lamellae. These deposits stain orange-red with Congo red and manifest green birefringence when viewed with the polarizing microscope. Dichroism occurs when the deposits are viewed with

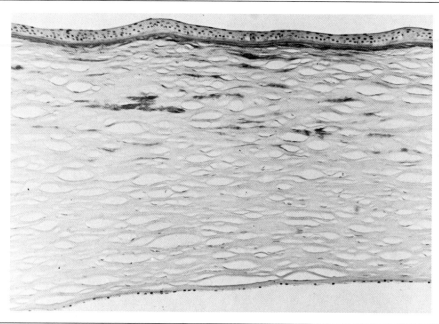

Fig. 12-29. *Lattice dystrophy. Congo-red-stained section demonstrates fusiform lesions in the anterior stroma. Similarly staining material is also seen forming a subepithelial layer. (×125 before 30% reduction.)*

Fig. 12-30. *Lattice dystrophy. Transmission electron micrograph shows mass of amyloid filaments 10 nm in diameter (arrow) and adjacent normal stromal collagen fibrils (box). (×45,000 before 35% reduction.) Inset, Fusiform stromal lesion that distorts normal lamellar architecture. (Congo red, ×500 before 35% reduction.) (From G. O. Waring, M. M. Rodrigues, and P. R. Laibson [410].)*

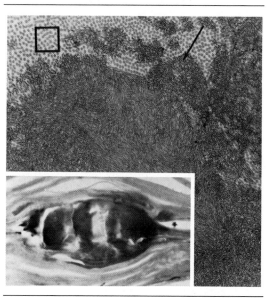

polarization and a green filter [123]. Increased fluorescence is present with thioflavine-T staining and ultraviolet light. When stained with crystal violet, metachromasia is usually apparent. Immunofluorescence studies have shown positive staining with antisera to human amyloid [30]. Polarization microscopy may demonstrate epithelial or Bowman's layer involvement that is not apparent on initial histologic examination.

Electron microscopy shows the amyloid lesions to consist of extracellular masses of fine, electron-dense fibrils 80 to 100 Å in diameter (Fig. 12-30) [127, 270]. Many of the fibrils are highly aligned, which explains the birefringence and dichroism; however, they do not show periodicity. Normal or electron-dense collagen fibrils may admix with the finer amyloid fibrils. Elastotic material may be present in more advanced cases [93]. Keratocytes in the involved areas are decreased in number and show cytoplasmic vacuolation and degeneration. Others appear metabolically active with prominent dilated endoplasmic reticulum and Golgi apparatus [179, 220, 270]. Descemet's membrane is usually normal but sometimes contains amyloid deposits. The endothelium is usually found to be normal [123, 220].

Amyloid is a glycoprotein with a fibrous component differing from collagen in amino acid content and fiber character. Amyloidosis is classified into two basic groups: systemic and localized. Each group is subdivided into primary and secondary amyloidosis [43]. In primary systemic amyloidosis, the amyloid contains fragments of immunoglobulin light chains, and a similar component (M component) is found in the serum or urine. However, in secondary amyloidosis, the main amyloid component is a nonimmunoglobulin protein (protein AA) usually occurring in association with an elevated serum amyloid A–related protein (SAA). The deposits in both of these conditions are associated with a structural protein (protein AP) that is also present in normal serum [293]. Evaluation of typical lattice dystrophy has shown the presence of protein AP in characteristic lattice lesions. Staining with anti-AA antiserum was initially reported as positive [280, 418], but other investigators have not been able to corroborate these findings [269, 327].

Typical lattice dystrophy (type I) is considered a localized primary form of amyloidosis. Amyloid deposits have not been found in other excised tissues from these patients [220, 275]. However, systemic amyloidosis may be associated with lattice dystrophy (latticelike dystrophy or lattice dystrophy type II) [275]. In this generalized amyloidosis, the onset of clinical corneal changes is later, erosive symptoms are less frequent, and the visual outcome is more favorable than in typical lattice dystrophy [218]. Systemic manifestations of cranial and peripheral neuropathies and dermatologic involvement become prominent with age. Amyloid deposits are found in arteries, basement membranes, skin, peripheral nerves, sclera, and other tissues throughout the body. Open-angle glaucoma and pseudoexfoliation are frequently present [277]. Clinically there are fewer lattice lines in the cornea, and they are more radially oriented in the peripheral cornea with relative central sparing. The more amorphous dots are fewer than in typical lattice dystrophy. An amyloid layer forms beneath a normal-appearing Bowman's membrane, in contrast to the disrupted Bowman's membrane encountered in lattice dystrophy type I. Fewer but similar stromal lesions are present in type II; these share the same staining characteristics as the amyloid in type I [275]. The amyloid in type II lattice dystrophy shows no reactivity to anti–protein AA antiserum and demonstrates

loss of Congo red staining after treatment with permanganate [276, 418]. Amyloid deposits may occur in the cornea in other disorders including primary familial amyloidosis of the cornea [214, 369] (also called gelatinous-drop-like dystrophy [4, 413]) and polymorphic amyloid degeneration [261] and in association with local ocular diseases or injury [136].

The treatment of typical lattice dystrophy includes management of recurrent epithelial erosions with patching or soft contact lenses. Penetrating keratoplasty is employed in the later stages of the disease, but recurrence within the graft is more common than with granular or macular dystrophy [274]. Elevated subepithelial opacities and fine lattice lines in the anterior stroma may appear both centrally and in the periphery of grafts. Electron microscopy has confirmed the amyloid nature of these deposits even when typical staining has not been present using light microscopy [240].

The origin of the amyloid deposits in lattice dystrophy remains unknown, but it is probably not related to degenerating nerve fibers or systemic amyloidosis. Theories of local pathogenesis include degeneration of collagen or ground substance and production of amyloid from affected keratocytes [223, 410].

GELATINOUS-DROP-LIKE DYSTROPHY

Gelatinous-drop-like dystrophy is a rare familial disorder well documented in the Japanese literature since the first report by Nakaizumi [282]. Early investigators in the United States termed the condition *primary familial amyloidosis of the cornea* [214, 369]. A report of a similar condition appeared in the European literature in 1930 [244]. The inheritance of this disorder is unclear, but it is probably autosomal recessive [369].

This bilateral dystrophy presents in the first decade of life with photophobia, lacrimation, and decreased visual acuity. Erosive symptoms have been prominent in some patients. Early in the progression the changes may resemble those of primary band-shaped keratopathy. Examination reveals a central "mulberry-like" opacity with protuberant subepithelial mounds that appear white on focal illumination and semitransparent on retroillumination. The opacities increase in number and depth with age. Surrounding the moundlike excrescences, flat, often dense subepithelial opacities are seen. Vascularization, if present, is usually minimal. Anterior and posterior cortical lens changes have been reported [369].

Multiple subepithelial deposits with staining and polarization findings typical of amyloid are present [4, 214, 369, 413]. A flat, more uniform layer of a similar material may surround the nodular masses. Bowman's membrane is usually absent. Ultrastructural examination clearly demonstrates the amyloid nature of these deposits. Fusiform stromal amyloid deposits resembling those found in lattice dystrophy have also been seen. Rapid superficial recurrence of this dystrophy after keratoplasty has been reported [262, 281].

CENTRAL CRYSTALLINE DYSTROPHY

In 1924 van Went and Wibaut described three generations of a pedigree with hereditary stromal crystalline dystrophy [398]. Schnyder clarified the entity and documented its stable and asymptomatic initial clinical course and autosomal dominant inheritance [346, 347]. This bilaterally symmetrical dystrophy produces an axial, ring-shaped, yellow-white opacity evident at birth or in early life [98, 162, 204]. The opacity has a regular border and consists of numerous fine polychromatic crystals. It is located in the anterior stroma and involves Bowman's membrane, although the epithelium is usually normal (Fig. 12-31). Five morphologic appearances of the central opacity have been described: (1) a discoid central opacity without crystals, (2) a central crystalline opacity with an ill-defined margin, (3) a discoid central crys-

Fig. 12-31. *Slit-lamp photograph of characteristic axial opacity in central crystalline dystrophy. The anterior location of the pattern is demonstrated in slit-beam section, and a crisp light reflex is seen from the overlying smooth epithelial surface.*

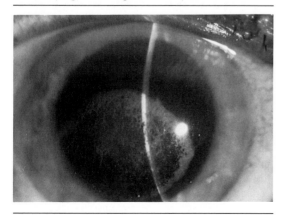

talline opacity with a garlandlike margin, (4) a ring opacity of crystal aggregates with a clear center, and (5) an annular crystalline opacity with fine crystals and a clear center [83]. A single pedigree may have any combination of these various morphologies, and there may be great variation in the extent of the involvement within a single pedigree. The opacities usually stabilize later in life.

Corneal arcus and limbal girdles are frequent accompaniments of the central opacities and may appear early in life [83]. They should be considered a feature of the dystrophy although they are not present in all cases. Xanthelasmas have been reported less frequently [133, 255]. Chondrodystrophy and genu valgum have appeared in certain pedigrees [41, 83, 255]. Hyperlipidemia has been reported in a significant percentage of patients with central crystalline dystrophy, although no correlation between presence or extent of the dystrophy and type of lipid elevation exists [41, 199, 255]. In one case the clinically observed corneal lesions lessened in a patient with hypercholesterolemia on a modified lipid diet [379]. However, other cases that have required keratoplasty because of severe corneal involvement have shown repeated documentation of normal blood lipid levels.

Slit-lamp examination shows numerous minute needlelike crystals that appear polychromatic on focal and indirect illumination. Palisades, aggregates, or meshwork clumps of these crystals in the anterior stroma have various shapes. The intervening stroma is usually clear, but in some cases a haziness is present because of smaller, white, punctate stromal opacities. Crystals may variably extend to the deeper stroma and cause a milkly opalescence of the cornea [41]. Arcus and limbal girdles are usually present and may be dense. In some cases these seem to blend with the stroma crystals. The peripheral stroma remains clear in most cases but may be diffusely involved with an atypical appearance. Corneal sensation is usually normal but may be diminished over the lesion or diffusely [41].

Frozen histopathologic specimens show birefringent cholesterol crystals and globular neutral fats thought to correspond to the crystals and dot opacities seen clinically [139, 416]. Noncrystalline cholesterol and cholesterol esters have also been demonstrated [41, 139, 416]. Stains for triglycerides and free fatty acids are negative. The epithelium is usually normal, although cholesterol clefts and fat-laden macrophages have been noted [10, 140]. Subepithelial glycogen deposits may be present, and epithelial glycogen content may be increased [139]. The basement membrane may be focally absent. Bowman's membrane is usually partially or totally destroyed.

On electron microscopy characteristic trapezoidal or oblong spaces disrupt the normal stromal architecture and may be associated with multilamellar bodies [416]. Small round empty spaces are also present within the stroma [10]. Patches of a fine granular or fibrillar electron-dense material may be present near the crystal spaces (Fig. 12-32). In one instance similar deposits in the deep stroma were characterized as amyloid by staining and electron microscopy [99].

The cause of the typical cholesterol deposits is unclear. This disorder probably represents a localized abnormality of cholesterol metabolism in the cornea, which may become modified by systemic hyperlipidemia [41, 48]. All patients with crystalline dystrophy should be investigated for systemic hyperlipoproteinemia with appropriate fasting blood studies. In those with normal serum cholesterol and triglyceride levels, a lipoprotein electrophoresis should also be obtained.

Keratoplasties have been performed in a minority of patients with this disorder. Recurrences have occurred in both penetrating [83] and lamellar keratoplasties [83, 139].

Other corneal conditions can produce similar polychromatic crystalline corneal changes. Marginal crystalline dystrophy (of Bietti) was described in two brothers who had fine crystalline opacities in the anterior stroma of the paralimbal cornea. In addition, both brothers had fundus albipunctatus. Vision was unaffected in this disorder [11]. A similar appearance of peripheral crystalline deposits was present in three members of a family described by Offret and coauthors. Ultrastructural findings in this instance documented extensive accumulation of electron-dense polygonal crystals in the extracellular spaces [286].

Corneal crystals are also seen in some patients with dysproteinemia [12, 222, 287]. Examples are patients with multiple myeloma, Waldenström's macroglobulinemia, benign monoclonal gammopathy, Hodgkin's disease, and cryoglobulinemia. Cystine corneal crystals may be seen in all three forms (infantile, adolescent, and adult) of cystinosis [90, 338]. Other disorders rarely causing crystals in the cornea include gout [356], porphyria [57], familial lecithin-cholesterol acyltransferase deficiency [145], and the Richner-Hanhart syndrome [20]. Very unusual causes of a much less typical appearance of corneal crystals include hyperbilirubinemia, Tangier disease, lipid keratopathy, rhubarb gluttony, and botanical exposure, especially to the Dieffenbachia plant [101].

FLECK DYSTROPHY

François and Neetens described fleck dystrophy (dystrophie mouchetée) in 31 members of one family [129]. This rare, autosomal dominant dystrophy may be congenital and is usually noted as an incidental finding [7, 375]. It is generally bilateral but may be asymmetric [375]. Unilateral cases have been reported [150, 290]. The vision is not affected, and no symptoms of erosion are present, but an occasional patient may have mild photophobia. This disorder is stable or slowly progressive once noted and is characterized by small, gray-white, discrete opacities throughout the stroma extending to the limbus (Fig. 12-33).

The corneal changes are subtle and are seen only with careful slit-lamp examination. The opacities vary in size, configuration, depth, and

Fig. 12-32. *Transmission electron micrograph of stromal lesions in crystalline dystrophy. Characteristic geometric crystal spaces* (arrow) *are surrounded by fine electron-dense fibrillogranular deposits* (f). *The surrounding stroma is punctuated by round empty spaces* (asterisk). *(×45,000 before 38% reduction.) (From G. O. Waring, M. M. Rodrigues, and P. R. Laibson [410].)*

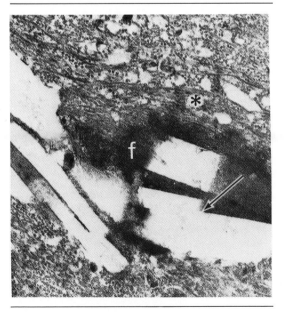

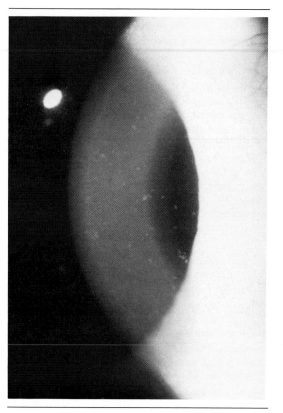

Fig. 12-33. *Fleck dystrophy. Fine irregularly shaped opacities appear gray-white with focal and retroillumination and extend to the limbus.*

number and are seen best in retroillumination. Homogeneous dots and flecks or comma-shaped, stellate, circular, and wreathlike opacities with relatively clear centers are present. High magnification most often shows a doughnutlike opacity with sharp peripheral borders and a relatively clear center. The surrounding stroma is clear. Bowman's membrane and the epithelium are not involved. Corneal sensation is usually normal.

Associated ocular conditions have included esotropia [129], central cloudy corneal dystrophy [66, 129, 142], keratoconus [308], limbal dermoid [308], papillitis [308], angioid streaks [308], punctate cortical lens opacities [367], and familial decreased corneal sensation [22]. It is unlikely that these are truly part of the dystrophy. Extensive systemic evaluation has failed to demonstrate any generalized mucopolysaccharide disorder [290]. One pedigree had two family members with homocystinuria, but this was felt to be a random occurrence [150].

Light microscopy demonstrates abnormally distended keratocytes at all stromal levels. The intervening stroma appears normal, as do the epithelium, Bowman's membrane, Descemet's

Fig. 12-34. *Transmission electron micrograph of cornea in fleck dystrophy. Large membrane-limited intracytoplasmic vacuoles* (asterisk) *contain a fine fibrillogranular material. Surrounding collagen fibrils* (C) *appear normal.*

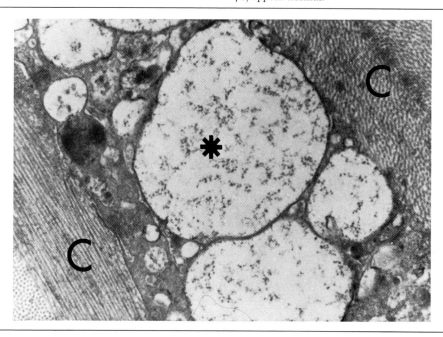

membrane, and endothelium. Lipid stains including Sudan black B and oil red O, and glycosaminoglycan stains including alcian blue and colloidal iron are positive and correspond to the involved keratocytes [215, 285]. Congo red staining for amyloid is negative [285]. No significant staining for glycosaminoglycan is present in conjunctival cells.

Ultrastructural examination shows extensive membrane-limited cytoplasmic vacuolations within the involved keratocytes (Fig. 12-34). Most of the vacuoles contain a fibrillogranular material, while others contain smaller vesicles [215]. Both of these types of vacuoles contain occasional membranous inclusions and pleomorphic electron-dense deposits [215, 285]. In keratocytes with lesser involvement, the vacuoles appear to be associated principally with prominent Golgi complexes. Rarely they seem to be derived from the rough endoplasmic reticulum [285]. Nonspecific changes can be seen in the surrounding stroma, but no specific extracellular material is present. The histopathologic specimens differ from those in macular dystrophy by showing only isolated keratocyte involvement without extracellular glycosaminoglycan accumulation.

Based on these histologic findings, fleck dystrophy represents an inherited storage disorder involving glycosaminoglycans and complex lipids that is limited entirely to the cornea. This is a unique situation genetically since metabolic disorders typically show recessive inheritance rather than the dominant hereditary pattern of fleck dystrophy [150].

POLYMORPHIC STROMAL "DYSTROPHY"

Pillat described two elderly sisters with deep, punctate, heterogeneous stromal opacities [298]. One had fine radial lines in the anterior peripheral cornea, and both had minimally decreased visual acuity. Much later, 10 additional unrelated patients with a spectrum of similar changes were collected under the appellation *polymorphic stromal dystrophy* [374, 386]. A larger, more recent series further defined this clinical entity with histopathology confirming the amyloid nature of the deposits [261]. However, family studies have failed to demonstrate this disorder in more than one generation, and this condition has not been found in younger individuals. Therefore, unless the heritability is demonstrated, this "dystrophy" may best be termed polymorphic amyloid degeneration [231].

CENTRAL CLOUDY DYSTROPHY

François described a rare bilateral condition consisting of faint deep opacification in the axial stroma occurring in 2 siblings and 6 unrelated additional patients [122]. Subsequent reports have documented the familial nature of this entity, and autosomal dominant inheritance has been suggested [32, 373]. Unilateral cases have also been reported [21, 122]. Unusual patients have presented with other ocular disorders including fleck and pre-Descemet's dystrophies [67, 68, 129], spherophakia [21], and glaucoma [32]. One patient with pseudoxanthoma elasticum manifested both central cloudy and fleck dystrophies [68]. Although noted as young as 8 years of age, progression of central cloudy corneal dystrophy of François is minimal. Corneal sensation remains intact, and treatment is not indicated [231].

The lesions are not macroscopically visible and do not decrease visual acuity. Slit-lamp examination shows involvement of the axial two-thirds of the cornea with multiple, large, light gray opacities in the deep stroma separated by narrow lines of relatively clear stroma. This pattern is best seen with broad oblique illumination or scleral scatter. The margins of these lesions are fluffy and indistinct, but the cracklike clear areas lend a polygonal structure to the opacities (Fig. 12-35). Descemet's membrane and the endothelial mosaic are unaffected. Fainter, similar lesions may occur in the anterior stroma, giving a layered effect to the opacities but sparing Bowman's membrane.

This entity seems clinically identical to the condition termed posterior crocodile shagreen by Vogt [154, 231, 401]. It is probably more accurate

Fig. 12-35. *Central cloudy dystrophy. Axial portion of the cornea contains multiple gray-white opacities separated by relatively clear cracklike areas.*

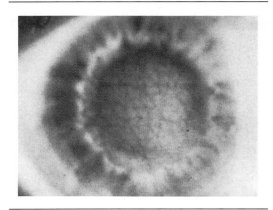

to use the term *posterior crocodile shagreen* for similar findings unless multiple family members, especially younger patients, manifest similar changes.

Transmission electron microscopic evaluation of one case of posterior crocodile shagreen demonstrated a distinctive "sawtooth" pattern with some of the collagen lamellae located at right angles to others [231]. Interspersed in these areas were patches of abnormal collagen with 100-nm banding. The uninvolved peripheral and anterior stromal architecture was normal. This histologic pattern is unique among known dystrophies and degenerations [231].

POSTERIOR AMORPHOUS CORNEAL DYSTROPHY

A distinct-appearing deep opacification appeared in three generations of a single pedigree as early as the first decade of life [51]. Vision was not markedly affected, vascularization and inflammation were not present, but stromal thinning was prominent. One affected individual had corectopia and an iridocorneal adhesion [51]. More recently, eight affected members spanning five generations of separate pedigrees have been evaluated with apparent autosomal dominant inheritance [95]. Additional features of the dystrophy, including extension to the limbus, flattened corneal topography, hypermetropia, and anterior iris anomalies, were elucidated. The presence of typical changes in a 6-month-old affected family member with clouding of the cornea noted from the age of 16 weeks suggested that these changes

Fig. 12-36. *Posterior amorphous corneal dystrophy. Diffuse gray-white deep stromal opacities impart a diffuse haziness to the cornea of this 6-month-old infant.*

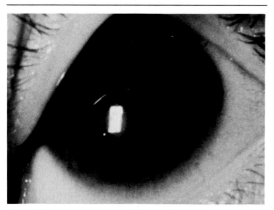

may be congenital (Fig. 12-36) [95]. No histopathologic data are yet available.

Layers of gray, amorphous, sheetlike opacities occur in axial, axial-peripheral, diffuse, and, less commonly, peripheral forms. These changes are most prominent in the deep stroma, but all stromal layers have been reported to be involved (Fig. 12-37). Irregularities and clear stromal breaks in these opacities are prominent. Descemet's membrane may be involved with posterior bowing and distortion of the endothelial pattern. Central, uniform corneal thinning with flattened keratometry readings is present in patients with the axial involvement.

Gonioscopy may demonstrate a prominent Schwalbe's line with numerous fine iris processes. However, there was no evidence of glaucoma in either reported pedigree. Various iris anomalies including prominent pupillary mem-

Fig. 12-37. *Slit-lamp photograph showing corneal involvement in posterior amorphous corneal dystrophy. Gray sheet of opacification (arrow) is seen in the posterior cornea on slit-beam section. Less-dense opacities are located in the more anterior stromal layers.*

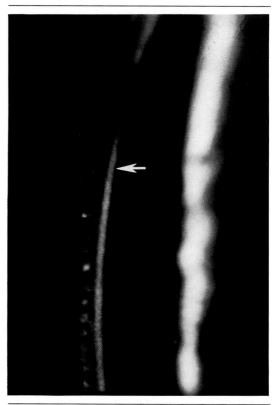

brane remnants [95], anterior stromal tags [95], corectopia [51], a large iridocorneal adhesion [51], and a generalized sponginess of the iris stroma have been noted. Iris atrophy has not been present. Horizontal strabismus was found in three family members [95].

The large amorphous nature of these opacities and the involvement of Descemet's membrane distinguish this entity from congenital hereditary stromal dystrophy [425], central cloudy dystrophy or posterior crocodile shagreen, and pre-Descemet's dystrophy. The corneal thinning differs dramatically from other posterior dystrophies including congenital hereditary endothelial dystrophy [210] and posterior polymorphous dystrophy [58]. The absence of ghost vessels in posterior amorphous stromal dystrophy distinguishes it from interstitial keratitis, although marked corneal thinning may be present in both conditions. The lack of progression, the possible congenital origin, and the presence of iris anomalies have raised the possibility that this condition may be a dysgenesis involving embryonic mesoderm [95].

CONGENITAL HEREDITARY STROMAL DYSTROPHY

Diffuse, bilateral, congenital corneal opacification has been classified in a number of different ways (Table 12-3). Most congenital corneal clouding has been linked to endothelial dysfunction. Recently, a dystrophy has been separated from other causes of congenital corneal opacification on the basis of unique clinical corneal findings and characteristic electron microscopic findings [425]. This disorder, termed congential hereditary

Table 12-3. *Causes of Congenital and Infantile Corneal Opacification*

Diagnosis	Differential Features
Congenital glaucoma	Bilateral in 75%; cornea enlarged; epithelium edematous, stroma often less so; tears in Descemet's membrane; raised intraocular pressure; recessive inheritance
Birth trauma	Usually unilateral; stroma edematous and thickened; tears in Descemet's membrane; normal corneal diameter; normal ocular pressure; negative family history
Congenital hereditary endothelial dystrophy	Bilateral; diffuse marked stromal edema and thickening; normal intraocular pressure; minimal progression; atrophic endothelium; usually recessive inheritance
Congenital hereditary stromal dystrophy	Bilateral; central stromal opacification with normal thickness; normal ocular pressure; nonprogressive; normal Descemet's membrane and endothelium; dominant inheritance
Posterior polymorphous dystrophy	Bilateral; diffuse corneal opacity; normal or increased corneal thickness; normal intraocular pressure; abnormal endothelium; dominant inheritance
Congenital rubella	Cataract, miosis, microphthalmos, retinopathy; systemic stigmata; viral culture from body fluids; raised rubella antibody titer
Congenital syphilis	Bilateral; corneal vascularization; choroidoretinopathy; systemic stigmata; positive serologic results
Mucopolysaccharidosis	Bilateral; some corneal thickening; ± optic atrophy; ± retinopathy; systemic stigmata; excess urinary mucopolysaccharide; mainly mucopolysaccharide storage; autosomal recessive inheritance except Hunter's, which is X-linked
Mucolipidosis	Bilateral; ± cherry-red macular spot; systemic stigmata; no excess urinary mucopolysaccharide; mucopolysaccharide and sphingolipid storage; recessive inheritance

± = finding may be present or absent.

stromal dystrophy (CHSD), appears to be a result of disordered stromal fibrogenesis. Only two pedigrees have been studied with typical electron microscopic findings although there may be other reports in the literature with similar clinical and light microscopic presentations [86, 425]. CHSD appears to be inherited in an autosomal dominant fashion.

A diffuse flaky or feathery haze is more pronounced in the central anterior stroma and less obvious in the deep peripheral stroma. In contrast to congenital hereditary endothelial dystrophy, the anterior and posterior layers of the cornea appear normal and central corneal thickness is not increased in CHSD. Opacification is present at birth and seems stationary with longitudinal observation for as long as 11 years. Corneal sensation remains unaffected, and epithelial edema and recurrent erosions do not occur. As with other congenital corneal opacities, decreased vision is eventually documented although nystagmus and strabismus are often present at an early age [425].

The epithelium and Bowman's membrane are normal by both light and electron microscopy [425]. The stroma shows clefting and fine layering of the lamellae. The characteristic and distinct ultrastructural picture consists of alternating layers of collagen fibrils approximately one-half the normal fibril diameter. These layers consist of lightly packed, aligned fibers in a lamella sandwiched by layers of smaller fibrils arranged in a more random or haphazard fashion. Although collagen fibrils of a similar diameter may be found in granular and lattice dystrophies, the aggregate morphologies are distinctly different. In CHSD Descemet's membrane lacks the anterior banding of the fetal portion but is of normal thickness. The posterior portion of Descemet's membrane is normal. In contrast to congenital hereditary endothelial dystrophy, which demonstrates a markedly abnormal endothelium and disorganization of the posterior portion of Descemet's membrane, the endothelium in CHSD is entirely normal [332].

Penetrating keratoplasty has been performed without known clinical recurrence of the dystrophy. However, vision depends on the extent of deprivation before keratoplasty. Early successful keratoplasty may help overcome the deprivation amblyopia.

The pathogenesis of CHSD remains unclear but involves disordered fibrogenesis of the stroma. The endothelium may play an early role in the production of this disorder as evidenced by the abnormal anterior portion of Descemet's membrane. Later endothelial function and morphology appear to be normal [425].

PRE-DESCEMET'S DYSTROPHY

A number of "dystrophies" have been reported with fine opacities limited to the extreme posterior stroma. Although some reported cases have occurred in families, heritability of these conditions has been questioned. Most of these probably represent a spectrum of degenerative changes since they have appeared in patients over 30 years of age, do not cause symptoms or reduce vision, and require no treatment. Previous descriptions of this group of heterogeneous disorders have included cornea farinata, deep filiform dystrophy [116, 258], posterior punctiform dystrophy [117], punctate pre-Descemet's dystrophy [69], and pre-Descemet's dystrophy [159].

Cornea farinata is the most common of these disorders and is thought to be an involutional change. A myriad of fine dustlike or flourlike opacities are found diffusely in the deep stroma. The spots are more prominent centrally and are best seen with retroillumination. Families in which cornea farinata was seen in several members have been described, but cornea farinata is generally held to be a degenerative process associated with aging [291, 300].

Pre-Descemet's dystrophy exhibits opacities at the same level, but they are larger and more polymorphous than those of cornea farinata (Fig. 12-38). However, these two entities have been reported to occur concomitantly in the same eye or as separate lesions in opposite eyes of the same patient [159]. Dendritic, boomerang, circular, dotlike, comma-shaped, linear, filiform, and semicircular discrete deposits have been described [74, 159]. These heterogeneous deposits were found axially, diffusely, or in an annular pattern sparing the central cornea and a small band of peripheral cornea adjacent to the limbus. More females than males have been reported with this condition. Inheritance over two generations was described in three pedigrees, and the disorder occurred in siblings in another family [159]. Pre-Descemet's dystrophy has been reported with other ocular conditions including keratoconus [65, 159, 258], epithelial basement membrane dystrophy [159], posterior polymorphous dystrophy [159], and central cloudy corneal dystrophy [67]. Identical lesions can be found in affected males and carriers of X-linked recessive ichthyosis [350].

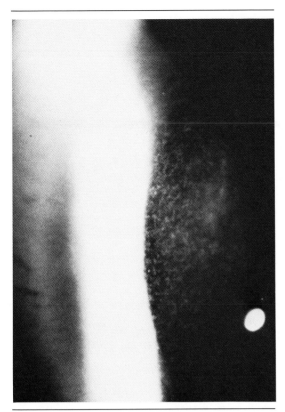

Fig. 12-38. *Pre-Descemet's dystrophy. Numerous, irregular, deep stromal opacities are highlighted well against the pupil with slit-lamp retroillumination.*

Histopathologic specimens obtained in one case with clinical pre-Descemet's dystrophy showed the involvement to be limited to the posterior stromal keratocytes without any changes in the endothelium, Descemet's membrane, stromal collagen, or anterior keratocytes [74]. Striking vacuolation and enlargement of the posterior keratocytes were present, with histochemical staining showing lipidlike material. Ultrastructural examination revealed a spectrum from a few to many cytoplasmic membrane-bound vacuoles within the posterior keratocytes. The vacuole contents included fibrillogranular material and electron-dense lamellar inclusions resembling lipofuscin. No extracellular deposition of a similar material was noted [74]. These pathologic findings tend to support the hypothesis that this "dystrophy" is actually an aging change, although there may be a genetic predisposition in certain pedigrees.

A related but clinically distinct disorder termed polychromatic dystrophy was more recently de-scribed [103]. Apparent autosomal dominant inheritance was observed in four generations of a single pedigree involving 8 of 46 family members. This disorder differed from pre-Descemet's dystrophy by exhibiting polychromatic, deep stromal filaments that were more uniform in size and present over the entire cornea including the limbus. No particular aggregations or annular patterns were appreciated, and Descemet's membrane and the endothelium were clinically unaffected. Some of the opacities were associated with optically clear spaces in the stroma. No histopathology has been done in this disorder [103].

Dystrophies of the Endothelium and Descemet's Membrane

FUCHS' DYSTROPHY AND CORNEA GUTTATA

Fuchs' dystrophy is a term that applies to the edematous stage of a progression of changes occurring in the cornea secondary to endothelial dysfunction (Fig. 12-39). As with some of the other dystrophies, such as epithelial basement membrane dystrophy, there is considerable overlap between changes that are common in the normal population and early dystrophic alterations that are more rare but ultimately more severe. This condition was initially termed *dystrophia epithelialis corneae* by Fuchs in a description of patients with epithelial edema, stromal clouding, and decreased corneal sensitivity [135]. Fuchs did not have the benefit of the biomicroscope and therefore was unaware of endothelial pathology. Later longitudinal observations documented that endothelial changes preceded the epithelial and stromal changes, often by many years.

Fuchs' dystrophy is bilateral but often asymmetric and involves women more than men, most frequently after the sixth decade of life [230]. Clinical changes, however, may be present much earlier in life. The dystrophy shows gradual progression over decades with three clinical stages:

1. Endothelial dystrophy (cornea guttata). Initially the patient is asymptomatic, and the findings are limited to multiple axial corneal guttae associated with a fine bronze stippling of pigment clumps on the posterior corneal surface. The guttae may be irregular and vary in size and configuration. By direct slit-lamp illumination, they appear as golden refractile mounds on the posterior corneal surface. Specular reflection discloses black holes in the endothelial mosiac (Fig. 12-40). On

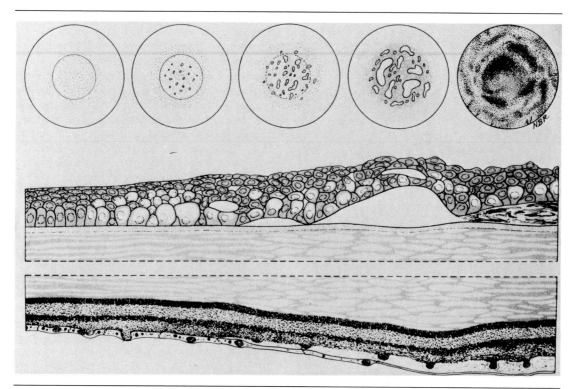

Fig. 12-39. *Composite drawing of the clinical and histopathologic changes in Fuchs' dystrophy. Beginning at the left, corneal guttae appear as focal excrescences posterior to Descemet's membrane. With endothelial decompensation, fluid accumulates in the basal epithelial cells and later in the entire epithelium and stroma. Descemet's membrane takes on a slate gray appearance owing to the production of an increasingly thick posterior collagenous layer. The endothelium phagocytoses pigment and gradually becomes more atrophic. Subepithelial bullae are followed by the appearance of an avascular collagenous layer in the subepithelial space. The late stages may show relatively less edema with increasing cicatrization. (From G. O. Waring, M. M. Rodrigues, and P. R. Laibson [411].)*

retroillumination, they appear as focal black spots against the red reflex. With time the guttae spread peripherally and may coalesce. Descemet's membrane takes on a beaten-metal appearance, thickens, and begins to show a faint gray opacification with irregularity most apparent with tangential focal illumination. At this stage the retinoscopic red reflex may take on a diffusely mottled appearance, and vision may be mildly affected. Cornea guttata characterized by typical, small spots on the posterior corneal surface is a common clinical diagnosis in patients of middle to older age groups. These excrescences of Descemet's membrane are identical to Hassal-Henle bodies, which are normally found in the corneal periphery even in younger individuals. Population studies show that up to 70 percent of patients over the age of 40 have at least one gutta [147, 279]. Confluent cornea guttata has been found in 3.9 percent of those over age 40 [254]. In spite of the clinical appearance of confluent guttae over most of the posterior corneal surface, the condition may not necessarily progress to the second or edematous stage. On the other hand, some patients have shown progression to corneal edema with few or even no guttae present [1]. Specular microscopy of the fel-

low eyes of some of these patients demonstrated decreased endothelial cell counts and cellular pleomorphism in spite of the absence of cornea guttata. Histology in these cases did, however, demonstrate diffuse thickening of Descemet's membrane, which is typical of Fuchs' dystrophy.

2. Fuchs' dystrophy (stromal dystrophy with or without epithelial edema). If endothelial function is not adequate to keep the cornea from becoming turgescent, then corneal edema occurs. Initially early morning epithelial edema resulting from decreased osmolarity of the nocturnal tears occurs.

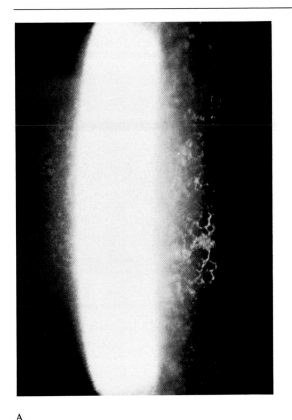

A

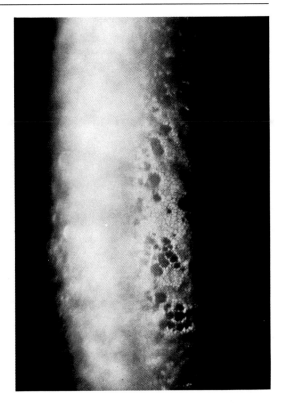

B

Fig. 12-40. *Specular photographs of the corneal endothelium of a patient with Fuchs' dystrophy. The characteristic black holes in the endothelial mosaic correspond to corneal guttae. These are confluent in the central cornea (A) and more scattered in more peripheral endothelium (B).*

This clears as the day progresses because the normal drying effect of the environment increases tear osmolarity. Symptoms of fluctuating visual acuity usually precede clinically apparent corneal epithelial edema. Early stromal edema creates a faint relucence just anterior to Descemet's membrane and later just posterior to Bowman's membrane. Early epithelial edema involves the basal epithelial layers and appears as fine bedewing. This creates a fine beaten-metal pattern on retroillumination and a pigskinlike texture to the corneal surface seen best with oblique illumination. With progressive edema small, isolated microcysts of clear fluid coalesce to become fusiform lakes or large epithelial or subepithelial bullae that severely diminish vision (Fig. 12-41). Shift lines similar to fingerprints may occur as linear or curvilinear shadows in the deep epithelium [37]. In-

Fig. 12-41. *Stromal edema, faint gray opacification, and subepithelial bullae in Fuchs' dystrophy.*

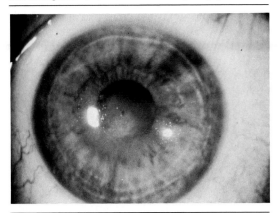

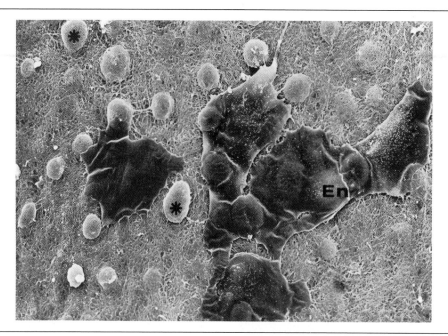

Fig. 12-42. *Scanning electron micrograph of the posterior corneal surface in Fuchs' dystrophy demonstrates a few remaining endothelial cells (En), the surrounding exposed surface of the posterior collagen layer, and many guttae (asterisk). (×300 before 30% reduction.) (Courtesy of Kenneth R. Kenyon.)*

creasing edema imparts a marbled look to the stroma and is seen best with sclerotic scatter. Normally the central cornea is thinner than the periphery. This relationship becomes reversed with central edema and may be appreciated by careful slit-lamp examination. Descemet's membrane is displaced posteriorly with irregular central folds and wrinkles. The initial changes usually occur axially and progress peripherally to involve the entire cornea but may also occur in an eccentric distribution. Bullous keratopathy with subsequent bullae and epithelial breakdown causes irritation, photophobia, scarring, and vascularization.

3. Subepithelial scarring. With chronic corneal edema a diffuse, subepithelial sheet of scar tissue is seen separating the stroma from the epithelium. At the time of the appearance of this swirling heterogeneous layer, corneal sensation is diminished and corneal edema may become less prominent, leading to end-stage cicatrization of the cornea. Secondary complications including erosions, ulcers, vascularization, and increased intraocular pressure may occur.

The heredity of this disorder has been the subject of few comprehensive studies, considering its frequency in the population relative to other, more rare, dystrophies [230, 233]. When the proband has confluent cornea guttata, family studies have shown nearly a 40 percent rate of confluent cornea guttata in members over 40 years of age. Women were more frequently and severely involved than men. No association was noted between severity of disease in parents and severity in the offspring. There was, however, no significant difference in endothelial cell counts or morphology by specular microscopy between unaffected family members and age-matched controls [345]. Initial inspection of the pedigrees of the involved families suggested an autosomal dominant mode of inheritance; however, a simple mendelian inheritance could not be demonstrated clearly by statistical methods so other factors must be involved [73, 230]. Corneal guttae are rarely present in early life, but individuals and families with congenital cornea guttata have been described [91, 382]. These cases, however, tended not to progress to corneal edema.

Corneal guttae are not specific for Fuchs' dystrophy. They represent an abnormal product of affected endothelial cells from a variety of conditions including aging and inflammation [408].

Secondary guttae can be confluent, forming hyaline ridges or geographic patterns, in contrast to the primary form. Transient pseudoguttae appear in cases of trauma or endotheliitis and may resemble typical guttae on specular microscopy [234]. However, experimentally and clinically they resolve when the inflammation abates. They have been found to represent focal edema of the endothelial cells. A similar transient pattern has been seen after normal endothelium was exposed to air [100].

The primary defect in Fuchs' dystrophy is thought to be in the corneal endothelial cell and is manifested by its production of a thickened, abnormal basement membrane. The most striking changes in the endothelium are present over guttae, where the endothelial cells may be markedly attenuated or absent. These cells may be morphologically altered from their normal hexagonal shape and contain numerous membrane-bound vacuoles and phagocytosed melanin granules. Cellular degeneration and increased cytoplasmic filaments are evident on electron microscopy [181, 186]. Some of these cells have been shown to take on fibroblast-like characteristics with production of collagen and glycosaminoglycans; others exhibit microvilli similar to those of epithelial cells. Scanning electron microscopy has demonstrated the unusual contour of the posterior surface and enlargement and pleomorphism of the endothelial cells (Fig. 12-42) [302].

The most characteristic histopathologic change in Fuchs' dystrophy is thickening of Descemet's membrane with a collagenous posterior layer and guttate excrescences [407]. Electron microscopy shows that the most anterior fetal portion of Descemet's membrane is normal with the characteristic 110-nm banding [28]. However, the nonbanded layer immediately posterior is thinned or absent. Most of the increased thickness is due to changes in the more posterior layers, which are laid down throughout life. These layers contain fibrils with 110-nm banding similar to fibrils of the anterior fetal zone but occurring in patches with a background of amorphous ground substance. Randomly oriented fusiform bundles of collagen fibrils with 64-nm periodicity are also present, as are fine 20-nm microfibrils. Smaller oxytalan microfibrils are most prominent around the posterior excrescences [5]. The layers adjacent to the endothelium show a more disorganized and fibrillar appearance. Posterior excrescences often contain material with 110-nm bands and may contain cellular debris (Fig. 12-43).

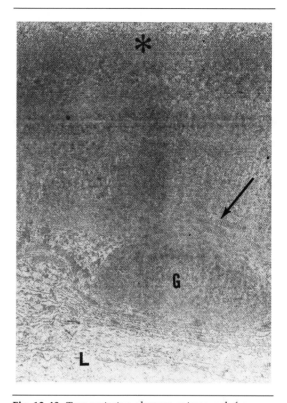

Fig. 12-43. *Transmission electron micrograph from a case of Fuchs' dystrophy. The anterior portion of Descemet's membrane (asterisk) is normal. The posterior layers contain patches of collagen fibrils with 110-nm bands (arrow) in a background of more amorphous appearance. Posterior and adjacent to a focal guttate excrescence (G) is a lamella of loose fibrillar material (L). (From G. O. Waring, M. M. Rodrigues, and P. R. Laibson [411].)*

In the early edematous stages fluid accumulates within the basal epithelial cells. The entire epithelium is later involved with thickening and separation from the underlying normal Bowman's layer and loss of hemidesmosomes. An avascular collagen layer accumulates in this space and contains active fibroblasts [186]. Changes in the stroma are secondary to edema with disruption of the lamellar architecture and accumulation of fine fibrillogranular material near the keratocytes. In later stages cicatrization with a more regular and compact architecture may occur.

Treatment of Fuchs' dystrophy depends on the stage of progression, the status of the fellow eye, and associated conditions such as increased intraocular pressure or concomitant cataract. Topical sodium chloride is used in the early stages to dehydrate the corneal epithelium and reduce fluctuations in visual acuity [88]. In patients complaining of blurred vision in the morning, bedtime hyperosmotic ointment, such as 5% sodium chloride, is helpful. A hair dryer can also be effective in reducing the morning edema. Soft contact lenses may be used to decrease the surface astigmatism and therefore can sometimes improve vision in the early stages of epithelial edema. When the edema is more severe, soft contact lenses can reduce erosive symptoms from bullous breakdown and act as a bandage protecting the corneal blisters from the lids. Superficial cauterization has been used in patients who do not tolerate contact lenses and are not candidates for surgery.

Penetrating keratoplasty is indicated when visual rehabilitation is desired. The long-term clarity of grafts in this disorder has been limited, possibly because of the aged, abnormal remaining host endothelium [371]. The intraocular pressure should be monitored and controlled at all stages of the disease because of the effect on stromal hydration. Combined cataract surgery and penetrating keratoplasty or a triple procedure with insertion of an intraocular lens is indicated in patients with significant lenticular opacities [8].

CONGENITAL HEREDITARY ENDOTHELIAL DYSTROPHY

The term *congenital hereditary corneal dystrophy* was used by Maumenee in a description of 8 patients with diffuse, bilateral corneal opacities apparent very early in life or at birth [264]. Later, the disorder became known as *congenital hereditary endothelial dystrophy* (CHED) when it became apparent that the corneal clouding was secondary to a dystrophy of the corneal endothelium [209]. Additional clinical, histochemical, and ultrastructural studies have helped to differentiate this disorder from other congenital corneal disorders including the systemic mucopolysaccharidoses, congenital glaucoma, macular dystrophy, posterior polymorphous dystrophy (PPMD), and congenital hereditary stromal dystrophy [55, 210, 243] (see Table 12-3).

Two distinct modes of inheritance have been described for CHED [197]. The autosomal recessive type presents with corneal clouding at birth or in the neonatal period, tends to remain stationary, and may be accompanied by nystagmus. Corneal clouding appears later in pedigrees with an autosomal dominant pattern and is often preceded by irritation and photophobia. The opacification is slowly progressive in some of these cases, and mystagmus is less frequently seen [197, 264, 292].

There may be considerable overlap between the dominant pattern of CHED and findings in younger, more severely affected individuals with PPMD. The wide spectrum of expression of disorders with autosomal dominant inheritance, especially PPMD, and the similarity in the pathologic findings have led certain investigators to conclude that some cases of CHED and PPMD are part of a spectrum of expression of a single genetic defect [55, 58].

We believe in most cases it is appropriate to diagnose these two dystrophies as two distinct clinical and pathologic conditions. One must wonder about the validity of the original diagnosis of CHED in probands who later had typical findings of PPMD described in both symptomatic and asymptomatic family members [243, 292]. It is probable that these cases actually represented more severely involved examples of the spectrum of PPMD. However, there remains a small portion of cases in which clinical, genetic, and histopathologic differentiation is not clear-cut [55, 58].

In CHED affected corneas are of normal diameter and show an irregular, ground-glass opacification of the stroma that may vary from a mild haze to a more confluent, milky opacification. This is prominent centrally but extends to the peripheral cornea. The result is diffuse, marked thickening of the corneal stroma. Small, more dense white stromal opacities and diffuse gray thickening of Descemet's membrane may be present. In cases with adequate visualization corneal guttae are not seen and the endothelial mosaic is abnormal or absent. Epithelial edema, with bedewing or microcysts, is apparent, although macrocystic changes with epithelial lakes and bullae are unusual [366]. Late stages may show superficial vascularization, scarring, and band keratopathy. The corneal stroma remains markedly thickened. Intraocular pressure is normal, and corneal sensation remains intact. Aside from nystagmus and esotropia, no other ocular or systemic findings are commonly encountered. Conjunctival biopsies and serum and blood studies have shown no evidence of increased glycosaminoglycans or protein abnormalities [210]. The vision varies with the degree of corneal clouding but usually deteriorates to the finger-counting range in fully affected individuals.

The most striking histopathologic findings are profound stromal edema, attenuation or absence of the endothelium, and changes in the posterior

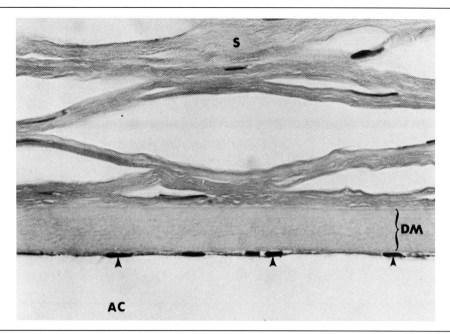

Fig. 12-44. *Light micrograph of cornea in congenital hereditary endothelial dystrophy shows markedly thickened Descemet's membrame (DM) and dystrophic endothelial cells (arrowheads). (S = posterior stroma, AC = anterior chamber.) (H&E ×600 before 30% reduction.) (From K. R. Kenyon and A. E. Maumenee. Published with permission from the* American Journal of Ophthalmology *76:419–439, 1973. Copyright by the Ophthalmic Publishing Company.)*

structure of Descemet's membrane (Fig. 12-44) [6, 55, 201, 202, 209, 210, 264, 292, 366]. The endothelial cells are markedly attenuated or totally absent; when present they show atrophy, cytoplasmic vacuolation, and the presence of myelin granules. The anterior banded portion of Descemet's membrane is usually normal, but the posterior layer is altered in all cases, with varying thickness and composition. A noncellular basement-membrane-like material with fine embedded small-diameter filaments usually occupies the midzone, while larger, more disordered collagen fibrils comprise the more posterior layers (Fig. 12-45). No guttate excrescences of this abnormal Descemet's membrane have been noted.

The stromal lamellae show large fluid clefts. The keratocytes are essentially normal. Some of the stromal collagen fibrils are larger than usually found in other conditions with corneal edema. Fibrils of different sizes up to 60 nm have been reported, while other reports show normal fiber

diameter [209, 210, 266]. Nonspecific changes were found in the epithelial and Bowman's layers secondary to chronic edema or other infectious, vascular, or calcific complications.

Endothelial cell cultures in CHED have not grown under standard conditions, and no biochemical or structural protein abnormalities have been identified [366]. The condition seems to result from loss of endothelial cells sometime after the fifth month of gestation; this conclusion is based on the normal appearance of the fetal zone of Descemet's membrane. The stromal or epithelial changes are thought to be secondary and are distinctive from the secondary changes occurring in Fuchs' dystrophy.

Treatment includes topical sodium chloride in the early stages and penetrating keratoplasty in the later stages or in cases of the congenital variety. Keratoplasty in infants or neonates is fraught with difficulty [342, 409]. The long-term prognosis for grafts in this condition is not favorable [292, 366].

POSTERIOR POLYMORPHOUS CORNEAL DYSTROPHY

A variety of names have been used to describe PPMD since some of its features were first reported by Koeppe [58, 227]. PPMD is a bilateral

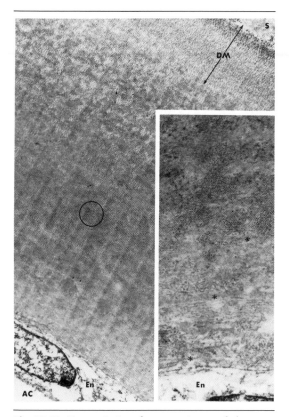

Fig. 12-45. *Transmission electron micrograph from a case of congenital hereditary endothelial dystrophy. The anterior zone of Descemet's membrame (DM) shows normal thickness and substructure. Both 55-nm and 110-nm bands (circle) are present in the extremely thickened abnormal posterior layer. (S = posterior stroma, En = endothelial cells, AC = anterior chamber.) (Originally ×9,200 before 38% reduction.) Inset, Higher magnification of the posterior zone demonstrates multiple lamellae of basement-membrane-like material (asterisks) and fine filaments. (En = endothelium.) (×41,600.) (From K. R. Kenyon and A. E. Maumenee. Published with permission from the* American Journal of Ophthalmology *76:419–439, 1973. Copyright by the Ophthalmic Publishing Company.)*

disorder of the corneal endothelium characterized by a spectrum of typical changes in the posterior cornea and less commonly in the angle and iris structures [157]. In the vast majority of cases, an autosomal dominant mode of inheritance can be demonstrated. There are, however, cases in which recessive inheritance is suggested [275]. A wide variation in expression within affected family members is often present in PPMD [58]. The disorder may be unilateral or seem to be unilateral

with only minimal involvement of the fellow eye. Ocular involvement may also be sectorial with only patches of cornea or iris clinically altered [58].

Most of the affected individuals are asymptomatic, which makes the age of onset difficult to determine. However, the fact that corneal edema and typical vesicles have been noted shortly after birth in families with PPMD suggests a congenital onset. This is also supported by evaluation of the ultrastructure of Descemet's membrane [26, 55, 303, 391].

Clinical slit-lamp examination shows vesicles, islands of abnormal endothelium, characteristic bands, or gray thickened sheets of Descemet's membrane as isolated findings or in various combinations with (Fig. 12-46) or without corneal edema. Vesicles appear as small excavations or blisters of Descemet's membrane with a scalloped margin surrounded by a mild haze. These may occur in cluster, linear, arborizing, or geographic configurations (Fig. 12-47). On specular microscopy they appear as blacked-out areas, often with septa and sometimes with a surrounding pleomorphic endothelial mosaic (Fig. 12-48) [176]. Similar vesicular lesions have been reported unilaterally in asymptomatic patients without a family history of PPMD [289].

Thickening of Descemet's membrane can create focal, geographic, or diffuse graying with a peau d'orange appearance on retroillumination. More prominent focal thickening of this membrane may create excrescences projecting into the anterior chamber or characteristic bandlike lesions with a scalloped irregular margin and non-

Fig. 12-46. *Diffuse corneal edema obscuring the more characteristic slit-lamp findings in posterior polymorphous dystrophy.*

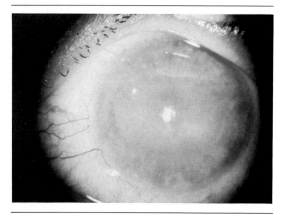

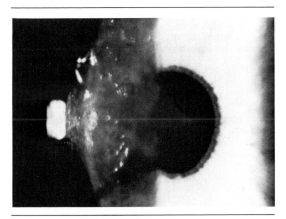

Fig. 12-47. *Slit-lamp examination of patient with posterior polymorphous dystrophy may reveal characteristic vesicles. Opacification at the level of Descemet's membrane is well seen highlighted against the pupil.*

Fig. 12-48. *Specular microscopy in a case of posterior polymorphous dystrophy showing abnormal dark areas in endothelial mosaic with internal fine septa.*

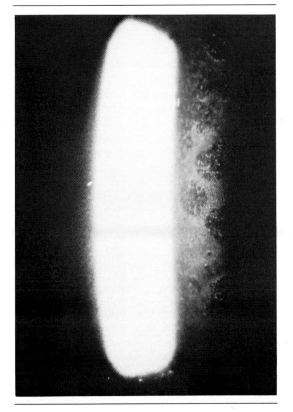

tapering terminations [59]. The nonparallel margins of these bands appear as linear white opacities with direct or tangential illumination.

Small, basal, iridocorneal adhesions visible only with gonioscopy or larger grossly visible lesions may be present in a minority of affected individuals and are always associated with other corneal findings of PPMD, which are usually more prominent in the area or sector of the adhesion [Fig. 12-49] [58, 328]. Ectropion uveae may occur, often in association with glassy membranes that extend from the iris to the back of the cornea [58]. Iris stromal atrophy is not present as it is in Chandler's syndrome or essential iris atrophy. An unusual variant of PPMD with ring-shaped corneal clouding has also been described [427]. Increased intraocular pressure is found in a significant percentage of patients with PPMD. The pressure should be monitored in edematous corneas with electronic applanation. Corneal sensation remains intact in this disorder [58].

Histopathologic specimens from advanced cases of PPMD show characteristic alterations in the endothelial cells. Scanning electron microscopy demonstrates that there are two different populations of endothelial cells [303, 330]. The first are typical hexagonal cells with scant microvilli and normal-appearing junctional complexes. These cells appear more pleomorphic bordering areas of endothelial cell loss or areas of more fibroblast-like or epithelium-like cells. The second type are larger and squamous with prominent microvilli. Light and transmission electron microscopy show these cells to occur in multiple layers with a stratified appearance [26, 55, 192, 303, 330, 332, 391].

Fig. 12-49. *Sectorial corneal edema and iridocorneal adhesion with associated ectropion uveae in posterior polymorphous dystrophy.*

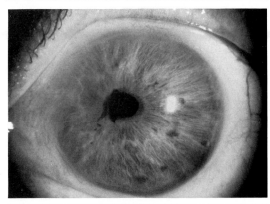

They have numerous prominent desmosomal attachments and microvilli and contain scattered cytoplasmic filaments 10 nm in diameter (Fig. 12-50). The mitochondria, ribosomes, and endoplasmic reticulum are more prominent in the anterior layers of these cells. Immunofluorescent staining of PPMD endothelium with antikeratin antiserum shows fluorescence corresponding to the areas of epithelium-like cells [332].

Descemet's membrane varies in thickness and may have a multilaminar appearance. The anterior layer with 110-nm bands is normal, but the uniform posterior granular layer is replaced by a variably thick or thin layer composed of fusiform bundles of collagen with 55- to 110-nm bands in

Fig. 12-50. *Transmission electron micrograph of cornea in posterior polymorphous dystrophy. The posterior portion of Descemet's membrane contains patches of broad-banded collagen* (black arrow). *Multiple layers of endothelial cells* (E) *contain increased keratofibrils and show numerous desmosomal attachments* (circles). *Microvilli project from the endothelial surface* (white arrow). (×13,000 *before 38% reduction.*) (*Courtesy of Thomas A. Weingeist.*)

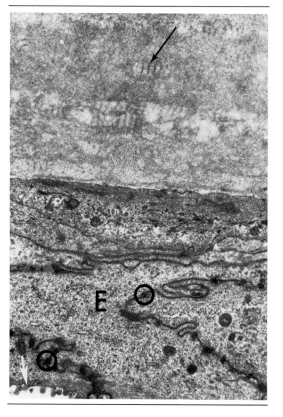

a matrix of basement-membrane-like material (Fig. 12-50). Excavations or excrescences of the posterior portion of this unusual Descemet's membrane have been described [171, 303]. Stromal and epithelial changes in transplanted corneas are related to the chronic corneal edema.

Trabecular and iris specimens from PPMD patients with glaucoma have shown that the epithelium-like cells may extend across the inner trabecular meshwork and onto the anterior surface of the iris [328]. This may be a factor in the production of iridocorneal adhesions and glassy membranes in this disorder. Other investigators have demonstrated a high iris insertion into the trabecular meshwork with associated collapse of the intertrabecular spaces [27].

The epithelial nature of the endothelial cells is a differentiating factor between PPMD and disorders comprising the iridocorneal endothelial (ICE) syndrome [96, 328]. These latter disorders present sporadically with unilateral, progressive ocular changes. Rieger's syndrome, like PPMD, is bilateral and dominantly inherited but includes an anteriorly placed Schwalbe's line, infantile glaucoma, and other systemic anomalies [198].

The pathogenesis of the epithelium-like cells in PPMD remains unclear, but theories of transformation of embryonal cells or abnormal differentiation of neural crest cells have been proposed. As in CHED, the histopathology of Descemet's membrane in PPMD points to a gestational onset [58, 331].

Treatment is usually not required for cases of PPMD. Mild corneal edema may be managed with topical sodium chloride. Severe or congenital cases may require penetrating keratoplasty. If glaucoma and iris pathology are not present, the results of penetrating keratoplasty are excellent. If epithelium-like endothelial cells have grown across the trabecular meshwork and glaucoma is present, the results are much worse and glaucoma management is very difficult [58].

Keratoconus

Keratoconus is a bilateral, noninflammatory condition that results in ectasia of the axial cornea with resultant progressive visual loss owing to irregular myopic astigmatism and scarring. It usually becomes manifest in adolescence with irregular corneal astigmatism and may follow a steadily progressive course, usually with stabilization after 10 or 20 years. Other cases have a more rapid and steady deterioration necessitating surgical treatment [232].

The incidence of keratoconus varies with the criteria for diagnosis and is probably approximately 1 to 2 per thousand population. Although most cases of keratoconus are sporadic, it sometimes shows a familial pattern [170]. Affected relatives of probands may show a broad spectrum of involvement with milder forms considered a forme fruste of the disorder. Occurrence in monozygotic twins has also been reported. However, the specific inheritance pattern in that portion of clinical cases that may be genetic remains unclear. The reported occurrence of keratoconus in successive generations has tended to support an autosomal dominant mode of inheritance [170]. Reports of parental consanguinity have been cited as evidence for a recessive mode. Multifactorial inheritance and modification by familial or environmental factors have been invoked by various investigators to explain the findings. Overall, there seems to be less than a 10 percent chance of keratoconus occurring in a blood relative of an affected proband [232].

In the typical case blurring of vision presents in the teens with increasing myopia, irregular astigmatism with distorted keratometry mires, inferior steepening of the keratometric readings, and irregularity of the retinoscopic light reflex. With progression glare and photophobia become more prominent, and spectacles do not fully correct visual acuity.

Slit-lamp examination reveals an ectasia or protrusion that is usually inferior and nasal to the geometric center of the cornea. Two distinct morphologies of this cone-shaped ectasia have been described [294]. The first is more round, smaller, and more central in location. Much less common is an oval or sagging configuration that is larger and displaced more inferiorly and temporally. The ectasia may be partially or totally surrounded by a faint brown epithelial pigment line (Fleischer's ring) that is highlighted with diffuse cobalt blue illumination against a dilated pupil (Fig. 12-51). Associated fine epithelial fibrillar lines can also be noted just inside or crossing the pigment ring with broad oblique illumination [40]. There may be increased visualization of corneal nerves in a reticular pattern, although decreased corneal sensation is usually a very late finding.

The area of ectasia shows corneal thinning that is especially prominent at the apex. Faint striae (Vogt's striae) may be present in the deep stroma and Descemet's membrane (Fig. 12-52). These

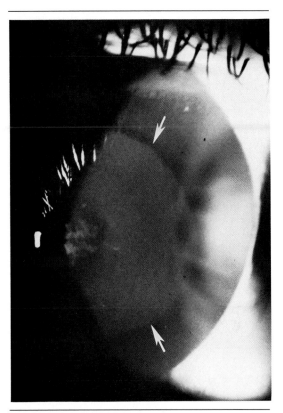

Fig. 12-51. *Diffuse slit-lamp photograph demonstrates the Fleischer ring (arrows) that surrounds the area of ectasia in this case of keratoconus. Apical scarring is also apparent in oblique illumination.*

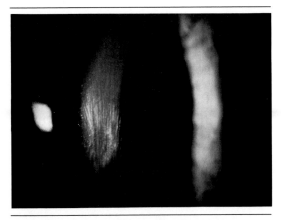

Fig. 12-52. *Slit-lamp photograph in keratoconus showing vertical striae near the apex of the cone. These striae are seen at the level of Descemet's membrane and the deep stroma. They disappear when external pressure is applied to the globe.*

consist of parallel, linear, or curvilinear opaque lines usually oriented along the meridian with the steepest curvature [336]. The fact that they disappear with any manuever that increases intraocular pressure demonstrates their mechanical rather than pathologic nature. Scar tissue at the level of Bowman's membrane near the apex of the cone may produce superficial linear opacities. Dark lines can also be present at that level. These probably represent unfilled breaks in Bowman's membrane [232].

With progression the protrusion of the cone may be prominent enough to distort the contour of the lower lid on down gaze (Munson's sign). Ruptures in Descemet's membrane can occur, creating an acute edematous condition termed *acute keratoconus* or *acute hydrops*. This gradually resolves in a matter of weeks to months without specific treatment and results in scarring and usually flattening of the conical apex [372]. Rarely, the cornea remains edematous. Cycloplegics and patching are used to reduce photophobia and discomfort.

Keratoconus can occur with a variety of systemic and ocular diseases, some of which are inherited [232]. Many of these associations may be coincidental, since keratoconus is a relatively common disorder. However, other diseases may modify the course of the keratoconus, possibly by inducing irritation and resultant eye rubbing. Especially in some of the systemic connective tissue disorders, a common tissue alteration may cause keratoconus. Keratoconus thus may be the end result or final common pathway of a number of disorders including systemic collagen disease, trauma, or preexisting abnormalities of corneal tissue [232].

Frequent associations between atopic disease and keratoconus have been reported [312]. Immunoglobulin E has often been found to be elevated in patients with keratoconus [312]. Keratoconus is reported to occur in up to 8 percent of patients with Down's syndrome. Acute hydrops is encountered more frequently in these patients, possibly because of repeated or prolonged ocular trauma [232].

Cases of Ehlers-Danlos syndrome, which is the result of abnormal cross-linkage of collagen, may include keratoconus [265]. Other systemic connective tissue disorders reported in association with keratoconus include Marfan's syndrome, Rieger's syndrome, anetoderma, focal dermal hypoplasia, nail-patella syndrome, Apert's disease, and Crouzon's disease [232]. Mitral valve prolapse

has also been reported in a significant percentage of keratoconus patients [16].

Associated ocular conditions include retinitis pigmentosa, Leber's congenital amaurosis, and vernal conjunctivitis. Rare associations with macular coloboma, retrolental fibroplasia, retinal aplasia, and other corneal dystrophies have been reported [232].

The histopathology of keratoconus is well described and varies with the stage of the disease. The Fleischer ring is formed by ferritin particles that accumulate in the basal epithelium, both within the cells and extracellularly. Early degenerative changes occur in the basal epithelial cells or anterior stroma with resultant alterations in Bowman's membrane. Disruption of this layer may be associated with invasion of the defects by epithelium anteriorly and collagen and fibroblast-like keratocytes posteriorly, creating typical Z-shaped areas [301]. Stromal collagen lamellae are decreased in number in the central area with resultant stromal thinning [306]. In advanced stages there is more disorganization of the lamellae and individual collagen fibrils. Granular and microfibrillar material is deposited in the stroma and may be associated with keratocytes. A spectrum of degenerating, normal, and fibroblast-like keratocytes has been described, with the last type accumulating in the anterior stroma surrounding areas of disrupted Bowman's layer [307]. Most authors feel that these anterior keratocytes play a primary role, possibly through a defect in fibrogenesis or increased collagenolysis [232].

Stromal scarring may occur at any level but is usually most prominent in the deeper layers. Ruptures in Descemet's membrane may occur with a scroll configuration to the free ends and production of new Descemet's material both in the scroll and bridging the defect [372].

The biochemistry of keratoconus remains unclear in spite of the increasing sophistication of the investigations. Recently, increased collagenolytic activity has been demonstrated in organ cultures from corneal buttons obtained at the time of keratoplasty [318].

Treatment in the early stages involves spectacle correction if tolerated. Associated ocular conditions should be controlled to reduce irritation and inflammation. This may secondarily reduce ocular trauma from eye rubbing, which is felt by some to be a modifying, if not causal, factor in this condition. An appropriately fit hard contact lens should be used if spectacles no longer give satisfactory vision. Regular reevaluation of contact lens wear is important to reduce contact lens–induced complications in the dynamic phase of the disorder. If lens fit or comfort becomes unsatisfactory, then penetrating keratoplasty is indicated. The prognosis in surgical cases is excellent, but endothelial rejection is relatively common and permanent mydriasis may occur even when no mydriatics have been used at the time of surgery. Other less frequently employed surgical treatments include thermokeratoplasty [9], lamellar keratoplasty [321], and epikeratophakia [206].

CORNEAL DISORDERS ASSOCIATED WITH INHERITED SYSTEMIC DISEASE

Because the cornea shares its ectodermal, mesodermal, and neural crest origin with other tissues involved in genetically determined metabolic and systemic diseases, corneal conditions may be seen among these disorders (Table 12-4). Some corneal findings may be so characteristic as to be pathognomonic of the specific disease; others are nonspecific. Corneal pathology can also be related to secondary complications or environmental factors. An attempt will be made to highlight some of the more common or characteristic disorders with emphasis on the corneal complications. Many of these conditions are covered in more depth elsewhere in this text.

Corneal Manifestations in Inherited Skin Disease

Genodermatosis is a term used to describe hereditary systemic skin disease. In many of these disorders corneal changes occur. In some the changes are a primary manifestation. Others show secondary scarring and vascularizing stages owing to involvement of the lids or lacrimal system (see Chap. 19, The Skin and the Eye).

ICHTHYOSIS

Ichthyosis is an inherited disorder in which hyperkeratosis of the horny layer produces thick, dry, scaly skin with cornification (Fig. 12-53). The condition is present at birth or shortly thereafter [205]. Dominant (ichthyosis vulgaris and congenital ichthyosiform erythroderma), recessive (lamellar ichthyosis), and X-linked recessive (X-linked ichthyosis) forms have been described. Corneal findings are most prominent in X-linked ich-

Table 12-4. *Selected Inherited Metabolic Disorders with Corneal Manifestations*

I. Disorders of carbohydrate metabolism
   A. Mucopolysaccharidoses
     1. Hurler's (I-H)
     2. Scheie's (I-S)
     3. Hunter's (IIA, IIB)
     4. Sanfilippo (IIIA, IIIB, IIIC, IIID)
     5. Morquio's (IV)
     6. Maroteaux-Lamy (VI)
     7. Sly (VII)
   B. Glycogen storage disease
     1. von Gierke's disease (type I)
     2. Pompe's disease (type II)

II. Disorders of lipid metabolism
   A. Hyperlipoproteinemias
     1. Familial hypercholesterolemia (type II)
     2. Familial hyperlipoproteinemia (type III)
   B. Familial plasma cholesterol ester deficiency
   C. Tangier disease
   D. Fish-eye disease
   E. Fabry's disease
   F. Niemann-Pick disease
   G. Gaucher's disease
   H. Fucosidosis

III. Combined disorders
   A. Mucolipidoses I, II, III, and IV
   B. GM_1 gangliosidosis type I
   C. Sulfatidosis
   D. Goldberg's syndrome

IV. Disorders of protein metabolism
   A. Cystinosis
   B. Richner-Hanhart syndrome
   C. Alkaptonuria

V. Disorders of mineral metabolism
   A. Wilson's disease
   B. Hemochromatosis

thyosis and are manifest in affected males and to a lesser extent in carrier females [350].

Nonspecific punctate keratitis and increased visibility of the corneal nerves may be present [132]. Gray, elevated, superficial nodules resembling Salzmann's nodular degeneration have been reported [396]. Small refractile bodies have also been seen in the endothelium, superficial stroma, and epithelium [341]. An unusual case showed a bilateral, central, superficial corneal opacity unassociated with lid abnormalities [337]. More characteristic have been small punctate or filiform opacities in the deep stroma identical to those of pre-Descemet's dystrophy (Fig. 12-54) [13, 350]. These diffuse opacities tend to increase with age in affected individuals, although they do not di-

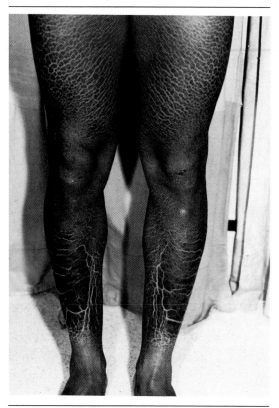

Fig. 12-53. Scaly skin of lower extremities in ichthyosis.

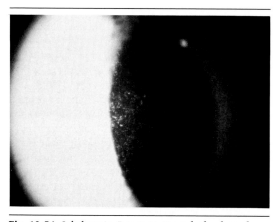

Fig. 12-54. Ichthyosis. Punctate irregularly shaped opacities in deep stroma.

minish visual acuity. Similar opacities have been seen in ichthyosis vulgaris. Other corneal findings may be secondary to lid involvement, especially in the dominant, nonbullous type (congenital ichthyosiform erythroderma) [13].

Vascularizing keratitis with corneal thinning, pannus formation, and stromal scarring has been described in patients with ichthyosis and neurosensory deafness. In these cases deafness is present at birth or develops at an early age. This triad of disorders has been termed the keratitis, ichthyosis, and deafness (KID) syndrome [355]. Approximately one-half of patients with KID syndrome have absent or scanty hair, eyebrows, and eyelashes. Visual loss in this disorder may be profound. This condition resembles hereditary hypohidrotic ectodermal dysplasia and may possibly be transmitted as a recessive trait [355].

EPIDERMOLYSIS BULLOSA

Epidermolysis bullosa is a term used for a group of chronic bullous skin and mucous membrane disorders. Recessive and dominant modes of inheritance have been described. Corneal involvement has been most frequent in the dominant dystrophic and recessive polydysplastic forms [115]. Diffuse granular clouding of the epithelium and Bowman's membrane, recurrent erosion with scarring, bullous keratitis, and ulceration have been described. Histopathology has shown epithelial vacuolation with poor epithelial adherence to an irregularly thickened Bowman's membrane [110].

Recently corneal findings were reported in two generations of a family with dominantly inherited epidermolysis bullosa simplex. These consisted of small cystic or bullous epithelial lesions in a ring pattern in the midperipheral cornea in the proband and similar lesions in the far corneal periphery of his mother [156].

KERATOSIS FOLLICULARIS SPINULOSA DECALVANS

Keratosis follicularis spinulosa decalvans, a rare disorder that is also termed Siemann's disease, keratosis pilaris decalvans, or follicular ichthyosis, is an inherited disorder of keratinization. There is generalized hyperkeratosis and roughness of the skin with spiny projections from the follicles that replace normal hairs and produce the texture of goose flesh. The eyebrows, eyelids, and lashes are frequently and prominently involved. Other features include atopy, hyperkeratosis of the palms and soles, and photophobia [314].

Punctate, farinaceous epithelial and subepithelial corneal opacities have occurred in some affected family members. Increased visibility of the corneal nerves, diminished tear production, a peripheral corneal pannus, and recurrent erosions in both fully involved individuals and carriers are reported [33]. Sex-linked inheritance has been proposed to explain the predominance of affected males.

Histopathology in 2 cases showed large vacuolated cells located principally in the superficial layers of the epithelium with eosinophilic contents and pyknotic nuclei. There was also thickening of the epithelial basement membrane with anterior extensions between the basal cells of the epithelium [115].

HEREDITARY HYPOHIDROTIC ECTODERMAL DYSPLASIA

Hypohidrotic ectodermal dysplasia, a rare skin disease, is inherited in a sex-linked recessive form in most pedigrees. It is manifest in males and less prominently in the female carriers. An autosomal recessive pattern may be the mode of inheritance in some kindreds [155]. The triad of hypohidrosis, hypotrichosis, and defective dentition is present in addition to other abnormalities [315].

A variety of nonspecific corneal changes including diffuse or sectorial punctate staining, erosions, Bowman's level and stromal opacification, corneal thinning, and pannus have been described in a minority of affected individuals [15, 420]. This disorder was also reported in association with granular dystrophy in one family [217].

Ectodermal dysplasia can occur in conjunction with cleft lip and palate and deformities of the hands and feet (EEC syndrome [ectrodactyly, ectodermal dysplasia, and cleft lip and palate]). The puncta and meibomian gland orifices are often absent in these individuals. Corneal changes may be secondary, but a primary dystrophic defect has been proposed to explain stromal opacification in some cases [15].

KYRLE'S DISEASE (HYPERKERATOSIS FOLLICULARIS ET PARAFOLLICULARIS IN CUTEM PENETRANS)

Kyrle's disease is a rare disorder manifested by scattered, flesh-colored, firm papules that spare the mucous membranes, palms, and soles. Characteristic histopathology shows a keratotic plug with basophilic cellular debris and abnormal keratinized epithelial cells beneath the plug [52]. Two siblings in one pedigree showed unusual corneal findings consisting of multiple, diffuse, punctate, yellow-brown opacities in the anterior stroma. These opacities were of greatest concentration and stromal depth near the limbus with a lucid interval. The patients also had subcapsular cataracts. The 19-year-old son of one of the patients had typical skin involvement and early posterior subcapsular cataracts but did not show corneal involvement [381].

KERATOSIS FOLLICULARIS (DARIER'S DISEASE)

Darier's disease is an autosomal dominant condition characterized by brown, scaly papules that are most prominent in the intertriginous areas, forehead, and scalp. Lesions may also be found on the palmar and plantar surfaces, and the mucous membranes, including the conjunctiva, can also become involved. Flat, nebular opacities of the epithelium with various configurations are seen in the peripheral cornea, usually separated from the limbus by a small lucid zone without vascularization. These are seen best with broad oblique illumination and occur over the entire periphery of the cornea without predilection for the palpebral zone. There seems to be no correlation between the presence of these lesions and the extent of the skin involvement. Another corneal finding is central epithelial irregularity with radiating cobweb patterns that can be outlined by using topical fluorescein [23].

Peripheral corneal biopsies in 2 patients showed epithelial edema, particularly of the basal cells, with a granular material beneath the basal epithelium. By electron microscopy, this material was found to be an electron-dense granular substance. A lack of hemidesmosomes and a multilaminar epithelial basement membrane were also noted [23].

Other, less common forms of corneal involvement in Darier's disease have included anterior stromal opacities, pannus formation, fine epithelial keratitis, and a limbal nodule [23, 118, 190]. Hyperkeratotic plaques involving the lids and lashes are frequently seen, and trichiasis may occur secondarily.

ROTHMUND'S SYNDROME (ROTHMUND-THOMSON SYNDROME)

Rothmund's syndrome is a recessive disorder characterized by congenital or infantile poikiloderma, rapidly developing cataracts, and hypogonadism. Females are affected twice as often as males. Partial loss of the eyelashes, eyebrows, and scalp hair occurs in half of the affected individuals. A band-shaped degeneration of the cornea has been noted in a minority of patients with this syndrome. Histopathologic findings did not differ from those in cases of primary band keratopathy [257, 353].

ACRODERMATITIS ENTEROPATHICA

Acrodermatitis enteropathica, a rare familial syndrome, is characterized by dermatitis of the distal extremities and around body orifices. It is associated with alopecia and chronic diarrhea. The dermatitis is usually vesicular or bullous in nature but later becomes more psoriasiform. If untreated, the disease is usually fatal before puberty. It is thought to show autosomal recessive inheritance [412].

Early photophobia with blepharitis and subsequent conjunctivitis are common. Loss of the brows and lashes may occur. Peripheral and central subepithelial corneal opacities have been described. Linear white or light brown opacities resembling corneal nerves and radiating to the limbus are associated with the more diffuse opacities. Erosions and punctate epithelial staining are intermittently present, but vascularization is usually not present. Corneal sensation is variable [263, 412]. In one case ultrastructural examination showed fragmentation and focal destruction of Bowman's layer and the epithelial basement membrane [412].

HEREDITARY MUCOEPITHELIAL DYSPLASIA

Mucoepithelial dysplasia, a recently recognized disorder, manifests panepithelial involvement with early conjunctival and corneal findings. Autosomal dominant inheritance has been observed in a three-pedigree study. Involved individuals show ocular symptoms in infancy including photophobia, tearing, and blepharospasm. Esotropia and horizontal nystagmus are often present. The conjunctiva displays diffuse vascular dilatation without a significant follicular or papillary response. The corneal epithelium, which contains microcysts, may become heaped up at the limbus, irregular, or opacified. Subsequent corneal pannus formation and advancing subcapsular cataracts usually lead to legal blindness within the first decade of life. Dermatologic manifestations include follicular keratosis, nonscarring alopecia,

and susceptibility to mucocutaneous infections, especially by *Candida*. Death usually occurs secondary to pulmonary complications [424].

Corneal histopathology shows varied thickness of the epithelial layer, intraepithelial dyskeratotic bodies, and lack of normal desmosomes and gap junctions. Lamellar and penetrating keratoplasties have not been successful in this disorder [424].

DERMOCHONDROCORNEAL DYSTROPHY

An extremely rare disorder is characterized by skeletal deformities, cutaneous xanthomatosis, and central corneal opacification. Deformities of the hands and feet appear in the first 5 years of life and may be associated with a period of hypercholesterolemia. The corneal changes appear within the first decade of life and are subepithelial and central in location. These hazy, white opacities elevate the overlying epithelium and show convex anterior and concave posterior margins. The periphery and deeper layers of the cornea are unaffected [121, 320].

MISCELLANEOUS DISORDERS

Corneal involvement has been observed in a variety of other inherited dermatologic disorders. In these diseases corneal changes are unusual and are often secondary findings. Some recessively inherited disorders in this category include xeroderma pigmentosum [316], familial dysautonomia (Riley-Day syndrome) [151], keratosis palmaris et plantaris with periodontopathy (Papillon-Lefèvre syndrome) [168], Werner's syndrome [46], and Cockayne's syndrome [34]. Dominantly inherited disorders include focal dermal hypoplasia (Goltz's syndrome) [385], benign acanthosis nigricans [239], Naegeli's syndrome [364], progeria (Hutchinson-Gilford syndrome) [82], cutis verticis gyrata (Rosenthal-Kloepfer syndrome) [335], pityriasis rubra pilaris [228], and the basal cell nevus syndrome, among others. Dyskeratosis congenita (Zinsser-Cole-Engman syndrome) is an X-linked disorder that rarely produces corneal changes [354].

Genetically Determined Metabolic Disorders Associated with Corneal Disease

DISORDERS OF CARBOHYDRATE METABOLISM— MUCOPOLYSACCHARIDOSES

The mucopolysaccharidoses are genetically determined deficiencies of lysosomal hydrolytic enzymes active in the breakdown of the protein complexes of acid mucopolysaccharides (or glycosaminoglycans). The result is tissue accumulation as well as urinary excretion of these partially degraded glycosaminoglycans. The deficient hydrolytic enzyme for each type of mucopolysaccharidosis has been determined by tissue culture studies [18]. Cross-culture studies have demonstrated that differing phenotypes may share the same enzymatic defect.

The extracellular matrix of the cornea contains three principal glycosaminoglycans. The most prevalent is keratan sulfate I, which is unique to the cornea; the others are chondroitin 6-sulfate and chondroitin 4-sulfate [71]. In the mucopolysaccharidoses keratan sulfate and an additional glycosaminoglycan, dermatan sulfate, accumulate in excess in the cornea. All of the major recognized types of mucopolysaccharidoses manifest histopathologic evidence of corneal accumulation, and most have characteristic clinical corneal opacification as a typical feature in addition to various degrees of skeletal dysplasia, facial dysmorphism, and mental retardation. Other ocular manifestations include retinal pigmentary degeneration and optic atrophy.

The appearance of the progressive corneal clouding is similar in most of these conditions. Usually there is a diffuse ground-glass nature to the opacity imparted by a myriad of fine, gray-yellow opacities (Fig. 12-55). Some cases demonstrate an annular pattern with relative central clearing and peripheral superficial and deep opacification imparting a gray hue to Descemet's membrane. There may be associated corneal edema,

Fig. 12-55. *Diffuse corneal opacification involving the entire cornea in a patient with mucopolysaccharidosis VIA (Maroteaux-Lamy).*

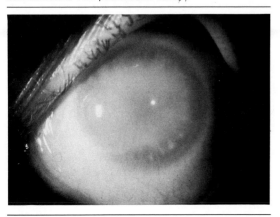

but it is usually much less than that found in congenital hereditary endothelial dystrophy.

The corneal histopathologic findings, which vary with the clinical involvement, include cytoplasmic vacuolation of the epithelial cells, subepithelial histiocytes, keratocytes, and some endothelial cells [119, 208]. Extracellular glycosaminoglycans are present in the stroma or in the subepithelial layers [149]. Bowman's membrane may be fragmented, especially in the peripheral cornea, because of the presence of numerous distended histiocytes [387]. Descemet's membrane remains unaffected.

Ultrastructural examination shows that the intracellular vacuoles are of two types. One contains a fine fibrillogranular sustance; the other, membranous lamellar vacuoles characteristic of glycolipid (Fig. 12-56). Individual keratocytes may be greatly distended by the intracytoplasmic vacuoles (Fig. 12-57). Various stages of edema have been noted with distortion of the lamellae. The individual collagen fibrils, however, remain unchanged.

Hurler's Syndrome. (Mucopolysaccharidosis I-H). Hurler's syndrome is characterized by moderate dwarfism, marked skeletal dysplasia and gargoylism, hepatosplenomegaly, severe mental retardation, and early death (Fig. 12-58). Progressive corneal clouding is a very early and consistent finding in this disorder and may be severe. The epithelium and endothelium appear normal. Corneal thickness may be increased. Pigmentary retinopathy and optic atrophy are frequent, and open-angle glaucoma has been seen [143, 365]. Short-term success of corneal tranplantation has been reported in this disorder [333].

Scheie's Syndrome. (Mucopolysaccharidosis I-S). Scheie's syndrome shares the same enzymatic defect as Hurler's, but the gross facial, skeletal, and mental defects are absent [343]. Corneal clouding may be present early in life or at birth and is slowly progressive. Acute glaucoma has also been reported in this condition. Retinal pigmentary degeneration and optic atrophy may be present. Penetrating keratoplasties have been performed in some cases with variable results [70, 310, 343].

Hunter's Syndrome. (Mucopolysaccharidosis IIA, IIB). In contrast to the other mucopolysaccharidoses, which are all inherited in an autosomal recessive manner, Hunter's syndrome is an X-linked recessive disorder. The features are similar to those of Hurler's syndrome with less promi-

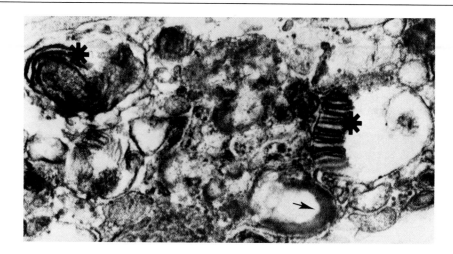

Fig. 12-56. *Transmission electron micrograph of keratocyte in mucopolysaccharidosis VIB (Maroteaux-Lamy) demonstrates membranous lamellar material (asterisks) within membrane-bound cytoplasmic vacuoles. A fine electron-lucent granular material accumulates in other vacuoles (arrow). (Original magnification ×67,000 before 30% reduction.) (Courtesy of Kenneth R. Kenyon.)*

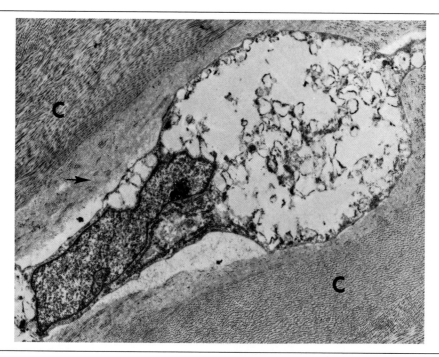

Fig. 12-57. *Transmission electron micrograph of stromal keratocyte in MPS mucopolysaccharidosis VIA (Maroteaux-Lamy) demonstrates massive distention by intracytoplasmic vacuoles. The keratocyte is surrounded by a fine fibrillogranular material (arrow), and the stromal collagen (C) is normal. (×67,000 before 24% reduction.) (Courtesy of Kenneth R. Kenyon.)*

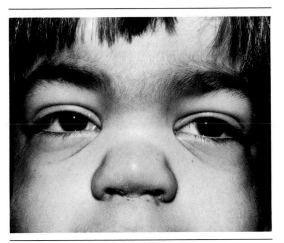

Fig. 12-58. *Facial features typical of mucopolysaccharidosis (I-H) (Hurler) including prominent brows with hypertrichosis, saddle nose, and chronic rhinorrhea. Progressive corneal opacification is usually present. (Courtesy of G. Frank Judisch.)*

nent skeletal and mental manifestations [149, 387]. Clinical corneal clouding is rare but may be present by slit-lamp examination of older affected individuals with the mild phenotype (IIB). A more severe phenotype (IIA) usually shows only histopathologic evidence of corneal involvement without clinical corneal opacification.

Sanfilippo's Syndrome. (Mucopolysaccharidosis IIIA, IIIB, IIIC, IIID). Four distinct enzymatic defects have been demonstrated in Sanfilippo's syndrome, which is characterized by severe retardation and early death [216]. The cornea is usually clear, but mild haze has been reported in rare cases [14, 339].

Morquio's Syndrome. (Mucopolysaccharidosis IV). Individuals with Morquio's syndrome are normal at birth but develop pronounced dwarfism with normal intelligence and characteristic facies. Corneal clouding may be clinically absent, mild, or severe, and retinal pigmentary changes are not present [403].

Maroteaux-Lamy Syndrome. (Mucopolysaccharidosis VI). Maroteaux-Lamy syndrome also resembles the Hurler phenotype, but affected persons retain normal intellect. A mild (VIB) or severe (VIA) phenotype can occur based on the extent of skeletal dysplasia, but these phenotypes share the same enzymatic defect (a deficiency of aryl-

sulfatase B). Diffuse corneal haze is present in both phenotypes, and corneal transplantation has been reported in one case [152, 378].

Sly's Syndrome. (Mucopolysaccharidosis VII). Sly's syndrome or β-glucuronidase deficiency demonstrates a regular association with corneal opacification in the majority of patients reported with the infantile variety of this extremely rare disorder [183]. The age at onset of clouding has varied from 7 months [17] to 8 years [357]. A milder adult form, which presents in the second decade of life, may be accompanied by less marked corneal opacification.

DISORDERS OF CARBOHYDRATE METABOLISM— GLYCOGEN STORAGE DISEASE

Glycogenosis type I (von Gierke's disease) is probably the most frequent form of glycogenosis. It results from a deficiency in glucose 6-phosphatase. In this autosomal recessive disorder, clinical signs appear in the first year of life with prominent hepatomegaly and episodes of severe hypoglycemia. A faint brown peripheral corneal infiltration was reported in one case [325].

Clinical corneal opacification has not been described in glycogenosis type II (Pompe's disease), but widespread accumulation of glycogen in the eye, including the cornea, has been demonstrated by histopathology [246].

Disorders of Lipid Metabolism

Genetically determined disorders involving lipid metabolism or lipid storage are associated with a variety of corneal disturbances. Some of the disorders in this category have been subclassified by the lipid component but are included in this broader classification for simplification.

THE FAMILIAL HYPERLIPOPROTEINEMIAS

Six distinct genetic conditions comprise the familial hyperlipoproteinemias. Each includes an elevation of plasma triglycerides or cholesterol [131]. In two of these disorders, familial hypercholesterolemia (type II) and familial hyperlipoproteinemia (type III), a presenile corneal arcus (arcus lipoides) may be a feature in addition to xanthelasmas and lipemia retinalis [362]. Arcus occurs much less frequently in hyperlipoproteinemia types IV and V.

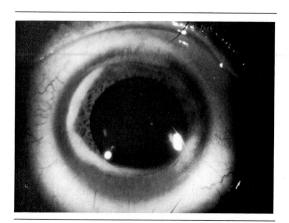

Fig. 12-59. *Dense presenile corneal arcus in a 46-year-old male. This opacification of the peripheral cornea had been noted in the first decade of life. A clear zone separates the arcus from the limbus.*

Familial Hypercholesterolemia (Type II). Familial hypercholesterolemia, an autosomal dominant condition, is present in approximately 1 in 500 births in North America and Europe and is characterized clinically by xanthomas, corneal arcus, and premature heart disease. Hypercholesterolemia is present with increased low-density lipoprotein (LDL) because of defects in the cell surface receptor that regulates both cholesterol synthesis and LDL degradation. Homozygous individuals have more severe manifestations of this disorder than do heterozygotes [362].

Premature corneal arcus may be the presenting finding in heterozygous individuals in the third or fourth decade of life. Its presence seems to correlate with patient age rather than with the absolute levels of lipid elevation [400, 421]. Arcus is present in 50 percent of the heterozygotes over age 30 and in 75 percent of the heterozygotes by the fifth decade [188]. It usually appears clinically in the first decade of life in homozygous individuals. Unilateral arcus may be seen in affected individuals with contralateral carotid stenosis, which indicates that other factors such as blood supply, intraocular pressure, and temperature may also have an effect on the presence and distribution of the arcus [352, 421].

The arcus begins as a mild haze involving initially the deep, and then the superficial, layers of the cornea. The early distribution is an arc in the inferior cornea followed by a similar pattern in the superior cornea. Later, these fuse to form a ring involving the entire periphery and including the more superficial layers. Although initially

separated from the limbus by a lucid zone, the arcus may become confluent with the limbus with progression and may have a more blurred central margin (Fig. 12-59). Histopathology has revealed deposition of phospholipids, cholesterol esters, and triglycerides in the corresponding corneal layers [352, 393].

Corneal arcus may be present in 15 to 50 percent of the middle-aged general population, depending on the criteria for its diagnosis. It is more evident in black patients at a younger age and may be related to age, serum cholesterol, and a variety of hereditary factors [256]. The presence of corneal arcus in patients younger than 50 years of age has been shown to be an independent risk factor for coronary artery disease [188, 334].

Familial Hyperlipoproteinemia Type III. Familial hyperlipoproteinemia type III, a rare, autosomal recessive trait, is characterized by the presence of abnormal lipoproteins termed very-low-density β-lipoprotein (β-VLDL). The exact metabolic defect in their genesis is unclear. Fortunately, a regimen of dietary control and various medications is usually effective in reducing their levels. The most striking clinical finding is the presence of palmar xanthomas that appear after the age of 20. Corneal arcus is reported in a minority of patients with this condition, although its incidence increases with age [131].

FAMILIAL PLASMA CHOLESTEROL ESTER
DEFICIENCY (LECITHIN-CHOLESTEROL
ACYLTRANSFERASE DEFICIENCY)

This rare autosomal recessive trait is characterized by diffuse corneal opacities in all cases and is usually accompanied by normochromic anemia and proteinuria. Very low levels of plasma lecithin-cholesterol acyltransferase (LCAT) activity and resultant markedly reduced levels of plasma cholesterol esters and lysolecithin are present. The structure and function of all lipoprotein classes are affected. Foam cells and typical sea-blue histiocytes are found in various tissues [144].

Corneal opacification appears in the first decade of life as numerous, fine, grayish dots throughout the entire stroma. These are concentrated centrally and more so in the periphery, creating a diffuse central haze and more dense peripheral arcuslike opacification. Sometimes a clear limbal zone is present. Vision is not significantly reduced in most cases. Corneal histopathology shows vacuoles in the anterior stroma and less prominently in Bowman's membrane. The vacuoles may contain phospholipids as well as nonesterified cholesterol [422, 423].

TANGIER DISEASE

Tangier disease, a rare autosomal recessive disorder is characterized by low plasma cholesterol and hyperplastic orange-yellow tonsils in conjunction with normal or elevated triglycerides. High-density α-lipoprotein (HDL) may be absent in homozygotes and decreased in heterozygotes. Clinical manifestations are secondary to widespread tissue deposition of cholesterol esters, especially in the reticuloendothelial system [175]. The course is relatively benign with increasing mild corneal opacification and relapsing neuropathy. By the fifth decade all involved patients have developed diffuse, fine opacities scattered throughout the stroma, although the opacities were apparent as early as 7 years of age in one patient [362]. These scattered opacities are especially prominent in the deep, axial cornea with a shagreenlike distribution usually without a peripheral arcus. Histopathology of the conjunctiva shows cholesterol deposition primarily in pericytes [56].

FISH-EYE DISEASE

An extremely rare dysproteinemia has recently been recognized and is characterized by increasing corneal opacification that makes the eyes resemble those of a boiled fish [50]. Fish-eye disease is distinguished from Tangier disease by normal HDL electrophoretic mobility. LCAT activity is also normal, in contrast to that found in familial plasma cholesterol ester deficiency [297].

Corneal clouding usually becomes apparent in the second decade and is progressive in all cases. The stromal haze is composed of numerous gray-yellow opacities in a mosaic pattern, which may appear more dense in the peripheral cornea. The epithelium is clinically unaffected. A yellow, superficial, arcuslike ring has been described in some patients. Successful corneal transplantation without short-term recurrence has been reported in fish-eye disease [297].

Histopathologic findings were limited to the stroma and Bowman's layer in two transplanted corneas. Numerous membrane-bound vacuoles with amorphous contents were found between the collagen fibrils of the stroma, apparently unas-

sociated with keratocytes. Histochemical staining disclosed a cholesterol-containing lipid material in these vacuoles, but the exact nature of the material remains unknown [297].

FABRY'S DISEASE (ANGIOKERATOMA CORPORIS DIFFUSUM UNIVERSALE)

Fabry's disease is an X-linked lysosomal storage disorder resulting from the absence or deficiency of the lysosomal enzyme ceramide trihexosidase, an α-galactosidase. There is progressive deposition of neutral glycosphingolipids in various fluids and tissues, including the eye. Affected males have the characteristic skin lesions of angiokeratoma coporis diffusum universale and a variety of other systemic manifestations in addition to corneal changes. Heterozygous carrier females generally show the characteristic corneal findings by the second decade of life and may manifest a systemic expression typical of the hemizygous state in some instances [85].

The corneal involvement in Fabry's disease is the most prominent ocular manifestation and may be diagnostic in both the hemizygous males and carrier females [351]. Clinical corneal changes have been noted as early as 6 months of age in a heterozygote carrier [363]. These changes do not diminish visual acuity over the course of the disease. However, detection and recognition of the carrier female is important because of the genetic implications of the X-linked inheritance.

On slit-lamp examination there is a fine whorl-like pattern of subepithelial lines radiating from a common point in the inferior, central cornea (Fig. 12-60). These lines or wedge-shaped bands vary from a faint white to brown but are most often described as cream colored [113, 351]. They are composed of focal aggregations of a multitude of small punctate opacities. These fine dots may also be scattered throughout the intervening epithelium, creating a mild, diffuse corneal haze that alone may be the presenting manifestation in younger individuals [351]. In the later stages the pattern spreads to involve the superior and more peripheral cornea. The deeper layers of the cornea remain uninvolved, but other ocular manifestations including lid edema, conjunctival vascular dilatations (Fig. 12-61), lenticular opacities, and retinal vascular anomalies are seen in the majority of hemizygotes and a minority of heterozygous female carriers [113].

Similar epithelial opacities have previously been

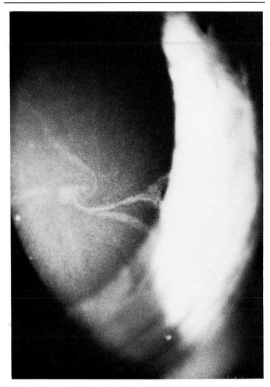

A

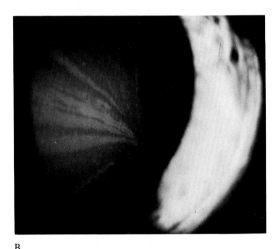

B

Fig. 12-60. *Subepithelial whorl opacities in Fabry's disease. A. Swirling pattern in an involved male. B. Less extensive involvement in his sister.*

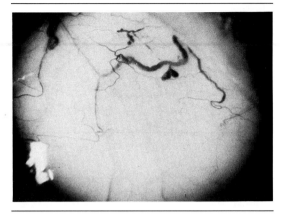

Fig. 12-61. *Fabry's disease. Tortuous conjunctival vessels with saccular dilatations.*

described as cornea verticillata or vortex corneal dystrophy [163]. However, it has since become apparent that the patients with these opacities were carriers of Fabry's disease [84]. A similar vortex pattern may occur with certain systemic medications including amiodarone, amodiaquine hydrochloride, quinacrine hydrochloride, chloroquine, hydroxychloroquine sulfate, chlorpromazine, and indomethacin [38, 77, 178]. Similar whorl-like configurations may also be seen in Tangier disease, Melkersson-Rosenthal syndrome, and striate melanokeratosis. Angiokeratoma corporis diffusum and conjunctival and retinal vascular anomalies have been noted in fucosidosis, but the corneal involvement differs from that in Fabry's disease [359].

Histochemical study of frozen sections has shown lipid material in the basal layer of the corneal epithelium in Fabry's disease [108]. Ultrastructural studies demonstrated intracytoplasmic lamellar inclusions with a periodicity of 4 to 6 nm in most ocular tissues, especially in the apical region of the basal epithelial cells [108, 126, 414]. Giant epithelial inclusion bodies were also present in a hemizygous individual [125]. Areas of reduplication of the epithelial basement membrane and accumulation of a subepithelial amorphous material were noted in both a carrier female and a hemizygous male [322, 414]. Bowman's membrane, stromal keratocytes, and the endothelium may occasionally show the typical osmiophilic inclusions, but none have been described in Descemet's membrane [322]. Histopathologic involvement of the conjunctiva may precede clinical presentation of the disease; however, the more convenient enzymatic analysis of serum, urine, tears, leukocytes, or cultured fibroblasts is usually employed for diagnosis in the absence of typical corneal findings [208, 299].

NIEMANN-PICK DISEASE

Sphingomyelinase is deficient in the infantile or type A subgroup of Niemann-Pick disease, a recessively inherited disorder. The ocular findings in the macular region predominate, but subtle, diffuse corneal opacification may also be present [406]. Ultrastructural examination reveals lamellar and membranous lipid cytosomes in the epithelium, stromal keratocytes, and endothelium [249, 323]. The presence of these structures in the cornea has also been demonstrated in an involved fetus [182].

GAUCHER'S DISEASE

Gaucher's disease, an autosomal recessive disorder, is the most frequently encountered sphingolipid storage disease and is especially common among Ashkenazic Jews. Three clinical forms share a lack or deficiency of the enzyme glucocerebrosidase. Enlarged lipid-laden histiocytes (Gaucher's cells) are found throughout the body, especially in the reticuloendothelial system [31].

In the chronic or adult form triangular brownish lesions occur in the interpalpebral conjunctiva. These may extend onto the cornea at both the temporal and nasal limbus at the level of Bowman's membrane. These lesions resemble pingueculae, but histopathology reveals typical Gaucher's cells [296].

FUCOSIDOSIS

Corneal opacification is usually not present in fucosidosis. However, a homogeneous central corneal opacity with geographic margins involving Bowman's zone was described in one case [359]. Tortuosity and saccular dilatation of the conjunctival vessels may also be apparent.

Combined Disorders

MUCOLIPIDOSES

The mucolipidoses are a group of inherited metabolic diseases characterized by the accumulation of glycosaminoglycans and glycolipids. They share features of both the mucopolysaccharidoses and lipidoses, but the urine glycosaminoglycan excretion is normal. Affected individuals have a vari-

able amount of psychomotor retardation in addition to skeletal and facial dysmorphism. Corneal opacification resembling that in the mucopolysaccharidoses is seen in some types. Optic atrophy and the cherry-red spot characteristic of the sphingolipidoses may be present. However, retinal pigment epithelial degeneration is usually not found.

Mucolipidosis I. Corneal opacification is occasionally seen in the recessively inherited group of phenotypically diverse disorders caused by the deficiency of the lysosomal hydrolase acid neuraminidase [207]. In some of the juvenile forms corneal clouding involving both the superficial and deep layers of the cornea may develop. Lamellar and penetrating keratoplasties have been performed, and histopathology shows the major site of involvement to be in the epithelium, with lesser stromal and endothelial changes [60]. Bowman's layer is relatively uninvolved. Conjunctival findings similar to those in Fabry's disease have also been noted, and a cherry-red macular spot may be present [248].

Mucolipidosis II (I-Cell Disease). Mucolipidosis II is characterized by a Hurler-like dysmorphism, severe growth and psychomotor retardation, hepatomegaly, and early death. Mild clinical corneal clouding has occurred in fewer than 50 percent of the cases, usually as a late finding. Congenital clouding has occurred in rare cases [119]. The periphery of Bowman's membrane may be involved clinically and histopathologically. Megalocornea with normal intraocular pressure or glaucoma has been reported. Macular cherry-red spots are not present [250].

Ultrastructural studies of the cornea have revealed basal epithelial edema and involvement of the subepithelial fibroblasts and anterior stromal keratocytes with numerous membrane-limited vacuoles [213, 247, 250]. Some vacuoles are filled with a fibrillogranular material or lamellar membranous inclusions, while other vacuoles appear clear. Bowman's layer may be replaced by these distended cells, but the posterior stroma, Descemet's membrane, and epithelium are relatively uninvolved [25]. Characteristic findings are also present in the conjunctiva, independent of the extent of corneal involvement [213, 250].

Mucolipidosis III. Mucolipidosis III resembles mucolipidosis II, but in the former the psychomotor deficits are less severe, hepatomegaly is not present, and the longevity is relatively normal.

Mild corneal opacification that may involve the deep stroma appears in the first decade of life. No corneal histopathologic data are available, but conjunctival pathologic changes are similar to those in the other mucolipidoses [245, 309].

Mucolipidosis IV. Mucolipidosis IV is characterized by psychomotor retardation without hepatosplenomegaly or gross facial and skeletal deformities [72]. Corneal opacification is a prominent sign and is present at birth or in early infancy. The clouding involves the central epithelial layers more than the periphery without significant stromal edema. Fluctuations in the degree of corneal opacification have been noted in some patients [278]. Epithelial debridement and lamellar keratoplasty have cleared the opacification for brief periods, but clouding subsequently recurred [211, 278]. Penetrating keratoplasty was performed in a mild variant with clinical recurrence in the grafted tissue [238]. Electron microscopy shows numerous vacuoles in the epithelial cells with relative preservation of Bowman's layer and a lesser involvement of the anterior stromal keratocytes [211, 238, 278]. This differs from mucolipidosis II and III, in which the involvement is principally subepithelial or anterior stromal. As with other mucolipidoses, the conjunctival epithelium is heavily involved [436].

G_{M1} GANGLIOSIDOSIS TYPE I

Corneal clouding is present in a minority of patients with G_{M1} gangliosidosis type I, a rare autosomal recessive disorder caused by a deficiency of acid β-galactosidase. Psychomotor retardation, Hurler-like skeletal dysmorphism, hepatosplenomegaly, and severe neurologic disturbances are present. Cherry-red spots occur in approximately one-half the patients, and death usually occurs before age 2.

Corneal histopathologic findings in G_{M1} gangliosidosis type I are similar to those in the mucopolysaccharidoses: membrane-bound vesicles, some of which contain dense spherical inclusions, in epithelial cells and keratocytes [102, 415].

SULFATIDOSIS (MULTIPLE SULFATASE DEFICIENCY)

In the Austin type of sulfatidosis there are combined features of both metachromatic leukodystrophy and a mucopolysaccharidosis. The gargoyle features are usually mild, but neurologic deterioration is rapid. Multiple mucopolysaccharide sulfatases are deficient. Corneal clouding may be present at a young age [64].

GOLDBERG'S SYNDROME

Both β-galactosidase and neuraminidase are deficient in Goldberg's syndrome, which combines the features of a mucopolysaccharidosis and a sphingolipidosis [384]. Gargoyle facies, dwarfism, moderate mental retardation, seizures, dysostosis multiplex, and hearing loss are present in addition to corneal clouding and a macular cherry-red spot in the initial pedigree [148]. Mucopolysacchariduria, vacuolation of blood cells, and visceromegaly, however, are not present.

Disorders of Protein Metabolism

CYSTINOSIS

Cystinosis is a rare recessive disorder characterized by the lysosomal accumulation of cystine crystals in the leukocytes, reticuloendothelial system, visceral organs, and, most typically, the eye. The clinical expression is extremely varied. Three forms have been described: an infantile nephropathic type, an adult benign form, and an intermediate adolescent type [344, 435].

Characteristic corneal changes occur in all three recognized forms and are the only clinical findings in the adult benign form [63]. They consist of fine, polychromatic, tinsel-like stromal crystals that are located principally in the superficial stroma over the entire cornea and in deeper stromal layers in the periphery (Fig. 12-62). The epithelial surface remains smooth, and corneal sensation is unaffected. Other cases have shown pre-Descemet's crystals with relative sparing of the middle stromal layers [76].

The crystals have been noted in the first decade of life in both the adolescent and adult forms and are usually present very early in the infantile nephropathic form, although they have been seen only histopathologically at birth. In all forms the crystals increase in density with age. A characteristic peripheral pigmentary retinopathy may precede the corneal crystals in the infantile form and is occasionally seen in the adolescent type [124, 429]. Photophobia is usually the only ocular symptom and is mild in the adult form, variable in the adolescent form, and extreme in the nephropathic form.

Corneal light microscopy has demonstrated fu-

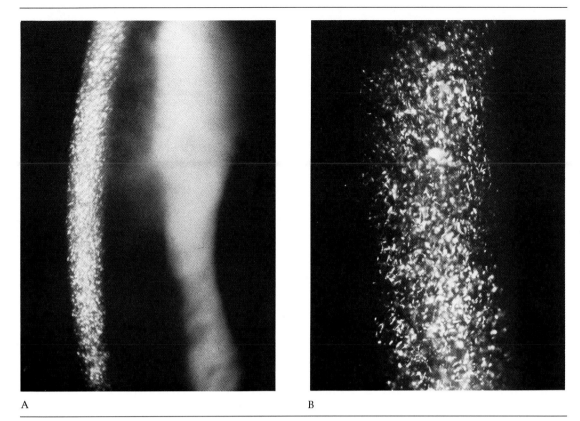

A   B

Fig. 12-62. *Slit-lamp appearance of the cornea in cystinosis. A. Diffuse fine crystals are present over* *the entire cornea. B. Higher magnification reveals the refractile nature of the individual stromal crystals.*

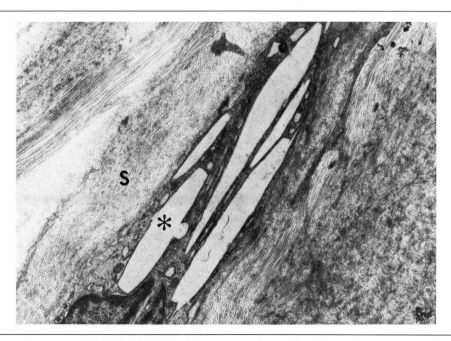

Fig. 12-63. *Transmission electron micrograph of a stromal keratocyte in cystinosis. Membrane-limited crystal spaces (asterisk) fill the keratocyte but are not* *evident in the stroma (S). (× 19,000 before 30% reduction.) (Courtesy of Kenneth R. Kenyon.)*

siform crystals in Bowman's membrane and in association with the stromal keratocytes of the central cornea, mixed with more rhomboid or polygonal crystals in the corneal periphery [124, 212]. Electron microscopy reveals that the crystals are intracellular and enclosed in a lysosome-like structure bound by a single or double membrane (Fig. 12-63). Crystals are not found in epithelial cells, but large perinuclear vacuoles are present [212].

RICHNER-HANHART SYNDROME

Richner-Hanhart syndrome, a rare autosomal recessive disorder, is characterized by herpetiform corneal lesions, palmar and plantar keratoses, and mental retardation. It has been known as the Oregon type of tyrosinosis, tyrosinemia type II, oculocutaneous tyrosinosis, or keratosis palmaris et plantaris with corneal dystrophy [267]. Soluble tyrosine aminotransferase is deficient in this condition and results in tyrosinemia.

Bilateral, herpetiform, fluorescein-staining, central epithelial corneal opacities appear very early. Recurrent episodes of marked photophobia and lacrimation may occur. The surrounding cornea shows a diffuse ground-glass haziness. Corneal sensation remains intact, and vascularization usually does not occur [18, 189]. Cases have been reported with the typical skin changes without clinical ocular involvement [184, 317].

Histopathology of the cornea demonstrated hyperplastic stratified epithelium with some intracellular edema [434]. Membrane-bound inclusion bodies were present in the superficial conjunctival epithelial cells, deeper fibrocytes, and capillary endothelial cells in one case [18].

ALKAPTONURIA

Alkaptonuria is a rare recessive disorder resulting from the absence of homogentisic acid oxidase. Oxidation of the homogentisic acid excreted in the urine will turn the urine darker with time. A dark pigmentation (ochronosis) occurs in various connective tissues including the sclera. Scleral pigmentation usually appears in the interpalpebral area near the insertions of the horizontal rectus muscles. Pigment particles or golden brown globules may appear in the peripheral interpalpebral cornea and usually darken and increase in number with age [119].

Disorders of Mineral Metabolism

WILSON'S DISEASE

Wilson's disease is a rare autosomal recessive disorder of copper metabolism characterized by degenerative changes in the brain, cirrhosis of the liver, and the presence of pigment rings in the cornea (Kayser-Fleischer rings). Clinical symptoms rarely occur before 6 years of age and may appear as late as the fifth decade. Serum levels of the copper-binding protein ceruloplasmin are decreased. The exact genetic defect remains unclear [340]. Early diagnosis is imperative because effective therapy is available in this once-fatal disease [53].

The Kayser-Fleischer ring is the single most diagnostic sign in Wilson's disease and is present clinically in 97 percent of cases with neurologic involvement, although it may be absent in young children with hepatic involvement alone [419]. It begins initially in the superior and later in the

Fig. 12-64. *Opacification and pigmentation at the level of Descemet's membrane (arrow) is demonstrated in this slit-lamp photograph of the Kayser-Fleischer ring in Wilson's disease.*

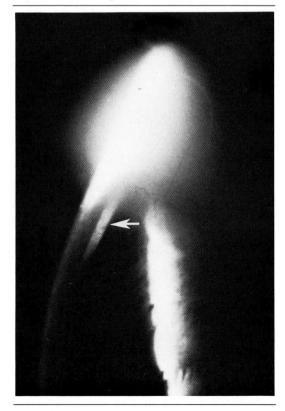

inferior poles of the cornea at the level of Descemet's membrane (Fig. 12-64). Subsequent circumferential spread involves the entire peripheral cornea. In the earliest stages the ring may be better visualized with gonioscopy, which shows peripheral extension to, and sometimes beyond, Schwalbe's line. The rings are generally brown or green-yellow. With differing illumination, however, they may appear red or even blue because of reflection and scattering of the incident light [395]. A similar deposition of pigment is present in the lens capsule in a minority of affected individuals [394].

Granular, copper-containing deposits have been demonstrated in Descemet's membrane corresponding to the clinical distribution of the pigment ring. By electron microscopy the deposits have been found in the middle and posterior portions of Descemet's membrane, sometimes occuring in layers [172, 394, 395]. They are always present in a gradient pattern with the larger granules located more anteriorly [191]. Similar deposits may be found in the stroma and cytoplasm of the endothelial cells. Recently, the use of x-ray spectroscopic methods has demonstrated copper in the central cornea where no granules have been identified [194].

The Kayser-Fleischer ring may diminish and serum laboratory values normalize after successful liver homotransplantation [348]. Pigmentation also diminishes or disappears in patients treated with D-penicillamine, but hypocupremia and hypoceruloplasminemia usually remain [177, 377, 419]. Similar pigment rings may also appear in primary biliary cirrhosis, chronic active hepatitis with cirrhosis, other chronic cholestatic syndromes, and exogenous chalcosis [105, 203].

HEMOCHROMATOSIS

Primary hemochromatosis is a genetically determined disorder of iron metabolism classically producing pigmentation of the skin, cirrhosis of the liver, and diabetes. There is widespread accumulation of iron as hemosiderin, which becomes clinically apparent usually after the fifth decade of life. The exact mode of inheritance has not been determined.

A brown pigmentation of the bulbar conjunctiva most marked at the inferior limbus and extending onto the cornea has been described in a minority of affected individuals studied [81]. Histopathology demonstrates traces of ferric iron in the corneal epithelium.

REFERENCES

1. Abbott, R. L., et al. Specular microscopic and histologic observations in nonguttate corneal endothelial degeneration. *Ophthalmology (Rochester)* 88:788, 1981.

2. Akiya, S., and Brown, S. I. The ultrastructure of Reis-Bücklers' dystrophy. *Am. J. Ophthalmol.* 72:549, 1973.

3. Akiya, S., and Brown, S. I. Granular dystrophy of the cornea. *Arch. Ophthalmol.* 84:179, 1970.

4. Akiya, S., Ito, I., and Matsui, M. Gelatinous droplike dystrophy of the cornea: Light and electron microscopic study of superficial stromal lesion. *Jpn. J. Clin. Ophthalmol.* 26:815, 1972.

5. Alexander, R. A., Grierson, I., and Garner, A. Oxytalan fibers in Fuchs' endothelial dystrophy. *Arch. Ophthalmol.* 99:1622, 1981.

6. Antine, B. Histology of congenital corneal dystrophy. *Am. J. Ophthalmol.* 69:964, 1970.

7. Aracena, T. Hereditary fleck dystrophy of the cornea: Report of a family. *J. Pediatr. Ophthalmol.* 12:223, 1975.

8. Arentsen, J. J., and Laibson, P. R. Penetrating keratoplasty and cataract extraction: Combined vs. nonsimultaneous surgery. *Arch. Ophthalmol.* 96:75, 1978.

9. Arentsen, J. J., and Laibson, P. R. Thermokeratoplasty for keratoconus. *Am. J. Ophthalmol.* 82:447, 1976.

10. Babel, J., Englert, U., and Ricci, A. La dystrophie cristalline de al cornée: Étude histologique et ultrastructurale. *Arch. Ophthalmol. (Paris)* 33:721, 1973.

11. Bagolini, B., and Ioli-Spada, G. Bietti's tapetoretinal degeneration with marginal corneal dystrophy. *Am. J. Ophthalmol.* 65:53, 1968.

12. Barr, C. C, Gelender, H., and Fout, R. L. Corneal crystalline deposits associated with dysproteinemia. *Arch. Ophthalmol.* 98:884, 1980.

13. Barrie, J., Blach, R. K., and Wells, R. S. Ocular manifestations of ichthyosis. *Br. J. Ophthalmol.* 52:217, 1968.

14. Bartocas, C., et al. San Filippo type C disease: Clinical findings in four patients with a new variant of mucopolysaccharidosis III. *Eur. J. Pediatr.* 130:251, 1979.

15. Baum, J. L., and Bull, M. J. Ocular manifestations of the ectodactyly, ectodermal dysplasia, cleft lip-palate syndrome. *Am. J. Ophthalmol.* 78:211, 1974.

16. Beardsley, R. L., and Foulks, G. N. An association of keratoconus and mitral valve prolapse. *Ophthalmology (Rochester)* 89:35, 1982.

17. Beaudet, A. L., et al. Variation in the phenotypic expression of beta glucuronidase deficiency. *J. Pediatr.* 86:388, 1975.

18. Berman, E. R. Diagnosis of metabolic eye disease by chemical analysis of serum, leukocytes and skin fibroblast tissue culture. *Birth Defects* 12(3):15, 1976.

19. Biber. Über einige seltene Hornhauterkrankungen. Dissertation, Zurich, 1890.

20. Bienfang, D. C., Kuwabara, T., and Pueschel, S. M. The Richner-Hanhart syndrome: Report of a case with associated tyrosinemia. *Arch. Ophthalmol.* 94:1133, 1976.

21. Bietti, G. B. Contribution à la connaissance des dégénérescenses cornéenes séniles. *Arch. Ophtalmol. (Paris)* 25:37, 1965.

22. Birndorf, L. A., and Ginsberg, S. P. Hereditary fleck dystrophy associated with decreased corneal sensitivity. *Am. J. Ophthalmol.* 73:670, 1972.

23. Blackman, H. J., Rodrigues, M. M., and Peck, G. L. Corneal epithelial lesions in keratosis follicularis (Darier's disease). *Ophthalmology (Rochester)* 87:931, 1980.

24. Boles-Carenini, B. Juvenile familial mosaic degeneration of the cornea associated with megalocornea. *Br. J. Ophthalmol.* 45:64, 1961.

25. Borit, A., Sugarman, G. I., and Spencer, W. H. Ocular involvement in I-cell disease (mucolipidosis II): Light and electron microscopic findings. *Albrecht von Graefes Arch. Klin. Exp. Ophthalmol.* 198:25, 1976.

26. Boruchoff, S. A., and Kuwabara, T. Electron microscopy of posterior polymorphous degeneration. *Am. J. Ophthalmol.* 72:879, 1971.

27. Bourgeois, J., Shields, M. B., and Thresher, B. S. Open-angle glaucoma associated with posterior polymorphous dystrophy: A clinicopathologic study. *Ophthalmology (Rochester)* 91:421, 1984.

28. Bourne, W. M., Johnson, D. H., and Campbell, R. J. The ultrastructure of Descemet's membrane: III. Fuchs' dystrophy. *Arch. Ophthalmol.* 100:1952, 1982.

29. Bourquin, J. B., Babel, J., and Klein, D. Nouvel arbre généalogique de dystrophie cornéenne granuleuse (Groenouw I). *J. Genet. Hum.* 3:137, 1954.

30. Bowen, R. A., et al. Lattice dystrophy of the cornea as a variety of amyloidosis. *Am. J. Ophthalmol.* 7:822, 1970.

31. Brady, R. O. Glucosyl Ceramide Lipidosis: Gaucher's Disease. In J. B. Stanbury, J. B. Wyngaarden, and D. S. Fredrickson (Eds.), *The Metabolic Basis of Inherited Disease* (4th ed.). New York: McGraw-Hill, 1978.

32. Bramsen, T., Ehlers, N., and Baggesen, L. H. Central cloudy corneal dystrophy of François. *Acta Ophthalmol. (Copenh.)* 54:221, 1976.

33. Britton, H., et al. Keratosis follicularis spinulosa decalvans. *Arch. Dermatol.* 114:761, 1978.

34. Broderick, J. D., and Dark, A. J. Corneal dystrophy in Cockayne's syndrome. *Br. J. Ophthalmol.* 57:391, 1973.

35. Broderick, J. D., Dark, A. J., and Peace, G. W. Fingerprint dystrophy of the cornea: A histologic study. *Arch. Ophthalmol.* 92:483, 1974.

36. Bron, A. J. Anterior corneal mosaic. *Br. J. Ophthalmol.* 52:659, 1968.

37. Bron, A. J. Superficial fibrillary lines: A feature of the normal cornea. *Br. J. Ophthalmol.* 59:133, 1975.

38. Bron, A. J. Vortex patterns of the corneal epithelium. *Trans. Ophthalmol. Soc. U.K.* 93:455, 1973.

39. Bron, A. J., and Brown, N. A. Some superficial corneal disorders. *Trans. Ophthalmol. Soc. U.K.* 91:13, 1971.

40. Bron, A. J., et al. Fibrillary lines of the cornea: A clinical sign in keratoconus. *Br. J. Ophthalmol.* 59:136, 1975.

41. Bron, A. J., Williams, H. P., and Carruthers, M. E. Hereditary crystalline stromal dystrophy of Schynder: I. clinical features of a family with hyperlipoproteinaemia. *Br. J. Ophthalmol.* 56:383, 1972.

42. Brown, N. A., and Bron, A. J. Recurrent erosion of the cornea. *Br. J. Ophthalmol.* 60:84, 1976.

43. Brownstein, M. H., Elliott, R., and Helwig, E. B. Ophthalmologic aspects of amyloidosis. *Am. J. Ophthalmol.* 69:423, 1970.

44. Bücklers, M. *Die erblichen Hornhautdystrophie: Dystrophiae corneae hereditariae.* Stuttgart: Ferdinaud Enke, 1938.

45. Bücklers, M. Über eine weitere familiäre Hornhautdystrophie (Reis). *Klin. Monatsbl. Augenheilkd.* 114:386, 1949.

46. Bullock, J., and Howard, R. Werner's syndrome. *Arch. Ophthalmol.* 90:53, 1973.

47. Burns, R. P. Meesman's corneal dystrophy. *Trans. Am. Ophthalmol. Soc.* 66:530, 1968.

48. Burns, R. P., Connor, W., and Gipson, I. Cholesterol turnover in hereditary crystalline corneal dystrophy of Schnyder. *Trans. Am. Ophthalmol. Soc.* 76:184, 1978.

49. Buxton, J. N., and Fox, M. L. Superficial epithelial keratectomy in the treatment of epithelial basement membrane dystrophy. *Arch. Ophthalmol.* 101:392, 1983.

50. Carlson, L. A., and Philipson, B. Fish-eye disease: A new familial condition with massive corneal opacities and dyslipoproteinaemia. *Lancet* 2:922, 1979.

51. Carpel, E. F., Sigelman, R. J., and Doughman, D. J. Posterior amorphous corneal dystrophy. *Am. J. Ophthalmol.* 83:629, 1977.

52. Carter, V. H., and Constantine, V. S. Kyrle's disease: II. Histopathologic findings in five cases and review of literature. *Arch. Dermatol.* 97:633, 1968.

53. Cartwright, G. E. Diagnosis of treatable Wilson's disease. *N. Engl. J. Med.* 298:1347, 1978.

54. Cavanaugh, D. W., et al. Pathogenesis and treatment of persistent epithelial defects. *Trans. Am. Acad. Ophthalmol. Otolaryngol.* 81:754, 1976.

55. Chan, C. C., et al. Similarities between posterior polymorphous and congenital hereditary endothelial dystrophies: A study of 14 buttons of 11 cases. *Cornea* 1:155, 1982.

56. Chu, F. C., et al. Ocular manifestations of familial high-density lipoprotein deficiency (Tangier disease). *Arch. Ophthalmol.* 97:1926, 1979.

57. Chumbley, L. C. Scleral involvement in symptomatic porphyria. *Am. J. Ophthalmol.* 84:729, 1977.

58. Cibis, G. W., et al. The clinical spectrum of posterior polymorphous dystrophy. *Arch. Ophthalmol.* 95:1529, 1977.

59. Cibis, G. W., and Tripathi, R. C. The differential diagnosis of Descemet's tears (Haab's striae) and posterior polymorphous dystrophy bands. *Ophthalmology (Rochester)* 89:614, 1982.

60. Cibis, G. W., Tripathi, R. C., and Harris, D. J. Mucolipidosis I. *Birth Defects* 18(6):359, 1982.

61. Cogan, D. G., et al. Microcystic dystrophy of the corneal epithelium. *Trans. Am. Ophthalmol. Soc.* 63:213, 1964.

62. Cogan, D. G., et al. Microcystic dystrophy of the cornea: A partial explanation for its pathogenesis. *Arch. Ophthalmol.* 92:470, 1974.

63. Cogan, D. G., et al. Cystinosis in an adult. *JAMA* 164:394, 1957.

64. Cogan, D. G., Kuwabara, T., and Moser, H. Metachromatic leukodystrophy. *Ophthalmologica* 160:2, 1970.

65. Collier, M. Dystrophie filiforme protonde de la cornée. *Bull. Soc. Ophthalmol. Fr.* 64:1034, 1964.

66. Collier, M. Dystrophie mouchetée parenchyme cornéen avec dystrophie nuageuse centrale. *Bull. Soc. Ophthalmol. Fr.* 64:608, 1964.

67. Collier, M. M. Dystrophie nuageuse centrale et dystrophie pontiforme prédescemétique dans une même famille. *Bull. Soc. Ophthalmol. Fr.* 66:575, 1966.

68. Collier, M. Élastorrhexie systématisée et dystrophies cornéennes chez deux soeurs. *Bull. Soc. Ophthalmol. Fr.* 65:301, 1965.

69. Collier, M. Hereditary nature of the punctate pre-Descemet dystrophy. *Bull. Mem. Soc. Fr. Ophthalmol.* 64:731, 1964.

70. Constantopoulos, G., Dekaban, A. S., and Scheie, H. G. Heterogeneity of disorders in patients with corneal clouding, normal intellect, and mucopolysaccharidosis. *Am. J. Ophthalmol.* 72:1106, 1971.

71. Cotlier, E. The Cornea. In R. A. Moses (Ed.), *Adler's Physiology of the Eye* (6th ed.). St. Louis: Mosby, 1975.

72. Crandall, B. F., et al. Review article: Mucolipidosis IV. *Am. J. Genet.* 12:301, 1982.

73. Cross, H. E., Maumenee, A. E., and Cantolino, S. J. Inheritance of Fuchs' endothelial dystrophy. *Arch. Ophthalmol.* 85:268, 1971.

74. Curran, R. E., Kenyon, K. R., and Green, W. R. Pre-Descemet's membrane corneal dystrophy. *Am. J. Ophthalmol.* 77:711, 1974.

75. Cursino, J. W., and Fine, B. S. A histologic study of calcific and noncalcific band keratopathies. *Am. J. Ophthalmol.* 82:395, 1976.

76. Dale, R. T., et al. Adolescent cystinosis: A clinical and specular microscopic study of an unusual sibship. *B. J. Ophthalmol.* 65:828, 1981.

77. D'Amico, D. J., Kenyon, K. R., and Ruskin, J. N. Amiodarone keratopathy: Drug-induced lipid storage disease. *Arch. Ophthalmol.* 99:257, 1981.

78. Dark, A. J. Bleb dystrophy of the cornea: Histochemistry and ultrastructure. *Br. J. Ophthalmol.* 61:65, 1977.

79. Dark, A. J. Cogan's microcystic dytrophy of the cornea: Ultrastructure and photomicroscopy. *Br. J. Ophthalmol.* 62:821, 1978.

80. Dark, A. J., and Thompson, D. S. Lattice dystrophy of the cornea: A clinical and microscopic study. *Br. J. Ophthalmol.* 44:257, 1960.

81. Davies, G., et al. Deposition of melanin and iron in ocular structures in haemochromatosis. *Br. J. Ophthalmol.* 56:338, 1972.

82. DeBusk, F. L. The Hutchinson-Gilford progeria syndrome. *J. Pediatr.* 80:697, 1972.

83. Delleman, J. W., and Winkelman, J. E. Degeneratio corneae cristallinea hereditaria: A clinical, genetical and histological study. *Ophthalmologica* 155:409, 1968.

84. Denden, A., and Franceschetti, A. T. Cornea verticillata: Ein Symptom des Morbus Fabry-Anderson. *Ber. Dtsch. Ophthalmol. Ges.* 69:145, 1969.

85. Desnick, R. J., Klionsky, B., and Sweeley, C. C. Fabry's Disease. In J. B. Stanbury, J. B. Wyngaarden, and D. S. Fredrickson (Eds.), *The Metabolic Basis of Inherited Disease* (4th ed.). New York: McGraw-Hill, 1978.

86. Desvignes, P., and Vigo, A. À propos d'un cas de dystrophie cornéenne parenchymateuse familiale à hérédité dominate. *Bull. Soc. Ophthalmol. Fr.* 55:220, 1955.

87. DeVoe, A. G. Certain abnormalities of Bowman's membrane with particular reference to fingerprint lines in the cornea. *Trans. Am. Ophthalmol. Soc.* 60:195, 1962.

88. DeVoe, A. G. The management of endothelial dystrophy of the cornea. *Am. J. Ophthalmol.* 61:1084, 1966.

89. Dimmer, F. Über oberflächliche gittrige Hornhauttrübung. *Z. Augenheilkd.* 2:354, 1899.

90. Dodd, M. J., Pusin, S. M., and Green, W. R. Adult cystinosis: A case report. *Arch. Ophthalmol.* 96:1054, 1978.

91. Dohlman, C. H. Familial congenital cornea guttata in association with anterior polar cataract. *Acta Ophthalmol. (Copenh.)* 29:445, 1951.

92. Dubord, P. J., and Krachmer, J. H. Diagnosis of early lattice corneal dystrophy. *Arch. Ophthalmol.* 100:788, 1982.

93. Dubord, P. J., Rodrigues, M. M., and Krachmer, J. H. Corneal elastosis in lattice corneal dystrophy. *Ophthalmology (Rochester)* 88:1239, 1981.

94. Duke-Elder, S. S., and Leigh, A. G. Diseases of the Outer Eye. In S. S. Duke-Elder (Ed.), *System of Ophthalmology*, Vol. 8, Part 2. St. Louis: Mosby, 1965.

95. Dunn, S. P., Krachmer, J. H., and Ching, S. S. New findings in posterior amorphous dystrophy. *Arch. Ophthalmol.* 102:236, 1984.

96. Eagle, R. C., et al. Proliferative endotheliopathy with iris abnormalities: The iridocorneal endothelial syndrome. *Arch. Ophthalmol.* 97:2104, 1979.

97. Ehlers, N., and Bramsen, T. Central thickness in corneal disorders. *Acta Ophthalmologica (Copenh.)* 56:412, 1978.

98. Ehlers, N., and Matthiessen, M. Hereditary crystalline corneal dystrophy of Schnyder. *Acta Ophthalmol. (Copenh.)* 51:316, 1973.

99. Eiferman, R. A., et al. Schnyder's crystalline dystrophy associated with amyloid deposition. *Metab. Pediatr. Ophthalmol.* 3:15, 1979.

100. Eiferman, R. A., and Wilkins, E. L. The effect of air on human corneal endothelium. *Am. J. Ophthalmol.* 92:328, 1981.

101. Ellis, W., Barfort, P., and Mastmon, G. J. Keratoconjunctivitis with corneal crystals caused by the Dieffenbachia plant. *Am. J. Ophthalmol.* 76:143, 1973.

102. Emery, J. M., et al. GM$_1$-gangliosidosis: Ocular and pathological manifestations. *Arch. Ophthalmol.* 85:177, 1971.

103. Fernandez-Sasso, D., Acosta, J. E. P., and Malbran, E. Punctiform and polychromatic pre-Descemet's dominant corneal dystrophy. *Br. J. Ophthalmol.* 63:336, 1979.

104. Fine, B. S., et al. Meesmann's epithelial dystrophy of the cornea. *Am. J. Ophthalmol.* 83:633, 1977.

105. Fleming, C. R., et al. Pigmented corneal rings in non-Wilsonian liver disease. *Ann. Intern. Med.* 86:285, 1977.

106. Fogle, J. A., Green, W. R., and Kenyon, K. R. Anterior corneal dystrophy. *Am. J. Ophthalmol.* 77:529, 1974.

107. Fogle, J. A., et al. Defective epithelial adhesion in anterior corneal dystrophies. *Am. J. Ophthalmol.* 79:925, 1975.

108. Font, R. L., and Fine, B. S. Ocular pathology in Fabry's disease. *Am. J. Ophthalmol.* 73:419, 1973.

109. Forgacs, J., and Franceschetti, A. Histologic aspect of corneal changes. *Am. J. Ophthalmol.* 47:191, 1951.

110. Forgacs, J., and Franceschetti, A. II. Histologic aspect of corneal changes due to hereditary metabolic and cutaneous affections. *Am. J. Ophthalmol.* 47:191, 1959.

111. Foulks, G. N. Treatment of recurrent corneal erosion and corneal edema with topical osmotic colloidal solution. *Ophthalmology (Rochester)* 88:801, 1981.

112. Franceschetti, A. Classification and treatment of hereditary corneal dystrophies. *Arch. Ophthalmol.* 52:1, 1954.

113. Franceschetti, A. T. Fabry disease: Ocular manifestations. *Birth Defects* 12(3):195, 1976.

114. Franceschetti, A. Hereditäre rezidivierende Erosion der Hornhaut. *Z. Augenheilkd.* 66:309, 1928.

115. Franceschetti, A. Hereditary Skin Diseases (Genodermatoses) and Corneal Affectations. In *Symposium on Surgical and Medical Management of Congenital Anomalies of the Eye,* Transactions of the New Orleans Academy of Ophthalmology. St. Louis: Mosby, 1968. Chap. 4.

116. Franceschetti, A., et al. Severe filiform dystrophy of the cornea. *Bull. Mem. Soc. Fr. Ophthalmol.* 70:175, 1957.

117. Franceschetti, A., and Maeder, G. Severe dystrophy of the cornea in a case of congenital ichthyosis. *Bull. Mem. Soc. Fr. Ophthalmol.* 64:146, 1954.

118. Franceschetti, A., and Thier, C. J. Über Hornhautdystrophien bei Genodermatosen unter besonderer Berücksichtigung der Palmöplantakeratosen (klinische, genetische und histologische Studien). *Albrecht von Graefes Arch. Klin. Exp. Ophthalmol.* 162:610, 1961.

119. François, J. Metabolic disorders and corneal changes. *Dev. Ophthalmol.* 4:1, 1981.

120. François, J. Érosion dystrophique récidivante de l'épithélium cornéen. *Ophthalmologica* 177:121, 1978.

121. François, J. Heredo-familial corneal dystrophies. *Trans. Ophthalmol. Soc. U.K.* 86:367, 1966.

122. François, J. Une nouvelle dystrophie hérédofamiliale de la cornée. *J. Genet. Hum.* 5:189, 1956.

123. François, J., and Feher, J. Light microscopy and polarization optical study of the lattice dystrophy of the cornea. *Ophthalmologica* 164:1, 1972.

124. François, J., et al. Cystinosis: A clinical and histopathological study. *Am. J. Ophthalmol.* 73:643, 1972.

125. François, J., Hanssens, M., and Teuchy, H. Corneal ultrastructural changes in Fabry's disease. *Ophthalmologica* 176:313, 1978.

126. François, J., Hanssens, M., and Teuchy, H. Corneal ultrastructural changes in Fabry's disease. *Bull. Soc. Belge Ophthalmol.* 179:7, 1977.

127. François, J., et al. Ultrastructural findings in corneal macular dystrophy (Groenouw II type). *Ophthalmic Res.* 7:80, 1975.

128. François, J., Hanssens, M., and Teuchy, H. Ultrastructural changes in lattice dystrophy of the cornea. *Ophthalmic Res.* 7:321, 1975.

129. François, J., and Neetens, A. Nouvelle dystrophie hérédo-familiale du parenchyme cornéen (hérédo-dystrophie mouchetée) *Bull. Soc. Belge Ophthalmol.* 114:641, 1957.

130. François, J., et al. Study of lysosomes by vital stains in normal keratocytes and in keratocytes from macular dystrophy of the cornea. *Invest. Ophthalmol.* 15:599, 1976.

131. Fredrickson, D. S., Goldstein, J. L., and Brown, M. S. The Familial Hyperlipoproteinemias. In J. B. Stanbury, J. B. Wyngaarden, and D. S. Fredrickson (Eds.), *The Metabolic Basis of Inherited Disease* (4th ed.). New York: McGraw-Hill, 1978.

132. Friedman, B. Corneal findings in ichthyosis. *Am. J. Ophthalmol.* 39:575, 1955.

133. Fry, W. E., and Pickett, W. E. Crystalline dystrophy

of the cornea. *Trans. Am. Ophthalmol. Soc.* 48:220, 1950.

134. Fuchs, A. Über primaere quertelfoermige Hornhauttrübung. *Klin. Monatsbl. Augenheilkd.* 103:300, 1939.

135. Fuchs, E. Dystrophia epithelialis corneae. *Albrecht von Graefes Arch. Klin. Exp. Ophthalmol.* 76:478, 1910.

136. Garner, A. Amyloidosis of the cornea. *Br. J. Ophthalmol.* 53:73, 1969.

137. Garner, A. Histochemistry of corneal granular dystrophy. *Br. J. Ophthalmol.* 53:799, 1969.

138. Garner, A. Histochemistry of corneal macular dystrophy. *Invest. Ophthalmol.* 8:475, 1969.

139. Garner, A., and Tripathi, R. C. Hereditary crystalline stromal dystrophy of Schnyder: II. Histopathology and ultrastructure. *Br. J. Ophthalmol.* 56:400, 1972.

140. Ghosh, M., and McCulloch, C. Crystalline dystrophy of the cornea: A light and electron microscopic study. *Can. J. Ophthalmol.* 12:321, 1977.

141. Ghosh, M., and McCulloch, C. Macular cornea dystrophy. *Can. J. Ophthalmol.* 8:515, 1973.

142. Gillespie, F., and Covelli, B. Fleck (mouchetée) dystrophy of the cornea: Report of a family. *South. Med. J.* 56:1265, 1963.

143. Gills, J. P., et al. Electroretinography and fundus oculi findings in Hurler's disease and allied mucopolysaccharidoses. *Arch. Ophthalmol.* 74:596, 1965.

144. Gjone, E. Familial lecithin: cholesterol acyltransferase (LCAT) deficiency. *Birth Defects* 18(6):423, 1982.

145. Gjone, E., and Bergaust, B. Corneal opacity in familial plasma cholesterol ester deficiency. *Acta Ophthalmol. (Copenh.)* 47:222, 1969.

146. Glees, M. Über familiaeres Auftreten der primaeren, bandfoermigen Hornhautdegeneration. *Klin. Monatsbl. Augenheilkd.* 116:185, 1950.

147. Goar, E. L. Dystrophy of the corneal endothelium (cornea guttata), with a report of a histological examination. *Am. J. Ophthalmol.* 17:215, 1934.

148. Goldberg, M. F., et al. Macular cherry-red spot, corneal clouding, and beta-galactosidase deficiency: Clinical, biochemical, and electron microscopic study of a new autosomal recessive storage disease. *Arch. Intern. Med.* 128:387, 1971.

149. Goldberg, M. F., and Duke, J. R. Ocular histopathology in Hunter's syndrome. *Arch. Ophthalmol.* 77:503, 1967.

150. Goldberg, M. F., et al. Variable expression in flecked (speckled) dystrophy of the cornea. *Ann. Ophthalmol.* 9:899, 1977.

151. Goldberg, M. F., Payne, J. W., and Brunt, P. W. Ophthalmic studies of familial dysautonomia: The Riley-Day syndrome. *Arch. Ophthalmol.* 80:732, 1968.

152. Goldberg, M. F., Scott, C. I., and McKusick, V. A. Hydrocephalus and papilledema in the Maroteaux-Lamy syndrome (mucopolysaccharidosis type VI). *Am. J. Ophthalmol.* 69:969, 1970.

153. Goldman, J. N., Dohlman, C. H., and Kravitt, B. A. The basement membrane of the human cornea in recurrent epithelial erosion syndrome. *Trans. Am. Acad. Ophthalmol. Otolaryngol.* 73:471, 1969.

154. Goodside, V. Posterior crocodile shagreen. *Am. J. Ophthalmol.* 46:748, 1958.

155. Gorlin, R. J., Old, T., and Anderson, V. E. Hypohidrotic ectodermal dysplasia in females: A critical analysis and argument for genetic heterogeneity. *Z. Kinderheilkd.* 108:1, 1970.

156. Granek, H., and Baden, H. P. Corneal involvement in epidermolysis bullosa simplex. *Arch. Ophthalmol.* 98:469, 1980.

157. Grayson, M. The nature of hereditary deep polymorphous dystrophy of the cornea: Its association with iris and anterior chamber dysgenesis. *Trans. Am. Ophthalmol. Soc.* 72:516, 1974.

158. Grayson, M., and Wilbrandt, H. Dystrophy of the anterior limiting membrane of the cornea (Reis-Bücklers type). *Am. J. Ophthalmol.* 61:345, 1966.

159. Grayson, M., and Wilbrandt, H. Pre-Descemet dystrophy. *Am. J. Ophthalmol.* 64:276, 1967.

160. Griffith, D. G., and Fine, B. S. Light and electron microscopic observations in a superficial corneal dystrophy: Probable early Reis-Bücklers' type. *Am. J. Ophthalmol.* 63:1659, 1967.

161. Groenouw, A. Knötchenförmige Hornhauttrübungen (noduli corneae). *Arch. Augenheilkd.* 21:281, 1890.

162. Grop, K. Clinical and histologic findings in crystalline corneal dystrophy. *Acta Ophthalmol. (Copenh.)* 120:52, 1973.

163. Gruber, M. Cornea verticillata: I. Eine einfachdominant Variante der Hornhaut des menoschlichen Auges. *Ophthalmologica* 11:120, 1946.

164. Guerry, D. Fingerprint lines in the cornea. *Am. J. Ophthalmol.* 33:724, 1950.

165. Guerry, D. Observations on Cogan's microcystic dystrophy of the corneal epithelium. *Trans. Am. Ophthalmol. Soc.* 63:320, 1965.

166. Haab, O. Die gittrige keratitis. *Z. Augenheilkd.* 2:235, 1899.

167. Haddad, R., Font, R. L., and Fine, B. S. Unusual superficial variant of granular dystrophy of the cornea. *Am. J. Ophthalmol.* 83:213, 1977.

168. Haim, S., and Munk, J. Keratosis palmoplantaris congenita with peridontosis, arachnodactyly and a peculiar deformity of the terminal phalanges. *Br. J. Dermatol.* 77:42, 1965.

169. Hall, P. Reis-Bücklers dystrophy. *Arch. Ophthalmol.* 91:170, 1974.

170. Hammerstein, W. Zur Genetik des Keratoconus. *Albrecht von Graefes Arch. Klin. Exp. Ophthalmol.* 190:293, 1974.

171. Hanselmayer, H. Zur Histopathologie der hinteren polymorphen Hornhautdystrophie nach schlichtin: II. Ultrastrukturelle Bef unde, pathogenetische und pathophysiologische Bernerkungen. *Albrecht von Graefes Arch. Klin. Exp. Ophthalmol.* 185:53, 1972.

172. Harry, J., and Tripathi, R. Kayser-Fleischer ring: A pathologic study. *Br. J. Ophthalmol.* 54:794, 1970.

173. Hassell, J. R., et al. Macular corneal dystrophy: Failure to synthesize a mature keratan sulfate proteoglycan *Proc. Natl. Acad. Sci. U.S.A.*77:3705,1980.

174. Hassell, J. R., et al. Defective Conversion of a Glycoprotein Precursor to Keratan Sulfate Proteoglycan in Macular Corneal Dystrophy. In S. Hawkes and J. L. Wang (Eds.), *Extracellular Matrix.* New York: Academic, 1982.

175. Herbert, P. N., Gotto, A. M., and Fredrickson, D. S. Familial Lipoprotein Deficiency. In J. B. Stanbury, J. B. Wyngaarden, and D. S. Fredrickson (Eds.), *The Metabolic Basis of Inherited Disease* (4th ed.). New York: McGraw-Hill, 1978.

176. Hirst, L. W., and Waring, G. O. Clinical specular microscopy of posterior polymorphous endothelial dystrophy. *Am. J. Ophthalmol.* 95:143, 1983.

177. Hiti, H., et al. Die ruckbildung eines Kayser-Fleischer ringes bei Morbus Wilson under penicillamintherapie. *Klin. Monatsbl. Augenheilkd.* 176:235, 1980.

178. Hobbs, H. E., Eadie, S. P., and Somerville, F. Ocular lesions after treatment with chloroquine. *Br. J. Ophthalmol.* 45:284, 1961.

179. Hogan, M. J., and Alvarado, J. Ultrastructure of lattice dystrophy of the cornea: A case report. *Am. J. Ophthalmol.* 64:656, 1967.

180. Hogan, M. J., and Wood, I. Reis-Bücklers' corneal dystrophy. *Trans. Ophthalmol. Soc. U.K.* 91:41, 1971.

181. Hogan, M. J., Wood, I., and Fine, M. Fuchs' endothelial dystrophy of the cornea. *Am. J. Ophthalmol.* 10:9, 1971.

182. Howes, E. L., et al. Ocular pathology of infantile Niemann-Pick disease: Study of fetus of 23 weeks' gestation. *Arch. Ophthalmol.* 93:494, 1975.

183. Hoyme, H. E., et al. Presentation of mucopolysaccharidosis VII (β-glucuronidase deficiency) in infancy. *J. Med. Genet.* 18:237, 1981.

184. Hunziker, E. Richner-Hanhart syndrome and tyrosinemia type II. *Dermatologica* 160:180, 1980.

185. Iwamoto, T., and DeVoe, A. Electron microscopic studies on Fuchs' combined dystrophy: I. Posterior portion of the cornea. *Invest. Ophthalmol.* 10:9, 1971.

186. Iwamoto, T., and DeVoe, A. Electron microscopic studies on Fuchs' combined dystrophy: II. Anterior portion of the cornea. *Invest. Ophthalmol.* 10:29, 1971.

187. Iwamoto, T., et al. Ultrastructural variations in granular dystrophy of the cornea. *Albrecht von Graefes Arch. Klin. Exp. Ophthalmol.* 194:1, 1975.

188. Jaeger, W., and Eisenhauer, G. G. Der diagnostische Wert des Arcus cornae als Hinweis auf Lipoidstoffwechselstorungen. *Klin. Monatsbl. Augenheilkd.* 171:321, 1977.

189. Jaeger, W., et al. Herpetiform bilateral epithelial corneal dystrophy caused by tyrosinemia (Richner-Hanhart syndrome). *Klin. Monatsbl. Augenheilkd.* 173:506, 1978.

190. Jaensch, C. Hornhautbefund bei Darierscher Dermatose. *Klin. Monatsbl. Augenheilkd.* 78:96, 1927.

191. Johnson, B. L. Ultrastructure of the Kayser-Fleischer ring. *Am. J. Ophthalmol.* 76:455, 1973.

192. Johnson, B. L., and Brown, S. I. Posterior polymorphous dystrophy: A light and electron microscopic study. *Br. J. Ophthalmol.* 62:89, 1978.

193. Johnson, B. L., Brown, S. I., and Zaidman, G. W. A light and electron microscopic study of recurrent granular dystrophy of the cornea. *Am. J. Ophthalmol.* 92:49, 1981.

194. Johnson, R. E., and Campbell, R. J. Wilson's disease: Electron microscopic, X-ray energy spectroscopic, and atomic absorption spectroscopic studies of corneal copper deposition and distribution. *Lab. Invest.* 46:564, 1982.

195. Jones, S. T., and Stauffer, L. H. Reis-Bücklers corneal dystrophy. *Trans. Am. Acad. Ophthalmol. Otolaryngol.* 74:417, 1970.

196. Jones, S. T., and Zimmerman, L. E. Histopathologic differentiation of granular, macular and lattice dystrophies of the cornea. *Am. J. Ophthalmol.* 51:394, 1961.

197. Judisch, G. F., and Maumenee, I. H. Clinical differentiation of recessive congenital hereditary endothelial dystrophy and dominant hereditary endothelial dystrophy. *Am. J. Ophthalmol.* 85:606, 1978.

198. Judisch, G. F., Phelps, C. D., and Hanson, J. Rieger's syndrome: A case report with 15-year follow-up. *Arch. Ophthalmol.* 97:2120, 1979.

199. Kaden, R., and Feurle, G. Schnydersche Hornhautdystrophie und hyperlipidämie. *Albrecht von Graefes Arch. Klin. Exp. Ophthalmol.* 198:129, 1976.

200. Kanai, A., and Kaufman, H. E. Electron microscopic studies of primary band-shaped keratopathy and gelatinous, drop-like corneal dystrophy in two brothers. *Ann. Ophthalmol.* 14:535, 1982.

201. Kanai, A., and Kaufman, H. E. Further electron microscopic study of hereditary corneal edema. *Invest. Ophthalmol.* 10:545, 1971.

202. Kanai, A., et al. Electron microscopic study of hereditary corneal edema. *Invest. Ophthalmol.* 10:89, 1971.

203. Kaplinsky, C., et al. Familial cholestatic cirrhosis associated with Kayser-Fleischer rings. *Pediatrics* 65:782, 1980.

204. Karseras, A., and Price, A. Central crystalline corneal dystrophy. *Br. J. Ophthalmol.* 54:659, 1970.

205. Katowitz, J., Yolles, E., and Yanoff, M. Ichthyosis congenita. *Arch. Ophthalmol.* 91:208, 1974.

206. Kaufman, H. E., and Werblin, T. P. Epikeratophakia for the treatment of keratoconus. *Am. J. Ophthalmol.* 93:342, 1982.

207. Kelley, T. E., et al. Mucolipidosis I (acid neuraminidase deficiency). *Am. J. Dis. Child.* 135:703, 1981.

208. Kenyon, K. R. Lysosomal Disorders Affecting the Ocular Anterior Segment. In D. H. Nicholson (Ed.), *Ocular Pathology Update.* New York: Masson, 1980.

209. Kenyon, K. R., and Antine, B. The pathogenesis of congenital hereditary endothelial dystrophy of the cornea. *Am. J. Ophthalmol.* 72:787, 1971.

210. Kenyon, K. R., and Maumenee, A. E. Further studies of congenital hereditary endothelial dystrophy of the cornea. *Am. J. Ophthalmol.* 76:419, 1973.

211. Kenyon, K. R., et al. Mucolipidosis IV: Histopathology of conjunctiva, cornea, and skin. *Arch. Ophthalmol.* 97:1106, 1979.

212. Kenyon, K. R., and Sensenbrenner, J. A. Electron microscopy of cornea and conjunctiva in childhood cystinosis. *Am. J. Ophthalmol.* 78:68, 1974.

213. Kenyon, K. R., and Sensenbrenner, J. A. Mucolipidosis II (I-cell disease): Ultrastructural observation of conjunctiva and skin. *Invest. Ophthalmol.* 10:555, 1971.

214. Kirk, H. Q., et al. Primary familial amyloidosis of the cornea. *Trans. Am. Acad. Ophthalmol. Otolaryngol.* 77:411, 1973.

215. Kiskaddon, B. M., et al. Fleck dystrophy of the cornea: Case report. *Ann. Ophthalmol.* 12:700, 1980.

216. Klein, U., et al. Sanfilippo syndrome type C: Assay for acetyl-CoA: α-glucosaminide *N*-acetyltransferase in leukocytes for detection of homozygous and heterozygous individuals. *Clin. Genet.* 20:55, 1981.

217. Kline, A. Occurrence of ectodermal dysplasia and corneal dysplasia in one family. *J. Pediatr.* 55:355, 1959.

218. Klintworth, G. K. Corneal Dystrophies. In D. H. Nicholson (Ed.), *Ocular Pathology Update.* New York: Masson, 1980.

219. Klintworth, G. K. Current concept of macular dystrophy. *Birth Defects* 18(6):463, 1982.

220. Klintworth, G. K. Lattice corneal dystrophy: An inherited variety of amyloidosis restricted to the cornea. *Am. J. Pathol.* 50:371, 1967.

221. Klintworth, G. K. Proteins in Ocular Disease. In A. Garner and G. K. Klintworth (Eds.), *Pathobiology of Ocular Disease: A Dynamic Approach,* Part B. New York: Dekker, 1982.

222. Klintworth, G. K., Bredehoeft, S. J., and Reed, J. W. Analysis of corneal crystalline deposits in multiple myeloma. *Am. J. Ophthalmol.* 86:303, 1978.

223. Klintworth, G. K., et al. Recurrence of lattice corneal dystrophy type I in the corneal grafts of two siblings. *Am. J. Ophthalmol.* 94:540, 1982.

224. Klintworth, G. K., et al. Recurrence of macular corneal dystrophy within grafts. *Am. J. Ophthalmol.* 95:60, 1983.

225. Klintworth, G. K., and Smith, C. F. Abnormal product of corneal explants from patients with macular corneal dystrophy. *Am. J. Path.* 101:143, 1980.

226. Klintworth, G. K., and Vogel, F. S. Macular corneal dystrophy: An inherited acid mucopolysaccharide storage disease of the corneal fibroblast. *Am. J. Pathol.* 45:565, 1964.

227. Koeppe, L. Klinische Beobachtungen mit der Nernstspaltlampe und dem Hornhautmikroskop: I. Mitteilung. Frühjahrskatarrh. Streifentrübung ohne Faltenbildung. Keratitis bullosa interna. Angeborene Dellenbildung der Hornhauthinterfläche. *Albrecht von Graefes Arch. Klin. Exp. Ophthalmol.* 91:363, 1916.

228. Komoto, J. Obereinen Fall von Keratosis der Kornea und der Bindehaut mit pathologisch-anatomischien Befund. *Klin. Monatsbl. Augenheilkd.* 47:259, 1909.

229. Kopsa, M., and Marusic, K. Contribution à l'étude de la dégénérescence en mosaïque del la membrane de Bowman de la cornée. *Ophthalmologica* 136:83, 1958.

230. Krachmer, J. H., et al. Inheritance of endothelial dystrophy of the cornea. *Ophthalmolgica* 181:301, 1980.

231. Krachmer, J. H., et al. Corneal posterior crocodile shagreen and polymorphic amyloid degeneration. *Arch. Ophthalmol.* 101:54, 1983.

232. Krachmer, J. H., Feder, R. S., and Belin, M. W. Keratoconus and related non-inflammatory corneal thinning disorders. *Surv. Ophthalmol.* 27:281, 1984.

233. Krachmer, J. H., et al. A study of sixty-four families with corneal endothelial dystrophy. *Arch. Ophthalmol.* 96:2036, 1978.

234. Krachmer, J. H., Schnitzer, J. I., and Fratkin, J. Cornea pseudoguttata: A clinical and histopathologic description of endothelial cell edema. *Arch. Ophthalmol.* 99:1377, 1981.

235. Kuwabara, T., and Ciccarelli, E. C. Meesmann's corneal dystrophy. *Arch. Ophthalmol.* 71:676, 1964.

236. Laibson, P. R. Microcystic corneal dystrophy. *Trans. Am. Ophthalmol. Soc.* 74:488, 1976.

237. Laibson, P. R., and Krachmer, J. H. Familial occurrence of dot (microcystic), map, fingerprint dystrophy of the cornea. *Invest. Ophthalmol.* 14:397, 1975.

238. Lake, B. D., et al. A mild variant of mucolipidosis type 4 (ML4). *Birth Defects* 18(6):391, 1982.

239. Lamba, P., and Lal, S. Ocular changes in benign acanthosis nigricans. *Dermatologica* 140:356, 1970.

240. Lanier, J. D., Fine, M., and Togni, B. Lattice corneal dystrophy. *Arch. Ophthalmol.* 94:921, 1976.

241. Lemp, M. A., and Ralph, R. A. Rapid development of band keratopathy in dry eyes. *Am. J. Ophthalmol.* 83:657, 1977.

242. Lempert, S. L., et al. A simple technique for re-

moval of recurring granular dystrophy in corneal grafts. *Am. J. Ophthalmol.* 86:89, 1978.

243. Levenson, J. E., Chandler, J. W., and Kaufman, H. E. Affected asymptomatic relatives in congenital hereditary endothelial dystrophy. *Am. J. Ophthalmol.* 76:967, 1973.

244. Lewkojewa, E. F. Über einen Fall primärer degenerationamyloidose der Kornea. *Klin. Monatsbl. Augenheilkd.* 85:117, 1930.

245. Libert, J., Kenyon, K. R., and Maumenee, I. H. Mucolipidosis III (pseudo-Hurler polydystrophy): Ultrastructure of conjunctival biopsies. *Metab. Ophthalmol.* 1:145, 1977.

246. Libert, J., et al. Ocular ultrastructural study in a fetus with type II glycogenosis. *Br. J. Ophthalmol.* 61:476, 1977.

247. Libert, J., Pohl-Mockel, S., and Toussaint, D. Mucolipidose type II: Étude ultrastructurale de la cornée. *Bull. Soc. Belge Ophtalmol.* 164:241, 1973.

248. Libert, J., and Toussaint, D. Tortuosities of retinal and conjunctival vessels in lysosomal storage diseases. *Birth Defects* 18(6):347, 1982.

249. Libert, J., Toussaint, D., and Guiselings, R. Ocular findings in Niemann-Pick disease. *Am. J. Ophthalmol.* 80:991, 1975.

250. Libert, J., et al. Ocular findings in I-cell disease (mucolipidosis type II). *Am. J. Ophthalmol.* 83:617, 1977.

251. Lisch, W. Kombiniertes Vorkommen von primärer bandförmiger Hornhautdegeneration, anderen degenerativen Hornhautveränderungen und Keratoconus in einer Familie. *Albrecht von Graefes Arch. Klin. Exp. Ophthalmol.* 191:37, 1974.

252. Livni, N., Abraham, F. A., and Zauberman, H. Groenouw's macular dystrophy: Histochemistry and ultrastructure of the cornea. *Doc. Ophthalmol.* 37:327, 1974.

253. Lorenzetti, D. W. C., and Kaufman, H. E. Macular and lattice dystrophies and their recurrences after keratoplasty. *Trans. Am. Acad. Ophthalmol. Otolaryngol.* 71:112, 1967.

254. Lorenzetti, D. W. C., et al. Central corneal guttata: Incidence in the general population. *Am. J. Ophthalmol.* 64:1155, 1967.

255. Luxenberg, M. Hereditary crystalline dystrophy of the cornea. *Am. J. Ophthalmol.* 63:507, 1967.

256. Macarey, P. V. J., Lasagna, L., and Snyder, B. Arcus not so senilis. *Ann. Intern. Med.* 68:345, 1968.

257. Maeder, G. Le syndrome de Rothmund et le syndrome de Werner (étude clinique et diagnostique). *Ann. Ocul. (Paris)* 182:809, 1949.

258. Maeder, G., and Danis, P. Sur une nouvelle forme de dystrophie cornéenne (dystrophia filimormis profunda corneae) associée à un kératŏcone. *Ophthalmologica* 114:246, 1947.

259. Malbran, E. S. Corneal dystrophies: A clinical, pathological and surgical approach. *Trans. Am. Acad. Ophthalmol. Otolaryngol.* 76:573, 1972.

260. Malbran, E., D'Alessandro, C., and Valenzuela, J. Megalocornea and mosaic dystrophy of the cornea. *Ophthalmologica* 149:161, 1965.

261. Mannis, M. J., et al. Polymorphic amyloid degeneration of the cornea. *Arch. Ophthalmol.* 99:1217, 1981.

262. Matsui, M., Ito, K., and Akiya, S. Histochemical and electron microscopic examinations on so-called gelatinous drop-like dystrophy of the cornea. *Folia Ophthalmol.* 23:466, 1972.

263. Matta, C. S., Felker, G. V., and Ide, C. H. Eye manifestations in acrodermatitis enteropathica. *Arch. Ophthalmol.* 93:140, 1975.

264. Maumenee, A. E. Congenital hereditary corneal dystrophy. *Am. J. Ophthalmol.* 50:1114, 1960.

265. Maumenee, I. H. The cornea in connective tissue disease. *Ophthalmology (Rochester)* 85:1014, 1978.

266. McGee, H. B., and Falls, H. F. Hereditary polymorphous deep degeneration of the cornea. *Arch. Ophthalmol.* 50:462, 1953.

267. McKusick, V. A. *Mendelian Inheritance in Man: Catalogs of Autosomal Dominant, Autosomal Recessive, and X-Linked Phenotypes.* Baltimore: Johns Hopkins Press, 1983. Pp. 963–964.

268. McKusick, V. A., Neufeld, E. F., and Kelly, T. E. The Mucopolysaccharide Storage Diseases. In J. B. Stanbury, J. B. Wyngaarden, and D. S. Fredrickson (Eds.). *The Metabolic Basis of Inherited Disease* (4th ed.). New York: McGraw-Hill, 1978.

269. McMullan, F. D., et al. Corneal amyloidosis: An immunohistochemical analysis. *Invest. Ophthalmol. Vis. Sci.*, 1984.

270. McTigue, J. W., and Fine, B. S. The stromal lesion in lattice dystrophy of the cornea: A light and electron microscopic study. *Invest. Ophthalmol.* 3:355, 1964.

271. Meesmann, A. Über eine bisher nicht beschriebene dominant vererbte Dystrophia epithelialis corneae. *Ber. Dtsch. Ophthalmol. Ges.* 52:154, 1938.

272. Meesmann, A., and Wilke, F. Klinische und anatomische Untersuchungen über eine bisher unbekannte, dominant vererbte Epitheldystrophie der Hornhaut. *Klin. Monatsbl. Augenheilkd.* 103:361, 1939.

273. Mehta, R. F. Unilateral lattice dystrophy of the cornea. *Br. J. Ophthalmol.* 64:53, 1980.

274. Meisler, D. M., and Fine, M. Recurrence of the clinical signs of lattice corneal dystrophy (type I) in corneal transplants. *Am. J. Ophthalmol.* 97:210, 1984.

275. Meretoja, J. Comparative histopathological and clinical findings in eyes with lattice corneal dystrophy of two different types. *Ophthalmologica* 165:15, 1972.

276. Meretoja, J., et al. Partial characterization of amyloid proteins in inherited amyloidosis with lattice corneal dystrophy and in secondary amyloidosis. *Med. Biol.* 56:17, 1978.

277. Meretoja, J., and Tarkkanen, A. Pseudoexfoliation

syndrome in familial systemic amyloidosis with lattice corneal dystrophy. *Ophthalmic Res.* 7:194, 1975.

278. Merin, S., et al. The cornea in mucolipidosis IV. *J. Pediatr. Ophthalmol.* 13:289, 1976.

279. Moeschler, H. Untersuchungen über Pigmentierung der Hornhautrueckflaeche bei 395 am Spaltlampenmikroskop untersuchten Augen gesunder Personen. *Z. Augenheilkd.* 48:195, 1922.

280. Mondino, B. J., et al. Protein AA and lattice corneal dystrophy. *Am. J. Ophthalmol.* 89:377, 1980.

281. Nagataki, S., Tanishima, T., and Sakomoto, T. A case of primary gelatinous drop-like corneal dystrophy. *Jpn. J. Ophthalmol.* 16:107, 1972.

282. Nakaizumi, K. A rare case of corneal dystrophy. *Acta Soc. Ophthalmol. Jpn.* 18:949, 1914.

283. Nakanishi, I., and Brown, S. I. Ultrastructure of the epithelial dystrophy of Meesmann. *Arch. Ophthalmol.* 93:259, 1975.

284. Newsome, D. A., et al. Biochemical and histological analysis of "recurrent" macular corneal dystrophy. *Arch. Ophthalmol.* 100:1125, 1982.

285. Nicholson, D. H., et al. A clinical and histopathological study of François-Neetens speckled corneal dystrophy. *Am. J. Ophthalmol.* 83:554, 1977.

286. Offret, G., Puoliquen, Y., and Coscas, G. Une dystrophie cornéenne familiale: Étude clinique, histologique et ultrastructurale. *Arch. Ophthalmol. (Paris)* 29:537, 1969.

287. Orellona, J., and Friedman, A. H. Ocular manifestations of multiple myeloma, Waldenström's and benign monoclonal gammopathy. *Surv. Ophthalmol.* 26:157, 1981.

288. Pameijer, J. K. Über eine fremdartige familiäre oberflachliche Hornhautveränderung. *Klin. Monatsbl. Augenheilkd.* 95:516, 1935.

289. Pardos, G. J., Krachmer, J. H., and Mannis, M. J. Posterior corneal vesicles. *Arch. Ophthalmol.* 99:1573, 1981.

290. Patten, J. T., et al. Fleck (mouchetée) dystrophy of the cornea. *Ann. Ophthalmol.* 8:25, 1976.

291. Paufigue, L., and Étienne, R. La "cornea farinata." *Bull. Soc. Ophthalmol. Fr.* 50:522, 1950.

292. Pearce, W. G., Tripathi, R. C., and Morgan, G. Congenital endothelial corneal dystrophy: Clinical, pathological and genetic study. *Br. J. Ophthalmol.* 53:577, 1969.

293. Pepys, M. B., et al. Isolation of amyloid P component (protein AP) from normal serum as a calcium-dependent binding protein. *Lancet* 1:1029, 1977.

294. Perry, H. D., Buxton, J. N., and Fine, B. S. Round and oval cones in keratoconus. *Ophthalmology (Rochester)* 87:905, 1980.

295. Perry, H. D., Fine, B. S., and Caldwell, D. R. Reis-Bücklers' dystrophy: A study of eight cases. *Arch. Ophthalmol.* 97:664, 1979.

296. Petrohelos, M., et al. Ocular manifestations of Gaucher's disease. *Am. J. Ophthalmol.* 80:1008, 1975.

297. Philipson, B. T. Fish eye disease. *Birth Defects* 18(6):441, 1982.

298. Pillat, A. Zur Frage der familiären Hornhautentartung: Über eine eigenartige tiefe schollige und periphere gittenförmige familiäre Hornhautdystrophie. *Klin. Monatsbl. Augenheilkd.* 104:571, 1939.

299. Pilz, H., Heipertz, R., and Seidel, D. Review article: Basic findings and current developments in sphingolipidoses. *Hum. Genet.* 47:113, 1979.

300. Pippow, G. Zur Erbbedingtheit der cornea farinata (mehlstaubartige Hornhautdegeneration). *Albrecht von Graefes Arch. Klin. Exp. Ophthalmol.* 144:276, 1941.

301. Polack, F. M. Contributions of electron microscopy to the study of corneal pathology. *Surv. Ophthalmol.* 20:375, 1976.

302. Polack, F. M. The posterior corneal surface in Fuchs' dystrophy: Scanning electron microscope study. *Invest. Ophthalmol.* 13:913, 1974.

303. Polack, F. M., et al. Scanning electron microscopy of posterior polymorphous corneal dystrophy. *Am. J. Ophthalmol.* 89:575, 1980.

304. Pouliquen, Y. Ultrastructure of band keratopathy. *Arch. Ophthalmol.* 27:149, 1967.

305. Pouliquen, Y., et al. Dégénérescence en chagrin de crocodile de Vogt ou dégénérescence en mosaïque de Valerio. *Arch. Ophtalmol. (Paris)* 36:395, 1976.

306. Pouliquen, Y., et al. Étude morphologique de kératocône: I. Étude morphologique. *Arch. Ophthalmol. (Paris)* 30:497, 1970.

307. Pouliquen, Y., et al. Fibrocytes in keratoconus: Morphological appearance and changes in the extracellular spaces. Optical and electron-microscopic study. *Arch. Ophthalmol. (Paris)* 32:571, 1972.

308. Purcell, J. J., Krachmer, J. H., and Weingeist, T. A. Fleck corneal dystrophy. *Arch. Ophthalmol.* 95:440, 1977.

309. Quigley, H. A., and Goldberg, M. F. Conjunctival ultrastructure in mucolipidosis III (pseudo-Hurler polydystrophy). *Invest. Ophthalmol.* 10:568, 1971.

310. Quigley, H. A., and Goldberg, M. F. Scheie syndrome and macular corneal dystrophy: An ultrastructural comparison of conjunctiva and skin. *Arch. Ophthalmol.* 85:553, 1971.

311. Raab, M. F., Blodi, F., and Boniuk, M. Unilateral lattice dystrophy of the cornea. *Trans. Am. Acad. Ophthalmol. Otolaryngol.* 78:440, 1974.

312. Rahi, A., et al. Keratoconus and coexisting atopic disease. *Br. J. Ophthalmol.* 61:761, 1977.

313. Ramsey, R. M. Familial corneal dystrophy lattice type. *Trans. Am. Ophthalmol. Soc.* 60:701, 1957.

314. Rand, R., and Baden, H. P. Keratosis follicularis spinulosa decalvans: Report of two cases and literature review. *Arch. Dermatol.* 119:22, 1983.

315. Reed, W. B., Lopez, D. A., and Landing, B. Clinical spectrum of anhidrotic ectodermal dysplasia. *Arch. Dermatol.* 102:134, 1970.

316. Reese, A., and Wilber, J. The eye manifestations of

xeroderma pigmentosum. *Am. J. Ophthalmol.* 26:901, 1943.

317. Rehak, A., Selim, M. M., and Yadav, G. Richner-Hanhart syndrome (tyrosinaemia-II): Report of four cases without ocular involvement. *Br. J. Dermatol.* 104:469, 1981.

318. Rehany, U., Lahav, M., and Shoshan, S. Collagenolytic activity in keratoconus. *Ann. Ophthalmol.* 14:751, 1982.

319. Reis, W. Familiäre fleckige Hornhautentartung. *Dtsch. Med. Wochenschr.* 43:575, 1917.

320. Remky, H., and Engelbrecht, G. Dytrophia dermo-chondro-cornealis (François). *Klin. Monatsbl. Augenheilkd.* 151:319, 1967.

321. Richard, J. M., Paton, D., and Gasset, A. R. A comparison of penetrating keratoplasty and lamellar keratoplasty in the surgical management of keratoconus. *Am. J. Ophthalmol.* 86:807, 1978.

322. Riegel, E. M., et al. Ocular pathology of Fabry's disease in a hemizygous male following renal transplantation. *Surv. Ophthalmol.* 26:247, 1982.

323. Robb, R. M., and Kuwabara, T. The ocular pathology of type A Niemann-Pick disease: A light and electron microscopic study. *Invest. Ophthalmol.* 12:366, 1973.

324. Robin, A. L., et al. Recurrence of macular corneal dystrophy after lamellar keratoplasty. *Am. J. Ophthalmol.* 84:457, 1977.

325. Rodger, F. C., and Sinclair, H. M. *Metabolic and Nutritional Eye Diseases.* Springfield, Ill.: Thomas, 1969.

326. Rodrigues, M. M., et al. Disorders of the corneal epithelium: A clinicopathologic study of dot, geographic, and fingerprint patterns. *Arch. Ophthalmol.* 92:475, 1974.

327. Rodrigues, M. M., et al. Lack of evidence of AA reactivity in amyloid deposits of lattice corneal dystrophy and corneal amyloid degeneration. *Invest. Ophthalmol. Vis. Sci.*, 1984.

328. Rodrigues, M. M., et al. Glaucoma due to endothelialization of the anterior chamber angle: A comparison of posterior polymorphous dystrophy of the cornea and Chandler's syndrome. *Arch. Ophthalmol.* 98:688, 1980.

329. Rodrigues, M. M., et al. Microfibrillar protein and phospholipid in granular corneal dystrophy. *Arch. Ophthalmol.* 101:802, 1983.

330. Rodrigues, M. M., et al. Epithelialization of the corneal endothelium in posterior polymorphous dystrophy. *Invest. Ophthalmol. Vis. Sci.* 19:832, 1980.

331. Rodrigues, M. M., et al. Posterior polymorphous corneal dystrophy: recent developments. *Birth Defects* 18(6):479, 1982.

332. Rodrigues, M. M., et al. Endothelial alterations in congenital corneal dystrophies. *Am. J. Ophthalmol.* 80:678, 1975.

333. Rosen, D. A., et al. Keratoplasty and electron microscopy of the cornea in systemic mucopolysac-charidosis (Hurler's disease). *Can. J. Ophthalmol.* 3:218, 1968.

334. Rosenman, R. H., et al. Relations of corneal arcus to cardiovascular risk factors and the incidence of coronary disease. *N. Engl. J. Med.* 291:1322, 1974.

335. Rosenthal, J. W., and Kloepfer, H. W. An acromegaloid, cutis verticis gyrata, corneal leukoma syndrome: A new medical entity. *Arch. Ophthalmol.* 68:777, 1962.

336. Rowsey, J. J., Reynolds, A. E., and Brown, R. Corneal topography: Corneascope. *Arch. Ophthalmol.* 99:1093, 1981.

337. Sammartino, A., et al. Superficial annual corneal dystrophy, ichthyosis nigrans, microcephaly and mild mental subnormality. *Ophthalmologica* 185:226, 1982.

338. Sanderson, P., et al. Cystinosis: A clinical, histological and ultrastructural study. *Arch. Ophthalmol.* 91:270, 1974.

339. Sanfilippo, S. J., et al. Mental retardation associated with acid mucopolysacchariduria (heparitin sulfate type). *J. Pediatr.* 63:837, 1963.

340. Sass-Kortsak, A., and Bearn, A. G. Hereditary Disorders of Copper Metabolism. In J. B. Stanbury, J. B. Wyngaarden, and D. S. Fredrickson (Eds.), *The Metabolic Basis of Inherited Disease* (4th ed.). New York: McGraw-Hill, 1978.

341. Savin, L. H. Corneal dystrophy associated with congenital ichthyosis and allergic manifestations in male members of a family. *Br. J. Ophthalmol.* 40:82, 1956.

342. Schanzlin, D. J., Goldberg, D. B., and Brown, S. I. Transplantation of congenitally opaque corneas. *Ophthalmology (Rochester)* 87:1253, 1980.

343. Scheie, H. G., Hambrick, G. W., and Barness, L. A. A newly recognized forme fruste of Hurler's disease (gargoylism) (the Sanford R. Gifford lecture). *Am. J. Ophthalmol.* 53:753, 1962.

344. Schneider, J. A., Schulman, J. D., and Seegmiller, J. E. Cystinosis and The Fanconi Syndrome. In J. B. Stanbury, J. B. Wyngaarden, and D. S. Fredrickson (Eds.), *The Metabolic Basis of Inherited Disease* (4th ed.). New York: McGraw-Hill, 1978.

345. Schnitzer, J. I., and Krachmer, J. H. A specular microscopic study of families with endothelial dystrophy. *Br. J. Ophthalmol.* 65:396, 1981.

346. Schnyder, W. F. Mitteilung über einen neuen Typus von familiärer Hornhauterkrankung. *Schweiz. Med. Wochenschr.* 59:559, 1929.

347. Schnyder, W. F. Scheibenformige Kristalleinlage-rungen in der Hornhautmitte als Erbleiden. *Klin. Monatsbl. Augenheilkd.* 103:494, 1939.

348. Schoenberger, M., and Ellis, P. P. Disappearance of Kayser-Fleischer rings after liver transplantation. *Arch. Ophthalmol.* 97:1914, 1979.

349. Schutz, S. Hereditary corneal dystrophy. *Arch. Ophthalmol.* 29:523, 1943.

350. Sever, R. J., Frost, P., and Weinstein, G. Eye changes in ichthyosis. *JAMA* 206:2283, 1968.

351. Sher, N. A., Letson, R. D., and Desnick, R. J. The

ocular manifestations in Fabry's disease. *Arch. Ophthalmol.* 97:671, 1979.

352. Sheraidah, G. A. K., Winder, A. F., and Fielder, A. R. Lipid-protein constituents of human corneal arcus. *Atherosclerosis* 40:91, 1981.

353. Silver, H. K. Rothmund-Thomson syndrome: An oculocutaneous disorder. *Am. J. Dis. Child.* 111:182, 1966.

354. Sirinavin, C., and Terowbridge, A. A. Dyskeratosis congenita: Clinical features and genetic aspects. Report of a family and review of the literature. *J. Med. Genet.* 12:339, 1975.

355. Skinner, B. A., Greist, M. C., and Norins, A. L. The keratitis, ichthyosis, and deafness (KID) syndrome. *Arch. Dermatol.* 117:285, 1981.

356. Slansky, H. H., and Kuwabara, T. Intranuclear urate crystals in corneal epithelium. *Arch. Ophthalmol.* 80:338, 1968.

357. Sly, W. S. The Mucopolysaccharidoses. In P. K. Bondy and L. E. Rosenberg (Eds.), *Metabolic Control and Disease* (8th ed.). Philadelphia: Saunders, 1980.

358. Snip, R., Kenyon, K., and Green, W. Macular corneal dystrophy: Ultrastructural pathology of corneal endothelium and Descemet's membrane. *Invest. Ophthalmol.* 12:88, 1973.

359. Snyder, R. D., et al. Ocular findings in fucosidosis. *Birth Defects* 12(3):241, 1976.

360. Snyder, W. B. Hereditary epithelial corneal dystrophy. *Am. J. Ophthalmol.* 55:56, 1963.

361. Sornson, E. T. Granular dystrophy of the cornea: An electron microscopic study. *Am. J. Ophthalmol.* 59:1001, 1965.

362. Spaeth, G. L. Ocular manifestations of lipoprotein disease. *J.C.E. Ophthalmol.* 41:11, 1979.

363. Spaeth, G. L., and Frost, P. Fabry's disease: Its ocular manifestations. *Arch. Ophthalmol.* 74:760, 1965.

364. Sparrow, G. P., Samman, P. D., and Wells, R. S. Hyperpigmentation and hypohidrosis (the Naegeli-Franceschetti-Jadassohn syndrome): Report of a family and review of the literature. *Clin. Exp. Dermatol.* 1:127, 1976.

365. Spellancy, E., et al. Glaucoma in a case of Hurler disease. *Br. J. Ophthalmol.* 64:773, 1980.

366. Stainer, G. A., et al. Correlative microscopy and tissue culture of congenital hereditary endothelial dystrophy. *Am. J. Ophthalmol.* 93:456, 1982.

367. Stankovic, I., and Stojanovic, D. L'hérédodystrophie mouchetée du parenchyme cornéen. *Ann. Ocul. Paris* 197:52, 1964.

368. Stansbury, F. C. Lattice type of hereditary corneal degeneration: Report of five cases, including one of a child of two years. *Arch. Ophthalmol.* 40:189, 1948.

369. Stock, E. L., and Kielar, R. A. Primary familial amyloidosis of the cornea. *Am. J. Ophthalmol.* 82:266, 1976.

370. Stocker, F. W., and Holt, L. B. Rare form of hereditary epithelial dystrophy. *Arch. Ophthalmol.* 53:536, 1955.

371. Stocker, F. W., and Irish, A. Fate of a successful cornea graft in Fuchs' endothelial dystrophy. *Am. J. Ophthalmol.* 68:820, 1969.

372. Stone, D. L., Kenyon, K. R., and Stark, W. J. Ultrastructure of keratoconus with healed hydrops. *Am. J. Ophthalmol.* 82:450, 1976.

373. Strachan, I. M. Cloudy central dystrophy of François. *Br. J. Ophthalmol.* 53:192, 1969.

374. Strachan, I. M. Pre-Descemetic corneal dystrophy. *Br. J. Ophthalmol.* 52:716, 1968.

375. Streeten, B. W., and Falls, H. F. Hereditary fleck dystrophy of the cornea. *Am. J. Ophthalmol.* 51:275, 1961.

376. Streiff, E. B., and Zwahlen, P. Une famille avec dégénérescence en bandelette de la cornée. *Ophthalmologica* 111:129, 1946.

377. Sussmann, W., and Scheinberg, I. J. Disappearance of Kayser-Fleischer rings. *Arch. Ophthalmol.* 82:738, 1969.

378. Suveges, I. Histological and ultrastructural studies of the cornea in Maroteaux-Lamy syndrome. *Albrecht von Graefes Arch. Klin. Exp. Ophthalmol.* 212:29, 1979.

379. Sysi, R. Xanthoma corneae as hereditary dystrophy. *Br. J. Ophthalmol.* 34:369, 1950.

380. Taylor, P. J., Coates, T., and Newhouse, M. L. Episkopi blindness: Hereditary blindness in a Greek Cypriot family. *Br. J. Ophthalmol.* 43:340, 1959.

381. Tessler, H. H., Apple, D. J., and Goldberg, M. F. Ocular findings in a kindred with Kyrle disease. *Arch. Ophthalmol.* 90:278, 1973.

382. Theodore, F. H. Congenital type of endothelial dystrophy. *Arch. Ophthalmol.* 21:626, 1939.

383. Thiel, H.-J., and Behnke, H. Eine bisher unbekannte subepitheliale hereditäre Hornhautdystrophie. *Klin. Monatsbl. Augenheilkd.* 150:862, 1967.

384. Thomas, G. H., et al. Neuraminidase deficiency in the original patient with the Goldberg syndrome. *Clin. Genet.* 16:323, 1979.

385. Thomas, J. V., et al. Ocular manifestations of focal dermal hypoplasia syndrome. *Arch. Ophthalmol.* 95:1997, 1977.

386. Thomsitt, J., and Bron, A. J. Polymorphic stromal dystrophy. *Br. J. Ophthalmol.* 59:125, 1975.

387. Topping, T. M., et al. The ultrastructural ocular pathology of Hunter's syndrome: Systemic mucopolysaccharidosis type II. *Arch. Ophthalmol.* 86:164, 1971.

388. Tremblay, M., and Dubé, I. Macular dystrophy of the cornea: Ultrastructure of two cases. *Can. J. Ophthalmol.* 8:47, 1973.

389. Tremblay, M., and Dubé, I. Meesmann's corneal dystrophy: Ultrastructural features. *Can. J. Ophthalmol.* 17:24, 1982.

390. Tripathi, R. C., and Bron, A. J. Secondary anterior crocodile shagreen of Vogt. *Br. J. Ophthalmol.* 59:59, 1975.

391. Tripathi, R. C., Casey, T. A., and Wise, E. G. Hereditary posterior polymorphous dystrophy: An ul-

trastructural and clinical report. *Trans. Ophthalmol. Soc. U.K.* 94:211, 1974.

392. Trobe, J. D., and Laibson, P. R. Dystrophic changes in the anterior cornea. *Arch. Ophthalmol.* 87:378, 1972.

393. Tscheetter, R. Lipid analysis of the human cornea with and without arcus senilis. *Arch. Ophthalmol.* 76:403, 1966.

394. Tso, M. O. M., Fine, B. S., and Thorpe, H. E. Kayser-Fleischer ring and associated cataract in Wilson's disease. *Am. J. Ophthalmol.* 79:479, 1975.

395. Uzman, L. L., and Jakus, M. A. The Kayser-Fleischer ring: A histochemical and electron microscope study. *Neurology (N.Y.)* 7:341, 1957.

396. Vail, D. Corneal involvement in congenital ichthyosis. *Arch. Ophthalmol.* 24:215, 1940.

397. Valerio, M. Due forme rare di degenerazione giovanile della cornea; degenerazione a mogaido della cornea; un novo tipo di degenerazione cristalloide della cornea. *Boll. Ocul.* 18:659, 1939.

398. van Went, J. M., and Wibaut, F. Een zeldzame erfelijke hoornulie-saandoening. *Ned. Tijdschr. Geneeskd.* 68:2996, 1924.

399. Velhagen, Über die primaäre bandförmige Hornhauttrübung. *Klin. Monatsbl. Augenheilkd.* 42:428, 1904.

400. Vinger, P. F., and Sachs, B. A. Ocular manifestations of hyperlipoproteinemia. *Am. J. Ophthalmol.* 70:563, 1970.

401. Vogt, A. Corneal Degenerations of Various Etiology. In *Textbook and Atlas of Slit Lamp Microscopy of the Living Eye*, Vol. 1, transl. by F. C. Blodi. Bonn: Wayenborgh, 1981. Pp. 120–121.

402. Vogt, A. *Lehrbuch und Atlas der Spaltlampenmikroskopie des Lebenden Auges*, Vol. 1. Berlin: Springer, 1930. P. 263.

403. von Noorden, G. K., Zellweger, H., and Ponseti, I. V. Ocular findings in Morquio-Ullrich's disease. *Arch. Ophthalmol.* 64:585, 1960.

404. Waardenburg, P. J., and Jonkers, G. A. A specific type of dominant progressive dystrophy of the cornea developing after birth. *Acta Ophthalmol. (Copenh.)* 39:919, 1961.

405. Wales, H. J. A family history of corneal erosions. *Trans. Ophthalmol. Soc. N.Z.* 8:77, 1955.

406. Walton, D. S., Robb, R. M., and Crocker, A. C. Ocular manifestations of group A Niemann-Pick disease. *Am. J. Ophthalmol.* 85:174, 1978.

407. Waring, G. O. Posterior collagenous layer (PCL) of the cornea. *Arch. Ophthalmol.* 100:122, 1982.

408. Waring, G. O., et al. Alterations of Descemet's membrane in interstitial keratitis. *Am. J. Ophthalmol.* 81:773, 1976.

409. Waring, G. O., and Laibson, P. R. Keratoplasty in infants and children. *Trans. Am. Acad. Ophthalmol. Otolaryngol.* 83:283, 1977.

410. Waring, G. O., Rodrigues, M. M., and Laibson, P. R. Corneal dystrophies: I. Dystrophies of the epithelium, Bowman's layer and stroma. *Surv. Ophthalmol.* 23:71, 1978.

411. Waring, G. O., Rodrigues, M. M., and Laibson, P. R. Corneal dystrophies: II. Endothelial dystrophies. *Surv. Ophthalmol.* 23:147, 1978.

412. Warshawky, R. S., et al. Acrodermatitis enteropathica: Corneal involvement with histochemical and electron micrographic studies. *Arch. Ophthalmol.* 93:194, 1975.

413. Weber, F. L., and Babel, J. Gelatinous drop-like dystrophy. *Arch. Ophthalmol.* 98:144, 1980.

414. Weingeist, T. A., and Blodi, F. C. Fabry's disease: Ocular findings in a female carrier. A light and electron microscopic study. *Arch. Ophthalmol.* 85:169, 1971.

415. Weiss, M. J., et al. GM$_1$ gangliosidosis type I. *Am. J. Ophthalmol.* 76:999, 1973.

416. Weller, R. O., and Rodger, F. C. Crystalline stromal dystrophy: Histochemistry and ultrastructure of the cornea. *Br. J. Ophthalmol.* 64:46, 1980.

417. Werblin, T. P., et al. Prevalence of map-dot-fingerprint changes in the cornea. *Br. J. Ophthalmol.* 65:401, 1981.

418. Wheeler, G. E., and Eiferman, R. A. Immunohistochemical identifications of the AA protein in lattice dystrophy. *Exp. Eye Res.* 36:181, 1983.

419. Wiebers, D. O., Hollenhorst, R. W., and Goldstein, N. P. The ophthalmic manifestations of Wilson's disease. *Mayo Clin. Proc.* 52:409, 1977.

420. Wilson, F. M., Grayson, M., and Pieroni, D. Corneal changes in ectodermal dysplasia. *Am. J. Ophthalmol.* 75:17, 1973.

421. Winder, A. F. Factors influencing the variable expression of xanthelasmata and corneal arcus in familial hypercholesterolaemia. *Birth Defects* 18(6):449, 1982.

422. Winder, A. F., and Borysiewicz, L. K. Corneal opacification and familial disorders affecting plasma high-density lipoprotein. *Birth Defects* 18(6):433, 1982.

423. Winder, A. F., and Bron, A. J. Lecithin: cholesterol acyltransferase deficiency presenting as visual impairment, with hypocholesterolemia and normal renal function. *Scand. J. Clin. Lab. Invest.* 38:151, 1978.

424. Witkop, C. J., White, J. G., and Waring, G. O. Hereditary mucoepithelial dysplasia, a disease of gap junction and desmosome formation. *Birth Defects* 18(6):493, 1982.

425. Witschel, H., et al. Congenital hereditary stromal dystrophy of the cornea. *Arch. Ophthalmol.* 96:1043, 1978.

426. Witschel, H., and Sundmacher, R. Bilateral recurrence of granular corneal dystrophy in the grafts. *Albrecht von Graefes Arch. Klin. Exp. Ophthalmol.* 209:179, 1979.

427. Witschel, H., et al. Posterior polymorphous dystrophy of the cornea (Schlichting): An unusual var-

iant. *Albrecht von Graefes Arch. Klin. Exp. Ophthalmol.* 214:15, 1980.

428. Wolter, J. R., and Fralick, F. B. Microcystic dystrophy of corneal epithelium. *Arch. Ophthalmol.* 75:380, 1966.

429. Wong, V. G., Lietman, P. S., and Seegmiller, J. E. Alterations of pigment epithelium in cystinosis. *Arch. Ophthalmol.* 77:361, 1967.

430. Wood, T. O., et al. Treatment of Reis-Bücklers' corneal dystrophy by removal of subepithelial fibrous tissue. *Am. J. Ophthalmol.* 85:360, 1978.

431. Yamaguchi, T., Polack, F. M., and Rowsey, J. J. Honeycomb-shaped corneal dystrophy: A variation of Reis-Bücklers' dystrophy. *Cornea* 1:71, 1982.

432. Yamaguchi, T., Polack, F. M., and Valenti, J. Electron microscopic study of recurrent Reis-Bücklers' corneal dystrophy. *Am. J. Ophthalmol.* 90:95, 1980.

433. Yanoff, M., et al. Lattice corneal dystrophy: Report of an unusual case. *Arch. Ophthalmol.* 95:651, 1977.

434. Zaleski, W. A., Hill, A., and Murray, R. G. Corneal erosions in tyrosinosis. *Can. J. Ophthalmol.* 8:556, 1973.

435. Zimmerman, T. J., Hood, I., and Gasset, A. R. "Adolescent" cystinosis. *Arch. Ophthalmol.* 92:265, 1974.

436. Zwaan, J., and Kenyon, K. R. Two brothers with presumed mucolipidosis IV. *Birth Defects* 18(6):381, 1982.

13

Congenital Cataracts

Saul Merin

Any review of hereditary congenital cataracts must of necessity include a description of congenital cataracts arising from other causes. In many cases the hereditary influence is only indirect and hidden, while in others the exact cause, regardless of whether or not it is hereditary, may never be known. Moreover, both the morphology and the management of hereditary and nonhereditary congenital cataracts are often similar.

Lens opacities in the form of isolated single or multiple dots are extremely common in children [127]; hence only opacities that interfere with normal vision should be called cataracts. I shall also apply the term *congenital cataract* to those that appear during the first year of life. The term will be used synonymously with the term *infantile cataract*, because the same factors causing lens opacities at birth may also be present during the first year of life and because most congenital cataracts are not discovered at birth but during the first year of life.

Congenital cataract is one of the most common major abnormalities of the eye and therefore is a relatively frequent cause of blindness. François reviewed the available statistics, which showed that between 10.0 and 38.8 percent of all blindness in children is from this cause [47]. The lower figure is probably more accurate, since Scheie and Albert claimed a figure of 11.5 percent [147]. My colleagues and I found 13.4 percent with congenital cataract among 112 blind children in Cyprus [110], and Fraser and Friedmann, in the largest series (776 blind children), found 13.8 percent [55]. The extent of the problem can best be appreciated by the fact that 1 in 250 newborn babies (0.4%) has some form of congenital cataract [47].

This chapter will discuss the causal factors in congenital cataracts, the morphologic types, their relation to a specific cause and, finally, the prognosis and management of individual cases.

ETIOLOGIC CONSIDERATIONS

When a child is born with a cataract in one or both eyes, its cause must be investigated. Sometimes, as in the case of a familial congenital cataract, the cause will be obvious. In other cases elaborate laboratory investigations are necessary to make the determination.

Until a few years ago the cause of most congenital cataracts remained unknown. Verrey found a causal factor in only 25 percent [163]; François, in about one-third of all cases [47]. However, if we take into consideration associated abnormal perinatal conditions in which a congenital cataract is a frequent finding, no more than about one-third of the cases will remain without a clear cause [55, 105], and these last cases include all new mutations, in which the true cause of the cataract can be discovered only when the following generation is born.

The basic approach to a new individual case of congenital cataract is to try to relate the patient to one of two groups. The first comprises cases in which the cataract is an isolated finding, with the patient otherwise normal. In the second group the congenital cataract is a part of a syndrome or systemic abnormality or is associated with some other ocular disease.

Congenital Cataract as an Isolated Finding

The group with congenital cataract as the only abnormal finding is subdivided into those with hereditary cataracts and those with sporadic cataracts (hereditary or not).

HEREDITARY CATARACTS

When several members of one family are affected by a congenital cataract, we may assume a hereditary origin.

At least three different genes cause congenital cataract: two on the autosomes (dominant and recessive) and one on the X chromosome. Judging by the different morphologic types of isolated hereditary congenital cataract and from comparison of intrafamilial with interfamilial similarities of these cataracts, the number of pathologic genes is much higher than three. Autosomal dominant cataracts may be caused by at least twelve different genes, autosomal recessive by at least five different genes, and X-linked cataract by at least one gene. It seems certain that each different gene causing cataracts is at a different locus and possibly on a different chromosome.

By now two human autosomal dominant congenital cataract genes have known assignments to loci and chromosomes. By linkage analysis the locus for pulverulent nuclear congenital cataract (the Coppock cataract described by Nettleship and Ogilvie at the turn of the century [115]) was confined to chromosome 1 with close linkage to the Duffy blood group [26, 86, 133]. Another cataract (autosomal dominant posterior polar congenital cataract) may be linked to haptoglobin on chromosome 16 [102].

Between 8.3 and 25 percent of all congenital cataracts are familial [41, 50, 55, 70, 105, 163]. Autosomal dominant heredity is the most frequent mode of transmission. This was already known in the nineteenth century, when several generations of families suffering from this disease were described [168]. The transmission is ordinarily very regular throughout the generations, because the penetrance of the disease is complete and its expressivity is more or less similar. The chances are that half of the children of an affected person, but none of the children of a normal member of the family, will be affected. Fig. 13-1 shows the pedigree of a typical family with autosomal dominant cataract.

Autosomal recessive congenital cataracts (Fig. 13-2) are less frequent than autosomal dominant. However, they are not uncommon in populations with a high rate of consanguineous marriages [113]. About one of four families with congenital hereditary cataract seen in the genetic service of the Haddassah eye department of Jerusalem, Israel, suffer from the recessive disease. We found a similar incidence of recessive cataracts in Cyprus, where the villagers are endogamous [110].

X-linked cataract is rare, and only a small number of such families have been described; all had X-linked recessive types. The cataract in the affected men may be nuclear at first and then may remain so or progress to maturation. In many cases it is associated with microcornea [15, 126]. The female carriers show sutural cataracts not affecting the vision [45, 65, 91, 126]. Occasionally such female carriers may show the full-blown disease in accordance with Lyon's theory [96]. This is probably the explanation for published pedigrees describing X-linked cataracts in affected females.

Some insight into the mechanisms of action of the abnormal genes causing a cataract can be obtained from animal experiments. Many types of hereditary congenital cataracts have been described in animals, including 30 mutations in-

Fig. 13-1. *Pedigree of a family with autosomal dominant congenital cataract. An unaffected member of the family will have normal children.*

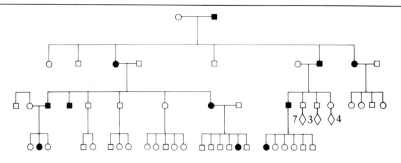

■ ● Congenital cataract

◊ Normal children of both sexes

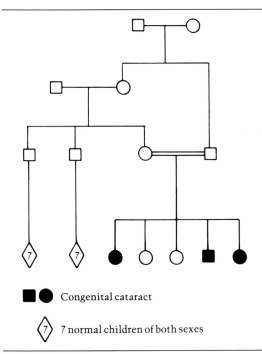

■● Congenital cataract

⟨7⟩ 7 normal children of both sexes

Fig. 13-2. *Pedigree of a family with autosomal recessive congenital cataract. The parents of the affected children are relatives, the father being an uncle of his wife.*

volving lens anomalies in mice [175], many in different breeds of dogs [4], in rats [82], and in many other animals. Three types of hereditary congenital cataracts have been described in the mouse and thoroughly investigated: an autosomal recessive type [114], an autosomal dominant type [54], and an autosomal intermediate type [16, 62]. In the dominant form disturbances in fiber formation, cellular replication, and capsular production lead to an anterior polar cataract. These changes, which start during gestational life and continue postnatally [176, 177], probably result from a specific defect in lenticular proteins. The whole class of γ-crystallins is decreased, and abnormal soluble proteins, not detectable in the normal lens, are present [58, 130]. In the recessive form a nuclear cataract is seen postnatally and slowly matures. Iwata and Kinoshita suggested that in the precataractous stage of the recessive form a defect in the cation pump mechanism is related to a 50 percent reduction in the activity of sodium-potassium ATPase [83]. This defect results in the accumulation of sodium in the lens, accompanied by an increase in water content. The defect in the activity of the enzyme is organ spe-

cific; that is, no other organ in the body of the affected mouse showed any abnormality in sodium-potassium ATPase activity. It was suggested that an abnormal lenticular polypeptide is the inhibitor of the sodium-potassium ATPase [56]. It is interesting, by comparison with human cataracts, that in a large number of homozygotic mice, about 10 percent showed a different phenotypic expression than the majority [94].

The Philly lens shows an autosomal dominant cataract with intermediate expression—homozygotes have a much faster appearance of the cataract than do heterozygotes. Absence of a functional messenger RNA results in failure to synthesize a β-crystallin polypeptide with a molecular weight of about 27,000 daltons [16, 162].

SPORADIC CATARACTS

It is usually difficult to determine the cause of a sporadic case of bilateral congenital cataract not associated with any other disease or ocular abnormality. Such cases make up about one-third of all cases of congenital cataracts [105]. Many of them are of hereditary origin, although this cannot be proved. Crawford and I estimated that in about a quarter of these cases the disorder is due to new autosomal dominant mutations [105]. Other cases in this group are due to autosomal recessive disease, appearing in only one of the siblings. Still others probably belong to the group of congenital cataracts associated with systemic disease; however, the systemic factor is too mild to be discovered.

Congenital Cataract as Part of a Syndrome or Systemic Disease

Congenital or infantile cataracts have been described in association with a large number of congenital anomalies. The description of all of them is beyond the scope of this chapter, especially because in many published cases the association remained doubtful. The present discussion will be limited to the confirmed syndromes, and the causal factors will be divided into hereditary (or those assumed to be genetic in origin) and nonhereditary.

HEREDITARY CATARACTS

With Renal Disease. Lowe's *oculocerebrorenal syndrome* [95], the best known association of cataract with renal disease, is caused by an X-linked recessive gene. The patient shows all or some of the following findings: mental retardation, aminoaciduria, hyperammonemia, tubular acidosis, dwarfism with rickets, congenital cataract, and congenital glaucoma [1]. Histologic studies have shown that the lens is small and thin, without differentiation into cortex and nucleus [29, 161]. The anterior capsule is hyperplastic, and the posterior capsule is adherent to the vitreous. The anterior chamber angle shows incomplete cleavage, the ciliary processes are pulled toward the lens by the zonules, and the retina extends far more anteriorly than usual. There is a segmental hypoplasia of the dilator pupillae, which causes miosis. Female carriers of the disease can frequently be recognized by spokelike or flakelike opacities in the posterior cortex [31, 87].

Alport's syndrome consists of hereditary hemorrhagic nephritis, sensorineural hearing loss, and ocular findings [145, 156]. Congenital cataract or a postnatally developing posterior cortical cataract can often be found. The mode of inheritance is not clear. It has been suggested that Alport's syndrome is X-linked dominant [171], but on review of the pedigrees, it seems more probable that it is autosomal dominant.

An *autosomal recessive syndrome* consisting of congenital cataracts, renal tubular necrosis, and encephalopathy was described by Crome and coworkers [28]. The affected girls were also mentally deficient, of small stature, and epileptic.

With Central Nervous System Disease. Marinesco-Sjögren syndrome, consisting of congenital spinocerebellar ataxia, mental retardation, and congenital cataract, is clearly an autosomal recessive disorder [99, 155]. Additional skeletal abnormalities, as well as epicanthus, nystagmus, and squint, are sometimes observed.

Sjögren's syndrome, described by Torsten Sjögren [154] (not to be confused with Sjögren's syndrome associated with keratoconjunctivitis sicca and described by Henrik Sjögren), consists of congenital cataracts and mental deficiency. It is assumed to be a hereditary autosomal recessive disease. However, a similar condition of congenital cataract and mental retardation is more often found to be nongenetic (see Nonhereditary Cataracts). I suggest using the term *T. Sjögren's syndrome* only for the genetic variety of this combination of congenital cataract and oligophrenia.

Smith-Lemli-Opitz syndrome is an autosomal recessive disorder in which microcephaly and mental retardation are associated with multiple other anomalies. Congenital cataract in 15 percent and various ocular abnormalities were described [90].

A large number of syndromes associating *congenital cataracts with various affections of the central nervous system such as convulsions or paraplegias* have been described. However, the evidence of their being genetic in origin is scanty, and the majority of them are probably due to intrauterine, nongenetic injurious factors.

With Skeletal Disease. Conradi's syndrome of congenital stippled epiphyses is frequently associated with congenital cataracts (see Chap. 19). The patient's roentgenograms show a typical radiologic picture of irregular calcification of the cartilage of the epiphyses. He or she may have contractures of limbs, kyphoscoliosis, or mental deficiency and often dies during the first 2 years of life from recurrent infection. The condition is not common. In one series 2 of 386 children with congenital cataract had this syndrome [105]. The eye may be normal except for the cataract, which is found in about 50 percent of the affected children, or the eye may also have one of the following: heterochromia iridis, optic atrophy, or optic hypoplasia [2]. The cataract may be unilateral or bilateral [160], but its presence indicates a worse prognosis for survival. Histologic studies have shown normal primary lens fibers but an abnormal equatorial lens epithelium [140]. The cells are swollen and proliferating but are not forming fibers. The time of appearance of the cataract is probably the fifth gestational month, when the nutrition of the lens changes from vascular to avascular. The genetic transmission is autosomal recessive.

Marfan's syndrome may show, in addition to the characteristic lens subluxation, a congenital cataract. In the various *chondrodystrophies* sporadic cases of congenital cataracts have been described; however, no firm association has been established.

In Mandibulofacial Syndromes. Three syndromes are included in this group. *Hallermann-Streiff syndrome* [68, 158], a term used frequently in the Western Hemisphere, and *François's dyscephalic syndrome* [46], a term used more in Europe, are most probably one and the same congenital disease. It shows seven cardinal signs: dyscephaly with bird's head, dental anomalies, proportional dwarfism, hypotrichosis, skin atrophy, bilateral microphthalmos, and, in most cases, bilateral congenital cataract [53]. The cataract has a peculiar "milky" content and in some patients undergoes a spontaneous resorption [51]. *Pierre Robin syndrome,* with its characteristic hypoplasia of the mandible and glossoptosis, is often associated with ocular anomalies such as congenital cataract, high myopia, and congenital glaucoma. Occasionally *mandibulofacial dysostosis,* or the *Treacher Collins syndrome,* is associated with congenital cataract [42].

The cause of the mandibulofacial syndromes is not clear, although a hereditary origin appears to apply to the Treacher Collins and Pierre Robin syndromes [42]. The Hallermann-Streiff-François syndrome appears sporadically, and, like Goldenhar's syndrome, it could be a developmental anomaly arising in the fifth to seventh gestational week (see Chapter 9) [98]. Familial occurrence may occur, but the mode of the hereditary transmission in these cases is not clear [51].

With Apical Malformations. A large number of cases associating various apical malformations, mainly polydactyly, with congenital cataracts have been described [47]. A truly repeatable syndrome is the *Rubinstein-Taybi syndrome* [139] of peculiar facies, mental retardation, broad thumbs and toes, and eye abnormalities, which occasionally includes congenital cataract [137]. The mode of inheritance is not clear.

With Skin Disease. Bloch-Sulzberger syndrome, or incontinentia pigmenti, consists of cutaneous pigmentation, dental anomalies, and alopecia and is frequently associated with ocular anomalies, including congenital cataract [151]. This cataract may be of "ocular origin" and secondary to retinal dysplasia with persistent hyperplastic primary vitreous. The mode of inheritance is not clear, but the disease has been observed only in females.

Congenital ectodermal dysplasia of the anhidrotic type is characterized by anhidrosis, hypotrichosis, and anodontia. It has occasionally been associated with microphthalmos, congenital cataract, and persistent hyperplastic primary vitreous.

Rothmund-Thomson syndrome consists of atrophic skin with patches of depigmentation and hyperpigmentation [136]. Telangiectases appear during the first year of life and may be associated with bilateral congenital cataracts. The transmission is autosomal recessive.

Schäfer's syndrome, or dyskeratosis palmaris et plantaris, may be associated with congenital cataract and, in addition, such systemic anomalies

as mental deficiency, dwarfism, and hypogenitalism [144].

For detailed discussion of hereditary diseases affecting both skin and eyes, see Chapter 19.

With Chromosomal Disorders. Patau's syndrome, or trisomy 13, is often associated with apparent congenital anophthalmia [124]. Occasionally, microphthalmos and congenital cataracts have been described [81, 105]. This syndrome is always associated with severe systemic abnormalities involving the cardiovascular system and brain and with polydactyly and cleft lip and palate. The patient usually does not survive the first year of life.

Edwards' syndrome, or trisomy 18, is more frequent than trisomy 13 [38]. The infant fails to thrive and has psychomotor retardation and malformations of the ears, face, and eyes. The characteristic eye finding is a narrow palpebral fissure, but congenital cataracts have been described [62].

Down's syndrome (mongolism, trisomy 21) is well known to ophthalmologists because of its high incidence and its frequently associated eye abnormalities. Characteristically, a cataract develops toward the end of the first decade of life, but a congenital cataract is not uncommon. In our series 15 cases of congenital cataract associated with Down's syndrome were described [105].

Further details on chromosome-induced ocular diseases appear in Chapter 8.

With Other Conditions. Galactosemia is one of the inborn errors of metabolism caused by a single autosomal recessive gene. It is characterized by nutritional failure, hepatosplenomegaly, cirrhosis, mental retardation, galactosemia, galactosuria, and infantile cataracts that appear during the first year of life. The basic metabolic disturbance is a deficiency in the enzyme galactose 1-phosphate uridyl transferase. The lens opacity characteristically starts as an "oil-drop" cataract [125] and progresses through a nuclear cataract to maturity. In the lens galactose is reduced to dulcitol by the enzyme aldose reductase, and the abnormal accumulation of this sugar alcohol leads to the accumulation of water in the lens. The swelling that ensues causes the disruption of the lens fibers [89]. This theory was later confirmed by showing that aldose reductase inhibitors, such as sorbinil (CP-45,634), effectively prevent cataract [30, 79, 128]. Therefore, cataracts are preventable if the basic metabolic disease is treated in the early stages [116] by withholding galactose from the diet (see Chaps. 2 and 20). Galactosemia has been assigned to chromosome 9 [10].

Another inborn error of metabolism, *galacto-kinase deficiency*, has congenital cataract as its main or only manifestation [64, 93]. The gene for galactokinase deficiency has been assigned to band q21–22 on chromosome 17 [39]. Congenital cataract was described in offspring of heterozygous mothers with low levels of galactokinase activity during pregnancy [71, 172]. This cataract can probably be prevented by dietary restriction of galactose during pregnancy.

Congenital hemolytic jaundice, an autosomal dominant disease with irregular penetrance, is frequently associated with congenital cataracts [37].

Multiple congenital malformations not included in one of the recognizable syndromes may be associated with congenital cataracts [105]. It has been suggested that such cases of multiple congenital malformations are hereditary and transmitted multifactorially [17].

NONHEREDITARY CATARACTS

In the category of nonhereditary cataracts are included cases that are definitely nongenetic and cases presumably nongenetic in origin. Usually the causal factor acts during the gestational period, but it may be active after birth, during the first year of life.

Prenatal Causes. Rubella syndrome, caused by the virus of rubella acting during the first trimester of pregnancy, is the most frequent single cause of congenital cataracts. It is responsible for about 20 percent of all such cases [70, 105], and in some series an even higher proportion has been found [81]. The cataract is caused by a direct invasion of the lens by the virus [174]. Rubella syndrome may occur anywhere in the world and is known to be a cause of congenital cataract in Africa, for example [117]. However, its incidence is much higher in the developed countries, where the better hygiene results in women being infected by "children's diseases" much later in life. The incidence of rubella cataract is invariably increased after each epidemic [3, 101, 152].

Large-scale immunization programs held in the last 10 years in many developed countries resulted in a drastic decrease in morbidity of rubella. As a result, the incidence of rubella cataract was greatly reduced. The dreadful periodic epidemics of rubella and congenital rubella cataracts of the 1950s and 1960s are no longer seen.

Other infectious diseases, such as toxoplasmosis, mumps, measles, influenza, chickenpox, herpes simplex, herpes zoster, cytomegalovirus disease, and echovirus type 3 have all been described as causative factors of congenital cataracts [75]. However, if such cataracts do appear as primary disorders, they are rarities. According to François, the infantile cataract seen not infrequently in toxoplasmosis is secondary to uveitis [47].

Developmental disturbances in the last trimester of pregnancy are probably one of the most frequent causes of congenital cataract. The typical child of this group is premature or, rather, dysmature (low birth weight for date) and suffers from birth anoxia, bilateral congenital cataract, and associated central nervous system (CNS) involvement. The most frequent CNS involvement is mental retardation, followed by convulsions, paraplegia or hemiplegia, and cerebral palsy [105]. The cause of this association of cataracts, dysmaturity, and CNS abnormalities could be intrauterine anoxia or hypoxia and the malnutrition that is claimed to be responsible for the dysmaturity of these neonates [36]. Anoxia has been shown in animal experiments to cause cataracts [7]. The incompleteness of this clinical picture is responsible for the large volume of literature on such associations as, for example, cataracts and prematurity, cataracts and mental retardation, cataracts and convulsive disorder, and cataracts and diplegia. Such cases are responsible for about one-fifth to one-third of all congenital cataracts [54, 105].

Perinatal and Postnatal Causes. Retrolental fibroplasia is the chief cause of blindness acquired in the early postnatal period. Sometimes it results in an infantile cataract, appearing during the first few months of life.

Hypoglycemia in one of its forms (neonatal hypoglycemia, ketotic or idiopathic hypoglycemia) may be associated with infantile cataracts [57, 103, 106, 148]. The frequency of cataract in ketotic hypoglycemia has been reported to be 37.5 percent [170]. The typical patient is a male infant, born after a complicated pregnancy, who is small for his gestational age and has some mental retardation. The cataract is characteristically lamellar and can be congenital, or it may appear later in life, in which case it may be preventable by early diagnosis and treatment [106]. It has been suggested that the formation of cataract in hypoglycemia is due to deactivation of lenticular hexokinase after the depletion of its substrates ATP and glucose [21, 22].

Neonatal hypocalcemia may be responsible for some cases of infantile cataract associated with neonatal tetany. In one series 30 percent of 142 patients treated for tetany had cataracts [92]. Goldmann produced cataracts in experimental animals by destroying the parathyroid gland and administering a calcium-deficient diet [66].

Congenital Cataract in Association with Another Ocular Abnormality

An infantile cataract, including cataracts present at birth or appearing during early life, may appear as a result of another ocular abnormality. Persistent hyperplastic primary vitreous is the most common cause of cataract in this group. The disease is usually unilateral. Also in this group are gross congenital defects of the retina, such as retinal dysplasia, congenital retinal detachment, and some conditions previously mentioned (trisomy 13, incontinentia pigmenti, congenital ectodermal dysplasia, and retrolental fibroplasia). To this group should also be added Norrie's disease, a recessive X-linked disorder, in which congenital microphthalmos, retinal dysplasia, and cataract are often associated with mental retardation and sometimes with deafness [169].

Congenital cataracts may be seen in congenital anomalies of the anterior segment of the eye, such as aniridia or Rieger's anomaly.

A number of eye conditions have been described in association with congenital cataract. Some of them, such as nystagmus, are probably caused by the cataract itself; others, such as microphthalmos, appear simultaneously. The association with microphthalmos is important because of the poor visual prognosis in such cases [55]. François found microphthalmos in 11 percent of his bilateral cases and in 23 percent of his unilateral cases of congenital cataract, and 31 percent of both types had nystagmus [47]. Other associated ocular anomalies are squint (frequent in unilateral cases), myopia, and retinopathies.

MORPHOLOGIC CLASSIFICATION OF CONGENITAL CATARACTS

Simplified Classification Scheme

With the introduction of the slit lamp into routine use in ophthalmology, a voluminous amount of literature has appeared on the subject of morphologic types of congenital cataracts. Every ophthalmologist could then, with great ease, "discover" a new cataract. Often, such descriptions remained isolated, but, because of the bizarre or unique lens opacities, these descriptions have been republished in standard textbooks for decades [37]. Adding to the confusion of the reader is the improper terminology used by some authors. For example, the term *zonular cataract* has been used synonymously with, or instead of, the term *lamellar cataract*.

A congenital cataract should be classified as being either total (complete) or partial (incomplete). A further subdivision of the incomplete type is necessary for a better understanding of each case, mainly from the etiologic and prognostic standpoints. Such a subdivision should, however, be kept as simple as possible. Slit-lamp examination is essential for classifying the problem in each patient, and it should be performed on each affected person regardless of his or her age.

In the scheme I use, congenital cataracts are classified into one of four main types: polar cataract, in which one of the poles of the lens, anterior or posterior, is affected, and the capsule and the underlying lens are involved; zonular cataract, in which a zone of the lens proper of any form or shape is opaque, while other parts of the lens are transparent; total cataract, in which the whole lens or almost the whole lens is opaque; and membranous cataract, in which the lens is completely opaque but is very thin and fibrotic.

The Morphologic Types of Congenital Cataracts and Their Relationship to Causation

POLAR CATARACTS

A localized opacity of the posterior capsule is not uncommon as a vestigial remnant of the hyaloid artery on the posterior lens capsule. It does not affect vision and so is not a true cataract. When the capsule of the lens and the underlying lens fibers are opaque, vision is practically always affected, although usually only to a slight extent. In my experience most polar cataracts, whether anterior or posterior, are unilateral, although in hereditary cases and in some sporadic cases, bilateral polar cataracts occur.

Congenital Anterior Polar Cataracts. Anterior polar cataracts may be familial or sporadic. In the familial form autosomal dominant heredity is the rule, and the cataract may take one of three forms:

1. Anterior polar cataract associated with other zonular lens opacities, mainly in lamellar form [173].
2. Anterior polar cataract associated with microphthalmus [72].
3. Anterior polar cataract associated with hyperplastic persistent pupillary membrane, a thick membrane covering the whole or most of the pupil. In three of the four families described, this membrane was attached to the lens, causing an anterior polar cataract [18, 109, 119, 167].

In the sporadic cases an anterior polar cataract may be associated with corneal opacities (possibly indicating the past existence of an intrauterine inflammation) or with simple remnants of the pupillary membrane attached to the anterior capsule of the lens [164]. Sporadic anterior polar cataracts may also be associated with lamellar opacities or with anterior lenticonus. Sometimes the thickened anterior capsule protrudes anteriorly, forming a pyramidal cataract. Most anterior polar cataracts are very small, not exceeding 1 to 2 mm in diameter. Because of the very small size of the cataract, visual acuity is usually good even in unilateral cases, and as the cataract is stationary and nonprogressive, the prognosis is also good. However, a remarkably high incidence of strabismus, refractive anisometropia, and poor visual acuity (more than one-third) was reported in one recent study of 63 patients [84]. In patients in whom the cataract is associated with other ocular changes, the visual prognosis must be judged according to the other abnormalities present.

Congenital Posterior Polar Cataracts. Like the anterior type, posterior polar cataracts may be familial or sporadic. The familial type is usually inherited as an autosomal dominant disease [52, 73] and rarely as an autosomal recessive condition [143]. It may also be seen in familial syndromes such as Alport's syndrome [156]. The sporadic type is often unilateral and associated with remnants of the hyaloid artery or with posterior lenticonus [153]. The posterior capsule and cortex are affected, and the opacity may extend forward to involve the whole or part of the nucleus. The diameter of the posterior polar cataract is usually larger than that of the anterior polar type, ranging, in my patients, between 0.7 and 4.5 mm. The visual acuity is much lower than in similar cases

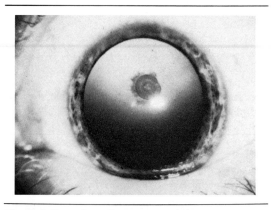

Fig. 13-3. *Posterior polar cataract of the stationary type. The pupil has been dilated with drops.*

of anterior polar cataracts, often necessitating surgical treatment. Posterior polar cataracts are usually stationary (Fig. 13-3), but progressive familial cases have been described [52]. In this progressive type spokes of posterior cortical opacity radiate from the center.

ZONULAR CATARACTS

A zonular cataract is an opacity of one zone or area of the lens proper, the rest of the lens being transparent. Zonular cataracts may be classified according to the zone involved, that is, nuclear, lamellar, and other types.

Nuclear Cataracts. As seen in infancy, nuclear cataract is always congenital. It may involve the embryonic nucleus or both the embryonic and fetal nucleus. Biomicroscopically, it may consist of fine grains, distinct dots (central pulverulent cataract), or small lines, or it may be chalky white. Nuclear cataracts are usually bilateral, ranging in size from 2.7 to 4.1 mm [107]. Visual acuity is usually more affected than in the other types of zonular cataracts.

Autosomal dominant, autosomal recessive, or X-linked hereditary transmission is the chief cause of nuclear cataracts.

Lamellar Cataracts. Lamellar cataract is the most common type of infantile cataract. Falls found this type in 40 percent of all his patients, as compared with nuclear cataract in 25 percent [41]. The typical lamellar cataract shows a circle of opacity around a clear nucleus. It is often associated with "riders," which are projections of opacities from the opacified lamella (Fig. 13-4).

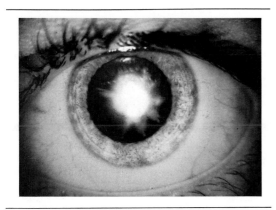

Fig. 13-4. *Nuclear and lamellar cataract with multiple riders.*

Lamellar cataracts may be congenital (prenatal) or may appear during postnatal development. Of the prenatal causes, heredity is the most important. The transmission characteristically is autosomal dominant, and some of the largest pedigrees were described in families with this cataract [168]. Congenital rubella cataract, although usually total, may not infrequently be of the lamellar type. Lamellar cataracts are also seen in the congenital cataract associated with disorders of the central nervous system and as early postnatal cataracts.

Lamellar cataracts are a result of a noxious factor active for a certain period during the development of the lens. They have been produced experimentally by irradiation [8], parathyroidectomy with resultant hypocalcemia [66], and an antirachitic diet combined with hypocalcemic tetany [165]. Several opaque lamellae with normal lens fibers between them were found when the noxious factor was active periodically and repeatedly. This can be seen experimentally [66] and in human diseases such as hypoglycemia [106].

The size of the lamellar opacity may indicate the time of its formation, as the lens at birth has a frontal diameter of 5.75 mm [25], and its postnatal changes can also be measured [6]; von Bahr reported that the most frequent size of lamellar cataract is 5 to 8 mm [165]. In our material the diameter of lamellar cataracts ranged from 2.6 to 6.9 mm, the most frequent size being 5.0 to 5.8 mm [107]. A postnatal cataract smaller than 5.75 mm may be due to later compression of the lens fibers and condensation of the nucleus.

Lamellar cataracts may be associated with other forms of zonular cataracts such as nuclear, fusiform, and sutural cataracts. The association of nuclear and lamellar cataracts is especially common. Sometimes what seems to be a nuclear cataract shows riders exactly like those of a lamellar cataract.

The visual acuity of an eye with lamellar cataract differs according to the density of the opacity [108]. When the cataract is translucent, the visual acuity may be almost normal, but when it is dense, visual acuity may be as low as 20/400.

Other Zonular Cataracts. Many forms of isolated opacities in a zone of the lens have been seen and have been given different names. Sutural cataracts affecting the anterior sutures are common, but other forms such as stellate (anterior and posterior sutures), spearlike (dispersed lines and needles), coralliform, and floriform are rare. In all these forms the visual acuity is little affected. When the cataract is hereditary, the transmission is autosomal dominant. To this group also belongs an autosomal dominant "ant-egg" cataract, in which egglike bodies may be scattered into the anterior chamber [134].

TOTAL CATARACTS

In the group of total cataracts are included all congenital cataracts with complete or almost complete congenital opacification of the lens or those incomplete congenital opacification of the lens or those with incomplete cataracts that mature rapidly in the first year after birth. Although rare, total cataracts may be transmitted as a hereditary isolated abnormality by an autosomal dominant or autosomal recessive gene [168]. The majority of congenital total cataracts are seen in cases associated with hereditary and nonhereditary systemic disease. Such is the case in Norrie's disease, Lowe's syndrome, T. Sjögren's syndrome, and in cataracts associated with CNS disorders. The characteristic rubella cataract is almost mature, with a small part of the lens in the periphery remaining transparent (Fig. 13-5), although in a minority of cases a rubella cataract may be lamellar. Congenital total cataracts are also seen in hereditary microcornea or microphthalmos.

Some congenital cataracts start as partial cataracts and then mature rapidly. Typical of this group is the galactosemic cataract, which starts as a small localized opacity and then matures. Maturation of an incomplete cataract is also seen in cataracts associated with skin disorders, although this usually occurs later in life.

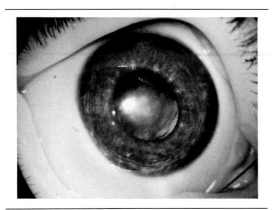

Fig. 13-5. *Cataract in congenital rubella syndrome. The cataract is almost total, a part of the periphery remaining transparent.*

Visual acuity in total cataracts not surgically treated is very low, and nystagmus is common.

MEMBRANOUS CATARACTS

Membranous cataracts (Fig. 13-6) are thin cataracts that are usually very dense and large in area and sometimes contain fibrous tissue. They may be congenital or develop from total cataracts. Most are unilateral and associated with some other ocular abnormality such as persistent hyperplastic primary vitreous.

Intrafamilial Similiarities and Differences in Hereditary Congenital Cataracts

When several members of one family are affected by a congenital cataract, it may be of the same basic morphologic type in all of them. Sometimes

Fig. 13-6. *Congenital membranous cataract.*

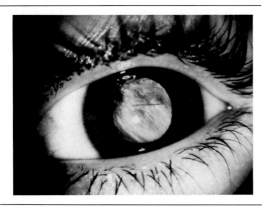

it may be strikingly similar in two members of a family (Fig. 13-7). In other cases various types of cataracts are seen in different members of one family [23, 24, 131]. This variety is observed most frequently in zonular cataracts of the sutural or axial type, with or without lamellar opacities (Fig. 13-8).

The most important intrafamilial similarity is the rate of progression of the cataract. If it is stationary (as it usually is), it will be so in all affected members of the family. And if it is progressive, it will be progressive in other affected relatives.

PROGNOSIS AND MANAGEMENT

From the standpoint of visual prognosis and management, congenital cataracts should be classified as total or partial, unilateral or bilateral, and with or without other ocular abnormalities. Although treatment in each case must be considered individually, it is possible to make generalizations based on experience and present trends in ophthalmology.

Prognosis in Untreated Cases and Indications for Treatment

The visual prognosis in any untreated case of congenital cataract depends on the type of cataract. In considering the indication for active treatment, the expected visual acuity of the eye is the most important factor. Some ophthalmologists are conservative in the approach to cases with bad visual prognosis, in which the functional surgical results are not promising. However, it seems to me that with the ease and relative lack of complications of present-day surgery, an eye with a congenital cataract should be actively treated whenever the expected visual acuity of the untreated eye is poor, as such treatment, administered early, yields better results than if no surgery is done.

UNILATERAL CONGENITAL CATARACT

The visual prognosis of a unilateral congenital cataract, if untreated, is poor, except in cases of very small polar cataracts [108]. In complete cataracts a deprivation amblyopia occurs. In incomplete cataracts a deep strabismic amblyopia develops and, even in this type, may also be combined with some deprivation or form of amblyopia, since such a unilateral cataract is usually very dense [108]. In untreated patients with unilateral com-

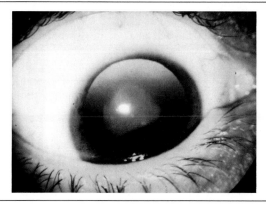
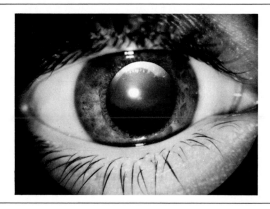

Fig. 13-7. *Similar congenital cataracts of the lamellar type in a father* (left) *and daughter* (right).

plete congenital cataracts, the resulting visual acuity is light perception only; it is less than 20/400 in untreated incomplete congenital cataracts. As functional surgical results are poor, investigators advocate no treatment for unilateral congenital cataracts [19, 88]. However, in such cases the eye is lost for practical vision. Unilateral congenital cataracts should thus be treated unless they are very small and slight in density. Surgery should be performed in the first year of life [69], or possibly in the first few days of life [166], and should be followed by vigorous antiamblyopia treatment.

BILATERAL COMPLETE (TOTAL)
CONGENITAL CATARACTS

When the congenital cataract is total or almost total, a deep deprivation amblyopia occurs. This

Fig. 13-8. *Sutural and lamellar congenital cataracts in a mother* (left), *son* (center), *and daughter* (right). *The sutural opacity was dense and the lamellar mild in the daughter, while the reverse was true for the mother and son.*

will happen in both eyes in bilateral cases. Surgical treatment is absolutely indicated and should be done as early as possible [142]. The second eye should be operated on soon after the first eye.

BILATERAL INCOMPLETE (PARTIAL)
CONGENITAL CATARACTS

The treatment of bilateral incomplete congenital cataract is the most controversial. Many eyes with incomplete cataracts will have useful vision. However, some patients may have a visual acuity of 20/200 or less in both eyes, and many others will have poor visual acuity (20/400 or less) in one eye, owing to deep strabismic amblyopia. Because of the uncertainty about the functional outcome, many ophthalmologists advise postponing the decision whether to treat or not until an age when visual acuity can be measured; if it is found to be 20/70 or less, operation is then recommended. Crawford and I found that the density of the incomplete cataract determines the visual outcome of the eye, and the size of the cataract (except when less than 2 mm) and its type are of minor importance only [108]. We have also devised a

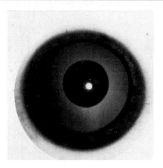
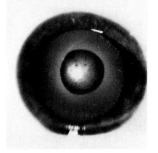
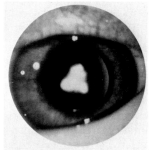

method of predicting future visual acuity from the density of the cataract.

Incomplete cataracts dense enough to prevent visualization of the fundus should be operated on. The expected visual acuity of such an eye, if untreated, is no more than about 20/100, and often is much less. When one eye is operated on, it is important to operate on the other eye also to prevent anisometropic amblyopia.

In some cases of bilateral incomplete cataracts, unilateral strabismus and amblyopia are seen. This may be the result of a difference in density of the cataract, the eye with the denser cataract being amblyopic.

CONGENITAL CATARACTS WITH ASSOCIATED OCULAR DEFECTS

According to all available statistics, patients with congenital cataracts with associated ocular defects have a poor visual prognosis, whether treated or untreated. The cataract is usually complete. The most frequent associated defect in this group is nystagmus, found in the bilateral cases. It is not clear whether this nystagmus is secondary to the cataract or is a primary defect of the foveal area. The latter possibility cannot be excluded, as in many of these cases the nystagmus can be seen in the first few days of life. Accepted opinion, however, is that the nystagmus is a result of the visual deprivation caused by the cataract. This opinion is based on two observations, namely, that in many cases the nystagmus appears only at the age of several months, and that nystagmus existing from birth can diminish or disappear after successful treatment [166]. Thus one must conclude that nystagmus does not contraindicate surgery but rather emphasizes the necessity of early treatment if surgery is indicated by the criteria that have been mentioned.

The visual prognosis of an eye with cataract and microphthalmos is poor. Treatment is useless in extreme cases and is not indicated.

If untreated, monocular strabismus and amblyopia as a result of a congenital cataract always cause very poor visual acuity in the affected eye. Early surgery is urged. Congenital cataract associated with persistent hyperplastic primary vitreous usually results in an eye with visual acuity ranging from light perception to hand movements. Ultrasound examinations should be performed, and if the vitreous membranes are not very thick, surgery is indicated, as it improves the chances for vision.

The decision whether or not to operate on a congenital cataract associated with other ocular abnormalities, such as glaucoma or other anterior segment abnormalities, must be based on the findings in each case, and no generalization is possible.

Management and Surgical Techniques

The accepted treatment for congenital cataracts is surgical. Different techniques have been advised over the years, but many of them are only of historical interest today. Management of congenital cataract and the relevant surgical techniques will be discussed in the following five sections.

OPTICAL IRIDECTOMY AND MEDICAL MANAGEMENT

Optical iridectomy and the use of mydriatics provide temporary treatment in cases of incomplete congenital cataracts. The rationale of the iridectomy is to allow better visual acuity through the clear periphery of the lens (around the cataract). Similarly, constant use of mydriatics keeps the pupil dilated, which enables peripheral rays of light to enter the eye through the lens. Such surgical or medical treatment has been advocated by several investigators as a temporary measure until the child is old enough to have his or her visual acuity tested. Then the decision is made whether or not to remove the lens [27, 69].

The optical iridectomy should be performed as a large sector iridectomy; some have advocated that it be done in the upper temporal or upper nasal quadrant [35]. However, optical iridectomy as treatment for congenital cataract is questionable [108], and even in Europe, where it was popular in the past, iridectomy has now generally been abandoned [67]. Its main value lay in its safety at a time when congenital cataract surgery was accompanied by many complications. Today iridectomy should probably be used only in exceptional cases. Similarly, mydriactics probably have little value as treatment for incomplete congenital cataracts. In addition, their mydriatic action is reduced with time, and I have seen complications such as obstruction of the lacrimal canaliculi from their use. On the other hand, it must be admitted that the long-term results of nonsurgical treatment consisting of mydriatics in the affected eye combined with proper and vigorous antiamblyopia patching of the good eye are not well enough known.

DISCISSION

Until the 1970s discission (or "needling") was a popular method of treating congenital cataract. In this operation a knife needle is introduced through the cornea or through the limbus into the lens to enable the cataract to be absorbed by the aqueous. Its value lies in its simplicity and in its few complications. However, it necessitates repeated operations, and a perfect optical result is difficult to obtain because of lens remnants and secondary membranes. It is of little use today as a primary procedure except in some cases of membranous cataracts. However, it is often used as a secondary procedure when, after aspiration, a thick posterior capsule remains or a secondary cataract develops. In such cases I incise the posterior capsule to enable a small mushroom of vitreous to enter the anterior chamber and keep the incision open.

The modern counterpart of the classic discission is the YAG-Neodymium laser capsulotomy, which can be performed with ease, with better results and fewer complications than a knife discission. The laser capsulotomy is extensively used in senile cataract and can certainly be used for congenital cataract with some modifications for anesthetized patients.

An operation that is between classic discission and aspiration was suggested by Moncreiff [111, 112]. In this procedure multiple incisions are made into the lens, and lens fragments are displaced into the anterior chamber by irrigation.

LINEAR EXTRACTION

In linear extraction an opening of no more than a quarter of the circumference of the limbus allows the lens to be grasped with a toothed capsular forceps and, subsequently, part of the anterior capsule to be removed. This is followed by irrigating or expressing out the lens material by means of a spoon. This method, popular for two centuries, is not used anymore today, mainly because of associated complications, the most common being pupillary block. To minimize the risk

of this complication, Chandler advised a linear extraction with a sector iridectomy, two peripheral iridectomies, and sphincterotomy at the 3-, 6-, and 9-o'clock meridians [20].

ASPIRATION AND IRRIGATION-ASPIRATION

Popularized by Scheie [146], aspiration became in the 1960s the method of choice for treatment of congenital cataract. It is simple, safe, and closest to the ideal congenital cataract procedure, as Ryan and von Noorden have stated [142]. The technique was based on the following procedure: opening of the anterior capsule with a knife needle, introduction of a needle into the lens material, and irrigation-suction of this material by a push-pull technique. Some surgeons preferred a corneal incision [69, 123, 142]; others preferred a limbal incision under a flap [149]. The operating microscope must be used, since it is the best way to avoid opening of the posterior capsule and aspiration of vitreous. The needle is usually an 18 or 19 gauge with a short, rounded tip, but a much smaller needle [77] with a side opening [59] or a modified Fuchs' syringe [43] may be used. A second needle may be introduced into the anterior chamber to supply a constant influx of irrigation fluid. An iridectomy may be performed through the corneal or limbal incision but is often not needed.

The pupil must be well dilated at the beginning of the operation. If it does not dilate, Franceschetti's cryopraxy is performed, as suggested by Maumenee and Goldberg [101].

In the decade 1965–1975 the use of more "advanced" manual methods for irrigation, such as the McIntyre system, and the various mechanical phacoemulsifiers used for irrigation and suction only, largely replaced the "simple" manual method of Scheie. It seems that in this decade 1975–1985 such methods continued to be preferred for removal of congenital cataract [157].

CATARACT EXTRACTION WITH
POSTERIOR CAPSULECTOMY

Intracapsular extraction as a one-stage procedure is not used in the surgical treatment of congenital cataract because of associated vitreous loss. Escapini suggested an intracapsular extraction in two stages: aspiration followed by extraction of the capsule by capsular forceps after using chymotrypsin [40]. However, with the excellent results achieved by aspiration only, such an operation seems unnecessary.

The major problem related to irrigation-aspiration is the frequent postoperative clouding of the posterior capsule [159]. As a result several surgeons suggested removal of the posterior capsule together with an anterior vitrectomy in one procedure. The approach may be through the limbus [122] or through the pars plana or pars plicata [33, 63, 129].

Capsulotomy, excision of the capsule under "open sky," may be used in cases with thick capsular remnants or in some thick membranous cataracts.

Congenital cataract associated with persistent hyperplastic primary vitreous was treated, before the mechanized vitrectomy era, in two stages by a limbal approach [60]. With mechanized vitrectomy instruments, such as the Ocutome [157] or a similar instrument, the operation may be performed in one stage using a pars plana or limbal approach.

POSTOPERATIVE TREATMENT AND
OPTICAL CORRECTION

Postoperative treatment is an essential part of congenital cataract surgery. Mydriatics and anti-inflammatory topical treatment should be given. Antiamblyopic treatment by occlusion of the good eye is essential and urgent in every case of suspected amblyopia. The postoperative optical defect must be corrected as early as possible and certainly not later than a few days after surgery. In patients with unilateral aphakia, the eye that was operated on may be fitted with a contact lens; good results have been claimed for this approach [5, 74, 78]. However, contact lenses have been advocated and used with various degrees of success in bilateral cases as well, providing an optical correction superior to that of glasses [34, 120, 123, 138, 166]. In infants distance vision involves objects at very close range. Thus for the first few postoperative months in the very young, an extra correction of at least +1.50 diopters (more for smaller babies) should be added to provide the child with an optical correction for close objects. This additional hyperopic correction must be increased whenever the eye is microphthalmic.

Intraocular lens implanation for congenital cataract, suggested by Binkhorst in the early 1970s [11, 12, 77], remains a controversial topic. It was probably used mainly in unilateral cases with both disappointing [97, 104] and encouraging results [9, 76]. The use of scleral lenses [44] never became popular, and glued-on contact lenses [32] never passed the experimental stage.

Results of Surgical Treatment of Congenital Cataract

The functional prognosis of an eye operated on for congenital cataract depends very much on the preoperative state of both the eye and the cataract. Results are far better in bilateral incomplete cataracts than in bilateral complete cataracts. Results are generally poor in unilateral cases. Two reviews of the results after conventional surgery (e.g., discissions, lamellar extraction) were made by François [48, 49]. According to various statistics, in patients with complete bilateral cataracts, 11 to 43 percent have visual acuity better than 20/100, while 40 to 75 percent have visual acuity less than 20/200. In bilateral incomplete cataracts 35 to 85 percent have good visual acuity (20/60 or better). However, the newer techniques yield better results [61]. Ryan and von Noorden compared aspiration with the conventional methods and showed that a visual acuity of 20/40 or better is found in 55 percent of all patients with congenital cataract after aspiration and in only 40 percent after conventional surgery [142]. Surgery of unilateral congenital cataracts yields far poorer results, although some outstanding successes have been claimed [100]. Intensive postoperative treatment with a contact lens in the aphakic eye and occlusion (possibly by an occluder contact lens [120]) of the good eye are necessary. With such vigorous treatment and frequent adjustment of the optical correction, results are surprisingly good [5, 78].

Another controversial problem is the question of visual results in rubella cataract. Scheie and associates stated that poor results have to be expected, especially if the operation is performed early in life [150]. Others, however, have reported good results and suggested operating early and in a one-stage procedure [13, 120]. With the modern methods, results are not different from those with other congenital cataracts.

The question of visual results according to age at operation is also controversial. In the past there have been many claims that better visual results are obtained if the operation is performed when the patient is older [80, 118, 141]. Broendstrup [14] and others asserted that age at operation is not important. However, as early as 1970 François pointed out that there is a clear bias in these statistics, as total cataracts and cataracts accompanied by other ocular anomalies such as nystagmus tend to be operated on earlier in life. More and more evidence is accumulating that early surgery, possibly as early as 2 to 4 months of age is important for better results [121, 135].

It may be said that congenital cataract surgery has now become a safe and reliable procedure with generally good results, if surgery is performed early, followed by vigorous antiamblyopic treatment and proper correction by the appropriate optical means [132], which should be periodically adjusted, possibly by follow-up of the actual visual acuity of the baby [85].

REFERENCES

1. Abbassi, V., Lowe, C. U., and Calcagno, P. L. Oculo-cerebro-renal syndrome: A review. *Am. J. Dis. Child.* 115:145, 1968.
2. Abedi, S. Syndromes with congenital cataract (Conradi-Hünerman syndrome): A case report. *Ann. Ophthalmol.* 14:595, 1982.
3. Alfano, J. E. Increased incidence of congenital cataracts (letter to the editor). *Am. J. Ophthalmol.* 59:723, 1965.
4. Barnett, K. C. Lens opacities in the dog as models for human eye disease. *Trans. Ophthalmol. Soc. U.K.* 102:346, 1982.
5. Beller, R., et al. Good visual function after neonatal surgery for congenital monocular cataracts. *Am. J. Ophthalmol.* 91:559, 1981.
6. Bellows, J. G. Phakochronology: The study of dating structural changes in the lens. *Br. J. Ophthalmol.* 52:540, 1968.
7. Bellows, J. G., and Nelson, D. Cataract produced by anoxia. *Arch. Ophthalmol.* 31:250, 1944.
8. Benedict, W. H. Development of x-ray-induced lamellar cataract in the newborn mouse in relation to age and time of irradiation. *Trans. Am. Ophthalmol. Soc.* 60:373, 1962.
9. Ben-Ezra, D., and Paez, J. H. Congenital cataract and intraocular lenses. *Am. J. Ophthalmol.* 96:311, 1983.
10. Benn, P. A., et al. Confirmation of the assignment of the gene for galactose-1-phosphate uridyltransferase (E.C. 2.7.7.12) to human chromosome 9. *Cytogenet. Cell Genet.* 24:37, 1979.
11. Binkhorst, C. D., and Gobin, M. H. Treatment of congenital and juvenile cataract with intraocular lens implants (pseudophakoi). *Br. J. Ophthalmol.* 54:759, 1970.
12. Binkhorst, C. D. The iridocapsular (two loop) lens and the iris clip (four loop) lens in pseudophakia. *Trans. Am. Acad. Ophthalmol. Otolaryngol.* 77:589, 1973.
13. Boniuk, V., and Boniuk, M. The incidence of phthisis bulbi as a complication of cataract surgery in the congenital rubella syndrome. *Trans. Am. Acad. Ophthalmol. Otolaryngol.* 74:360, 1970.
14. Broendstrup, P. Operation results obtained in bilateral infantile cataract. *Acta Ophthalmol.* [Suppl.] Copenh. 23:175, 1945.
15. Capella, J. A., et al. Hereditary cataracts and microphthalmia. *Am. J. Ophthalmol.* 56:454, 1963.
16. Carper, D., et al. Deficiency of functional messenger RNA for a developmentally regulated β-crystallin polypeptide in a hereditary cataract. *Science* 217:463, 1982.
17. Carter, C. O. Genetics of common disorders. *Br. Med. Bull.* 25:52, 1969.
18. Cassady, J. R., and Light, A. Familial persistent pupillary membranes. *Arch. Ophthalmol.* 58:438, 1957.
19. Chandler, P. A. Surgery of the lens in infancy and childhood. *Arch. Ophthalmol.* 45:125, 1951.
20. Chandler, P. A. Surgery of congenital cataract. *Am. J. Ophthalmol.* 65:663, 1968.
21. Chylack, L. T. Mechanism of hypoglycemia cataract formation in the rat lens: I. The role of hexokinase instability. *Invest. Ophthalmol.* 14:746, 1975.
22. Chylack, L. T., and Schaefer, F. L. Mechanism of "hypoglycemic" cataract formation in the rat lens: II. Further studies on the role of hexokinase instability. *Invest. Ophthalmol.* 15:519, 1976.
23. Collier, M. Variabilité des types de cataracte congénitale dans une même famille. *Bull. Soc. Ophtalmol. Fr.* 64:1043, 1964.
24. Collier, M. Nouvel exemple de variabilité dans une même famille. *Bull. Soc. Ophtalmol. Fr.* 68:910, 1968.
25. Collins, E. T. The aetiology of lamellar cataract. *Trans. Ophthalmol. Soc. U.K.* 40:406, 1920.
26. Conneally, P. M., et al. Confirmation of genetic heterogeneity in autosomal dominant forms of congenital cataract from linkage studies. *Cytogenet. Cell Genet.* 22:295, 1978.
27. Costenbader, F. D., and Albert, D. G. Conservatism in the management of congenital cataract. *Arch. Ophthalmol.* 58:426, 1957.
28. Crome, L., Duckett, S., and Franklin, A. W. Congenital cataracts, renal tubular necrosis and encephalopathy in two sisters. *Arch. Dis. Child.* 38:505, 1963.
29. Curtin, V. T., Joyce, E. E., and Ballin, N. Ocular pathology in the oculo-cerebro-renal syndrome of Lowe. *Am. J. Ophthalmol.* 64:533, 1967.
30. Datiles, M., Fukui, H., and Kinoshita, J. H. Galactose cataract prevention with sorbinil, an aldose reductase inhibitor: A light microscopic study. *Invest. Ophthalmol. Vis. Sci.* 22:174, 1982.
31. Delleman, J. W., Beekers-Wagemakers, E. M., and van Veelen, A. W. C. Opacities of the lens indicating carrier status of the oculo-cerebro-renal (Lowe) syndrome. *J. Pediatr. Ophthalmol.* 14:205, 1977.
32. Dohlman, C. H., et al. Further experience with glued-

on contact lenses (artificial epithelium). *Arch. Ophthalmol.* 83:10, 1970.

33. Douvas, N. G. Phakectomy with shallow anterior vitrectomy in congenital and juvenile cataracts. *Dev. Ophthalmol.* 2:163, 1981.

34. Dreifus, M. Klinische Erfahrungen mit hydrophilen Kontaktlinesen bei einseitig aphaken Kindern. *Ophthalmologica* 161:279, 1970.

35. Drews, L. C., and Drews, R. C. Optical iridectomy. *Am. J. Ophthalmol.* 58:789, 1964.

36. Drillien, C. M. Prognosis of infants of very low birth weight (letter to the editor). *Lancet* 1:697, 1971.

37. Duke-Elder, S. *System of Ophthalmology, Vol. 3: Normal and Abnormal Development.* London: Kimpton, 1964.

38. Edwards, J. H., et al. A new trisomic syndrome. *Lancet* 1:787, 1960.

39. Elsevier, S. M., et al. Assignment of the gene for galactokinase to human chromosome 17 and its regional localization to band q 21–22. *Nature* 251:633, 1974.

40. Escapini, H. Intracapsular extraction of congenital cataract: Technique in two successive stages. *Am. J. Ophthalmol.* 66:683, 1968.

41. Falls, H. F. Developmental cataracts. *Arch. Ophthalmol.* 29:210, 1943.

42. Feingold, M., and Gellis, S. S. Ocular abnormalities associated with first and second arch syndromes. *Surv. Ophthalmol.* 14:30, 1968.

43. Fink, A. I. Congenital cataract surgery: With a modification of the Fuchs syringe. *Am. J. Ophthalmol.* 60:1090, 1965.

44. Flom, L., Caldwell, J., and Kline, L. Minimal clearance scleral lenses in infants and children. *J. Pediatr. Ophthalmol.* 7:41, 1970.

45. Fraccaro, M., et al. X-linked cataract. *Ann. Hum. Genet.* 31:45, 1967.

46. François, J. A new syndrome: Dyscephalia with bird face and dental anomalies, nanism, hypotrichosis, cutaneous atrophy, microphthalmia and congenital cataract. *Arch. Ophthalmol.* 60:842, 1958.

47. François, J. *Congenital Cataracts.* Assen, Netherlands: van Gorcum, 1963.

48. François, J. Late results of congenital cataract surgery. *J. Pediatr. Ophthalmol.* 7:139, 1970.

49. François, J. Late results of congenital cataract surgery. *Ophthalmology (Rochester)* 86:1586, 1979.

50. François, J. Genetics of cataract. *Ophthalmologica* 184:61, 1982.

51. François, J. François dyscephalic syndrome. *Dev. Ophthalmol.* 7:13, 1983.

52. François, J., and Lambrechts, J. Cataracte polaire postérieure congénitale et évolutive à hérédité dominante. *Ann. Ocul. (Paris)* 184:423, 1951.

53. François, J., and Pierard, J. The Francois dyscephalic syndrome and skin manifestations. *Am. J. Ophthalmol.* 71:1241, 1971.

54. Fraser, F. C., and Schabtach, G. "Shrivelled": A hereditary degeneration of the lens in the house mouse. *Genet. Res.* 3:383, 1962.

55. Fraser, G. R., and Friedmann, A. I. *The Causes of Blindness in Childhood: A Study of 776 Children with Severe Visual Handicaps.* Baltimore: Johns Hopkins Press, 1967.

56. Fukui, H. N., Merola, L. O., and Kinoshita, J. H. A possible cataractogenic factor in the Nakano mouse lens. *Exp. Eye Res.* 26:633, 1969.

57. Gabilan, J. C., and Chaussain, J. L. L'association hypoglycémie idiopathique et cataracte chez l'enfant. *Arch. Fr. Pediatr.* 26:633, 1969.

58. Garber, A. T., Stirk, L., and Gold, R. J. M. Abnormalities of crystallins in the lens of the Cat Fraser mouse. *Exp. Eye Res.* 36:165, 1983.

59. Gass, J. D. M. Lens aspiration using a side-opening needle. *Arch. Ophthalmol.* 82:87, 1969.

60. Gass, J. D. M. Surgical excision of persistent hyperplastic primary vitreous. *Arch. Ophthalmol.* 8:163, 1970.

61. Gelbart, S. S., et al. Long-term visual results in bilateral congenital cataract. *Am. J. Ophthalmol.* 93:615, 1982.

62. Ginsberg, J., Perrin, E. V., and Sueoka, W. T. Ocular manifestations of trisomy 18. *Am. J. Ophthalmol.* 66:59, 1968.

63. Girard, L. J. Lensectomy through the pars plana by ultrasonic fragmentation (USF). *Ophthalmology (Rochester)* 86:1985, 1979.

64. Gitzelman, R. Hereditary galactokinase deficiency, a newly recognized cause of juvenile cataracts. *Pediatr. Res.* 1:14, 1967.

65. Goldberg, M. F., and Hardy, J. X-linked cataract. *Birth Defects* 7(3):164, 1971.

66. Goldmann, H. Experimentelle Tetaniekatarakt. *Albrecht von Graefes Arch. Ophthalmol.* 122:146, 1929.

67. Guillaumat, L. Les cataractes congénitales. *Bull. Soc. Ophtalmol. Fr.* 70:65, 1970.

68. Hallermann, W. Vogelgesicht und Cataracta congenita. *Klin. Monatsbl. Augenheilkd.* 113:315, 1948.

69. Harcourt, B., and Wybar, K. Congenital cataract: Surgical aspects. *Proc. R. Soc. Med.* 62:689, 1969.

70. Harley, J. D., and Hertzberg, R. Etiology of cataracts in childhood. *Lancet* 1:1084, 1965.

71. Harley, J. D., et al. Maternal enzymes of galactose metabolism and the inexplicable infantile cataract. *Lancet* 2:259, 1974.

72. Harman, N. B. Hereditary anterior polar cataract and microphthalmia. *Trans. Ophthalmol. Soc. U.K.* 30:139, 1910.

73. Harman, N. B. Hereditary posterior polar cataract. *Trans. Ophthalmol. Soc. U.K.* 30:140, 1910.

74. Helveston, E. M., Saunders, R. A., and Ellis, F. D. Unilateral cataracts in children. *Ophthalmic Surg.* 11:102, 1980.

75. Hertzberg, R. Rubella and virus-induced cataracts. *Trans. Ophthalmol. Soc. U.K.* 102:355, 1982.

76. Hiles, D. A. The need for intraocular lens implantation in children. *Ophthalmic Surg.* 8(3):162, 1977.

77. Hogan, M. J. Congenital cataract surgery. *Am. J. Ophthalmol.* 63:821, 1967.

78. Hoyt, C. S. Monocular congenital cataract (editorial). *J. Pediatr. Ophthalmol. Strabimus* 19:127, 1982.

79. Hu, T. S., Datiles, M., and Kinoshita, J. H. Reversal of galactose cataracts with sorbinil in rats. *Invest. Ophthalmol. Vis. Sci.* 24:640, 1983.

80. Hughes, W. F. Congenital cataracts. *Highlights Ophthalmol.* 1:97, 1957–1958.

81. Hull, D. Cataracts associated with metabolic disorders in infancy. *Proc. R. Soc. Med.* 62:694, 1969.

82. Ihara, N. A new strain of rat with an inherited cataract. *Experientia* 15:39, 909, 1983.

83. Iwata, S., and Kinoshita, J. H. Mechanism of development of hereditary cataract in mice. *Invest. Ophthalmol.* 10:504, 1971.

84. Jaafar, M. S., and Robb, R. M. Congenital anterior polar cataract: A review of 63 cases. *Ophthalmology (Rochester)* 91:249, 1984.

85. Jacobson, S. G., Mohinora, I., and Held, R. Development of visual acuity in infants with congenital cataracts. *Br. J. Ophthalmol.* 65:727, 1981.

86. Jay, M. Linkage and chromosomal studies in congenital cataract. *Trans. Ophthalmol. Soc. U.K.* 102:350, 1982.

87. Johnston, S. S., and Nevin, N. C. Ocular manifestations in patients and female relatives of families with the oculo-cerebro-renal syndrome of Lowe. *Birth Defects* 12(3):569, 1976.

88. Keith, C. G. In discussion: The visually handicapped child. *Proc. R. Soc. Med.* 62:570, 1969.

89. Kinoshita, J. H. Cataracts in galactosemia. *Invest. Ophthalmol.* 4:786, 1965.

90. Kretzer, F. L., Hittner, H. M., and Mehta, R. S. Ocular manifestations of the Smith-Lemli-Opitz syndrome. *Arch. Ophthalmol.* 99:2000, 1981.

91. Krill, A. E., Woodbury, G., and Bowman, J. E. X-chromosomal-linked sutural cataracts. *Am. J. Ophthalmol.* 68:867, 1969.

92. Kugelberg, I. Spasmophilie und Katarakt. *Acta Ophthalmol. [Suppl.] (Copenh.)* 14:220, 1936.

93. Levy, N. S., Krill, A. E., and Beutler, E. Galactokinase deficiency and cataracts. *Am. J. Ophthalmol.* 74:41, 1972.

94. Lipman, R. D., Muggleton-Harris, A. L., and Aroian, M. A. Phenotypic variation of cataractogenesis the Nakano mouse. *Exp. Eye Res.* 32:255, 1981.

95. Lowe, C. U., Terrey, M., and MacLachlan, E. A. Organic-aciduria, decreased renal ammonia production, hydrophthalmos and mental retardation: A clinical entity. *Am. J. Dis. Child.* 83:164, 1952.

96. Lyon, M. F. Sex chromatin and gene action in the mammalian X-chromosome. *Am. J. Hum. Genet.* 14:135, 1952.

97. Maida, J. W., and Sheets, J. H. Pseudophakia in children: A review of results of eighteen implant surgeons. *Ophthalmic Surg.* 10(12):61, 1979.

98. Mandelcorn, M. S., Merin, S., and Cardarelli, J. Goldenhar's syndrome and phocomelia: Case report and etiologic considerations. *Am. J. Ophthalmol.* 72:618, 1971.

99. Marinesco, G., Draganesco, S., and Vasiliu, D. Nouvelle maladie familiale caractérisée par une cataracte congénitale et un arrêt du développement somato-neuro-psychique. *Encephale* 26:97, 1931.

100. Marquardt, R. Behandlungsmöglichkeiten der einseitigen kongenitalen Katarakt. *Ber. Dtsch. Ophthalmol. Ges.* 69:305, 1969.

101. Maumenee, A. E., and Goldberg, M. F. Push-pull cataract aspiration and Franceschetti corepraxy. *Arch. Ophthalmol.* 74:72, 1965.

102. Maumenee, I. H. Classification of hereditary cataracts in children by linkage analysis. *Ophthalmology (Rochester)* 86:1554, 1979.

103. McKinna, A. J. Neonatal hypoglycemia: some ophthalmic observations. *Can. J. Ophthalmol.* 1:56, 1966.

104. Menezo, J. L., and Taboada, J. Assessment of intraocular lens implantation in children. *J. Am. Intraocul. Implant Soc.* 8:131, 1982.

105. Merin, S., and Crawford, J. S. The etiology of congenital cataracts: A survey of 386 cases. *Can. J. Ophthalmol.* 6:178, 1971.

106. Merin, S., and Crawford, J. S. Hypoglycemia and infantile cataract. *Arch. Ophthalmol.* 86:495, 1971.

107. Merin, S., and Crawford, J. S. Unpublished data, 1971.

108. Merin, S., and Crawford, J. S. Assessment of incomplete congenital cataract. *Can. J. Ophthalmol.* 7:56, 1972.

109. Merin, S., Crawford, J. S., and Cardarelli, J. Hyperplastic persistent pupillary membrane. *Am. J. Ophthalmol.* 72:717, 1971.

110. Merin, S., et al. Childhood blindness in Cyprus. *Am. J. Ophthalmol.* 74:538, 1972.

111. Moncreiff, W. F. Contributions to the surgery of congenital cataract: I. Modification of discission in the preschool age group. *Am. J. Ophthalmol.* 29:1513, 1946.

112. Moncreiff, W. F. Congenital cataract: Surgical and visual problems. Two decades of developments. *Ophthalmologica* 160:239, 1970.

113. Mostafa, M. S. E., et al. Genetic studies of congenital cataract. *Metab. Pediatr. Ophthalmol.* 5:233, 1981.

114. Nakano, K., et al. Hereditary cataract in mice. *Jpn. J. Clin. Ophthalmol.* 14:196, 1960.

115. Nettleship, E., and Ogilvie, F. M. A peculiar form of hereditary congenital cataract. *Trans. Ophthalmol. Soc. U.K.* 26:191, 1906.

116. Nordmann, J. Early postnatal cataracts. *Am. J. Ophthalmol.* 61:1256, 1966.

117. Olurin, O. Etiology of blindness in Nigerian children. *Am. J. Ophthalmol.* 70:533, 1970.

118. Owens, W. C., and Hughes, W. F. Results of surgical treatment of congenital cataract. *Arch. Ophthalmol.* 39:339, 1948.

119. Pagenstecher, A. Irismissbildung in drei Generationen (Teilweise Verdoppelung des mesodermalen Teiles der Iris). *Klin. Monatsbl. Augenheilkd.* 74:128, 1925.

120. Parks, M. M. In discussion. *Trans. Am. Acad. Ophthalmol. Otolaryngol.* 74:358, 1970.

121. Parks, M. M. Visual results in aphakic children. *Am. J. Ophthalmol.* 94:441, 1982.

122. Parks, M. M. Posterior lens capsulectomy during primary cataract surgery in children. *Ophthalmology (Rochester)* 90:344, 1983.

123. Parks, M. M., and Hiles, D. A. Management of infantile cataracts. *Am. J. Ophthalmol.* 63:10, 1967.

124. Patau, K., et al. Multiple congenital anomaly caused by an extra autosome. *Lancet* 1:790, 1960.

125. Patz, A. Cataracts in galactosemia: Observations in three cases. *Am. J. Ophthalmol.* 36:453, 1953.

126. Pavone, L., et al. Ocular manifestations in a family with probable X-linked cataracts. *Clin. Genet.* 20:243, 1981.

127. Pellaton, R. Die physiologischen Linsentrübungen im Kindesalter nach Spaltlampenuntersuchung an 164 normalen Kinderaugen. *Albrecht von Graefes Arch. Ophthalmol.* 36:453, 1953.

128. Peterson, M. J., et al. CP-45, 634: A novel aldose reductase inhibitor that inhibits polyol pathway activity in diabetic galactosemic rats. *Metabolism* 28 (Suppl. 1):456, 1979.

129. Peyman, G. A., et al. Pars plicata lensectomy and vitrectomy in the management of congenital cataracts. *Ophthalmology (Rochester)* 88:437, 1981.

130. Piatigorsky, J., et al. A molecular genetic approach to vision research: Crystallin gene expression in the lens. *Ophthalmol. Pediatr. Genet.* 3:61, 1983.

131. Poos, F. Über eine familiär aufgetretene besondere Schichtstarform: "Cataracta zonularis pulverulenta." *Klin. Monatsbl. Augenheilkd.* 76:502, 1926.

132. Pratt-Johnson, J. A., and Tillson, G. Visual results after removal of congenital cataracts before the age of one year. *Can. J. Ophthalmol.* 16:19, 1981.

133. Renwick, J. H., and Lawler, S. D. Probable linkage between a congenital cataract locus and the duffy blood group locus. *Ann. Hum. Genet.* 27:67, 1963.

134. Riise, R. Hereditary "ant-egg-cataract." *Acta Ophthalmol. [Suppl.] (Copenh.)* 45:341, 1967.

135. Rogers, G. L., et al. Visual acuities in infants with congenital cataracts operated on prior to six months of age. *Arch. Ophthalmol.* 99:999, 1981.

136. Rothmund, A. Über Cataracten in Verbindung mit einer eigenthümlichen Hautdegeneration. *Albrecht von Graefes Arch. Ophthalmol.* 14:159, 1868.

137. Roy, F. H., et al. Ocular manifestations of the Rubinstein-Taybi syndrome: Case report and review of the literature. *Arch. Ophthalmol.* 79:272, 1968.

138. Ruben, M. Role of contact lenses in aphakia in infants and young children. *Proc. R. Soc. Med.* 62:696, 1969.

139. Rubinstein, J. H., and Taybi, H. Broad thumbs and toes and facial abnormalities. *Am. J. Dis. Child.* 105:588, 1963.

140. Ryan, H. Cataracts of dysplasia epiphysealis punctata. *Br. J. Ophthalmol.* 54:197, 1970.

141. Ryan, S. J., Blanton, F. M., and von Noorden, G. K. Surgery of congenital cataract. *Am. J. Ophthalmol.* 60:583, 1965.

142. Ryan, S. J., and von Noorden, G. K. Further observations on the aspiration technique in cataract surgery. *Am. J. Ophthalmol.* 71:626, 1971.

143. Saebo, J. An investigation into the mode of heredity of congenital and juvenile cataracts. *Br. J. Ophthalmol.* 33:601, 1949.

144. Schäfer, E. Zur Lehre von den congenitalen Dyskeratosen. *Arch. Dermatol. Syphil.* 148:425, 1925.

145. Schatz, H. Alport's syndrome in a Negro kindred. *Am. J. Ophthalmol.* 71:1236, 1971.

146. Scheie, H. G. Aspiration of congenital or soft cataracts: A new technique. *Am. J. Ophthalmol.* 50:1048, 1960.

147. Scheie, H. G., and Albert, D. M. *Adler's Textbook of Ophthalmology* (8th ed.) Philadelphia: Saunders, 1969.

148. Scheie, H. G., Rubenstein, R. A., and Albert, D. M. Congenital glaucoma and other ocular abnormalities with idiopathic infantile hypoglycemia. *J. Pediatr. Ophthalmol.* 1:45, 1964.

149. Scheie, H. G., Rubenstein, R. A., and Kent, R. B. Aspiration of congenital or soft cataracts: Further experience. *Am. J. Ophthalmol.* 63:3, 1967.

150. Scheie, H. G., et al. Congenital rubella cataracts: Surgical results and virus recovery from intraocular tissue. *Arch. Ophthalmol.* 77:440, 1967.

151. Scott, J. G., et al. Ocular changes in the Bloch-Sulzberger syndrome (incontinentia pigmenti). *Br. J. Ophthalmol.* 39:276, 1955.

152. Sever, J. L. The epidemiology of rubella. *Arch. Ophthalmol.* 77:427, 1967.

153. Singh, D., and Singh, D. Posterior lenticonus with involvement of foetal nucleus. *Br. J. Ophthalmol.* 54:136, 1970.

154. Sjögren, T. Klinische und vererbungmedizinische Untersuchungen über Oligophrenie mit kongenitaler Katarakt. *Z. Ges. Neurol. Psychiatr.* 152:263, 1970.

155. Sjögren, T. Hereditary congenital spinocerebellar ataxia accompanied by congenital cataract and oligophrenia: A genetic and clinical investigation. *Confin. Neurol.* 10:293, 1950.

156. Sohar, E. Renal disease, inner ear deafness and ocular changes: A new heredofamilial syndrome. *Arch. Intern. Med.* 97:627, 1956.

157. Stark, W. J., et al. Management of congenital cataracts. *Ophthalmology (Rochester)* 86:1571, 1979.

158. Streiff, E. B. Dysmorphie mandibulofaciale (tête d'oiseau) et altérations oculaires. *Ophthalmologica* 120:79, 1950.

159. Taylor, D. S. I. Choice of surgical technique in the management of congenital cataract. *Trans. Ophthalmol. Soc. U.K.* 101:114, 1981.

160. Thiel, H.-J., Manzke, H., and Gunschera, H. Katarakt bei Chondrodystrophia calcificans connata (Conradi-Hünermann Syndrome). *Klin. Monatsbl. Augenheilkd.* 154:536, 1969.

161. Tripathi, R. C., et al. Lowe's syndrome. *Birth Defects* 18(6):629, 1982.

162. Uga, S., Kador, P. F., and Kuwabara, T. Cytological study of Philly mouse cataract. *Exp. Eye Res.* 30:79, 1980.

163. Verrey, F. Über Cataracta congenita. *Ophthalmologica* 133:302, 1957.

164. Vogt, A. Weitere Ergebnisse der Spaltlampenmikroskopie des vorderen Bulbusabschnittes. V. *Albrecht von Graefes Arch. Ophthalmol.* 108:219, 1922.

165. von Bahr, G. Studies on the aetiology and pathogenesis of cataracta zonularis. *Acta Ophthalmol. [Suppl.] (Copenh.)* 11, 1936.

166. von Noorden, G. K., Ryan, S. J., and Maumenee, A. E. Management of congenital cataracts. *Trans. Am. Acad. Ophthalmol. Otolaryngol.* 74:352, 1970.

167. Waardenburg, P. J. Gross remnants of the pupillary membrane, anterior polar cataract and microcornea in a mother and her children. *Ophthalmologica* 118:828, 1949.

168. Waardenburg, P. J., Franceschetti, A., and Klein, D. *Genetics and Ophthalmology*, Vol. 1. Assen, Netherlands: van Gorcum, 1961.

169. Warburg, M. Norrie's disease: A congenital progressive oculo-acoustico-cerebral degeneration. *Acta Ophthalmol. [Suppl.] (Copenh.)* 89, 1966.

170. Wets, B., et al. Cataracts and ketotic hypoglycemia. *Ophthalmology (Rochester)* 89:999, 1982.

171. Williamson, D. A. J. Alport's syndrome of hereditary nephritis with deafness. *Lancet* 2:1321, 1961.

172. Winder, A. F. Laboratory screening in the assessment of human cataracts. *Trans. Ophthalmol. Soc. U.K.* 101:127, 1981.

173. Wolfsohn-Jeffé, E. Hereditäre vordere Kapselkatarakt. *Klin. Monatsbl. Augenheilkd.* 91:236, 1933.

174. Zimmerman, L. E. Pathogenesis of rubella cataract: Greegg's syndrome. *Arch. Ophthalmol.* 73:761, 1965.

175. Zwaan, J. Genetically Determined Lens Abnormalities. In S. K. Srivastava (Ed.) *Red Blood Cell and Lens Metabolism.* 1980. Amsterdam: Elsevier, Pp. 415–422.

176. Zwaan, J., and Williams, R. M. Cataracts and abnormal proliferation of the lens epithelium in mice carrying the cat FR gene. *Exp. Eye Res.* 8:161, 1969.

177. Zwaan, J., and Williams, R. M. A comparison of lens development in normal mice and in mice with hereditary cataracts (abstract). *Exp. Eye Res.* 8:232, 1969.

14 Ectopia Lentis

Leonard B. Nelson
Irene H. Maumenee

The dislocated lens was probably first described by Berryat in 1749 [40]. A century later the term *ectopia lentis* was introduced by Stellwag to describe congenital dislocations [40]. But it was many years before ectopia lentis became recognized as an important diagnostic clue to the possible presence of other ocular or systemic disorders.

The most significant ocular manifestation of ectopia lentis is a reduction in visual acuity. The amount of visual disturbance varies with the type and degree of dislocation and the presence of associated ocular abnormalities. Minimal subluxation of a lens may cause no visual symptoms. But when the zonules are disrupted, causing increased curvature of the lens, the result may be lenticular myopia and astigmatism. If an eye with a dislocated lens has glaucoma, cataract, or retinal detachment, then the visual consequences are more serious, including permanent loss of vision.

Ectopia lentis continues to be a diagnostic and therapeutic challenge for most ophthalmologists. A thorough systemic and ocular evaluation is necessary to establish the etiology and to initiate the appropriate therapeutic and prophylactic measures. This chapter will review the approach to the patient with ectopia lentis, the differential diagnosis, the possible complications and overall management.

Modified from L. B. Nelson and I. H. Maumenee, Ectopia lentis. *Surv. Ophthalmol.* 27 : 143, 1982.

This work was made possible in part by grants from Fight for Sight, Inc. of New York to the Fight for Sight Children's Eye Center of Wills Eye Hospital, the Children's Eye Care Foundation of Washington, D.C. (Nelson), and grant number EY01773 of the National Eye Institute (Maumenee); and in part by support from the Wills Eye Hospital Research Department. Portions of this chapter were included in a thesis for the American Ophthalmological Association (Maumenee).

DIAGNOSTIC EVALUATION

The diagnosis of ectopia lentis usually requires a thorough evaluation with wide dilatation of the pupil. The lens may be minimally dislocated, bisecting the pupil, totally dislocated into the anterior chamber, or free-floating in the vitreous. An accurate evaluation of the patient with ectopia lentis can usually be made by following a sequential approach, as described in the following paragraphs and outlined in Table 14-1.

Family History

A complete and detailed history from either the patient or the parents should be obtained prior to the ocular evaluation. Specific inquiry should be made as to the possibility of cardiovascular disease and complications, skeletal abnormalities, and visual disturbances. A history of consanguinity, early family deaths, and mental retardation should also be obtained.

Physical Examination

A detailed physical examination of patients with ectopia lentis should be performed by a pediatric or medical consultant. However, there are certain physical signs that may help the ophthalmologist in the diagnostic evaluation. On inspection of the ocular adnexae, a clinical appearance of enophthalmos caused by reduced subcutaneous fat, combined with flat malar areas and hypoplastic facial muscles, gives a characteristic facial "myopathic" appearance. This appearance is often found in patients with the Marfan syndrome. In homocystinuria, the hair is often coarse and lightly colored. A high narrow palate similar to that found in the Marfan syndrome is frequently present.

Table 14-1. *Diagnostic Evaluation*

Family history
Physical examination
Visual acuity
External ocular
    examination
Slit-lamp examination
Retinoscopy and refraction
Ophthalmoscopy
Keratometry readings
Axial length measurements

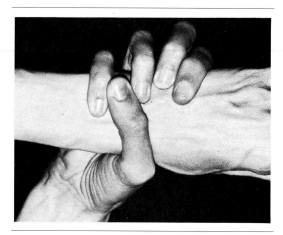

Fig. 14-2. *Overlap of the thumb and fifth finger when clasped around the opposite wrist.*

One should examine the extremities, looking for the particularly short hands and feet of the Weill-Marchesani syndrome or the excessively long and distal limbs (arachnodactyly) of the Marfan syndrome. In the thumb sign, a combination of a narrow hand, long digits, and loose-jointedness allows the thumb to extend well beyond the ulnar surface of the hand (Fig. 14-1) [179]. In the wrist sign, the combination of a thin wrist and long digits results in overlap of the thumb and fifth finger when they clasp the opposite wrist (Fig. 14-2) [191]. Both of these signs are found quite frequently in the Marfan syndrome.

Visual Acuity

Since ectopia lentis is potentially disastrous to visual function, it is important to establish a visual acuity early. It has been our experience that

Fig. 14-1. *Extension of thumb beyond the ulnar surface of the hand.*

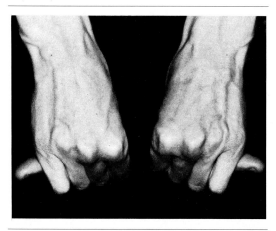

amblyopia is the most common cause for decreased vision in ectopia lentis, and should be treated with occlusion therapy. A careful refraction is of paramount importance. If anisometropia is present, it should be corrected optically. A close follow-up of the visual acuity and/or the binocular fixation pattern is necessary.

External Ocular Examination

The diagnosis of ectopia lentis rests on the observation of a lens that is either (1) out of place or (2) loose. Thus, attention to these two matters is of utmost importance. Phakokinesis is frequently overlooked unless it is specifically sought out as a possible finding. The corneal diameter in the Marfan syndrome is classically increased, giving the appearance of megalocornea [115]. The high incidence of strabismus in patients with ectopia lentis may be explained on the basis of amblyopia.

Slit-Lamp Examination

The slit-lamp examination should include an evaluation of the depth of the anterior chamber and the appearance of the iris and pupil; it should also determine whether transillumination, iridodonesis, or both exist. An evaluation of the lens position and shape before and after dilatation, as well as of the zonular complement, should be performed. It is important to assess the adequacy of the pupillary space for a possible aphakic correction. Phakokinesis can be best observed by having the patient change gaze from one objective of the slit lamp to the other while the examiner views the eye through the lowest power of the slit lamp. Because anomalies of the iridocorneal angle may be present in association with ectopia lentis, a careful gonioscopy is indicated as well.

Retinoscopy and Refraction

Retinoscopy (or examination with a hand-held slit lamp) may be the only way the diagnosis of ectopia lentis can be made in an infant without subjecting the patient to general anesthesia. Using this technique, the edge of the dislocated lens may be identified in the pupillary space.

Retinoscopy may reveal a significant refractive error, usually myopia and astigmatism. Occasionally an accurate refraction may be extremely difficult because of tilting or dislocation of the lens. In these cases an aphakic refraction may be performed. If an aphakic refraction improves visual acuity, then either aphakic contact lenses or spectacles should be considered. We have not hesitated to give aphakic contact lenses or spectacles to children as young as 2 years old in order to achieve development of good visual acuity. In cases where the dislocation is asymmetric in both eyes, it may be advantageous to refract one eye for distance with an aphakia correction and the other eye for near with a phakic correction [130b].

Ophthalmoscopy

Ophthalmoscopy is important in the evaluation of the patient with ectopia lentis. The most deleterious cause of visual reduction in these patients is a retinal detachment. Peripheral retinal findings may include prominent white without pressure, lattice degeneration, and retinal holes. Other retinal abnormalities, such as retinoschisis, optic atrophy, and central retinal artery occlusion, occur less frequently.

Keratometry

A keratometric reading prior to retinoscopy may assist in determining the refraction of these patients. We have found that astigmatism in many patients is mainly corneal. Keratometric readings have been performed on 137 eyes of patients with

the Marfan syndrome [115]. These important findings will be discussed in the section on ocular manifestations of the Marfan syndrome.

Axial Length Measurements

The first histopathologic report on the eyes of a patient with the Marfan syndrome demonstrated extreme size of the globe [51]. Further pathologic reports have confirmed this observation [12, 190]. Axial length measurements have been taken only in the Marfan syndrome [115]. The important prognostic indications of the measurements will be discussed below in the section on the Marfan syndrome.

DIFFERENTIAL DIAGNOSIS

Genetic ectopia lentis has been described in which no other ocular or systemic abnormalities (simple ectopia lentis, either congenital or of delayed onset, and ectopia lentis et pupillae). It may also occur as a common manifestation of systemic hereditary disorders, including Marfan syndrome, homocystinuria, Weill-Marchesani syndrome, hyperlysinemia, and sulfite oxidase deficiency. A number of ocular conditions have been associated with dislocation of the lens, and these are listed in Table 14-2.

Genetic Ectopia Lentis without Systemic Manifestations

SIMPLE ECTOPIA LENTIS

Simple ectopia lentis occurs either as a congenital disorder or as a spontaneous disorder of late onset [60, 189]. Both are inherited in the majority of

Table 14-2. *Ocular Disorders with Ectopia Lentis*

Trauma [91,131]

Retinitis pigmentosa [7,72,74]

Persistent pupillary membrane [37]

Aniridia [22,44a,130a]

Rieger's syndrome [101,105,178]

Megalocornea [92]

Dominantly inherited blepharoptosis and high myopia [68]

Congenital glaucoma

cases as autosomal dominant conditions without associated systemic abnormalities [53]. Recessive inheritance is rare, usually occurring in families in which consanguinity has been documented [53]. The ocular anomaly in simple ectopia lentis is usually manifested as a bilateral, symmetric, upward, and temporal displacement of the lens. Occasionally, the degree of displacement varies considerably between the two eyes.

Spontaneous late subluxation of the lens occurs between the ages of 20 and 65 years [189]. There is often marked irregularity and degeneration of the zonular fibers with subluxation of the lens inferiorly. Herniation of the vitreous associated with zonular degeneration may occur through the zonular defect into the anterior chamber. Both types of ectopia lentis are associated with cataracts and retinal detachment [92]. Glaucoma usually occurs more frequently in spontaneous late subluxation of the lens than in the congenital type [77, 123].

Seland described the changes in the zonular fibers from a patient with congenital simple ectopia lentis [164]. Although the ultrastructure of the lens capsule was normal, it was completely devoid of zonular fibers in most areas. The remaining capsular attachments were underdeveloped. Farnsworth and co-workers examined the lens from a patient who had presumably an identical diagnosis and found similar zonular abnormalities [54]. However, they also found a reduction of the lens fibers to 20 percent of their normal cross-sectional area.

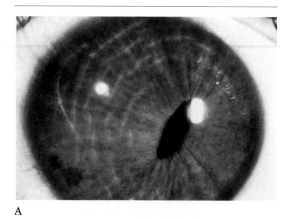

A

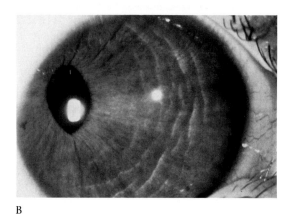

B

Fig. 14-3. *Ectopia lentis et pupillae. Note the eccentrically placed pupil of each eye.*

ECTOPIA LENTIS ET PUPILLAE

Ectopia lentis et pupillae is a rare congenital disorder in which there are combined anomalies of the lens with pupillary displacement (Fig.14-3). In two studies in which ectopia lentis occurred without systemic abnormalities, 81 to 93 percent had simple ectopia lentis and 7 to 19 percent had ectopia lentis et pupillae [34, 109].

The pupils are characteristically oval or slit shaped and ectopic, and they frequently dilate poorly [42]. The condition is usually bilateral, commonly not symmetrical but with the lenses and pupils displaced in the opposite direction from each other. Microspherophakia has been documented histopathologically [108].

Marked transillumination of the iris periphery has been reported in six patients with ectopia lentis et pupillae [108]. We have seen well-documented cases with this condition which do not have iris transillumination. The Marfan syndrome, in which ectopia lentis is commonly present, is another disorder in which iris transillumination has been documented clinically [115]. As with simple ectopia lentis, cataract formation, glaucoma, and retinal detachment can occur.

Ectopia of the lens and pupil follows a recessive mode of inheritance. However, there has been one report suggesting dominant inheritance [108]. Another description of a family showing dominant transmission was clinically atypical for this disorder [192]. Consanguinity is frequently reported [42, 59] or suspected [169].

Systemic Disorders Commonly Associated with Ectopia Lentis

MARFAN SYNDROME

General Comments. The first description of a family with the Marfan syndrome was probably made by an ophthalmologist, Elkanoh Williams, in 1895 [199]. He described several members of a family as having upwardly displaced lenses and generalized loose-jointedness. One patient had a spontaneous unilateral retinal detachment at age 28. The author unfortunately did not include any pictures of the patients, which may explain why his description went largely unnoticed.

The eponym "Marfan syndrome" has been used instead of "Williams syndrome" after Marfan, in 1896, described a 5½-year-old who had long thin extremities [112]. Boerger, a pediatrician, was the first to point out that ectopia lentis is part of the clinical manifestation of this syndrome [12].

The prevalence of the Marfan syndrome is from four to six per 100,000 people, without racial or ethnic predilection [143]. It is an autosomal dominant condition with variable expressivity and it is characterized by skeletal, cardiovascular, and ocular anomalies. Approximately 15 percent of cases have no family history and are presumably derived from a new mutation [143]. An elevated paternal age may be a significant factor in the occurrence of these new mutations. In one study of 23 sporadic cases, there was an increased mean paternal age of almost 7 years [130].

The basic defect of the Marfan syndrome is still unknown. Prockop and Sjoerdsma found an elevated excretion in the urine of hydroxyproline in three patients with the Marfan syndrome [142]. Because hydroxyproline is an amino acid unique to collagen, these findings in the Marfan syndrome may be of fundamental importance, suggesting a primary defect involving collagen. The increased hydroxyproline excretion may indicate increased amounts and a rapid rate of breakdown of soluble collagen.

Subsequently, a higher ratio of soluble to insoluble collagen in skin and fibroblast cultures from Marfan patients has been demonstrated [140]. Several investigators have found a decrease of type I collagen synthesis in aortic explants obtained at surgery for repair of a dissecting aneurysm [73a, 104]. Biochemical evaluation has provided evidence that the increase in soluble collagen is due to a defect in the biosynthesis of type I collagen, resulting from a qualitative and quantitative change

of the $\alpha 2$ chain [159]. The early cross-links of type I collagen require the $\alpha 2$ chain. The alteration of this chain results in increased collagen solubility, decreased collagen linking, and thus a reduction in its overall tensile strength. A low content of type I collagen in the media and adventitia of the aorta causes a reduction in its strength, which is necessary to withstand the pulsating blood pressure from the heart. As a result, the aorta may expand and dilate, leading to the gradual development of an aneurysm.

Recently, reduced tissue levels of dihydroxylysinonorleucine (skin) and 3-hydroxy-pyridinium (aorta) were demonstrated in Marfan patients [12a]. These abnormalities may result in a malalignment of some of the collagen fibrils involving the $\alpha 2$ chain of type I collagen. The defect in the $\alpha 2$ chain may cause a disturbance in the specific intermolecular cross-linking during the organization of type I : III collagens.

Several investigators have demonstrated a decreased content of elastin in the aorta of patients with the Marfan syndrome (1, 74a). Because of the close interrelations between elastin and collagen in the aorta, it is possible that a mutation that alters the function of either of these macromolecules can change the function of the other [141a].

Skeletal Manifestations. Abnormalities of the skeletal system include excessive height caused by increased length of the distal limbs (arachnodactyly), loose-jointedness, scoliosis, and anterior chest deformities. The skeletal proportions demonstrate an increased arm span in relation to body height and an elongated lower segment (pubis to sole) as compared to the upper segment (pubis to vertex) [122, 143]. The absolute height is not as important as the patient's relative height given the family background. These patients tend to be the tallest in their families.

Scoliosis is often severe and the most disabling skeletal complication. It generally worsens rapidly during the adolescent growth spurt. An attempt has been made to shorten this rapid growth to prevent progression of scoliosis and to reduce body height. In female patients, this reduction requires the administration of estrogen on a daily basis with progesterone for 5 days each month to prevent dysfunctional bleeding [170]. No conclusive data are available yet to show whether this therapy is effective. Other forms of therapy, all having varied success, include mechanical bracing with physical therapy and spinal fusion [156].

dren, may be caused by reduced or absent retrobulbar fat. Many patients present with a facial diopulmonary compromise. The age when the pectus excavatum can be repaired and the long-term results have not been established.

Cardiovascular Manifestations. The major cardiovascular complications of aortic dilatation, dissecting aortic aneurysm, and "floppy mitral valve" were first described clearly in 1943 [4, 52]. The vascular tissues mainly involved are those under high vasodynamic stress, such as the ascending aorta and the mitral valves. The aortic dilatation usually begins at the base and may be progressive. This simulates the course seen in syphilitic aortitis [122].

Magnetic resonance imaging can serve as the initial imaging test in clinically suspected cases of aortic dissection, and the information provided is sufficient to manage many cases [1b]. Additionally, magnetic resonance obviates the use of iodinated contrast media.

The average life expectancy is halved in the Marfan syndrome. In over 95 percent of the cases in which a cause of death can be established, a cardiovascular problem is at fault [129]. An echocardiogram should be obtained annually [143]. If aortic dilatation is demonstrated, prophylactic propranolol is recommended to reduce myocardial contractility in an attempt to stay progression of aortic dilatation and to prevent acute dissection of the aorta [143]. Although the initial trials of propranolol treatment were disappointing (partly because they were begun too late in the aortic disease process [133]), new randomized prospective protocols have begun [143]. Finally, improved prosthesis and surgical techniques for the cardiovascular complications have lowered the morbidity and mortality [36a, 45].

Patients with the Marfan syndrome are at increased risk of endocarditis and should receive antibiotic prophylaxis with dental or surgical procedures [13, 203]. It is recommended by some investigators that patients not participate in contact sports, isometric exercises, and weight lifting [143]. Since there apparently is an increased risk of vascular rupture during and shortly after pregnancy, women with echocardiographic evidence of aortic dilatation are advised against pregnancy [56a, 143, 143a].

Ocular Manifestations. An appearance of enophthalmos, especially in severely affected chil-

Corrections of the deformity of the anterior thorax should be performed only if there is car-"myopathic" appearance as a result of reduced subcutaneous fat, flat malar areas, hypoplastic facial muscles, and some degree of frontal bossing.

In the young age group, reduced visual acuity often results from delayed and inadequate refraction with the inevitable development of amblyopia, which is often bilateral. Among the Marfan patients there is a much wider distribution of refractive power, as well as a higher proportion of extreme refractive errors, than is found in the normal population [115]. Moderate-to-high myopia, however, is most frequently seen.

The corneal diameter may be increased, measuring up to 14 mm without incidence of increased intraocular pressure [115, 180]. The iris morphology is often striking. The anterior iris surface is commonly homogeneous with a decreased number of circumferential ridges, furrows, and crypts; thus it has a smooth, velvety appearance [1]. Iris transillumination, more marked at its base, occurs in approximately 10 percent of patients [115]. Commonly the pupil is miotic and difficult to dilate; occasionally, it is eccentric.

The presence of angle abnormalities—bridging pectinate strands, inconspicuous Schwalbe's line, and irregularity and fraying of the iris root—has been described by several investigators [17, 188]. These angle changes, however, are not pathognomonic of the Marfan syndrome because they have been found in a variety of connective-tissue disorders [19], as well as in the normal population. Gonioscopy will help demonstrate iridodonesis even if it is not appreciated on slit-lamp examination.

Ectopia lentis occurs in 50 to 80 percent of patients with the Marfan syndrome [43, 82, 115, 122]. It is almost always bilateral and symmetrical. Usually the amount of dislocation is stable from early childhood. In 193 eyes of Marfan patients with ectopia lentis, progression was personally observed in 7.5 percent [115].

The direction of dislocation is most commonly superotemporal (Fig. 14-4). The lens may be dislocated slightly backwards, as well as vertically and horizontally. This leaves a gap between the pupillary border and the anterior lens surface. In patients with even marked dislocation of the lens, a numerically good zonular complement can often be observed in the area of dislocation. This finding corresponds to the surgical observation that the zonular fibers do not break readily if a subluxed lens in a Marfan patient has to be removed. Chem-

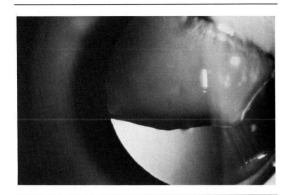

Fig. 14-4. *Superotemporal dislocation of the lens in a Marfan patient. Note the parallel alignment of the zonular fibers.*

ical studies to date have shown no evidence of collagen in the zonules [181a]. The deficiency in collagen cross-linking demonstrated in the aorta of Marfan patients does not help to explain lens dislocation in this disorder.

Myopic changes and retinal detachments are the two main retinal findings in Marfan patients. The choroid may be thin with various degrees of scleral crescents. Posterior staphylomata are uncommon in the Marfan patient. One patient with an anterior intercalary staphyloma required a scleral graft [70]. The peripheral retinal changes include lattice degeneration and retinal holes. In eyes with dislocated lenses, retinal detachments have occurred both spontaneously and following intraocular surgery [31, 43, 91].

Keratometric readings in a large series of Marfan patients demonstrated flatter corneas than are normal [115]. The steepest corneal curve often corresponds to the direction of the dislocation of the lens. Marfan patients with dislocated lenses had much flatter corneas than those without ectopia lentis. Also, patients who developed retinal detachments showed a trend towards more marked flattening of the cornea [115].

The mean axial length measurements for Marfan patients without ectopia lentis was 23.39 mm and for those with dislocation, 25.96 mm. The mean axial length of patients with a retinal detachment was 28.47 mm, versus a mean of 24.90 mm for all Marfan patients with or without dislocation of the lens but without a retinal detachment. Finally, no patient with a normal axial length developed a spontaneous retinal detachment [115].

Few histopathologic studies of the eyes of Marfan patients have been reported [51, 110, 147, 150].

Hypopigmentation of the posterior iris pigment epithelial layer was first observed by Dvorak-Theobald [51] and was confirmed by Ramsey and co-workers [147]. This histopathological finding helps explain the clinical observation of iris transillumination in the Marfan patient [110]. The iris has been demonstrated histologically to lack the usual circumferential ridges, furrows, and crypts and to have widespread patchy hypoplasia of the dilator muscle [147, 150]. The sparsely developed dilator muscle seems to account for the poor dilatation of the pupil.

The zonules and ciliary epithelium may appear normal by light microscopy [147]. However, on scanning electron microscopy, widespread separation of the zonular fibers into a fan of filaments with attenuation towards the lens capsule has been demonstrated. A second scanning electron microscopic evaluation showed abnormally large and grossly granular capsular fibers and zonular fibrils [55]. However, the zonular fibrils maintained the normal parallel orientation.

Abnormalities of the chamber angle include pectinate ligaments, interpreted as incomplete separation of iris and trabecular meshwork and scarcity of the circular fibers of the ciliary body. Anomalies in the outflow channel consist of changes in the configuration, size, and position of Schlemm's canal [18, 51, 150].

The most striking feature of the Marfan syndrome on many pathologic evaluations is the extreme size of the globe [1a, 51, 190]. Although there may be an extremely thin choroid and sclera, a staphyloma has not been demonstrated histopathologically. The common finding of ocular enlargement in histopathologic cases is consistent with the clinical findings obtained by axial length measurements [115].

HOMOCYSTINURIA

General Comments. Homocystinuria is an inborn error of metabolism of the sulfur-containing amino acids. Carson and Neill first detected homocystinuria using urine chromatography in patients with ectopia lentis while systematically searching for metabolic abnormalities in mentally retarded institutionalized individuals in Northern Ireland [25, 27]. Simultaneously and independently, Gerritsen and associates [64, 65] in Madison, Wisconsin, found the same metabolic defect in an infant thought to have cerebral palsy.

The frequency of the condition is about 0.021 percent in the mentally retarded, 0.17 percent in

Table 14-4. *Causes of Homocystinuria*

Cystathionine-B-synthetase deficiency [126]
  Pyridoxine responsive [5,63]
  Pyridoxine unresponsive [86,134,167]
N-5-methyltetrahydrofolate-homocysteine
  methyltransferase deficiency [84,106]
N-5-10-methyltetrahydrofolate reductase deficiency
  [61,168]
Secondary to treatment with 6-azauridine [88]

the mentally retarded with ocular abnormalities, and about 5 percent of all cases with nontraumatic dislocated lenses [176]. While screening 41,800 well babies, one case of homocystinuria was detected [197].

Homocystinuria is an autosomal recessive condition. Like the Marfan syndrome, it is characterized by skeletal, cardiovascular, and ocular abnormalities. Mental retardation occurs in approximately 50 percent of cases and may be progressive. Homocystinuria with recurrent episodes of pyridoxine- and folic-acid responsive, "schizophrenic-like" behavior was documented in a mildly retarded adolescent girl [61]. It is one of three hereditary systemic disorders associated with ectopia lentis that can be diagnosed biochemically. (Hyperlysinemia and sulfate oxidase deficiency are the others.)

Homocysteine is not normally detected in either urine or plasma. Cystathionine-β-synthase deficiency is the most common cause of homocystinuria. However, homocystinuria may be a manifestation of several other enzyme deficiencies in the same metabolic pathways (Table 14-4). The important biochemical pathways are illustrated in Figure 14-5.

The sodium-nitroprusside test is used to screen for homocysteine in the urine. In the test, 5 ml of urine is mixed with 2 ml of 5% sodium cyanide. After 10 minutes, two to four drops of 5% sodium nitroprusside are added, which causes a bright red color in the presence of homocysteine or cystine. Because the test will be positive in many conditions in which sulfur-containing metabolites are excreted, such as cystinuria, urine chromatography or high-voltage electrophoresis is necessary for a definitive diagnosis. The silver-nitroprusside test is more specific for homocysteine or cystine.

Thrombotic vascular occlusions constitute the main threat to survival in patients with homocystinuria. However, the pathophysiologic mechanism of homocystinuric thrombotic tendency remains unsettled. The platelets may be involved in the pathogenesis of this disorder. Increased platelet adhesiveness was produced by adding

Fig. 14-5. *Biochemical reactions in homocysteine metabolism. Several of the involved enzymes are indicated by numbers: (1) methionine adenosyltransferase; (2) betaine-homocysteine methyltransferase; (3) N-5-methyltetrahydrofolate-homocysteine methyltransferase; (4) N-5-10-methylene tetra-hydrofolate reductase; (5) cystathionine-β-synthetase; (6) cystathionase. (Modified from G. L. Spaeth, The usefulness of pyridoxine in the treatment of homocystinuria: A review of postulated mechanisms of action and a new hypothesis.* Birth Defects *12:347, 1976.)*

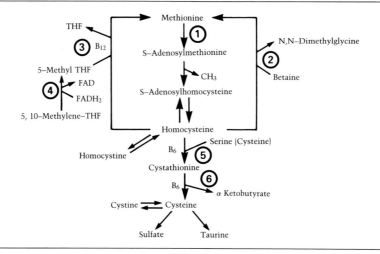

homocystine to normal whole blood in vitro in concentrations similar to those found in the blood of patients with homocystinuria [118]. Since this study, several reports have confirmed the abnormally increased adhesiveness of the platelets [6, 35]. Others have indicated the platelets to be normally adhesive [33, 80].

Platelet kinetics in patients with homocystinuria have demonstrated discrepant results. Harker and colleagues noted a decrease in platelet survival and an increase in platelet consumption using [51]Crplatelets in four homocystinuric patients [76]. By experimental induction of homocystinuria in baboons, the authors showed the formation of platelet thrombi on altered nonendothelialized vascular surfaces. The chronic injury to endothelium by homocystine seems to have created the conditions for early atherosclerotic lesions. Two subsequent studies have found the platelet survival to be within normal limits in patients with homocystinuria [81, 185]. Apart from such factors as genetic heterogeneity or differences in plasma homocysteine levels, the discrepancy in platelet survival time may be due to differences in methods of investigation.

Homocystine has been demonstrated to accelerate clotting in vitro [149]. This was shown to occur through the activation of the Hageman factor, which has the capacity to initiate clotting. It was suggested that perhaps the strategically localized deposition of homocysteine in the intima of blood vessels may be responsible for the unusual frequency of thrombosis in the homocystinuric patient.

Finally, homocysteine may produce changes in the arteries and other connective tissues by altering the state of aggregation and the normal fibrillar structure of proteoglycan molecules [117]. The effect of homocysteine on proteoglycan synthesis has been considered to be an important factor in the initiation of arteriosclerotic lesions, but little evidence has been accumulated to support this hypothesis.

One treatment of homocystinuria to correct the metabolic defect has involved a low-methionine and high-cystine diet, which has not been uniformly successful [14, 24, 26, 50, 134]. This diet has not only failed to normalize completely the abnormal biochemical findings, but it is difficult to prescribe (all eggs, meat, and cow's milk are forbidden) [6]. When this diet is prescribed to infants, failure to gain weight may be a serious complication [135].

Another approach to therapy is the supplementation with coenzymes. Pyridoxine (vitamin B_6) is the coenzyme necessary to activate the enzyme cystathionine-β-synthetase, which is the most common enzymatic deficiency in homocystinuric patients [125]. Barber and Spaeth were the first to demonstrate that certain homocystinuric patients respond biochemically to oral pyridoxine by lowering plasma homocysteine and methionine concentrations [5]. Some authors have confirmed the beneficial effect of pyridoxine [62, 63], while others have not [63, 126]. Approximately half of the cases seem to respond biochemically to pyridoxine [174]. The effect of pyridoxine follows a dose-response curve; some cases which are unresponsive at low doses will respond when given up to 500 mg daily [6]. It may be that some of the unresponsive cases would respond to doses larger than those presently employed.

In one of our patients, homocystinuria was detected at birth by the sodium-nitroprusside test, with later proof by chromatography. She had the test performed at that time because two older siblings had confirmed homocystinuria, one with a dislocated lens in the anterior chamber requiring extraction. At age 3 days, our patient was started on pyridoxine. She is now 23 years old with normal intelligence (recent college graduate), moderate myopia, and mild generalized osteoporosis. There has been no evidence of ectopia lentis or a previous thromboembolic episode.

Because elevated homocysteine may cause vascular injury with secondary platelet thromboemboli, a rational approach to prevent this phenomenon is necessary. In the homocystinuric patient who is unresponsive to pyridoxine, the use of a combination of antiplatelet utilization drugs, dipyridamole, and acetylsalicylic acid may provide protection against thrombus formation [76].

Recently betaine has been used in the treatment of homocystinuria that is not responsive to pyridoxine [171a, 197a]. All patients had a substantial decrease in plasma total homocystemia levels. There were also striking clinical changes after betaine treatments in some patients. Further clinical trial with betaine in patients with homocystinuria are still necessary.

Anesthesia may present significant risks to the homocystinuric patient [15, 39, 151]. Besides the phenomenon of frequent episodes of thromboemboli, the homocystinuric patient may develop hypoglycemia secondary to hyperinsulinemia [85]. It is postulated that the pancreatic islet cell is sensitive to the hypermethionemia associated with homocystinuria and causes hypoglycemia by inducing hyperinsulinemia. Finally, it is probably best to avoid drugs that may predispose to a hypercoagulable state, such as oral contraceptives [154].

Skeletal Manifestations. Excessive height and low ratio of upper segment to lower segment are common skeletal findings in the homocystinuric patient [161]. These findings are similar to those of the Marfan syndrome. Generalized osteoporosis with vertebral collapse, scoliosis, deformities of the anterior chest, and a modest degree of limitation of joint mobility are other skeletal anomalies in homocystinuria [122]. Many of the patients have a toes-out "Charlie Chaplin" gait.

Cardiovascular Manifestations. The etiology of cardiovascular disease in homocystinuria involves intimal and endothelial changes, disruption of the elastic lamillae, and partial or complete obstruction of all-size vessels in various organs [26, 67, 98, 161]. Cardiac murmurs, cardiomegaly, and hypertension are often present. Fatal coronary occlusion has occurred in several adolescents, with one described in an 11-year-old [23]. Thrombosis in the arteries is manifested by arterial bruits, loss of pulses, and ischemic symptoms. Acute gangrene of the leg requiring amputation occurred in an 18-year-old homocystinuric patient [58]. Dilatation of the aorta, which is commonly found in the Marfan syndrome, is not a characteristic cardiac abnormality in patients with homocystinuria.

Ocular Manifestations. Ectopia lentis is the ocular hallmark of homocystinuria and can be detected in approximately 90% of patients [43, 175]. The dislocation is bilateral and symmetrical, with the lens usually migrating either inferiorly or inferonasally (Fig. 14-6). The lens in homocystinuria is much more mobile than in the Marfan syndrome. This may be related to the clinical observation of progressive irregularity of the zonular fibers and the appearance of a fringe of white zonular remnants at the equator of the lens and on the surface of the ciliary body [145, 146].

Ectopia lentis is an acquired and progressive abnormality in this disorder. The earliest detection of ectopia lentis was in a 3-year-old [122]. It was not recognized in another patient until 28 years of age [35]. Myopia is common and may

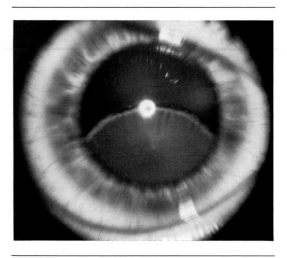

Fig. 14-6. *Inferior dislocation of the lens in a homocystinuric patient. Note the absence of most zonular fibers.*

precede the detection of ectopia lentis by several years [103]. The development of progressive lenticular myopia is often the first sign of a lens dislocation.

The concentration of cystine, an amino acid, may be low in the urine and plasma of homocystinuric patients [174a]. Zonular fibers normally have a high content of cystine [71a]. In homocystinuria, a deficiency of cystine may affect normal zonular development and consequently predispose to lens dislocation [3, 175].

Although microphthalmos has been reported in homocystinuria, no axial length measurements were taken [3, 139]. Most patients have blue irides. Aniridia was reported in one case, in which the mother and brother of the patient also had aniridia [138, 139]. Albinism was described in seven patients, although a detailed description was not provided [3].

Retinal detachment is usually a complication of lens surgery, although it may occur spontaneously [43]. Optic atrophy has been observed, usually on the basis of glaucoma [138, 175]. Reports on the changes in the retinal vasculature are limited. Wilson and Ruiz described a 6-year-old boy with homocystinuria who developed acute glaucoma and later revealed bilateral central retinal artery occlusions with optic disc pallor [200]. Another homocystinuric patient demonstrated sclerotic changes of a retinal artery that may well have represented a branch arterial occlusion [128].

Henkind and Ashton first reported the histo-

Table 14-5. *Systemic Features of the Marfan Syndrome, Homocystinuria, and the Weill-Marchesani Syndrome*

Systemic feature	Marfan syndrome	Homocystinuria	Weill-Marchesani syndrome
Inheritance	Autosomal dominant	Autosomal recessive	Unsettled but probably autosomal recessive
Skeletal	Arachnodactyly Joint laxity Sternal deformity	Occasional arachnodactyly Osteoporosis Sternal deformity	Stocky build Short digits Tight joints Brachycephaly
Vascular	Dilatation and/or dissection of aorta. Aortic and mitral valve disease	Dilatation with thrombosis in medium-sized arteries and veins	None
Mental retardation	Absent	Frequent	Absent
Skin	Striae distensae	Malar flush Livedo reticulosis	None
Gait	Normal	"Charlie Chaplin" gait	Normal

pathologic ocular findings in four eyes of three homocystinuric patients [79]. They found the zonular fibers deficient adjacent to the lens. There zonules had recoiled to the surface of the ciliary body and were matted and retracted into a felt-work that fused with a greatly thickened basement membrane of the nonpigmented epithelium.

The greatly thickened basement membrane overlying the ciliary body in homocystinuria has subsequently been shown by electron microscopy to be composed of degenerate zonular material [148]. In addition, Ramsey and co-workers noted that the degree of zonular abnormality was related to age; the younger the patient, the more normal appeared the zonular fragments composed of oriented filaments [148].

WEILL-MARCHESANI SYNDROME

General Comments. In 1932, Weill found, among eight cases with presumed Marfan syndrome, a patient who was short in stature and had "short swollen fingers" with limited range of motion [195]. Seven years later, Marchesani recognized the combination of short fingers (brachydactyly) and microspherophakia as a syndrome [111]. The Weill-Marchesani syndrome is rarer than either the Marfan syndrome or homocystinuria. Mental retardation is not a characteristic of this disorder and no metabolic defect has been found (Table 14-5).

Although the Weill-Marchesani syndrome is

unequivocally familial, the precise hereditary pattern remains unclear. Among parents and relatives, various features such as brachydactyly and short stature have been described, suggesting an autosomal dominant mode of inheritance [102, 141, 177]. One family with successive generations of presumed Weill-Marchesani syndrome was reinvestigated by McKusick and shown to represent a generally short-statured family with simple autosomal dominant ectopia lentis [119, 120, 122]. The syndrome has also been considered to be a recessive disorder with partial expression in the heterozygote. The high rate of consanguinity in this syndrome supports the latter pattern of inheritance [48, 124, 204].

Skeletal Manifestations. The skeletal features of the Weill-Marchesani patient are the antithesis of those found in the Marfan patient. Weill-Marchesani patients are short, with a large thorax and stubby spade-like hands with increased subcutaneous tissue. The head is often brachycephalic with a depressed nasal bridge. Many of the patients have marked limitation of mobility upon both active and passive motion of their fingers and wrists. Seeleman described the fingers and toes of a 3-year-old boy as capable of only minimal flexion [163]. Generalized joint stiffness and reduced mobility are also commonly observed in these patients [152].

Ocular Manifestations. Although lenticular abnormalities may be absent in the Marfan syndrome and homocystinuria, the presence of mi-

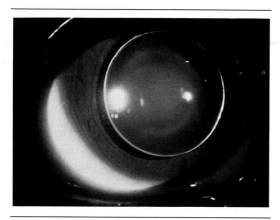

Fig. 14-7. *Microspherophakic lens following dilatation in a Weill-Marchesani patient. Note the central position with identification of the lens edge. (Courtesy of the Scheie Eye Institute Library).*

crospherophakia is considered a prerequisite to the diagnosis of the Weill-Marchesani syndrome (Fig. 14-7)[94]. Microspherophakia, however, may occur as an isolated familial anomaly in either an autosomal dominant or a recessive pattern [96]. It has also been described in a pedigree of primordial dwarfism with features unlike those of the Weill-Marchesani syndrome [121]. Microspherophakia has been reported in association with such systemic syndromes as the Marfan syndrome and homocystinuria [43], Alport's syndrome [172], and Klinefelter's syndrome [10].

Microspherophakia is commonly present prior to dislocation of the lens [94]. It may be progressive and responsible for the significant myopia that develops in these patients. Jones described two children whose myopia progressed by 7 and 15 diopters within one year as the lens of each gradually assumed a more spherical shape [97].

The lens may maintain a central position with identification of its equator following dilatation. With time, subluxation of the lens develops, usually in an inferior direction. In one series, the frequency of ectopia lentis was approximately 84 percent; 18.2 years was the mean age at diagnosis [94]. The zonules, which frequently appear abnormally elongated and lax, may contribute to the development of spherophakia and ectopia lentis [31]. However, there is no histologic evidence to confirm this clinical observation. The overall lenticular mass itself has been shown to be reduced by approximately 25 percent [94].

The elongated zonules do permit the lens to move forward, increasing its area of contact with

the iris [187]. The sequence of progressive shallowing of the anterior chamber eventually results in pupillary-block glaucoma. The observation, in which miotics increase the pupillary block whereas mydriatics relieve it, was referred to as "inverse glaucoma" by Urbanek [186] and has since been confirmed by others [11, 83, 95, 165, 198].

Parasympathomimetic agents cause contraction of the ciliary muscle and further loosening of the zonules support. Cycloplegic agents, on the other hand, relax the ciliary muscle, which results in tightening of the zonular support and posterior movement of the lens. If a miotic does not cause a rise in pressure in the microspherophakic eye, then it may be assumed that the lens is dislocated, with a poor zonular complement [11]. Recently Wright and Chrousos reported a case of cyclopentolate-induced bilateral acute-angled closure glaucoma associated with the Weill-Marchesani syndrome without lens subluxation [202a]. The mechanism of the cyclopentolate-induced glaucoma, proposed by the authors, was most likely due to mid-dilatation, which caused a relaxation of peripheral iris. This allowed the peripheral iris to bow anteriorly, closing an already crowded angle.

Feiler-Ofry and co-workers described a family with abnormalities of the anterior chamber angles, one of which had the Weill-Marchesani syndrome with glaucoma [56]. These chamber angle anomalies, which include bridging pectinate strands, numerous iris processes, fraying of the iris root, and anomalous angle vessels, have been described in other disorders of connective tissue and, therefore, are not specific for this disorder [19]. Other ocular abnormalities rarely reported in the Weill-Marchesani syndrome include megalocornea [97], eccentric pupil [144], nonspecific chorioretinal degeneration [144], and scleral staphyloma [107].

HYPERLYSINEMIA

Hyperlysinemia is a rare disorder due to an inborn error of metabolism of the essential amino acid lysine [202]. The diagnosis is made by demonstration of elevated plasma levels of lysine using paper chromatography [162] and is confirmed by either ion exchange [173] or spectrophotometric methods [47]. Lysine-ketoglutamate reductase, which converts lysine to saccharopine, was found to be reduced considerably in patients with hyperlysinemia [44]. The role of lysine metabolism in the extraocular muscles, zonules, and nervous tissue is incomplete. Therefore, the pathogenesis of the associated anomalies in hyperlysinemia is unknown.

There are seven recorded cases of this metabolic disorder with some clinical findings in common. Four of the patients had profound mental retardation and three had hypotonic muscles. Consanguinity was commonly reported, suggesting a recessive mode of inheritance [2, 66, 171].

Ocular abnormalities have been found in two patients with hyperlysinemia. One patient had bilateral subluxated lenses and lateral rectus muscle paresis and another had bilateral spherophakia [171]. Neither patient had any systemic abnormalities, which casts doubt on the possibility of a single gene defect. Although more patients are needed to prove that these ocular findings may be the result of the same gene that causes hyperlysinemia, they should be considered in the differential diagnosis of ectopia lentis.

SULFITE OXIDASE DEFICIENCY

Sulfite oxidase deficiency is an extremely rare metabolic disorder in sulfur metabolism that leads to increased urinary excretion of S-sulfocysteine, taurine, sulfite, and thiosulfate [9, 89, 166]. A deficiency of sulfite oxidase activity, resulting in an inability to convert sulfite to sulfate, has been considered responsible for abnormal urinary metabolites and an inability to excrete inorganic sulfate [127]. The metabolic defect responsible for loss of enzyme activity may be due to low hepatic levels of the molybdenum cofactor [95a]. A diagnosis may be made by finding an increased urinary thiosulfate through quantitative determination and the presence of S-sulfocysteine by means of two-dimensional separation of urinary amino acids [89].

The main clinical features of the three reported cases of sulfite oxidase deficiency are the involvement of the central nervous system and the development of ectopia lentis. One patient was born with neurological abnormalities including severe mental retardation and seizures. The patient deteriorated to a virtually decorticate state by 9 months [89]. Bilateral ectopia lentis was discovered when the patient was 1 year old. Another patient demonstrated similar neurologic abnormalities at birth, except that ectopia lentis was noted at 3 weeks of age [9]. The third patient was normal until 18 months of age, when the neurologic symptoms developed; ectopia lentis was

not diagnosed until the patient was 4 years old. Sulfite oxidase deficiency was demonstrated in cultured skin fibroblasts from one patient whose parents both had intermediate levels of enzyme activity [166]. This observation indicates a genetic basis of the disorder and suggests an autosomal recessive inheritance pattern.

The progressive neurologic abnormalities in sulfite oxidase deficiency have been investigated. The neuropathology of one patient demonstrated cortical atrophy, which was most severe in the parietal area [158]. Histologic changes showed severe and widespread loss of neurons, myelin, and axons, with surrounding glial proliferation. When S-sulfocysteine was injected into rat brain, neuronal degeneration and swelling of dendritic processes were induced [132]. Although the mechanism of brain damage and ectopia lentis remains unknown, the association of these two findings should alert the ophthalmologist to the possibility of this rare syndrome.

Ocular Disorders with Ectopia Lentis

There are various ocular disorders that have been reported to occur with ectopia lentis. The most common is ocular trauma, which was the cause of ectopia lentis in 53 percent of cases in one series [91]. In other series, the incidence of trauma resulting in a displaced lens ranged from 22 to 56 percent [131]. Most of the other associated ocular disorders are cited in individual case reports, some of which lack adequate clinical and laboratory information. These ocular disorders include retinitis pigmentosa [7, 72, 74], persistent pupillary membrane [37], aniridia [22, 44a, 130a], Rieger's syndrome, [101, 105, 178], megalocornea [92], and dominantly inherited blepharoptosis, high myopia, and ectopia lentis [68]. We have observed ectopia lentis in several patients with congenital glaucoma.

Systemic Disorders with Rarely Associated Ectopia Lentis

Ectopia lentis has been associated with other systemic disorders. It was described in a Marfan-like syndrome with hyaloideoretinal degeneration [36]. Syphilitics have been found to have dislocated lenses, often with a history of trauma [71, 157a, 170a]. Whether the treponemal infection or the trauma directly affects the zonules is not clear. Other systemic diseases in which ectopia lentis has rarely been reported include Sturge-Weber syndrome [46, 57], mandibulofacial dysostosis [100], Ehlers-Danlos syndrome [183, 184], Crouzon's syndrome [136], Refsum's syndrome [99], and scleroderma [155]. We have observed ectopia lentis in a patient with the Kniest syndrome. It seems unlikely that ectopia lentis would escape detection in a majority of these conditions. In our 55 patients with Ehlers-Danlos syndrome, and the 22 with Crouzon's syndrome, not one had a dislocated lens. However, it would be advantageous to obtain dilated slit-lamp examinations on more of these patients to document the presence of a displaced lens.

COMPLICATIONS

The patient with ectopia lentis may be followed for many years without significant ocular problems. However, ocular complications associated with displacement of the lens are unfortunately frequent and often serious. The associated abnormalities include amblyopia, uveitis, glaucoma, cataract formation, and retinal detachment.

Ectopia lentis may cause visual symptoms that vary in severity, depending on the position of the lens. The lens may remain in its normal central position, dislocated slightly backwards, with minimal refractive error. Lenticular myopia may result from increased curvature of the lens because of relaxation of or poor complement of the zonules. A displaced lens may be tilted, causing a significant myopia and astigmatism which are difficult to correct optically. Finally, if the lens is sufficiently displaced so that it occupies only a portion of the pupillary aperture, an aphakic correction will be necessary. These refractive errors in ectopia lentis may play a role in the development of amblyopia [69, 87]. Therefore, early and careful refraction is necessary to avoid the occurrence of amblyopia.

Uveitis may occur in ectopia lentis by two different mechanisms. Iridocyclitis, the most common complication in one series of displaced lenses, may be due to contact irritation of the ciliary body or iris [131]. This type of uveitis is often acute, temporary, and recurrent and is usually responsive to topical steroids. A posterior dislocation is usually well tolerated for years, provided the lens capsule does not become permeable or rupture, allowing lens protein to escape [116]. If this occurs, a phacolytic uveitis with or without a secondary glaucoma may result, requiring a cataract extraction [30, 90].

Glaucoma is a common and often serious complication of ectopia lentis. The mechanism of glaucoma in these eyes varies greatly. In post-traumatic cases, glaucoma is frequently caused by a post-concussion deformity characterized by degeneration and sclerosis of the ciliary body and trabeculae and recession of the iris root [157, 201]. These pathologic findings indicate that glaucoma is not caused directly by the displaced lens and that it would have occurred in these traumatized eyes even if the lens had not dislocated. Glaucoma may result from outflow obstruction by chronic inflammatory cells from a lens-induced uveitis [78], macrophages from a phacolytic glaucoma [29, 30], pigment particles released by trauma [49], or vitreous forced into the anterior chamber angle [32]. Finally, it may occur from pupillary block, as described in the Weill-Marchesani syndrome, or by dislocation of the lens into the anterior chamber. Iridectomy is often the treatment of choice; it can prevent or cure the pupillary block glaucoma and simultaneously provide a clear optical area.

Although the lens in ectopia lentis may remain clear for many years, the gradual development of a cataract is frequent. The lens opacity may be partial or complete with eventual morgagnian changes if it becomes totally dislocated posteriorly in the vitreous. Besides causing a visual disturbance, a hypermature cataract may also be responsible for phacolytic glaucoma [116].

Retinal detachments are common and often disastrous complications in the eye with ectopia lentis. They have been reported spontaneously in cases of congenital dislocation of the lens regardless of surgery [16, 28, 205]. Jensen and Cross described retinal detachments in the Marfan syndrome and homocystinuria only in eyes with aphakia or ectopia lentis [93]. However, they found no significant difference in the frequency of retinal detachment before or after lens surgery. Treatment of retinal detachment is often difficult because the dislocated lens may interfere with visualization of areas of degeneration or tears responsible for the condition. Jarrett found that of 38 retinal detachments in a series of 166 cases of ectopia lentis, only 14 were successfully repaired [91].

MANAGEMENT

Ectopia lentis continues to be a perplexing management problem for the ophthalmologist. Emphasis should be directed toward improvement of vision and the preservation of the globe through prevention or amelioration of complications. Trauma may precede the migration of a previously subluxated lens into the anterior chamber or vitreous. These patients more commonly have retinal detachments following trauma; therefore, they should be advised against participation in contact sports [41].

The patient with ectopia lentis may have one of the hereditary disorders with potentially serious systemic abnormalities. Hence it is mandatory for the ophthalmologist to refer all these patients to the appropriate pediatric or medical consultant for evaluation. If one of the hereditary disorders is discovered, then the family must be counseled about the risks of having subsequent affected children. It is important that all relatives at risk be identified and have a thorough examination.

Early diagnosis of ectopia lentis, with the proper optical correction either through a phakic or aphakic zone of the pupillary area, may decrease the incidence of amblyopia. If the edge of the subluxated lens crosses the pupil, a patient may use the aphakic part for distance and the phakic for near vision. Manipulation of the iris may be necessary to create a larger area for an aphakic correction. A mydriatic instilled at regular intervals may improve the vision and also test whether a surgical or laser manipulation of the iris is worthwhile. If chronic mydriasis is difficult, as in the Marfan patient with a hypoplastic iris dilator muscle, then an optical iridectomy may increase the aphakic pupillary space adequately [196].

Straatsma and associates have used photocoagulation of the iris to provide a larger pupillary opening [181]. We have also successfully used the argon laser. However, a long-term follow-up of these patients is necessary to determine whether this method of creating a larger pupillary opening is satisfactory.

The treatment of glaucoma in ectopia lentis depends on the type of glaucoma present. In pupillary block due to microspherophakia, peripheral iridectomy has been suggested as the safest procedure [31]. However, surgical complications are common with frequent vitreous loss because of the lack of protection of the vitreous face by the lens periphery. Laser iridectomy, preferably performed prior to the development of glaucoma, has been proposed as a safer treatment [153]. This may be combined with thymoxamine [153], a specific α-adrenergic blocking agent [194]. Thymoxamine causes miosis with little or no effect on

ciliary muscle [73], depth of the anterior chamber [182], or facility of outflow [193]. Finally, a lens in the anterior chamber should be vigorously treated initially with cycloplegic and mydriatic agents that may relieve the pupillary block and allow the lens to fall back behind the iris [51a, 77, 206]. Massage on the cornea through a closed lid may help the lens return to its original position. These maneuvers should be attempted prior to surgical intervention, especially in patients with homocystinuria who are at increased risk with general anesthesia.

Lens surgery in ectopia lentis can be difficult and may lead to both intraoperative and postoperative complications. One author feels that the mere presence of a subluxated lens is reason to remove it [8], while others feel that specific indications are necessary [20, 31, 75, 88a, 115]. These indications for lens surgery include [1] the presence of a lens in the anterior chamber, especially with lens touch of the corneal endothelium, [2] a lens opacity that is mature or hypermature, [3] evidence of lens-induced uveitis, [4] an inadequate visual acuity that is uncorrectable by refraction and iris manipulation, and [5] imminent complete luxation of the lens. Only the first three are true indications.

The surgical techniques for the removal of a dislocated lens are numerous and there is much disagreement about which procedure is the most desirable. In one method, a double-pronged needle is passed through the pars plana to trap and support the dislocated lens [21]. The lens is then removed with capsule forceps or an erysiphake. This procedure involves much manipulation and may be traumatic to the eye; it can no longer be recommended.

Open-sky vitrectomy with successful cryoextraction of 22 dislocated lenses has been reported [38]. Included in the series were patients with the Marfan syndrome, homocystinuria, and simple ectopia lentis. In 21 cases, the dislocated lenses were removed intracapsularly. In the other case, the lens nucleus had been dislocated in a previous operation and secondary glaucoma had developed. The authors state that all patients had "useful vision" postoperatively. A long-term follow-up of these patients is needed.

Jensen and Cross reported the results of surgery on 115 patients with the Marfan syndrome and 42 patients with homocystinuria [93]. Surgical techniques included discission, aspiration, and intra- or extracapsular extraction. Vitreous loss occurred in 30 percent of patients with either syndrome. In the Marfan patients, 25 percent of the eyes subsequently developed retinal detachment, while this complication occurred in 11 percent of homocystinuric patients. Sixty-eight percent of the Marfan patients and 54 percent of the homocystinuric patients benefited from lens surgery.

In a long-term study of 46 eyes with ectopia lentis that underwent surgery, intracapsular extraction was performed in 31 cases (69.5%) [186a]. The indication for surgery was poor visual acuity with best optical correction. Diagnoses in these patients included simple ectopia lentis, Marfan syndrome or homocystinuria (one patient only). An improvement in visual acuity as tested five years postoperatively ranged from 38.6 percent in Marfan patients to 50 percent of the simple ectopia lentis patients. Complications, including retinal detachment and glaucoma, occurred in 64 percent of the Marfan patients and in 10 percent of patients with simple ectopia lentis.

Discission and aspiration has been associated with a low incidence of complications [114, 160]. In one series of eight patients with ectopia lentis, the preoperative visual acuities ranged from 20/40 to 20/200 [114]. Postoperatively, the visual acuities ranged from 20/25 to 20/70. In three of the four eyes in which lens aspiration was performed because of elevated pressure, the intraocular pressure was controlled postoperatively without medication. However, two of the four eyes required repeated discission. Three of the nine eyes operated for reduced visual acuity required a subsequent single discission. No significant intraoperative or postoperative complications occurred in this small series, but a long-term follow-up is needed.

With the availability of automated vitrectomy instruments, vitreous loss and its sequelae can be avoided. Peyman and co-workers reported on 32 eyes with ectopia lentis surgically managed with the vitrophage [137]. These patients were followed for a period ranging from 5 to 45 months. In 12 cases caused by trauma, good surgical results were obtained in 10 eyes. Except for minimal intraocular bleeding and transient corneal edema, there were no significant operative complications in the traumatic cases. Those eyes with phacolytic glaucoma returned to normal intraocular pressure following lensectomy and vitrectomy. In one case, a lens with a hard nucleus and dislocation into the vitreous was successfully removed through a clear corneal incision while the vitrophage tip was maintained in the vitreous through a sclerotomy. In this case, no significant

adverse changes were noted in the late follow-up period.

Poor visual results did occur in Peyman's series when lens dislocation was associated with perforating injuries [137]. In these cases, vitrectomy and lensectomy helped clear the media and reform the globes, but inoperable retinal detachments and ciliary body damage was common.

If a markedly dislocated lens is cataractous, we would not remove the cataract but would give the patient an aphakic prescription. When a cataractous lens is minimally dislocated and an adequate aphakic pupillary space cannot be achieved, we have successfully performed a planned extracapsular cataract extraction [115]. In Marfan patients, the cataract is commonly nucleosclerotic. The nucleus, therefore, is usually removed easily with a cryoprobe after an anterior capsulotomy. The residual cortical material is then irrigated and aspirated. Our postoperative results have been good.

It is not rare for dislocated lenses to become hypermature and leak lens material, leading to a uveitis or even phacolytic glaucoma. Examination of the anterior chamber aqueous for macrophages can help clarify the diagnosis where questionable. Totally dislocated, leaking lenses should be removed after the intraocular pressure is lowered and the eye is quieted with topical steroids. The lens can be extracted with a cryoprobe or with a vitreous cutting instrument after the anterior vitreous has been removed with a vitreous cutting device.

REFERENCES

1. Abraham, P. A., Peregda, A. J., Carnes, W. H., et al. Marfan syndrome: demonstration of abnormal elastin in aorta. *J. Clin. Invest.* 70:1245, 1982.

1a. Allen, R. A., Straatsma, B. R., Apt, L., and Hall, M. O. Ocular manifestations of the Marfan syndrome. *Trans. Am. Acad. Ophthalmol. Otolaryngol.* 71:18, 1967.

1b. Amparo, E. G., Higgins, C. B., Hricak, H., et al. Aortic dissection; magnetic resonance imaging. *Radiology* 155:399, 1985.

2. Armstrong, M. D., and Robinow, M. A case of hyperlysinemia: Biochemical and clinical observations. *Pediatrics* 39:546, 1967.

3. Arnott, E. J., and Greaves, D. P. Ocular involvement in homocystinuria. *Br. J. Ophthalmol.* 48:688, 1964.

4. Baer, R. W., Taussig, H. B., and Oppenheimer, E. H.

Congenital aneurysmal dilatation of the aorta associated with arachnodactyly. *Bull. Hopkins Hosp.* 72:309, 1943.

5. Barber, G. W., and Spaeth, G. L. Pyridoxine therapy in homocystinuria. *Lancet* 1:337, 1967.

6. Barber, G. W., and Spaeth, G. L. The successful treatment of homocystinuria with pyridoxine. *J. Pediatr.* 75:463, 1969.

7. Bardelle, A. M., and Cardete, P. Ectopia iristallina e retinopatia pigmentaria. *Minerva Oftalmol.* 10:197, 1968.

8. Barraquer, J. I. Surgical treatment of the lens displacements. *Arch. Soc. Am. Oftalmol. Opt.* 1:30, 1958.

9. Beemer, F. A., and Deileman, J. W. Combined deficiency of xanthene oxidase and sulfite oxidase; ophthalmological findings in a 3-week-old girl. *Metab. Pediat. Ophthalmol.* 4:49, 1980.

10. Bessiere, E., Riviere, J., and Leuret, J. P. Le rebeller, an association of Klinefelter's disease and congenital anomalies, comptodactyly, microphakia. *Bull. Soc. Ophtalmol. Fr.* 62:197, 1962.

11. Blaxter, P. L. Spherophakia. *Trans. Ophthalmol. Soc. UK* 88:621, 1969.

12. Boerger, F. Ueber zwei Faelle von Arachnodaktylie. *Z. Kinderheilkd.* 12:16, 1914.

12a. Boucek, R. J., Noble, N. L., Gunta-Smith, Z., and Butler, W. T. The Marfan syndrome: a deficiency in chemically stable collagen crosslinks. *N. Engl. J. Med.* 305:988, 1981.

13. Bowers, D., and Lim, D. W. Subacute bacterial endocarditis and Marfan's syndrome. *Can. Med. Assoc. J.* 86:455, 1962.

14. Brenton, D. P., Cusworth, D. C., Dent, C. E., et al. Homocystinuria, clinical and dietary studies. *Q.J.* 139:325, 1966.

15. Brown, R. B., Watson, P. D., and Taussig, L. M. Congenital metabolic diseases of pediatric patients: Anesthesiologyia implications. *Anesthesiology* 43:197, 1975.

16. Burch, F. E. Association of ectopia lentis and arachnodactyly. *Arch. Ophthalmol.* 15:645, 1936.

17. Burian, H. M. Chamber angle studies in developmental glaucoma. Marfan's syndrome and high myopia. *J. Missouri Med. Assoc.* 55:1088, 1958.

18. Burian, H. M., and Allen, L. Histologic study of the chamber angle of patients with Marfan's syndrome. *Arch. Ophthalmol.* 65:323, 1961.

19. Burian, H. M., Von Noorden, G. K., and Ponseti, I. V. Chamber angle anomalies in systemic connective tissue disorders. *Arch. Ophthalmol.* 64:671, 1960.

20. Calhoun, F. P., and Hagler, W. S. Experience with the José Barraquer method of extracting a dislocated lens. *Trans. Am. Ophthalmol. Soc.* 57:221, 1959.

21. Calhoun, F. P., and Hagler, W. S. Experience with the José Barraquer method of extracting a dislocated lens. *Am. J. Ophthalmol.* 50:701, 1960.

22. Callahan, A. Aniridia with ectopia lentis and secondary glaucoma. Genetic, pathologic and surgical considerations. *Am. J. Ophthalmol.* 32:28, 1949.

23. Carey, M. C., Donovan, D. E., and Fitzgerald, O. Homocystinuria. A clinical and pathological study of nine subjects in six families. *Am. J. Med.* 45:7, 1968.

24. Carson, N. A. J. Homocystinuria. Trial treatment of a 5-year-old severely retarded child with a natural diet low in methionine. *Am. J. Dis. Child.* 113:95, 1967.

25. Carson, N. A. J., Cusworth, D. C., Dent, C. E., et al. A new inborn error of metabolism associated with mental deficiency. *Arch. Dis. Child.* 38:425, 1963.

26. Carson, N. A. J., Dent, C. E., and Field, C. M. B., et al. Homocystinuria. Clinical and pathological review of ten cases. *J. Pediatr.* 66:5, 1965.

27. Carson, N. A. J., and Neill, D. W. Metabolic abnormalities detected in a survey of mentally backward individuals in Northern Ireland. *Arch. Dis. Child.* 37:505, 1962.

28. Chandler, P. A. Surgery of the lens in infancy and childhood. *Arch. Ophthalmol.* 45:125, 1951.

29. Chandler, P. A. Problems in the diagnosis and treatment of lens-induced uveitis and glaucoma. *Arch. Ophthalmol.* 60:828, 1958.

30. Chandler, P. A. Completely dislocated hypermature cataract and glaucoma. *Trans. Am. Ophthalmol. Soc.* 57:242, 1959.

31. Chandler, P. A. Choice of treatment in dislocation of the lens. *Arch. Ophthalmol.* 71:765, 1964.

32. Chandler, P. A., and Johnson, C. C. A neglected cause of secondary glaucoma in eyes in which the lens is absent or subluxated. *Arch. Ophthalmol.* 47:740, 1947.

33. Chase, H. P., Goodman, S. I., and O'Brien, D. Treatment of homocystinuria. *Arch. Dis. Child.* 42:514, 1967.

34. Clark, C. C., Ectopia lentis. A pathologic and clinical study. *Arch. Ophthalmol.* 21:124, 1939.

35. Cline, J. W., Goyer, R. A., Lipton, J., et al. Adult homocystinuria with ectopia lentis. *South. Med. J.* 64:613, 1971.

36. Cotlier, E., and Reinglass, H. Marfan-like syndrome with lens involvement. *Arch. Ophthalmol.* 93:93, 1975.

36a. Crawford, E. F., Crawford, J. C., Stowe, C. L., et al. Total aortic replacement for chronic aortic dissection occurring in patients with and without Marfan's syndrome. *Ann. Surg.* 195:358, 1984.

37. Crebain, A. R. Persistent pupillary membrane and congenital ectopia lentis. *Am. J. Ophthalmol.* 12:87, 1929.

38. Croll, M., and Croll, L. S. Cryoextraction of dislocated lenses. *Ann. Ophthalmol.* 7:1245, 1975.

39. Crooke, J. W., Towers, J. F., and Taylor, W. H. Management of patients with homocystinuria requiring surgery under general anesthesia. *Br. J. Anaesthesiol.* 43:96, 1971.

40. Cross, H. E. Ectopia lentis in systemic heritable disorders. *Birth Defects* 10:113, 1974.

41. Cross, H. E. Differential diagnosis and treatment of dislocated lenses. *Birth Defects* 12:335, 1976.

42. Cross, H. E. Ectopia lentis et pupillae. *Am. J. Ophthalmol.* 88:381, 1979.

43. Cross, H. E., and Jensen, A. D. Ocular manifestations in the Marfan syndrome and homocystinuria. *Am. J. Ophthalmol.* 75:405, 1973.

44. Dancis, J., Hutzler, J., Cox, R. P., et al. Familial hyperlysinemia with lysine-ketoglutarate reductase insufficiency. *J. Clin. Invest.* 48:1447, 1969.

44a. David, R., MacBeath, L., and Jenkins, T. Aniridia associated with micro-cornea and subluxated lenses. *Br. J. Ophthalmol.* 62:118, 1978.

45. Davis, Z., Pluth, J. R., and Giuliani, E. R. The Marfan syndrome and cardiac surgery. *J. Thorac. Cardiovasc. Surg.* 75:505, 1978.

46. Del Buono, G., and Brogi, M. Un caso di sindromi de Sturge Weber Krabbe con sublussazione bilaterale del cristallino. *G. Ital. Oftalmol.* 15:123, 1962.

47. Dickerman, H. W., and Carter, M. L. A spectrophotometric method for the determination of lysine utilizing bacterial lysine decarboxylase. *Anal. Biochem.* 3:195, 1962.

48. Drethelm, W. Uber Ectopia lentis ohne Arachnodaktylie und ihre Beziehungen zur Ectopia lentis et pupillae. *Ophthalmologica* 114:16, 1947.

49. Dryden, J. S., Perraut, L. E., and Seward, W. H. Sclerocorneal transfixation method for the removal of posteriorly dislocated lenses. *Am. J. Ophthalmol.* 52:468, 1961.

50. Dunn, N. G., Perry, T. L., and Dolman, C. L. Homocystinuria: A recently discovered cause of mental defect and cerebrovascular thrombosis. *Neurology* 16:407, 1966.

51. Dvorak-Theobald, G. Histologic eye findings in arachnodactyly. *Am. J. Ophthalmol.* 24:1132, 1941.

51a. Elkington, A. R., Freedman, S. S., Joy, B., and Wright, P. Anterior dislocation of the lens in homocystinuria. *Br. J. Ophthalmol.* 57:325, 1973.

52. Etter, L. E., and Glover, L. P. Arachnodactyly complicated by dislocated lens and death from rupture of dissecting aneurysm of the aorta. *J.A.M.A.* 123:88, 1943.

53. Falls, H. F., and Cotterman, C. W. Genetic studies on ectopia lentis. *Arch. Ophthalmol.* 30:610, 1943.

54. Farnsworth, P. N., Burke, P. A., Blanco, J., et al. Ultrastructural abnormalities in a microspherical ectopic lens. *Exp. Eye Res.* 27:399, 1978.

55. Farnsworth, P. N., Burke, P. A., Dotto, M. E., et al. Ultrastructural abnormalities in a Marfan's syndrome lens. *Arch. Ophthalmol.* 95:1601, 1977.

56. Feiler-Ofry, V., Stein, R., and Godel, V. Marchesani's syndrome and chamber angle anomalies. *Am. J. Ophthalmol.* 66:862, 1968.

56a. Fergusen, J. E., Ueland, K., Stinson, E. B., et al. Marfan's syndrome: acute aortic dissection during labor, resulting in fetal stress and cesarean section followed by successful surgical repair. *Am. J. Obstet. Gynecol.* 147:759, 1985.

57. Ferry, A. P., and Font, R. L. The Phakomatoses. In A. P. Ferry (ed): *Ocular and Adnexal Tumors, Int. Ophthalmol. Clin.* Boston: Little Brown, 1972, pp. 1–50.

58. Finkelstein, J. D., Fenichel, G. M., and Reichmister, J. Homocystinuria. *Clin. Proc. Child. Hosp. (Washington)* 25:291, 1969.

59. Franceschetti, A. Ectopia lentis et pupillae congenita als rezessives Erblerden und ihre Manifestierung durch Konsanguinitat. *Klin. Monatsbl. Augenheilkd.* 78:351, 1927.

60. François, J. *Heredity in Ophthalmology.* St. Louis: Mosby, 1961, pp. 161–164.

61. Freeman, J. M., Finkelstein, J. D., and Mudd, S. H. Folate-responsive homocystinuria and "schizophrenia." A defect in methylation due to deficient 5, 10-methylenetetrahydrofolate reductase activity. *N. Engl. J. Med.* 292:491, 1975.

62. Garston, J. B., Gordon, R. R., Hart, C. T., et al. An unusual case of homocystinuria. *Br. J. Ophthalmol.* 54:248, 1970.

63. Gaull, G. F., Rassin, D. K., and Sturman, J. A. Pyridoxine-dependency in homocystinuria. *Lancet* 2:1302, 1968.

64. Gerritsen, T., Vaughn, J. G., and Waisman, H. A. The identification of homocystine in the urine. *Biochem. Biophys. Res. Commun.* 9:493, 1962.

65. Gerritsen, T., and Waisman, H. A. Homocystinuria: Absence of cystathionine in the brain. *Science* 145:588, 1964.

66. Ghadimi, H., Binnington, V. I., and Pecora, P. Hyperlysinemia associated with retardation. *N. Engl. J. Med.* 273:723, 1965.

67. Gibson, J. B., Carson, R. A. J., and Neill, D. W. Pathological findings in homocystinuria. *J. Clin. Pathol.* 17:427, 1964.

68. Gillum, W. N., and Anderson, R. L. Dominantly inherited blepharoptosis, high myopia and ectopia lentis. *Arch. Ophthalmol.* 100:282, 1982.

69. Giri, D. V. A case of ectopia lentis with coloboma. *Br. J. Ophthalmol.* 8:275, 1924.

70. Goldberg, M. E., and Ryan, S. J. Intercalary staphyloma in Marfan's syndrome. *Am. J. Ophthalmol.* 67:329, 1969.

71. Golden, B., and Thompson, H. S. Implication of spiral forms in the eye. *Surv. Ophthalmol.* 14:179, 1969.

71a. Graymore, C. N. Biochemistry of the Eye. London: Academic Press, 1970, p. 391.

72. Guillaumat, L. Lemartre: Muyopie forte, retinite pigmentaire, luxation congenitale des deux cristallins chez une jeune fille issue d'un mariage consanguin. Probleme pathogenique. *Bull. Soc. Ophtalmol. Fr.* 3:90, 1948.

73. Haddad, N. J., Moyer, N. J., and Riley, F. C. Mydriatic effect of phenylephrine hydrochloride on the miotic-treated eye. *Am. J. Ophthalmol.* 70:729, 1970.

73a. Halbritter, R., Aumailey, M., Rackwitz, R., et al. Case report and study of collagen metabolism in Marfan syndrome. *Klin. Wochenschr.* 59:83, 1981.

74. Halpern, B. L., and Sugar, A. Retinitis pigmentosa associated with bilateral ectopia lentis. *Ann. Ophthalmol.* 13:823, 1981.

74a. Halme, T., Vihersari, T., Savonen, T., et al. Desmosines in aneurysms of the ascending aorta (annulo-aortic ectasia). *Biochim. Biophys. Acta* 717:105, 1982.

75. Hark, G. M., Kalil, H. M., Ferry, J. F., et al. Subluxations and luxations of the lens: With a special note on the Barraquer operation and on Marfan's and Marchesani's syndromes. *South. Med. J.* 54:642, 1961.

76. Harker, L. A., Slichter, S. J., Scott, C. R., et al. Homocystinemia vascular injury and arterial thrombosis. *N. Engl. J. Med.* 291:537, 1974.

77. Harshman, J. P. Glaucoma associated with subluxation of the lens in several members of a family. *Am. J. Ophthalmol.* 31:833, 1948.

78. Heath, P. Secondary glaucoma due to the lens. *Arch. Ophthalmol.* 25:424, 1941.

79. Henkind, P., and Ashton, N. Ocular pathology in homocystinuria. *Trans. Ophthalmol. Soc. U.K.* 85:21, 1965.

80. Hilden, M., Brandt, N. Y., Nilsson, I. M., et al. Investigations of coagulation and fibrinolysis in homocystinuria. *Acta Med. Scand.* 195:533, 1974.

81. Hill-Zobel, R. L., Pyeritz, R. F., Scheffel, V., et al. Kinetics and biodistribution of III In-Oxine labeled platelets in homocystinuria. *N. Engl. J. Med.* 307:781, 1982.

82. Hindle, N. W., and Crawford, J. S. Dislocation of the lens in Marfan's syndrome. *Can. J. Ophthalmol.* 4:128, 1969.

83. Hobbs, I. A. The spherophakia-brachymorphia syndrome: Two cases among five brothers. *Med. J. Aust.* 1:80, 1965.

84. Hollowell, J. G., Hall, W. K., Coryell, J. D., et al. Homocystinuria and organic aciduria in a patient with vitamin-B12 deficiency. *Lancet* 2:1428, 1969.

85. Holmgren, G., Falkmer, S., and Hambaeus, L. Plasma insulin content and glucose tolerance in homocystinuria. *Ups. J. Med. Sci.* 78:215, 1973.

86. Hooft, C., Rassin, D. K., and Sturman, J. A. Pyridoxine treatment in homocystinuria. *Lancet* 1:1384, 1967.

87. Horner, W. D., and Maisler, S. Ectopia lentis, with report of a case of total dislocation directly downward. *Trans. Sect. Ophthalmol. AMA.* 126, 1933.

88. Hyanek, J., Bremer, H. J., and Slavik, M. "Homocystinuria" and urinary excretion of B-amino acids in patients treated with 6-azauridine. *Clin. Chem. Acta* 25:288, 1969.

88a. Iliff, C. E., and Kramar, P. A working guide for the management of dislocated lenses. *Ophthalmol. Surg.* 2:251, 1971.

89. Irreverre, F., Mudd, S. H., Heizer, W. D., et al. Sulfite oxidase deficiency: Studies of a patient with mental retardation, dislocated lenses and abnormal urinary excretion of S-sulfocysteine, sulfite and theosulfate. *Biochem. Med.* 1:187, 1967.

90. Irvine, S. R., and Irvine, A. R. Lenses induced uveitis and glaucoma. *Am. J. Ophthalmol.* 35:370, 1952.

91. Jarrett, W. H., Jr. Dislocation of the lens: A study of 166 hospitalized cases. *Arch. Ophthalmol.* 78:289, 1967.

92. Jensen, A. D. Heritable Ectopia Lentis. *Genetic and Metabolic Eye Disease.* Boston, Little Brown, 1974, pp. 325–336.

93. Jensen, A. D., and Cross, H. E. Surgical treatment of dislocated lenses in the Marfan syndrome and homocystinuria. *Trans. Am. Acad. Ophthalmol. Otolaryngol.* 76:1491, 1972.

94. Jensen, A. D., Cross, H. E., and Paton, D. Ocular complications in the Weill-Marchesani syndrome. *Am. J. Ophthalmol.* 77:261, 1974.

95. Jezegabel, C., Rossazza, C., and Rogez, J. L'hypertonic oculaire au cours du syndrome de Weill-Marchesani. *Bull. Soc. Ophtalmol. Fr.* 71:359, 1971.

95a. Johnson, J. L., Waud, W. R., Rajagopalan, K. V., et al. Inborn errors of molybdenum metabolism: Combined deficiencies of sulfite oxidase and xanthine dehydiogenase in a patient lacking the molybdenum cofactor. *Proc. Natl. Acad. Sci.* 77:3715, 1980.

96. Johnson, V. P., Grayson, M., Christian, J. C., et al. Dominant microspherophakia. *Arch. Ophthalmol.* 85:534, 1971.

97. Jones, R. F. The syndrome of Marchesani. *Br. J. Ophthalmol.* 45:377, 1961.

98. Kanwar, Y. S., Manaligod, J. R., and Wong, P. W. K. Morphologic studies in a patient with homocystinuria due to 5, 10-methylenetetra-hydrofolate reductase deficiency. *Pediatr. Res.* 10:598, 1976.

99. Karyofilis, A., Berneaud-Kotz, G., and Jacobs, I. Heredopathia Atactica polyneuritiformis. *Fortschr. Neurol. Psychiatr.* 38:321, 1970.

100. Kirkham, T. H. Mandibulofacial dysostosis with ectopia lentis. *Am. J. Ophthalmol.* 70:947, 1970.

101. Kittel, V. Beobachtungen bei familiar aufretender Iris-atrophie mit Drucksteigerung. *Klin. Monatsbl. Augenheilkd.* 129:464, 1956.

102. Kloepfer, H. W., and Rosenthal, J. W. Possible genetic carriers in the spherophakia-brachymorphia syndrome. *Am. J. Hum. Genet.* 7:398, 1975.

103. Komrower, G. M. Dietary treatment of homocystinuria. *Am. J. Dis. Child.* 113:98, 1967.

104. Krieg, T., and Muller, P. K. The Marfan's syndrome. In vitro study of collagen metabolism in tissue specimens of the aorta. *Exp. Cell. Biol.* 45:207, 1977.

105. Lemmingson, W., and Riethe, P. Beobachtungen bei Dysgenesis mesodermalis corneae et iridis in Konbination mit Oligodontie. *Klin. Monatsbl. Augenheilkd.* 133:877, 1958.

106. Levy, H. L., Mudd, S. H., Schulman, J. D., et al. A derangement in B^{12} metabolism associated with homocystinuria cystathioninemia, hypermethioninemia and methylmalonic aciduria. *Am. J. Med.* 48:390, 1970.

107. Levy, J., and Anderson, P. E. Marchesani's syndrome. *Br. J. Ophthalmol.* 45:223, 1961.

108. Luebbers, J. A., Goldberg, M. F., Herbst, R., Hattenbauer, J., and Maumenee, A. E. Iris transillumination and variable expression in ectopia lentis et pupillae. *Am. J. Ophthalmol.* 83:647, 1977.

109. Lund, A., and Stontoft, F. Congenital ectopia lentis. *Acta Ophthalmol.* 29:33, 1950.

110. Lutman, F. C., and Neel, J. B. Inheritance of arachnodactyly, ectopia lentis and other congenital anomalies (Marfan's syndrome) in the E. family. *Arch. Ophthalmol.* 41:276, 1949.

111. Marchesani, O. Brachydaktylie und angeborene Kugellinseals Systemerkrankung. *Klin. Monatsbl. Augenheilkd.* 103:392, 1939.

112. Marfan, A. B. Un cas de deformation congenitale desquatyre members, plus pronocee aux extremities, characterisee par l'allongement des os avec un certain degre d'amincessement. *Bull. Soc. Med. Hop., Paris* 13:220, 1896.

113. Mash, A. J., Hegmann, J. P., and Spivey, B. E. Genetic analysis of indices of corneal power and corneal astigmatism in human populations with varying incidences of strabismus. *Invest. Ophthalmol.* 14:826, 1975.

114. Maumenee, A. E., and Ryan, S. J. Aspiration technique in the management of the dislocated lens. *Am. J. Ophthalmol.* 68:808, 1969.

115. Maumenee, I. H. The eye in the Marfan syndrome. *Trans. Am. Ophthalmol. Soc.* 79:684, 1981.

116. Maxwell, E. M. Case of traumatic dislocation of lens. *Trans. Ophthalmol. Soc. U.K.* 71:780, 1951.

117. McCully, K. S. Importance of homocysteine-induced abnormalities of proteoglycan structure in arteriosclerosis. *Am. J. Pathol.* 59:181, 1970.

118. McDonald, L., Brace, C., Field, C., et al. Homocystinuria, thrombosis and the blood-platelets. *Lancet* 1:745, 1964.

119. McGavic, J. S. Marchesani's syndrome. *Am. J. Ophthalmol.* 47:413, 1959.

120. McGavic, J. S. Weill-Marchesani syndrome, brachymorphism and ectopia lentis. *Am. J. Ophthalmol.* 62:820, 1966.

121. McKusick, V. A. Primordial dwarfism and ectopia lentis. *Am. J. Hum. Genet.* 7:189, 1955.

122. McKusick, V. A. *Heritable Disorders of Connective Tissue.* St. Louis: Mosby, 1972, pp. 61–223.

123. Meyer, E. T. Familial ectopia lentis and its complications. *Br. J. Ophthalmol.* 38:163, 1954.

124. Meyer, S. J., and Holstein, T. Spherophakia with glaucoma and brachydactyly. *Am. J. Ophthalmol.* 24:247, 1941.

125. Mudd, S. H., Edwards, W. A., Loeb, P. M., et al. Homoycystinuria due to cystathionine synthetase deficiency: The effect of pyridoxine. *J. Clin. Invest.* 49:1762, 1970.

126. Mudd, S. H., Finklestein, J. D., Irreverre, F., et al. Homocystinuria: An enzymatic defect. *Science* 143:1443, 1964.

127. Mudd, S. H., Irreverre, F., and Laster, L. Sulfite oxidase deficiency in man: Demonstration of the enzymatic defect. *Science* 156:1599, 1967.

128. Mukuno, K., Matsui, K., and Haraguchi, H. Ocular manifestation of homocystinuria: Report of two cases. *Acta Soc. Ophthalmol. Jap.* 71:66, 1967.

129. Murdoch, J. L., Walker, B. A., Halpern, B. L., et al. Life expectancy and causes of death in the Marfan syndrome. *N. Engl. J. Med.* 286:804, 1972.

130. Murdoch, J. L., Walker, B. A., and McKusick, V. A. Parental age effects on the occurrence of new mutations for the Marfan syndrome. *Ann. Hum. Genet.* 35:331, 1972.

130a. Nelson, L. B., Spaeth, G. L., and Nowinsky, T. S. et al. "Aniridia." *Surv. Ophthalmol.* 28:621, 1984.

130b. Nelson, L. B., and Szmyd, S. M. Aphakic correction in ectopial lentis. *Ann. Ophthalmol.* 17:445, 1985.

131. Nirankari, M. S., and Chaddah, M. R. Displaced lens. *Am. J. Ophthalmol.* 63:1719, 1967.

132. Olney, J. W., Misra, C. H., and deGubareff, T. Cysteine-S-sulfate: Brain damaging metabolite in sulfite oxidase deficiency. *J. Neuropathol. Exp. Neurol.* 34:167, 1975.

133. Ose, L., and McKusick, V. A. Prophylactic use of propranolol in the Marfan syndrome to prevent aortic dissection. *Birth Defects* 13(3C):163, 1977.

134. Perry, T. L., Hansen, S., Love, D. L., and Crawford, L. E. Treatment of homocystinuria with a low-methionine diet, supplemental cystine and methyl donor. *Lancet* 2:474, 1968.

135. Perry, T. L., Hansen, S., and MacDougall, L. Sulfur-containing amino acids in the plasma and urine of homocystinurics. *Clin. Chim. Acta* 15:409, 1967.

136. Pesme, Verger, Montoux. Dysostose craniofaciale avec ectopie du crystallin. *Arch. Fr. Pediatr.* 7:348, 1950.

137. Peyman, G. A., Rauchand, M., Goldberg, M. F., and Ritacia, D. Management of subluxated and dislocated lenses with the vitriophage. *Br. J. Ophthalmol.* 63:771, 1979.

138. Presley, G. D., and Sidbury, J. B. Homocystinuria and ocular defects. *Am. J. Ophthalmol.* 63:1723, 1967.

139. Presley, G. D., Stinson, I. N., and Sidbury, J. B. Homocystinuria at the North Carolina State School for the Blind. *Am. J. Ophthalmol.* 66:884, 1968.

140. Priest, R. E., Moinaddin, J. F., and Priest, S. H. Collagen of Marfan syndrome is abnormally soluble. *Nature* 245:264, 1973.

141. Probert, L. A. Spherophakia with brachydactyly. Comparison with Marfan's syndrome. *Am. J. Ophthalmol.* 36:1571, 1953.

141a. Prockop, D. J., and Kivirikko, K. I. Heritable diseases of collagen. *N. Engl. J. Med.* 311:376, 1984.

142. Prockop, D. J., and Sjoerdsma, A. Significance of urinary hydroxyproline in man. *J. Clin. Invest.* 40:843, 1961.

143. Pyeritz, R. E., and McKusick, V. A. The Marfan syndrome: Diagnosis and management. *N. Engl. J. Med.* 300:772, 1979.

143a. Pseitz, R. E. Maternal and fetal complications of pregnancy in the Marfan syndrome. *Am. J. Med.* 71:784, 1981.

144. Rahman, M., and Rahman, S. Marchesani's syndrome. *Br. J. Ophthalmol.* 47:182, 1963.

145. Ramsey, M. S., Dartz, L. D., and Beaton, J. W. Lens fringe in homocystinuria. *Arch. Ophthalmol.* 93:318, 1975.

146. Ramsey, M. S., and Dickson, D. H. Lens fringe in homocystinuria. *Br. J. Ophthalmol.* 59:338, 1975.

147. Ramsey, M. S., Fine, B. S., Shields, J. A., et al. The Marfan syndrome: A histopathologic study of ocular findings. *Am. J. Ophthalmol.* 76:102, 1973.

148. Ramsey, M. S., Yanoff, M., and Fine, B. S. The ocular histopathology of homocystinuria. *Am. J. Ophthalmol.* 74:377, 1972.

149. Ratnoff, O. D. Activation of Hageman fractor by L-Homocystine. *Science* 162:1107, 1968.

150. Rech, M. J., and Lehman, W. I. Marfan's syndrome: (arachnodactyly) with ectopia lentis. *Trans. Am. Acad. Ophthalmol. Otolaryngol.* 58:212, 1954.

151. Regenbogen, I., Ilie, S., and Elian, I. Homocystinuria—A surgical and anesthetic risk. *Metabol. Pediatr. Ophthalmol.* 4:209, 1980.

152. Rennert, O. M. The Marchesani syndrome; A brief review. *Am. J. Dis. Child.* 117:703, 1969.

153. Ritch, R., and Wand, M. Treatment of the Weil-Marchesani syndrome. *Ann. Ophthalmol.* 13:665, 1981.

154. Ritchie, J. W. K., and Carson, N. A. J. Pregnancy and homocystinuria. *J. Obstet. Gynecol. Br. Commton.* 80:661, 1973.

155. Rizzuti, A. B. Complications in the surgical management of the displaced lens. *Int. Ophthalmol. Clin.* 5:3, 1965.

156. Robins, P. R., Moe, J. M., and Winter, R. B. Scoliosis in Marfan's syndrome. Its characteristics and results of treatment in thirty-five patients. *J. Bone Joint Surg.* 57:358, 1975.

157. Rodman, H. I. Chronic open-angle glaucoma associated with traumatic dislocation of the lens. *Am. J. Ophthalmol.* 63:445, 1963.

157a. Rosenbaum, I. J., and Podos, S. M. Traumatic ectopia lentis. Some relationships to syphilis and glaucoma. *Am. J. Ophthalmol.* 64:1095, 1967.

158. Rosenblum, W. I. Neuropathologic changes in a case of sulfite oxidase deficiency. *Neurology* 18:1187, 1968.

159. Scheck, M., Siegel, R. C., Parker, J., Chang, Y., and Fu, J. C. C. Aortic aneurysm in Marfan's syndrome: Changes in the ultrastructure and composition of collagen. *J. Anat.* 129:645, 1979.

160. Scheie, H. G., Rubenstein, R. A., and Kent, R. B. Aspiration of congenital or soft cataracts: Further experience. *Am. J. Ophthalmol.* 63:3, 1967.

161. Schimke, R. N., McKusick, V. A., Huang, T., et al. Homocystinuria. Studies of 20 families with 38 affected members. *J.A.M.A.* 193:711, 1965.

162. Scriver, C. R., Davies, E., and Cullen, A. M. Application of a simple micromethod to the screening of plasma for a variety of aminoacidopathies. *Lancet* 2:230, 1964.

163. Seeleman, K. Brachydaktylie und angeborene Kugellinse. *Z. Kinderheilkd.* 67:1, 1949.

164. Seland, J. H. The lenticular attachment of the zonular apparatus in congenital simple ectopia lentis. *Acta Ophthalmol.* 51:520, 1973.

165. Shapera, T. M. Micro- and spherophakia with glaucoma. *Am. J. Ophthalmol.* 17:726, 1934.

166. Shih, V. E., Abrams, I. F., Johnson, I. L., et al. Sulfite oxidase deficiency. Biochemical and clinical investigations of a hereditary metabolic disorder in sulfur metabolism. *N. Engl. J. Med.* 297:1022, 1977.

167. Shih, V. E., and Efron, M. L. Pyridoxine-unresponsive homocystinuria. *N. Engl. J. Med.* 283:1206, 1970.

168. Shih, V. E., Salam, M. Z., Mudd, S. H., et al. A new form of homocystinuria due to N5–10 methylene tetrahydrofolate deficiency. *Pediatr. Res.* 6:395, 1972.

169. Siemens, H. W. Ueber die Aetiologie der Ectopia lentis et pupillae. *Albrecht von Graefes Arch. Klin. Exp. Ophthalmol.* 109:359, 1920.

170. Skovby, F., and McKusick, V. A. Estrogen treatment of tall stature in girls with the Marfan syndrome. *Birth Defects* 13(3C):155, 1977.

170a. Smith, J. L., and Taylor, W. H. The FTA-ABS test in ocular and neurosyphilis. *Am. J. Ophthalmol.* 60:653, 1965.

171. Smith, T. H., Holland, M. G., and Woody, N. C. Ocular manifestations of familial hyperlysinemia. *Trans. Am. Acad. Ophthalmol. Otolaryngol.* 75:355, 1971.

171a. Smolin, L. A., Benerenga, N. J., and Berlow, S. The use of betaine for the treatment of homocystinuria. *J. Pediatr.* 99:467, 1981.

172. Sohar, E. Renal disease, inner ear deafness and ocular changes. A new heredofamilial syndrome. *Arch. Intern. Med.* 97:627, 1956.

173. Spackman, D. H., Stein, W. H., and Moore, S. Automatic recording apparatus for use in the chromatography of amino acids. *Anal. Chem.* 30:1190, 1958.

174. Spaeth, G. L. The usefulness of pyridoxine in the treatment of homocystinuria: A review of postulated mechanisms of action and a new hypothesis. *Birth Defects* 12:347, 1976.

174a. Spaeth, G. L., and Barber, G. W. Homocystinuria: In a mentally retarded child and her normal cousin. *Trans. Am. Acad. Ophthalmol. Otolaryngol.* 69:912, 1965.

175. Spaeth, G. L., and Barber, G. W. Homocystinuria—Its ocular manifestations. *J. Pediatr. Ophthalmol.* 3:42, 1966.

176. Spaeth, G. L., and Barber, G. W. Prevalence of homocystinuria among the mentally retarded: Evaluation of a specific screening test. *Pediatrics* 40:586, 1967.

177. Stadlin, W., and Klein, D. Ectopie congenitale du crystallin avec spherophaquie et brachymorphie accompagnee de paresis due regard. *Ann. Oculist* 181:692, 1948.

178. Starke, H. Zur Pathogenese des Marfan-Syndromes. *Albrecht von Graefes Arch. Klin. Exp. Ophthalmol.* 151:384, 1951.

179. Steinberg, I. A simple screening test for the Marfan syndrome. *Am. J. Roentgenol.* 97:118, 1966.

180. Stephenson, W. V. Anterior megalophthalmos and arachnodactyly. *Am. J. Ophthalmol.* 8:315, 1954.

181. Straatsma, B. R., Allen, R. A., Pettit, T. H., and Michael, M. O. Subluxation of the lens treated with iris photocoagulation. *Am. J. Ophthalmol.* 61:1312, 1966.

181a. Streeten, B. W., Swann, D., Licari, P. A., et al. The protein composition of the ocular zonules. *Invest. Ophthalmol.* 24:19, 1983.

182. Susanna, R., Drance, S., Schirlzer, M., and Douglas, G. The effects of thymoxamine on anterior chamber depth in human eyes. *Can. J. Ophthalmol.* 13:250, 1978.

183. Thomas, C., Cordier, J., and Algan, B. Une etiologie nouvelle du syndrome de luxation spontanee des cristallins: La maladie d'Ehlers-Danlos. *Bull. Doc. Belge. Ophthalmol.* 100:375, 1952.

184. Thomas, C., Cordier, J., and Algan, B. Les alterations oculaires de la maladie d'Ehlers-Danlos. *Arch. Ophthalmol.* (Paris) 14:691, 1954.

185. Uhleman, E. R., Ten Pas, J. H., Lucky, A. W., et al. Platelet survival and morphology in homocystinuria due to cystathionine synthatase deficiency. *N. Engl. J. Med.* 295:1283, 1976.

186. Urbanek, J. Glaucoma juvenile inversum. *Z. Augenheilkd.* 77:171, 1930.

186a. Varga, B. The results of my operations improving visual acuity of ectopia lentis. *Ophthalmologica* 162:98, 1971.

187. Vogt, A. Cited by S. J. Meyer and T. Holstein. Spherophakia with glaucoma and brachydactyly. *Am. J. Ophthalmol.* 24:247, 1941.

188. Von Noorden, G. K., and Schultz, R. O. A gonioscopic study of the chamber angle in Marfan's syndrome. *Arch. Ophthalmol.* 64:929, 1960.

189. Waardenburg, P. J., Franceschetti, A., and Klein, D. *Genetics and Ophthalmology.* Netherlands, Royal Von Gorcum, 1961, pp. 954–957.

190. Wachtel, J. G. The ocular pathology of Marfan's syndrome. *Arch. Ophthalmol.* 76:512, 1966.

191. Walker, B. A., and Murdoch, J. L. The wrist sign: A useful physical finding in the Marfan syndrome. *Arch. Intern. Med.* 126:276, 1970.

192. Walls, G. L., and Heath, G. G. Dominant ectopia lentis et pupillae. *Am. J. Hum. Genet.* 11:166, 1959.

193. Wand, M., and Grant, W. M. Thymoxamine hydrochloride: Effects on the facility of outflow and intraocular pressure. *Invest. Ophthalmol.* 15:400, 1976.

194. Wand, M., and Grant, W. M. Thymoxamine hydrochloride: An alpha-adrenergic blocker. *Surv. Ophthalmol.* 25:75, 1980.

195. Weill, G. Ectopie des cristallins et malformations generales. *Ann. Ocul.* 169:21, 1932.

196. Whiting, M. Congenital dislocation of the lens. *Br. J. Ophthalmol.* 47:54, 1963.

197. Wilcken, B. Incidence of homocystinuria. *Lancet* 1:273, 1975.

197a. Wilcken, D. E. L., Wilcken, B., Dudman, N. P. B., et al. Homocystinemia—the effects of betaine in the treatment of patients not responsive to pyridoxine. *N. Engl. J. Med.* 309:448, 1983.

198. Willi, M., Kut, L., and Cotlier, E. Pupillary-block glaucoma in the Marchesani syndrome. *Arch. Ophthalmol.* 90:504, 1973.

199. Williams, E. Rare cases, with practical remarks. *Trans. Ophthalmol. Soc.* 2:291, 1873–1879.

200. Wilson, R. S., and Ruiz, R. S. Bilateral central retinal artery occlusion in homocystinuria. *Arch. Ophthalmol.* 82:267, 1969.

201. Wolf, S. M., and Zimmerman, L. E. Chronic secondary glaucoma associated with retrodisplacement of iris root and deepening of the anterior chamber angle secondary to contusion. *Am. J. Ophthalmol.* 54:547, 1962.

202. Woody, N. C. Hyperlysinemia. *Am. J. Dis. Child.* 108:543, 1964.

202a. Wright, K. W., and Chrousos, G. A. Weill-Marchesani syndrome in bilateral angle closure glaucoma. *J. Pediatr. Ophthalmol. Strab.* 22:129, 1985.

203. Wunsch, C. M., Steinmetz, E. F., and Fisch, C. Marfan's syndrome and subacute bacterial endocarditis. *Am. J. Cardiol.* 15:102, 1965.

204. Zabriskie, J., and Riesman, M. Marchesani syndrome. *J. Pediatr.* 52:159, 1958.

205. Zeeman, W. P. C. Ueber ectopia pupillae et lentis congenita. *Klin. Monatsbl. Augenheilkd.* 74:325, 1925.

206. Zeeman, W. P. C. Ectopia lentis congenita. *Acta Ophthalmol.* 20:1, 1942.

15

Hereditary Retinal Detachment and Vitreoretinal Dysplasias

Joel A. Kaplan
Frank P. LaFranco
Ira Garoon

"Hereditary" retinal detachment is infrequent and not truly inherited as a primary disease. Detachments occurring in patients with myopia, sickle cell hemoglobinopathy, or Ehlers-Danlos syndrome are really secondary in origin. Retinal detachments can also be associated with hereditary vitreoretinal dysplasia. Five such syndromes that produce detachments are congenital retinoschisis, Wagner-Stickler syndrome, Favre's syndrome, familial exudative vitreoretinopathy, and the median clefting syndrome.

MYOPIA

The relationship between inherited high myopia and retinal detachment has always been a confusing one. Although the two entities are frequently associated, they may be caused by at least two different factors. Detachments occur more frequently in eyes with vitreoretinal degeneration, and, since such degeneration is prevalent in high myopia, these eyes have more detachments than nonmyopic eyes. Most of these detachments, however, can be classified as "developmental" rather than primary, hereditary ones.

Several reports discussing the relationship of myopia to familial retinal detachments do attempt to establish a hereditary pattern for the detachment itself [9, 12, 13, 28, 36]. Most families show an autosomal dominant pattern, but there is often skipping of a generation, which creates an irregular pattern of transmission. Edmund also reported one family with a recessive pattern [9]. Thus it would appear that there are enough reported pedigrees to substantiate the belief that detachments of the retina can sometimes be ge-

netically transmitted independently of myopia. François raises the question whether or not there are two independent genes, one for the myopia and the other for the detachment [10, 11]. He suggests that these two genes are close together on the same autosomal chromosome, thus causing the frequent association. However, he also feels that crossing over may occur and may explain the occasional dissociation when a regular pattern is not observed (Figs. 15-1 through 15-3) (see Chap. 3).

SICKLE CELL HEMOGLOBINOPATHY

Sickle cell hemoglobin (hemoglobin S) is inherited through the action of a mutant gene. The molecular defect is a single amino acid substitution (valine for glutamic acid) on the β chain of the hemoglobin molecule through mechanisms that are as yet imperfectly understood. This single amino acid difference between normal adult hemoglobin (hemoglobin A) and hemoglobin S confers a change in the three-dimensional molecular configuration of the hemoglobin molecule, which in turn results in a crescentic, sickled appearance of the red blood cell, especially under conditions of hypoxia. The sickled red blood cell is prematurely destroyed in the body, giving rise to hemolytic anemia. It is also considerably more rigid than the normal erythrocyte and tends to cause increased viscosity of the blood and to occlude small retinal arterioles. Systemically, the hemolytic component often predominates, whereas in the retina the infarcted and ischemic components tend to be paramount.

When sickle hemoglobin is inherited from one

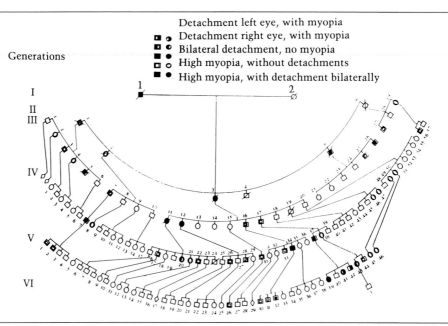

Fig. 15-1. *Pedigree of six generations with high myopia associated with retinal detachment. (From F. Gillespie and B. Covelli,* Arch. Ophthalmol. 69 : 733, 1963. *Copyright 1963, American Medical Association. Reproduced by permission.)*

Fig. 15-2. *Pedigree of family with retinal detachment. (From A. I. Friedmann and E. Epstein [12]. Reproduced by permission.)*

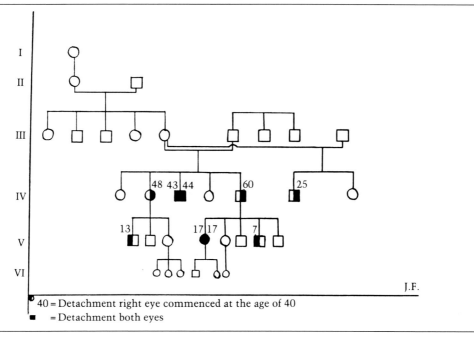

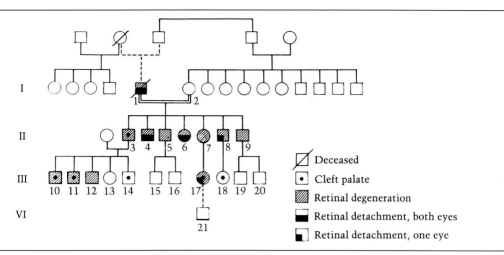

Fig. 15-3. *Pedigree of three generations with retinal degeneration and detachments. This may be an example of retinal detachments associated with the facial clefting syndrome [26] (see Median Clefting Syndrome, in text). (From W. V. Delaney, Jr. et al., Arch. Ophthalmol. 69 : 44, 1963. Copyright 1963, American Medical Association. Reproduced by permission.)*

parent only, the combination of abnormal plus normal hemoglobin is called sickle cell trait (hemoglobin AS). Generally, both systemic and ocular complications are infrequent in these heterozygous carriers of sickle cell trait, and when they do occur they are usually mild. When sickle cell hemoglobin is inherited from both parents, the homozygous state (hemoglobin SS) is often responsible for severe systemic manifestations but is only rarely responsible for significant retinal abnormalities. Another mutant hemoglobin (hemoglobin C) is allelic to hemoglobin S. When hemoglobin C is inherited from one parent and hemoglobin S is inherited from the other, the doubly heterozygous condition called sickle cell hemoglobin disease (hemoglobin CS) is the result of the abnormal codominately functioning hemoglobins. CS disease has different and sometimes milder systemic manifestations than does the SS state and different and sometimes more severe systemic manifestations than the AS condition. However, the retinal manifestations of the CS disease are characteristically more severe than in either the AS or the SS combinations.

The discrepancy between ocular and systemic manifestations of the various sickle cell hemoglobinopathies is intriguing; however, no clearly documented explanation has been provided for the repeatedly observed lower incidence of proliferative sickle retinopathy in the most systemically severe type of hemoglobinopathy (SS).

It is possible that the proliferative sickle retinopathy is most severe in CS disease because the combined effect of only mild anemia (less severe than in SS) with more pronounced sickling (more severe than in AS) results in a higher blood viscosity than in either the AS or the SS condition. Higher total hemoglobin levels, lower fetal hemoglobin levels, and higher levels of irreversibly sickled cells have all been implicated as high-risk factors, but their precise roles have not been elucidated.

Proliferative sickle retinopathy begins as arteriolar occlusions (stage I) in the temporal periphery of the retina caused by microemboli, frequently at Y-shaped arteriolar bifurcations, by rigid sickled erythrocytes (Figs. 15-4 and 15-5). This stage is followed by the development of arteriolar-venular anastomosis (stage II). Neovascularization (stage III) then spontaneously develops, seemingly as an attempt to revascularize the ischemic peripheral retina (Fig. 15-6). The neovascular growth frequently takes on a fan-shaped form that resembles marine sea fans; hence the name *sea fans*. Sea fans occur in almost all electrophoretic varieties of sickle cell disease. They are most frequently seen in sickle cell hemoglobin C (SC) disease but are also common in sickle cell β-thalassemia (SB-thal). The sea fans often bleed into the vitreous (stage IV). As a result, vitreous traction, when coupled with thin atrophic retina, often results in retinal holes and tears and eventually rhegmatogenous retinal detachment (Fig. 15-7).

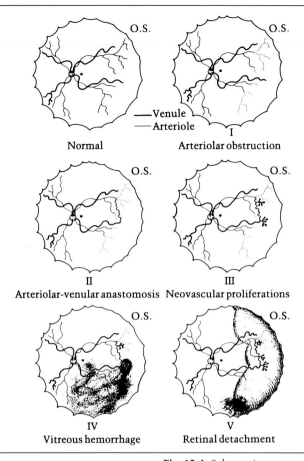

Fig. 15-4. *Schematic sequence of events in proliferative sickle retinopathy. (From M. F. Goldberg [16]. Reproduced by permission.)*

Fortunately, the natural course of proliferative sickle retinopathy shows autoinfarction of sea fans in 20 to 60 percent of patients. The cause of autoinfarction has not been clearly established but could involve repetitive sickling and thrombosis of the sea fan itself, traction with kinking of the neovascularization, avulsion of the sea fan by increased vitreous traction, and possibly the cessation of production of an angiogenic factor.

Treatment of proliferative sickle retinopathy is divided into photocoagulation therapy of the sea fan neovascularization, scleral buckling of rhegmatogenous retinal detachments, and pars plana vitrectomy for nonclearing vitreous hemorrhage.

Photocoagulation therapy has been used to close sea fan neovascularization and decrease the incidence of vitreous hemorrhage. The 20 to 60 percent incidence of autoinfarction suggests that photocoagulation should be reserved for those patients who have bilateral proliferative disease or have lost one eye to proliferative sickle retinop-

athy. In patients with early sea fan neovascularization in only one eye, follow-up study without treatment is reasonable. Focal treatment of small sea fans can be performed with xenon or argon laser coagulation. Feeder vessel techniques are more effective when the sea fan is large or elevated; however, choroidal neovascularization is a serious complication of feeder vessel coagulation. Scatter-type photocoagulation as used in panablation therapy for diabetic retinopathy has been effective in preliminary studies in treating early, but not advanced, proliferative sickle retinopathy.

Scleral buckling techniques for the treatment of rhegmatogenous retinal detachments in proliferative sickle retinopathy patients are accompanied by a significant incidence of complications (both ocular and systemic) that can threaten sight or life. The major ocular complication of anterior segment necrosis accompanying standard seg-

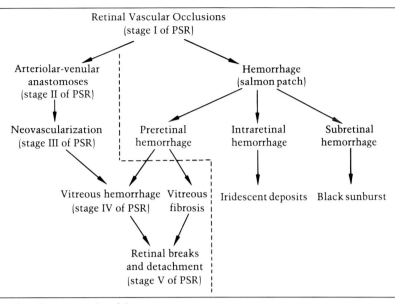

Fig. 15-5. *Presumed pathogenesis of proliferative sickle retinopathy (PSR).*

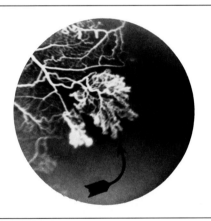

Fig. 15-6. *Fluorescein angiogram of retinal periphery in sickling. Arrow indicates typical neovascular "sea fan" growing into nonperfused area of retina.*

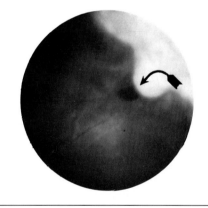

Fig. 15-7. *Retinal hole with retinal detachment (arrow).*

mental or encircling buckles can be avoided by preoperatively replacing about half the circulating sickle cell blood with transfused blood from normal donors. Intraoperative oxygen levels should be maintained at as high a level as possible, and postoperatively the continuous use of supplemental oxygen by face mask has proven useful.

Pars plana vitrectomy in sickle cell hemoglobinopathy is accompanied by a higher incidence of intraoperative and postoperative complications than in the diabetic population undergoing the same procedure. For this reason 6 months should be allowed to elapse after the onset of a visually disabling vitreous hemorrhage in one eye, the goal of surgery being clarification of the media and release of vitreous traction on the sea fans and retina. The postoperative glaucoma analogous to ghost cell glaucoma is caused by rigid sickled erythrocytes being trapped in the trabecular meshwork. Timolol maleate has been used to help control this serious complication.

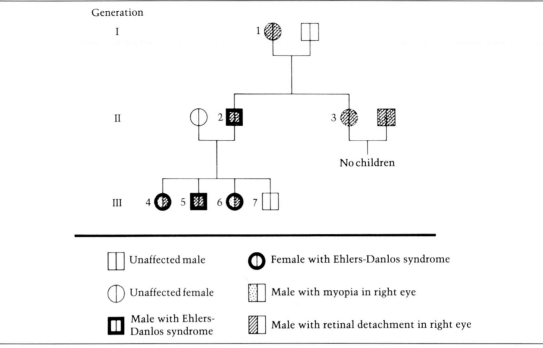

Generation

I

II

III

No children

☐ Unaffected male   ◑ Female with Ehlers-Danlos syndrome

◑ Unaffected female   ▨ Male with myopia in right eye

■ Male with Ehlers-Danlos syndrome   ▧ Male with retinal detachment in right eye

EHLERS-DANLOS SYNDROME

Ehlers-Danlos syndrome is a connective tissue disorder that is inherited as an autosomal dominant trait of variable penetrance. It has been reported mainly in whites. Clinically the disease is characterized by hyperelastic, fragile skin and hyperlaxity of the joints. It is present at birth but is usually not evident until the child begins to walk. The laxity of the joints causes frequent falls and repeated dislocations of many joints throughout the body. In addition to the joint and cutaneous manifestations, there are also abnormalities in the supporting tissue of the blood vessels or their walls. The ocular manifestations of the syndrome include vitreous hemorrhages and membranes, angioid streaks, and rhegmatogenous retinal detachments.

Pemberton and colleagues in 1966 described the association of familial retinal detachment and Ehlers-Danlos syndrome [31]. They reported three generations of a family in which 6 members were afflicted with myopia and retinal detachment (Fig. 15-8). Of the 6 patients with detachment, 4 had systemic manifestations of Ehlers-Danlos syndrome. Retinal breaks were present in six eyes of the 4 patients. All the breaks were located temporally and were accompanied by evidence of strong

Fig. 15-8. *Pedigree of a family with inherited retinal detachment and Ehlers-Danlos syndrome. (From J. W. Pemberton, H. M. Freeman, and C. L. Schepens, Arch. Ophthalmol. 76 : 817, 1966. Copyright 1966, American Medical Association. Reproduced by permission.)*

vitreous traction, such as rolled edges, areas of white without pressure, and horseshoe tears with visible adherent vitreous membranes. Premature degeneration and collapse of the vitreous body were present in all eyes. The premature degeneration may be a local manifestation of a generalized abnormality of the extracellular substance in this syndrome.

The management of a detachment associated with Ehlers-Danlos syndrome requires some considerations peculiar to the syndrome. Scleral buckling is preferable, because of the vitreous traction that is usually present. However, the excessively thin sclera may complicate this type of procedure, and often only photocoagulation or cryosurgery can be used in an attempt to obtain reattachment. The tendency for vitreous hemorrhage to occur dictates that only light diathermy, photocoagulation, or cryotherapy be used. Frequent postoperative examinations should be performed to detect additional retinal breaks, which may continue to form.

CONGENITAL RETINOSCHISIS

Congenital retinoschisis is a familial condition inherited as an X-linked recessive trait. The developmental defect is characterized by an actual splitting of the retina into an inner and outer layer, frequent vitreous hemorrhage, translucent membranes in the vitreous cavity, and a very characteristic macular appearance.

With the development of indirect ophthalmoscopy, fundus biomicroscopy, and fluorescein angiography, the diagnosis of X-linked retinoschisis has become frequent. It is no longer considered a rare condition, although its expression and penetrance is variable and many patients exhibit only certain characteristics of the disease. There are a few detailed clinical studies involving several cases of congenital retinoschisis, and these, along with comprehensive evaluations of some isolated cases, have contributed greatly to a more thorough understanding of this vitreoretinal dystrophy. The following description refers mainly to two series, one of 40 patients (Boston) [26] and the other of 48 patients (Chile) [38]. These are not to be confused with the pedigree of a family presented by Yassur and co-workers with autosomal dominant hereditary retinoschisis not associated with retinal detachment [41].

Congenital retinoschisis has been seen in children as young as 7 weeks old, but often it is not detected until the patients are of school age and present with signs and symptoms associated with poor visual acuity, strabismus, or both. In the Boston study the average age at diagnosis was just over 10 years, with an age range from 7 weeks to 28 years. The Chilean series contained patients first diagnosed at age 16 months to 55 years. The wide variation in the age at detection is related to the time when the macula becomes involved in the process with a resultant change in visual acuity. None of the patients in these two studies was reported as premature; none had a complicated gestation or delivery. There were no significant associated systemic diseases, although one of the patients in the Boston study was mentally retarded.

The typical sex-linked recessive pattern was definitely observed in both of these large studies as well as in other reported cases. There was a familial history in 39 of the 48 patients in the Chilean group and 15 of the 40 patients in the Boston study. The Boston series had a definite familial clustering with four brothers in one family, three in another, and four other separate pairs of brothers. The family histories of the others included one affected maternal uncle, four affected maternal cousins, one brother with retinal detachment, and three brothers and one uncle with chorioretinal scars. There were also four cousins with strabismus. Deutman has suggested that female carriers show a predilection for male brethren [7]. There has been one reported case with the typical clinical findings in a female. She was the daughter of an affected man and his second cousin.

The entity is definitely bilateral, and all but four of the eyes in the Boston group showed some degree of involvement; 47 percent of the eyes showed involvement in two retinal quadrants, with the inferotemporal the most commonly affected. The superonasal quadrant was least involved.

A common finding is ballooning of the retinoschisis with large, round, or oval breaks in the inner layer. Only 26 percent of the eyes did not have breaks in the inner retinal layer. This layer is extremely thin and transparent, forming a convex elevation. The defects in this inner layer may be of such magnitude that they extend from the region of the optic disc to the posterior vitreous base, involving one or more quadrants, with only narrow strands of tissue adherent to the elevated vessels bridging the breaks. The inner layer of the cavity usually contains the retinal vessels, although in some cases they are in the outer layer. This confirms the feeling that the splitting takes place in the nerve fiber layer as shown by Yanoff and associates [40] and Manschot. In this feature congenital retinoschisis differs from acquired, or senile, retinoschisis, in which the splitting occurs in the outer plexiform layer. Also the region of the ora serrata is not involved in congenital retinoschisis as it is in the acquired type. The staining properties of the fluid in the retinoschisis cavity in the congenital type do not show the presence of acid mucopolysaccharide as seen in acquired retinoschisis.

The outer layer of the retinoschisis can be identified by a faint gray haze over the retinal pigment epithelium and choroid. When breaks are present in this layer, the red color of the choroid is seen through them in sharp contrast to the haze of the surrounding area. Only 16 percent of the eyes studied had outer-layer breaks. They were small (less than two disc diameters), round or oval, and located near the posterior edge of the retinoschisis cavity. Some of them were horseshoe shaped, with rolled edges. Nine of the twelve eyes with outer-layer breaks had associated inner-layer holes and retinal detachments.

Delicate white strands may be seen extending from the inner wall to the outer wall of the retinoschisis cavity, causing a "frosted" appearance in the outer layer where the strands are attached. The retinal veins remained in the outer layer in 3 of the eyes, creating the appearance of a reduplicated vessel pattern, one in the inner layer, and one in the outer layer.

Macular changes are present in all cases of congenital retinoschisis. Seldom does the actual large retinoschisis cavity extend into the macular region, but a foveal retinoschisis appears to be present in all patients. These findings are bilateral and consist of small cysts arranged in a radial pattern with tiny folds in the internal limiting membrane. There may be pigment epithelial atrophy, and cases of bilateral eccentricity of the fovea above the medial raphe have been reported. For a more complete discussion of the macular pathophysiology and fluorescein angiogram findings in X-linked retinoschisis, see Chapter 17.

Retinal detachment in association with congenital retinoschisis was seen in 22 percent of the eyes in the Boston study [26]. This contrasts with the 5.2 percent in the Chilean group [38] and in the cases studied by Deutman [7]. Detachment occurs when there is either a hole in full-thickness retina, as in the usual rhegmatogenous detachment, or when there are breaks in both the inner and outer layer of the retinoschisis. Detachment usually involved both the affected retina and the retina unaffected by the retinoschisis process.

Vitreous changes are common in congenital retinoschisis, with approximately one-half of the eyes showing either vitreous hemorrhage or membranes. The bleeding seems to originate from the retinal vessels bridging the gaps across the large inner breaks and occurs from traction on the vessel itself or from enlargement of the inner layer defect. The origin of the membranes is not certain. They probably are secondary to the vitreous hemorrhage or else represent the thickening of the hyaloid membrane formed from adhesions of the inner limiting membrane of the retina to the hyaloid. With vitreous syneresis the membranes are then dragged anteriorly into the vitreous cavity.

Several of the involved eyes showed a translucent, whitish, cellophane-like membrane, felt to be a mesodermal remnant bridging the anterior chamber angle from the iris to Schwalbe's line. There was also peripheral iris atrophy.

Interestingly, in patients with congenital retinoschisis observed over a period of time, little actual progression was noted in the disease process. In cases that did show advancement, the changes were limited to the quadrants of the fundus already involved, and little if any progressive visual field defect was noted. Rapid progression of the disease probably occurs during the first 5 years of life, and by age 20 most cases are stationary. If the retinoschisis process has been limited to the periphery, reasonably good central vision can be maintained for several decades.

Regressive findings occur in approximately one-quarter of the involved eyes. These changes are usually limited to collapse of the retinoschisis bulla, shrinkage of the vitreous membrane, and improvement of visual acuity.

Since most cases of congenital retinoschisis are stationary or relatively nonprogressive, treatment is not indicated unless (1) progression is such that the macula is threatened, (2) associated retinal detachment is present, or (3) there are bleeding retinal vessels causing repeated vitreous hemorrhage. The patient should be observed at frequent intervals, and if any of these conditions exist, specific treatment should then be undertaken. The best form of treatment for either rapid progression or associated retinal detachment is a scleral buckling procedure. Photocoagulation should not be considered, except as a possible means of sealing off bleeding retinal vessels, and this is not very effective. Coagulating over the cyst itself has resulted in a high percentage of retinal detachments after the procedure. Delimiting the cyst with a barrage along its posterior border has never been shown to be more advantageous than just allowing the natural progression of the disease. Photocoagulation or cyrotherapy of outer-layer holes without detachment is of debatable value, depending on the specific location of the retinal break. Vitrectomy may be indicated in those eyes with persistent vitreous hemorrhage, but care must be taken not to destroy the elevated retina (inner layer) in the process. We know of no case in which a vitrectomy has actually been performed.

WAGNER-STICKLER SYNDROME

Wagner first described a vitreoretinal degeneration in 1938 based on his findings in three generations of a large Swiss family in which 23 members were affected. The hereditary pattern was autosomal dominant. His original description included presenile cataracts as the major cause of visual loss with involvement of the vitreous and retina. This same family was restudied in 1959 by Boehringer, Dieterle, and Landolt, and 20 additional cases were added. Finally, in 1961 Ricci again reviewed the same family and added 5 more additional cases for a total of 48 afflicted members. None of these patients was noted to have a retinal detachment. Since then, many authors have described a hyaloideoretinal degeneration with retinal detachment as the most common ocular feature and called it Wagner's syndrome.

The important features of Wagner's syndrome, which is an inherited hyaloideoretinopathy, may be summarized as Wagner first described them. Myopia is the most common refractive error. Alexander and Shea noted that the myopia is not axial, with no posterior staphylomas being found [1]. In Wagner's original family the decreased visual acuity was caused mainly by the development of cataracts that had their onset in the third decade. In those individuals with decreased vision and clear lenses, marked choroidal atrophy with loss of choriocapillaris and pigment epithelium in the posterior pole was apparently the cause of the visual loss. Syneresis of the vitreous gel was the most commonly reported ocular manifestation. The onset of the vitreous change occurs quite early, having been reported by Jansen in a 2 1/2-year-old patient [23]. Degeneration of the vitreous gel is accompanied by the development of large optically empty areas within the gel and the formation of mobile fenestrated membranes within the gel with multiple attachments to the retina near the equator. The retina itself frequently exhibits equatorially oriented lattice degeneration and characteristic areas of atrophy of the pigment epithelium and choriocapillaris oriented radially along the retinal veins and occasionally along the arteries.

The important relationship between the ocular and nonocular manifestations of Wagner's syndrome was often overlooked until 1965 when Stickler and associates described a connective tissue dysplasia that they called hereditary progressive artho-ophthalmopathy [34]. The hereditary pattern was also autosomal dominant. The ocular findings have been described in the ophthalmic literature as Wagner's syndrome, while the nonocular features have been studied by geneticists as Stickler's syndrome. The main characteristics of these patients included all the ocular findings included in Wagner's syndrome and the nonocular findings of joint disease, a characteristic physiognomy, cleft palate, and hearing loss. Retinal de-

Table 15-1. *Wagner's Syndrome*

Autosomal dominant

Myopia: often moderate, but may be severe

Strabismus

Cataract, usually beginning around puberty; mainly posterior cortical punctate opacities, nuclear sclerosis, and complicated cataract

Vitreous degeneration with syneresis and liquefaction, which produces an optically empty vitreous except for some vitreous membranes, notably a whitish, translucent, avascular, often fenestrated, hand-shaped membrane, oriented circumferentially near the equator and extending into the vitreous cavity from the surface of the retina

Fundus changes
 Foci of choroidal atrophy
 Peripheral retinal pigmentation, which may be perivascular
 Vascular sheathing, sclerosis, and caliber changes

Subnormal electroretinogram

tachments caused by large circumferential tears were indeed noted frequently in this group of patients.

Tables 15-1 and 15-2 present the clinical manifestations of Wagner's syndrome and Stickler's syndrome. Most authors are in agreement that there is no significant difference in the hyaloideoretinopathy of Wagner and the ocular findings in the arthro-ophthalmopathy of Stickler.

The diagnosis of Wagner-Stickler syndrome at the earliest possible time can be of value by allowing the patient to obtain treatment for the open-angle glaucoma or prophylactic treatment of retinal breaks before vision is permanently lost. The Wagner-Stickler syndrome should be considered when evaluating patients with (1) congenital myopia; (2) vitreoretinopathies exhibiting radially oriented perivascular chorioretinal degeneration; (3) rhegmatogenous retinal detachment caused by giant tears, especially in the presence of a positive family history; (4) posterior cleft palate; (5) Pierre Robin malformation complex; (6) unexplained juvenile arthropathy; and (7) mild epiphyseal dysplasia.

FAVRE'S SYNDROME

Favre's syndrome, or macrofibrillar vitreoretinal degeneration, has a recessive mode of transmission and is not associated with any specific refractive error [10, 11]. There is extensive vitreous

Table 15-2. *Stickler's Syndrome*

Autosomal dominant

Ocular complex
  Myopia
  Strabismus
  Presenile cataract
  Open-angle glaucoma
  Vitreous degeneration with syneresis and
    liquefaction producing an optically empty
    vitreous with membranes including whitish
    translucent, circumferential, equatorial lines

Fundus changes
  Myopic changes and atrophic thinning
  White with pressure
  Perivascular retinal pigmentation overlying atrophic
    retinal pigment epithelium, which can extend far
    posteriorly with a radial orientation
  Lattice degeneration
  Retinal breaks that are often large, multiple, or
    both
  Rhegmatogenous retinal detachment with a
    relatively poor prognosis for repair
  Subnormal electroretinogram, visual-evoked
    response, and electro-oculogram

Orofacial complex
  Facial bone hypoplasia; the facial appearance is
    variable depending on the extent to which each
    facial bone is hypoplastic (for example, flat
    midface, depressed nasal bridge, maxillary
    hypoplasia, micrognathia)
  High-arched palate
  Bifid uvula
  Posterior cleft palate, which may take the form of
    frank cleft palate, submucous cleft palate
    (detectable by palpation), or abnormal palatal
    mobility with rhinolalia aperta; cleft lip is not
    present
  Pierre Robin malformation complex: palatoschisis,
    micrognathia, and glossoptosis
  Abnormal teeth, malocclusion

Generalized skeletal complex
  Joint hyperextensibility
  Enlarged joints
  Early-onset degenerative arthritis
  Hypotonia and relative muscle hypoplasia
  Various other bony anomalies, e.g., kyphosis,
    scoliosis, pectus carinatum, accessory carpal
    ossicles, hip dislocation, coxa valga, talipes
    equinovarus
  Radiographic changes including mild generalized
    spondyloepiphyseal dysplasia with flattening of
    the epiphyses, narrowing of the diaphyses, flaring
    or widening of the metaphyses, wedging of the
    tubular bones, and anterior maxillary and
    mandibular underdevelopment

Hearing loss, which may be sensorineural or caused
  by otitis media, associated with cleft palate

degeneration associated with peripheral retinal degeneration. Vitreoretinal adhesions are present, with pockets of liquefied vitreous scattered among fibrillar vitreous membranes. Favre described two families with the condition. Delaney and coauthors have described additional cases [6].

FAMILIAL EXUDATIVE VITREORETINOPATHY

Familial exudative vitreoretinopathy was first described by Criswick and Schepens in 1969 [5]. Since then there have been several other familial studies [30, 37]. The cause of the disease is unknown, although several hypotheses have been suggested. While no inheritance pattern was initially determined, evidence suggesting a pure genetic defect has been raised. The disorder follows a dominant inheritance pattern, which makes genetic counseling important for families affected by the disease, regardless of the exact cause [30]. Another suggestion as to the origin of familial exudative vitreoretinopathy involves a defect of the oxygen transport system with a resultant lower oxygen concentration to the retina, thereby causing a retrolental-fibroplasia-type pathophysiology [37].

The disease primarily affects the retinal vasculature with the vitreous being secondarily involved. In general the patients are unaffected by systemic abnormalities. However, some patients were found to have a form of mental retardation. All patients were products of normal deliveries and had normal gestational age and weight. In those patients with only minimal manifestations, the visual acuity was only slightly reduced. The more severe the disease the greater the visual loss. Many patients showed the disease in only one eye, with excellent visual acuity in the fellow eye.

The disease tends to progress in three stages. There is an early form with evidence of peripheral vitreoretinal traction only. This is manifested by white with and without pressure. The second stage has abnormal vessels in the temporal periphery. The third stage not only has the retinal vascular changes, but vitreoretinal proliferation develops with subsequent traction retinal detachment.

The retinal vascular changes found in the second and third stages resemble those seen in retrolental fibroplasia with tortuous vessels in the posterior segment as well as the peripheral fundus. Miyakubo and associates, using wide-angle photography and fluorescein angiography, found a consistent, wide, V-shaped avascular zone extending towards the temporal periphery [29]. Multiple arteriolar-venular shunts were identified in the peripheral retina with fluorescein angiography. Heterotropia of the macula resulting from traction on the temporal retinal vessels is a characteristic finding, but it is not always identified. Subretinal exudates along with localized retinal detachments are commonly seen [5]. Other retinal findings include peripheral retinal pigmentation, retinal hemorrhages, and retinoschisis. The vitreous itself appears to be secondarily involved. The most frequent findings are syneresis and vitreoretinal membranes. Posterior detachments of the vitreous are not common. A histopathologic study, described by Brockhurst and colleagues, found a prominent vitreoretinal membrane posterior to the ora serrata in 2 patients [4].

Criswick and Schepens presented an extensive differential diagnosis, comparing this entity to retrolental fibroplasia, peripheral uveitis, Coats' disease, heterotropia of the macula, congenital retinal septa, angiomatosis retinae, Eales' disease, congenital retinoschisis, Wagner's disease, and retinoblastoma [5]. These investigators differentiated this disorder from Coats' disease on the basis of the vitreous changes in the vitreoretinal adhesions. It was not felt to be a variation of peripheral uveitis, because the exudative lesions were more posterior, were not on the pars plana, and were not more pronounced in the inferior fundus. There was also no sheathing or obliteration of the blood vessels.

MEDIAN CLEFTING SYNDROME

Knobloch and Layer reported on 89 patients with clefting syndromes of the face associated with retinal detachment [24]. Recently, V. Feiler-Ofry and Godel and co-workers [14] described a family with a member afflicted with a retinal detachment and median cleft face syndrome. In both studies there was an autosomal dominant pattern of inheritance. In Knobloch and Layer's study there were 5 patients with a characteristic physiognomy consisting of maxillary hypoplasia, depressed nasal bridge, and midfacial flattening. Palatoschisis was associated with bifid uvula, variable myopia, and lattice degeneration of the retina.

Retinal detachment was observed in 13 of Knobloch and Layer's patients and in 1 sibling in V. Feiler-Ofry's family. In addition, many of the remaining patients in Knobloch and Layer's study exhibited vitreous syneresis and membrane formation, as well as an atrophic thin retina associated with lattice degeneration. The retinal detachments generally occurred at an early age and were similar to those reported by Stickler in his syndrome of hereditary progressive arthroophthalmopathy.

REFERENCES

1. Alexander, R. L., and Shea, M. Wagner's disease. *Arch. Ophthalmol.* 74 : 310, 1965.
2. Bird, A. C. (Ed.). *Symposium on Medical and Surgical Disease of the Retina and Vitreous,* Transactions of New Orleans Academy of Ophthalmology. St. Louis: Mosby, 1983.
3. Blair, N. P., et al. Hereditary progressive arthroophthalmopathy of Stickler. *Am. J. Ophthalmol.* 88 : 876, 1979.
4. Brockhurst, R. J., Albert, D. M., and Zakov, N. Pathologic findings in familial exudative vitreoretinopathy. *Arch. Ophthalmol.* 99 : 2146, 1981.
5. Criswick, V. G., and Schepens, C. L. Familial exudative vitreoretinopathy. *Am. J. Ophthalmol.* 68 : 578, 1969.
6. Delaney, W. V., Jr., Podedworny, W., and Havener, W. H. Inherited retinal detachment. *Arch. Ophthalmol.* 69 : 44, 1963.
7. Deutman, A. F. Vitreoretinal Dystrophies. In D. Archer (Ed.), *Krill's Hereditary Retinal and Choroidal Diseases, Vol. 2. Clinical Characteristics.* Hagerstown, Md.: Harper & Row, 1977. Pp. 1043–1062.
8. Eagle, R. C., Jr., Yanoff, M., and Morse, P. H. Anterior segment necrosis following scleral buckling in hemoglobin SC disease. *Am. J. Ophthalmol.* 75 : 426, 1973.
9. Edmund, J. Familial retinal detachment. *Acta Ophthalmol. (Copenh.)* 39 : 644, 1963.
10. François, J. The Role of Heredity in Retinal Detachment. In A. McPherson (Ed.), *New and Controversial Aspects of Retinal Detachment.* New York: Hoeber Med. Div., Harper & Row, 1968.
11. François, J. The role of heredity in retinal detachment. *Int. Ophthalmol. Clin.* 8 : 965, 1968.
12. Friedman, A. I., and Epstein, E. Familial retinal detachment. *Am. J. Ophthalmol.* 51 : 33, 1961.
13. Gillespie, F., and Covelli, B. Hereditary high myopia with retinal detachment: A family study. *Arch. Ophthalmol.* 69 : 733, 1963.
14. Godel, N. P., Nemet, P., and Lazar, M. The Wagner-Stickler syndrome complex. *Doc. Ophthalmol.* 52 : 179, 1981.
15. Goldbaum, M. H., et al. Acute choroidal ischemia as a complication of photocoagulation. *Arch. Ophthalmol.* 94 : 1025, 1976.
16. Goldberg, M. F. Proliferative sickle retinopathy: Classification and pathogenesis. *Am. J. Ophthalmol.* 71 : 649, 1971.
17. Goldberg, M. F. Retinal detachment associated with

proliferative retinopathies. *Ophthalmic Surg.* 2 : 222, 1971.

18. Goldberg, M. F., Charache, S., and Acacio, I. Ophthalmologic manifestations of sickle cell thalassemia. *Arch. Intern. Med.* 128 : 33, 1971.

19. Gow, J., and Oliver, L. Familial exudative retinopathy. *Arch. Ophthalmol.* 86 : 150, 1971.

20. Jampol, L. M., et al. A randomized clinical trial of feeder vessel photocoagulation of proliferative sickle cell retinopathy: I. Preliminary results. *Ophthalmol.* 90 : 540, 1983.

21. Jampol, L. M., et al. An update on vitrectomy surgery and retinal detachment repair in sickle cell disease. *Arch. Ophthalmol.* 100 : 591, 1982.

22. Jampol, L. M., and Goldberg, M. F. Retinal breaks after photocoagulation of proliferative sickle cell retinopathy. *Arch. Ophthalmol.* 98 : 676, 1980.

23. Jansen, L. M. Degeneratio hyaloideoretinalis hereditaria. *Ophthalmologica* 144 : 458, 1962.

24. Knobloch, W. H., and Layer, J. M. Clefting syndromes associated with retinal detachment. *Am. J. Ophthalmol.* 73 : 517, 1972.

25. Knobloch, W. H. Inherited hyaloideoretinopathy and skeletal dysplasia. *Trans. Am. Ophthalmol. Soc.* 73 : 417, 1976.

26. Kraushar, M. F., et al. Congenital Retinoschisis. In J. G. Bellows (Ed.), *Contemporary Ophthalmology, Honoring Sr. Steward Duke-Elder.* Baltimore: Williams & Wilkins, 1972.

27. Lagua, H. Familial exudative vitreoretinopathy. *Albrecht von Graefes Arch. Klin. Exp. Ophthalmol.* 213 : 121.

28. Levy, J. Inherited retinal detachment. *Br. J. Ophthalmol.* 36 : 626, 1952.

29. Miyakubo, H., Inohara, N., and Hashimoto, K. Retinal involvement in familial exudative vitreoretinopathy. *Ophthalmologica* 185 : 125, 1982.

30. Ober, R. R., et al. Autosomal dominant familial vitreoretinopathy. *Br. J. Ophthalmol.* 64 : 112, 1980.

31. Pemberton, J. W., Freeman, H. M., and Schepens, C. L. Familial retinal detachment and the Ehlers-Danlos syndrome. *Arch. Ophthalmol.* 76 : 817, 1966.

32. Ryan, S. J., and Goldberg, M. F. Anterior segment ischemia following scleral buckling in sickle cell hemoglobinopathy. *Am. J. Ophthalmol.* 72 : 35, 1971.

33. Steahly, L. P., and Jones, W. L. An unusual case of retinoschisis and retinal detachment. *Ann. Ophthalmol.* 6 : 593, 1982.

34. Stickler, G. B., Belau, P. G., and Farrell, F. J. Hereditary progressive arthro-ophthalmopathy. *Mayo Clin. Proc.* 40 : 433, 1965.

35. Tolentino, F. L., Schepens, C. L., and Freeman, H. M. *Vitreoretinal Disorders: Diagnosis and Management.* Philadelphia: Saunders, 1976.

36. van den Bergh, E. O. Hereditary disposition to retinal detachment in two families. *Ophthalmologica* 149 : 236, 1965.

37. van Nouhuys, C. E. *Dominant Exudative Vitreoretinopathy and Other Vascular Developmental Disorders of the Peripheral Retina.* Dr. W. Junk, 1982.

38. Verdaguer, J. T. Juvenile retinal detachment. *Am. J. Ophthalmol.* 93 : 145, 1982.

39. Wilhelm, J. L., Zakov, Z. N., and Hoeltge, G. A. Erythropheresis in treating retinal detachments secondary to sickle cell retinopathy. *Am. J. Ophthalmol.* 92 : 582, 1981.

40. Yanoff, M., Rahn, E. K., and Zimmerman, L. E. Histopathology of juvenile retinoschisis. *Arch. Ophthalmol.* 79 : 49, 1968.

41. Yassur, Y., et al. Autosomal dominant inheritance of retinoschisis. *Am. J. Ophthalmol.* 94 : 338, 1982.

42. Zinn, K. M. Vitreoretinal surgery in a patient with sickle cell retinopathy. *Mt. Sinai J. Med. (N.Y.)* 48 : 79, 1981.

16   Retinoblastoma

Maria Musarella
Brenda L. Gallie

Retinoblastoma, the most common primary ocular malignancy in children, is one of several heritable childhood cancers. The target cells are the primitive retinal cells, which undergo malignant transformation before their final differentiation. These primitive cells disappear within the first few years of life, so retinoblastoma seldom arises after 3 or 4 years of age.

The disease exhibits a hereditary and nonhereditary occurrence in addition to a deletional form involving human chromosome 13 band q14 (Fig. 16-1). Since most children with heritable retinoblastoma have no family history of retinoblastoma, the term *sporadic,* implying only the absence of family history, does not contribute genetic information and will not be used in this chapter. Sixty percent of all retinoblastoma tumors arise at the somatic level in a single retinal cell. These children have no heritable predisposition to retinoblastoma, develop only a single tumor, and will not have children with retinoblastoma. Eighty-five percent of patients with unilateral retinoblastoma fall into this category.

In 40 percent of all children with retinoblastoma, the tendency to develop the tumors is heritable: The primitive retinal cells are predisposed to malignant transformation by a germ line mutation that is highly penetrant and shows a pattern of autosomal dominant transmission. These patients are usually detected by having bilateral, multiple tumors (85%). However, 15 percent of heritable cases are unilateral, and 10 percent are in unaffected carriers who do not express the retinoblastoma mutation. Only 6 percent of new cases of retinoblastoma have a family history of retinoblastoma. The majority of children with heritable retinoblastoma have acquired the predisposition to retinoblastoma as a result of a new germ cell mutation, which will be transmitted to 50 percent of their offspring.

Deletion of chromosome 13 band q14 predisposes the child to the development of retinoblastoma in 1 to 3 percent of all cases. The deletion can be detected by sensitive cytogenetic studies or by quantitative measurements of an enzyme with a genetic locus in band 13q14, esterase D (ESD). Expression of retinoblastoma in this group is bilateral or unilateral, usually associated with developmental retardation and congenital abnormalities, the severity of which depends on the extent of the 13q14 deletion.

Whether the patient with retinoblastoma falls into the hereditary, nonhereditary, or deletional subgroup, the genetic events that have occurred in the tumor are the same (Fig. 16-2). The two critical changes both involve the retinoblastoma locus on chromosome 13q14. The first is a mutation or deletion on one chromosome abolishing the normal function of the retinoblastoma locus. This affects all constitutional cells of the hereditary and deletional patients, but when the mutation is heterozygous, there is no discernible cellular effect. In nonhereditary cases the retinoblastoma locus on one chromosome 13 is mutated in only a single retinal cell. The second critical genetic event that leads to actual tumor formation is the same in all cases: loss of the normal allele at 13q14 on the homologous, nonmutated chromosome. This occurs in the individual retinal cell that becomes malignant and results in homozygosity for the defective mutation at 13q14 with complete absence of the normal product of

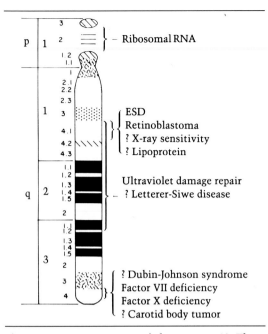

Fig. 16-1. *Human gene map of chromosome 13. The locations of disease mutations associated with chromosome 13 are indicated. Note proximal location of esterase D (ESD) to the retinoblastoma locus. The diseases not confirmed are indicated by question marks.*

the retinoblastoma locus in the retinoblastoma tumor cell.

The mortality rate in North America from treated retinoblastoma is 8 percent, in striking contrast to untreated cases, for which the mortality rate is close to 100 percent. Treatment includes surgery (enucleation of the eye), radiotherapy, cryotherapy, and photocoagulation. Chemotherapy is used as adjuvant prophylaxis or for known metastatic disease. Clinical features, pathology, and treatment are described elsewhere [36]. This chapter will deal specifically with the genetics of retinoblastoma.

FAMILY STUDIES

Autosomal Dominant Transmission

The first suggestion of the heritable tendency in retinoblastoma came from families in which more than one child developed retinoblastoma. Lerche documented a sibship in which 4 of 7 children had retinoblastoma, 3 unilaterally and 1 bilater-

Fig. 16-2. *Chromosomal mechanisms that would allow phenotypic expression of a recessive mutant allele at the retinoblastoma (RB) locus. Any of these events in a predisposed retinal cell will result in homozygosity for the mutant allele at the retinoblastoma locus on both chromosome 13 homologs. (M_1 = mutation 1; M_2 = mutation 2.)*

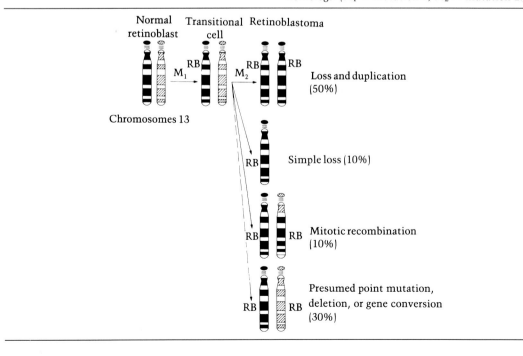

ally [59]. The parents were unaffected. Other reports from the older literature showed similar patterns of several affected sibs with unaffected parents [22, 47]. When surgery could effect a cure of retinoblastoma, transmission over two or more generations was observed [68], and an autosomal dominant pattern of transmission became evident [106]. Comprehensive statistics on family studies have determined the proportion of all retinoblastoma patients with secondary cases in their families. Kaelin collected 959 retinoblastoma cases from 13 series (1891–1953) [47]. In only 39 cases (4.1%) were there additionally affected family members. François and colleagues collected 2,995 published cases of retinoblastoma of which 6 percent were familial [31].

Chromosome Linkage Studies

The deletional form of retinoblastoma (described in more detail under Constitutional Chromosomal Changes below) focused attention on chromosome 13 as a likely site for the retinoblastoma mutation. ESD is the only polymorphic enzyme for which the genetic locus has been assigned to chromosome 13 (see Fig. 16-1) [104]. Since the quantitative amount of ESD produced by a cell depends on the number of copies of the ESD gene, cells from individuals with deletions of chromosome 13 have one-half the normal amount of ESD [93]. This characteristic is a feature of almost all patients with deletional retinoblastoma, even if the deletion is very small. Thus the ESD gene locus is within chromosome band 13q14. One case of deletional retinoblastoma with normal quantitative levels of ESD has now been reported [92], which shows that the ESD locus is not identical to the retinoblastoma locus, as was suggested by Howard [44].

ESD is genetically a polymorphic enzyme with at least three different phenotypes: ESD-1, ESD-1,2 and ESD-2. These phenotypes are determined by the codominant expression of two alleles, ESD-1 and ESD-2, segregating at the autosomal locus 13q14. The gene frequencies of the alleles differ for various populations. Eighty to ninety percent of all populations are homozygous for ESD-1, ten to twenty percent are heterozygous for ESD-1,2, and the remainder are ESD-2,2 or have rare alleles [110]. Informative families have been found in which parents with retinoblastoma are heterozygous for ESD, married homozygous individuals, and had both affected and unaffected offspring (Fig. 16-3) [19, 77, 90]. Linkage analysis of all families

reported with hereditary retinoblastoma with ESD isoenzymes to date have resulted in a lod (log odds) score for linkage of more than 3 (likelihood for linkage between the retinoblastoma and ESD loci more than 1,000 : 1) [77]. This is considered strong evidence that the genetic locus for autosomal dominantly inherited predisposition to retinoblastoma, or the retinoblastoma mutation, is located at chromosome 13q14. Studies of genetic changes in tumor cells have now shown that the nonheritable, somatic form of retinoblastoma also arises because of mutations at chromosome 13q14 (see Genetic Changes in Tumors, later in this chapter).

Penetrance and Expressivity

The penetrance and expressivity of the retinoblastoma mutation is variable in different families. Overall, 10 percent of obligate carriers do not exhibit clinical disease, but Bonaiti-Pellie and Briard-Guillemot have suggested from a segregation analysis of 211 nuclear families belonging to 166 pedigrees of hereditary retinoblastoma that there may be two types of retinoblastoma carriers, "high" and "low" transmittors [9]. The segregation ratio or proportion of offspring affected (penetrance) was found to be 0.49 when the transmitting parent was bilaterally affected, indicating almost complete penetrance of the dominant retinoblastoma mutation, but only 0.24 when the transmitting parent was unaffected or unilaterally affected. There was a correlation between expressivity (unilateral vs. bilateral retinoblastoma, retinoma, or no disease) and penetrance (proportion of offspring affected) that could be predicted from the proportion of bilaterally affected family members. In another study, when a carrier parent was unaffected, 54 percent of the affected children had bilateral tumors [62, 64]. If a parent had a unilateral tumor, 76 percent of the affected children had bilateral tumors. When both eyes of a parent were affected, 90 percent of the affected children had bilateral tumors. These figures have been used in the section on genetic counseling to derive risk figures for relatives of retinoblastoma patients of actually developing retinoblastoma tumors. Thus, penetrance and expressivity in a sibship were lowest when the parents were unaffected and highest when the parents were bilaterally affected [65].

However, within families there have been striking differences reported in retinoblastoma pene-

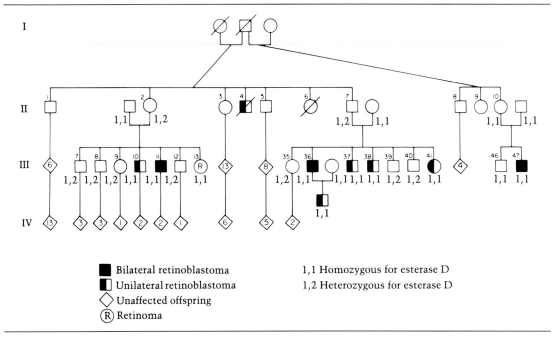

Fig. 16-3. *Pedigree of family demonstrating cosegregation of retinoblastoma and the esterase D-1 (ESD-1) allele. In generation III all affected, informative individuals are ESD-1 homozygotes. Individual 13 in generation III has retinoma (see Fig. 16-4 for description) and is also an ESD-1 homozygote. Unaffected individuals are ESD-1,2 heterozygotes. This family exhibits marked difference in retinoblastoma penetrance between generations II and III (retinoblastoma or retinoma and unilateral or bilateral).*

trance between generations. In a study of four generations with familial retinoblastoma, three forms of retinoblastoma gene expression occurred: unilateral, bilateral, retinoma (see Retinoma, later in chapter), or no clinical manifestation (Fig. 16-3) [19]. With each generation the penetrance and expressivity increased. Several models have been postulated to explain variability of penetrance and expressivity in familial cases of retinoblastoma: mutational mosaicism, multiple allelism, delayed mutation, host resistance, balanced translocation, and associated recessive lethal genes linked to the retinoblastoma locus [11, 12, 42, 54, 62–67, 72, 73, 75, 76, 96].

Motegi and co-workers have reported 5 cases of 13q14 deletion mosaicism in chromosomes of peripheral blood lymphocytes among 66 retinoblastoma patients [72, 73, 75]. Mosaicism occurs when the deletion occurs in only one cell of the mul-

ticell embryo. Thus, the deletion is present in only some of the patient's cells and is seen in only a percentage of the lymphocytes. If mosaicism is detected in a retinoblastoma individual, the parents could not be unaffected carriers of the retinoblastoma mutation, and the risk for future offspring would be zero. Mosaicism could also account for low penetrance (fewer than the usual 50% of offspring affected) in offspring of a mosaic patient since only a proportion of germ cells might carry the deletion. Mosaicism for a new mutation at the retinoblastoma locus without deletion could also theoretically occur but would be undetectable by presently available techniques.

Motegi and Minoda have observed a decrease in the proportion of 13q14 deleted cells as the patient gets older [76]. They suggested that the 13q14 mosaicism could disappear completely with age in some individuals.

Carlson and colleagues proposed that multiple allelism or heterozygosity in the expression of mutant alleles could explain the variability of penetrance and expressivity in familial cases of retinoblastoma [11, 12]. Mutational mosaicism arises when the mutation occurs after one or more cell divisions have taken place, so that only a portion of the cells of an individual have the mutation.

Delayed mutation occurs when the normal allele changes by premutation to an unstable intermediate premutated allele [42, 63]. This pre-mutated allele could be transmitted through several generations before undergoing a final rearrangement into a mutated allele in a somatic cell, which would lead to a tumor, or in germ cells, which would produce affected carriers. This theory would explain families with two or more affected siblings in the first affected generation.

Matsunaga proposes a host resistance model in which the three phenotypes (unaffected, unilaterally affected, and bilaterally affected) of gene carriers are determined largely by inherited tissue or host resistance to the major retinoblastoma mutation [63, 64, 66, 67]. In this model the unaffected carriers are inherently resistant to tumor formation, bilaterally affected persons are susceptible, and unilaterally affected carriers have intermediate susceptibility. Host resistance could be controlled by both genetic and environmental factors. Matsunaga theorizes that only one mutation may be required to produce retinoblastoma, the manifestation and expression of which depend on polygenic host resistance at gene loci other than chromosome 13q14. The second or crucial event initiating tumorigenesis would not be a true mutational event but an error in regulation of retinal differentiation. This error would be suppressed completely in the most resistant group of individuals, who would remain unaffected. Thus, the variability in expression or suppression of the normal differentiation of retinoblasts would depend on the degree of host resistance. Matsunaga postulates that neither of these events would involve chromosome 13. However, the retinoblastoma mutation leading to the hereditary form of retinoblastoma has been linked to chromosome 13 in all informative family studies [14, 77, 90], and somatic rearrangement of chromosome 13 has been shown to be important in retinoblastoma tumors [13]. This evidence strongly implicates chromosome 13 as the major site for genetic mutations leading to retinoblastoma.

Strong and co-workers have published an extensive pedigree showing a balanced translocation in unaffected carriers and sibs and unbalanced chromosome 13 deletion in affected individuals [96]. Thus in some pedigrees certain members who transmit the deletional form of retinoblastoma do not develop retinoblastoma because they are carriers of a balanced translocation. The number of families for which this mechanism accounts for variable penetrance and expressivity is likely to be small [87, 103].

A greater proportion of the deletion retinoblas-toma patients than of patients with the hereditary nondeletional form have unilateral disease. The excess of unilateral cases among the deletion patients suggests that deletion 13q14 has a lower carcinogenic potential than does the retinoblastoma mutation [54, 96]. The presence of essential genes on chromosome 13 near the retinoblastoma locus would explain reduced expressivity in deletion cases, since the second genetic event resulting in malignant retinoblastoma commonly involves loss of large parts of the normal chromosome 13 [13]. If all copies of essential genes were lost in the tumorigenic somatic rearrangement, the cell would not survive. A similar mechanism could explain decreased penetrance and expressivity in some nondeletion heritable cases, if recessive lethal genes were present on chromosome 13 [54]. Since homozygosity of an extensive region of chromosome 13 around the retinoblastoma locus is common in the tumors [13], in the presence of a recessive lethal gene only point mutation or gene conversion would succeed in producing a tumor. This would reduce the total number of tumors in individuals with such a recessive lethal gene and could result in families with reduced penetrance and expressivity.

New Germinal Mutations

Most cases of heritable retinoblastoma are new germinal mutations. Despite occasional reports of clusters of cases of retinoblastoma [97], it would appear that the incidence is constant in all parts of the world and in all races [29, 106]. One study compared the occurrence of nonfamilial bilateral retinoblastoma in an urban center to that in a rural area [98]. The results suggest that the incidences of retinoblastoma in a population could be used as an environmental monitor for mutagenic factors.

Several studies have identified a relationship between new germinal mutations resulting in retinoblastoma and paternal age [61, 83, 84]. Since spermatogonia are continuously dividing, older fathers may accumulate mutations. No such increase has been observed in unilateral cases. No maternal age effect has been seen in either bilateral or unilateral cases.

CONSTITUTIONAL CHROMOSOMAL CHANGES

Although most patients with retinoblastoma have normal constitutional karyotypes, 1 to 3 percent of patients have a deletion of the long arm of chromosome 13, involving specifically the q14 region. Nearly 100 deletional cases have been documented in the literature since the first report in 1963 by Lele and associates [58].

Simple deletion of the long arm of chromosome 13 is seen most often; however, mosaicism [101], ring chromosome [40], and more complex chromosome aberrations have also been reported [80, 102, 109]. No patient with deletion of the short arm of a D chromosome has had retinoblastoma. The smallest deletion of chromosome 13 associated with retinoblastoma has been shown by high-resolution techniques at prophase or prometaphase to involve sub-band of 13q14 [113]. Depending on the extent of the deletion, mental and developmental retardation and congenital malformations occur in addition to retinoblastoma.

Ophthalmologic abnormalities associated with deletion retinoblastoma have included hypertelorism, antimongoloid slant, epicanthus, blepharoptosis, microphthalmos, uveal colobomas, optic nerve hypoplasia, retinal dysplasia, and strabismus. Depending on the extent of the deletion, systemic malformations can include psychomotor retardation, microcephaly, trigonocephaly, frontal bossing, high-arched palate, cleft palate, micrognathia, flattened maxilla, protrusion of superior and maxillary incisors, ear malformations, absent or hypoplastic thumbs, prominent root of the nose, synostosis of fourth and fifth metacarpals, short stature, hirsutism, hypotonia, clubfoot, short fingers, agenesis of metacarpal bones, muscular defects, inguinal hernia, cardiomegaly, anogenital malformations, and skeletal defects. The typical facies with frontal bossing, epicanthal folds, and flattened maxilla has been noted by Motegi and coauthors [74].

Retinoblastoma has also been found in cases of aneuploidy involving chromosome 21 and chromosome X: translocation of 13qXp [20, 43, 78], trisomy 21 [8, 16, 30, 45, 69, 99], trisomy 21 with trisomy X [21], trisomy X [46], Klinefelter's syndrome XXY [30, 86, 111], and the XXXXY syndrome [100].

Lele and colleagues suggested that in the usual case of genetically predisposed retinoblastoma without a visible deletion, a submicroscopic mutation or deletion also on chromosome 13 might account for predisposition to retinoblastoma tumors [58]. The genetic locus for ESD has been localized to chromosomal region 13q14 by deletion mapping [93], since retinoblastoma patients with small deletions including 13q14 have 50 per-

cent of the normal levels of esterase D. Quantitative ESD determinations have been used to screen retinoblastoma patients for deletions. The proportion of all cases arising on the basis of deletion large enough to involve ESD must be less than 2 percent [23].

MANIFESTATIONS OF THE RETINOBLASTOMA MUTATION

Retinoblastoma

The usual manifestation of the retinoblastoma mutation is malignant tumors in both eyes. The number of tumors that individuals with the germinal mutation develop fits a Poisson distribution with a mean number of four tumors distributed between the two eyes [51, 53]. Therefore although both eyes are affected in 65 to 70 percent of cases, in 25 to 40 percent only one eye is affected, and in 1 to 10 percent no retinoblastoma tumors develop.

Retinoma

A small number of individuals with the retinoblastoma mutation (fewer than 2%) develop retinal lesions that do not demonstrate malignant progression. The word *retinoma* has been applied to these characteristic focal translucent retinal masses with "cottage cheese" calcification and underlying choroidal and pigment epithelial disturbance (Fig. 16-4) [33]. Many of the retinoma cases were discovered only when the patients' offspring developed malignant retinoblastoma; in others the presence of the retinoblastoma mutation in the individual with retinoma was subsequently demonstrated by the birth of affected offspring. Very little is known about the pathology of retinoma since there is no need to remove these eyes and only a few cases have been examined post mortem after a clinical course consistent with retinoma [88].

Retinoma has been considered, together with phthisis bulbi, to represent "spontaneous regression" of retinoblastoma. However, these are clearly quite different entities [35]. It is likely that phthisis bulbi arises when a large tumor outgrows or erodes its blood supply, whereas retinoma arises when the mutation that usually leads to malignancy of a retinoblast cell occurs in an almost terminally differentiated retinal cell. Insufficient cell divisions are available to allow more than limited abnormal retinoblast proliferation. A focal ab-

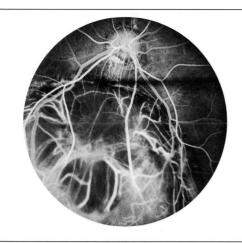

Fig. 16-4. *Fluorescein angiogram of one of three retinomas found in the left eye of a 64-year-old man when his granddaughter was found to have retinoblastoma. Two of his three children also had retinoblastoma. Two of the three characteristics of retinoma are evident: translucent mass and pigment epithelial disturbance. The other lesions showed the third characteristic, calcification.*

normality of retina forms, but malignant growth does not occur. Since there is evidence that the cell of origin of retinoblastoma is a very primitive multipotential cell, the pathology of different retinomas could include a wide range of nonproliferating cell types representing any of the neuronal or glial components of retina. The word *retinocytoma* has been applied to histologically benign-appearing lesions in the retina, often associated with retinoblastoma [60]. Retinocytomas have been observed in eyes enucleated because of presumedly inadequate response to therapy and will overlap with the biologically defined entity of retinoma [2]. The description of the histology of retinomas must await histologic examination in cases proven to be clinically benign [88].

Other Malignant Tumors

Retinoblastoma is only the first of a series of tumors that individuals with the heritable mutation may develop. The most common second primary tumors are osteogenic sarcoma and fibrosarcoma, while hematologic malignancies rarely occur. Abramson and colleagues applied life table analysis to 741 patients with heritable retinoblastoma, 91 of whom had developed second primary tumors [3]. They state that if radiation was used

to cure the retinoblastoma, 90 percent developed second malignancies within 32 years after the retinoblastoma, with a large fraction of tumors occurring within the radiation field. Even if no radiation was given, however, 50 percent developed second malignancies within the same period of time. More than three-quarters of all the second tumors, and most of the second tumors within the radiation field, were osteogenic sarcomas or fibrosarcomas. Patients with unilateral retinoblastoma without a family history, presumed not to have the retinoblastoma germ line mutation, have not developed second malignancies. Therefore, the retinoblastoma mutation induces susceptibility to malignancy primarily in retinoblasts, but also in other tissues. Ionizing radiation doubles the frequency of transformation in susceptible tissues. The retinoblastoma mutation appears to have no manifestations besides malignant tumor formation.

Cellular Effects

It has been suggested that fibroblasts from patients with deletion of 13q14 and retinoblastoma have abnormal radiation sensitivity, intermediate between normal sensitivity and the marked radiation sensitivity of ataxia telangiectasia [108, 109]. Nove and associates demonstrated segregation of retinoblastoma and radiation sensitivity in a series of patients with deletions of various portions of 13q and suggested that a radiation sensitivity locus was distal to the retinoblastoma locus (see Fig. 16-1) [79]. Increased radiation sensitivity in the nondeletional form of retinoblastoma has not been confirmed by other laboratories [26, 55, 71]. Repair of radiation-induced DNA breaks in retinoblastoma fibroblasts is also normal [112]. Cleaver and co-workers also found no DNA repair defect in heritable retinoblastoma fibroblasts but found abnormal DNA synthesis after irradiation with x-rays [18]. Since this effect was small, they concluded that it may not be an important factor in tumorigenesis in the presence of the germ line mutation.

Bloom's syndrome is characterized by a very high incidence of spontaneous exchange of DNA between sister chromatids (sister chromatid exchange, or SCE), which is presumed to be related to a high frequency of hematologic malignancies [17]. In heritable retinoblastoma spontaneous and chemically induced SCEs are normal [49], but radiation-induced SCEs of lymphocytes of bilaterally affected patients and their relatives demonstrate a dose-dependent two- to threefold increase compared with normal individuals [1]. This observation may be related to the tendency of individuals with the retinoblastoma germ line mutation to develop specific malignancies, but the small difference must be confirmed by further studies.

GENETIC CHANGES IN TUMORS

Knudson's Hypothesis

Knudson took advantage of the observation that bilateral cases were diagnosed earlier than unilateral cases to develop a hypothesis for oncogenesis of retinoblastoma [51]. When age at diagnosis in nonfamilial cases is plotted against the fraction of cases undiagnosed (Fig. 16-5), the bilateral cases fit an exponential curve, which suggests that only one event is required for tumor induction. The unilateral cases fit a second-order regression curve, which suggests that at least two events are necessary for tumor induction. Presumably, the hereditary tumors appear earlier because less time is required for one mutational event than for two. In the hereditary disease the first mutation (M_1) occurs in the germinal prezygotic cell, and the second (M_2) in the somatic retinal cells. In the nonheritable disease both mutations occur in a single somatic retinal cell (Fig. 16-6). Knudson and colleagues suggested that both mutations or events that were rate limiting in the generation of tumors could be identical for both hereditary and nonhereditary retinoblastoma [53]. They predicted that the first and second mutations could be at the same or adjacent sites in the same or homologous chromosomes or at nonhomologous sites.

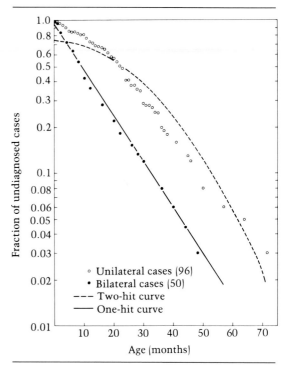

Fig. 16-5. Semilogarithmic plot of fraction of cases of retinoblastoma not yet diagnosed (S) versus age in months (t) from analysis of patients seen in Toronto. The bilateral cases fit a simple exponential curve, calculated from log $S = -t/33.3$, which implies that a single event in addition to the germ line mutation is required to produce tumors. The two-hit curve of the unilateral cases (log $S = -3.13 \times 10^{-4}t^2$) is convex, which suggests that tumor induction requires multiple events. This curve does not reach log 1.00 because 15–20% of unilateral cases are of the hereditary type and so contaminate the data.

Fig. 16-6. Knudson's hypothesis. Retinoblastoma has been shown to fit a two-mutation hypothesis for cancer initiation. The first mutation can be either germinal or somatic (retinal cell), while the second is always somatic.

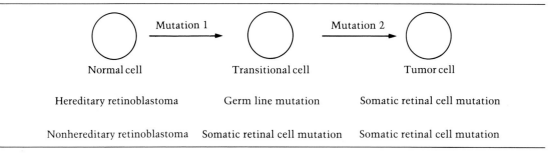

Tumor Chromosome Studies

All retinoblastoma tumor karyotype studies have shown abnormalities. Initial studies concentrated on the D group chromosomes and chromosome 13 abnormalities, as well as could be defined within existing technical limitations [41], since constitutional deletion of chromosome 13 was associated with retinoblastoma. Balaban and coauthors reported deletions of chromosome 13q14 in 5 of 6 retinoblastoma tumors, but the published karyotypes are difficult to assess [5]. Others have found a low frequency of deletion of 13q [6, 34, 38, 57].

Squire and associates examined the karyotype of 25 retinoblastoma tumors from patients with both unilateral and bilateral cases with normal peripheral blood karyotypes [95]. Every tumor contained either or both of two characteristic chromosomal rearrangements, isochromosome 6p or i(6p), and extra copies of chromosome 1q. The i(6p) abnormality occurred in 60 percent of retinoblastoma tumors but has not been observed frequently in other tumors and appears to be specific for retinoblastoma. Kusnetsova and colleagues observed a similar frequency of i(6p) by G-banding of retinoblastoma tumors examined directly after removal from patients [57]. Extra copies of chromosome 1q were found in 86 percent of the retinoblastoma tumors [95], with a common polysomic region distal to band 1q23. A similar region of chromosome 1q is frequently present in multiple copies in other malignancies [4].

When retinoblastoma cell lines were examined in more detail with high-resolution banding, nonrandom translocations were observed at three sites: 10q25, 17p13, and 14q32 [94]. Interestingly, 10q25 and 17p13 are reported fragile sites, and 14q32 is the site of the immunoglobin heavy chain locus and is the target site for rearrangements involving the c-*myc* oncogene in Burkitt's lymphoma. Recently, chromosomal translocations specific for different tumors have been linked to the chromosomal locations of human cellular oncogenes [48]. When DNA from an retinoblastoma tumor that had a translocation to 14q32 was probed with a DNA sequence that shows the rearrangements in Burkitt cells, no rearrangements were observed. Thus, the translocations at 14q32 in retinoblastoma do not involve the specific site associated with c-*myc* rearrangements described in lymphomas.

Benedict and co-workers reported one tumor with deletion of a chromosome 13 and retention of a deleted chromosome 13 [7]. The patient was suspected to have a submicroscopic deletion of chromosome 13 associated with retinoblastoma, on the basis of half-normal levels of the marker, ESD, in the blood. In the retinoblastoma tumor cells no ESD could be detected and only one chromosome 13 was present by karyotype analysis. The authors proposed that this tumor provided evidence that the retinoblastoma mutation is recessive at a cellular level: Only when the normal undeleted chromosome is lost from a somatic retinal cell does a tumor arise.

Since ESD is closely linked to the heritable retinoblastoma locus in band 13q14 [93, 105], ESD isoenzymes were used to study somatic genetic changes in that region in retinoblastoma tumors. Godbout and associates tested normal and tumor cells of hereditary and nonhereditary retinoblastoma patients who were heterozygous for isoenzymes of ESD [39]. Both alleles were expressed in normal cells, but 60 percent of the retinoblastoma tumors lost or failed to express one of the ESD isoenzymes. All these tumors had two normal-appearing chromosomes 13 on karyotype analysis. The authors concluded that "somatic inactivation" was most likely to account for the loss of ESD activity in the tumors and that somatic inactivation of normal genes in the region of the retinoblastoma locus was the second event leading to retinoblastoma tumor formation. Both unilateral and bilateral tumors showed loss of ESD, supporting Knudson's suggestion that the genetic changes for heritable and nonheritable retinoblastoma are the same.

Molecular Genetic Rearrangements

Heterozygosity of ESD occurs in less than 20 percent of the population, and no other polymorphic biochemical markers are known on chromosome 13 to permit other tumors to be studied [91]. Recombinant DNA technology, however, has provided the opportunity to find heterozygous DNA markers for any chromosomal region. These markers consist of heritable differences in the nucleotide sequence of genomic DNA (Fig. 16-7) [10]. Thus, when the gene itself is not detectable, the inheritance of the DNA fragment that is closely linked can be followed. Restriction enzymes cleave DNA at specific nucleotide sequences, yielding pieces of DNA of defined length called restriction fragments. These restriction fragments separate according to their molecular size when electro-

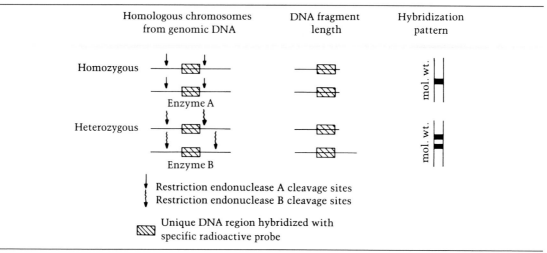

Fig. 16-7. *Restriction fragment length polymorphisms or DNA fragments from homologous chromosomes can be homozygous or heterozygous. Cuts are made in a pair of homologous chromosomes by enzyme A and enzyme B. Restriction enzyme A cleaves the homologous DNA sequences at identical locations, yielding only one fragment length homologous to specific probe and revealed as a single band on hybridization. Restriction enzyme B cleaves at different sites in both chromosomes yielding two fragment lengths generating the pattern of two bands when hybridized with the probe.*

phoresed in agarose gels. The DNA fragments can be detected using the method of Southern, by which DNA fragments from the agarose gel are transferred onto nitrocellulose paper and hybridized with selective radioactive DNA probe sequences, specific for unique single copy sequences within the chromosomal region of interest [89]. As illustrated in Fig. 16-7, if an individual is homozygous for a particular probe with a particular restriction enzyme, the DNA fragments from homologous chromosomes will be the same length and only one band will appear on the Southern gel. If the individual is heterozygous, the DNA fragments from homologous chromosomes will be different sizes and will migrate to different spots on the gel; the radioactive probe will hybridize to the DNA at two locations on the gel, yielding two bands. Thus, the identification of restriction fragment length polymorphisms (RFLPs) in the normal population allows the members of a pair of chromosomes to be distinguished.

Using recombinant DNA probes [14, 25] that identify RFLPs at sites above and below the segment containing the ESD and retinoblastoma loci, detailed analysis was made of the submicroscopic rearrangements of chromosome 13 in retinoblastoma tumors [13, 24]. RFLP markers on chromosome 13q that had been heterozygous in constitutional cells of the patient had become homozygous in 70 percent of retinoblastoma tumors studied. Three mechanisms to achieve this reduction to homozygosity were documented (see Fig. 16-2).

In 50 percent of tumors loss of one chromosome 13 appeared to be followed by duplication of the remaining chromosome. In one instance triplication of a remaining chromosome had occurred, resulting in trisomy 13, but in the other cases two karyotypically normal chromosomes 13 were present in the tumor.

One retinoblastoma tumor retained heteromorphism for a Q-banded karyotypic satellite marker on 13p and for an RFLP probe near the centromere but became homozygous for ESD and for markers distal to the 13q12 region. The chromosome 13 karyotype remained normal. The tumor is consistent with a mitotic recombination event resulting from a break and cross-over proximal to the 13q14. This tumor represents the first demonstration of mitotic recombination in mammalian cells.

The tumor with simple loss of chromosome 13 reported by Benedict and coauthors was confirmed to have lost one chromosome 13 by RFLP data [7].

Thirty percent of retinoblastoma tumors from individuals with informative heterozygous markers did not show any rearrangement of chromosome 13 with the RFLPs used. Point mutation, deletion, or gene conversion could result in homozygosity for mutations at the retinoblastoma locus that would not be detectable with present markers since none are exactly at the retinoblastoma locus.

We have incorporated the above recent data into an expansion of Knudson's model of oncogenesis in retinoblastoma [37]. The first event, M_1, results in an intermediate cell that is heterozygous for the mutation at the retinoblastoma locus. Heterozygosity at this locus has little if any effect on cellular function. Individuals with a germ line mutation are normal by parameters so far studied [32, 34]. The loss of the normal allele by random chromosomal rearrangements of chromosome 13 (simple loss, loss and duplication, mitotic recombination, point mutations, deletions, or gene conversion) results in homozygosity for the defective q14 region of chromosome 13. This may be the critical second event (M_2) in oncogenesis of retinoblastoma.

The retinoblastoma cancer gene is, therefore, recessive at the cellular level. Malignancy results only when both alleles are lost or inactivated and the retinal cell becomes homozygous at the 13q14 locus. This second event occurs usually in at least one retinoblast, accounting for the dominant pattern of tumor inheritance observed clinically.

Like retinoblastoma, Wilms' tumor occurs in childhood in both hereditary and nonhereditary forms [52]. Aniridia, genitourinary abnormalities, and mental retardation may be associated in a small percentage of children with Wilms' tumor with a specific deletion of band p13 of chromosome 11. It has been suggested that the germ line deletion of 11p13 is the first of two or more steps of tumorigenesis in these children, a similar deletion arising somatically in the more common isolated Wilms' tumor in children without other abnormalities. Using RFLPs, four groups of workers have shown that gross chromosomal changes result in homozygosity of all or part of chromosome 11 in a significant number of Wilms' tumors [28, 56, 81, 85], similar to the changes seen in chromosome 13 in retinoblastoma. The studies of Wilms' tumor failed to produce evidence of mitotic recombination.

GENETIC COUNSELING

Precise genetic counseling will be possible only when the retinoblastoma mutation can be detected in nonmalignant cells in the laboratory,

rather than inferred clinically by the presence of bilateral or multiple tumors or family history. Presently counseling must be based on analyses of populations of patients with retinoblastoma to determine risk estimates (Table 16-1).

All bilateral cases, whether familial or not, are considered to be heritable since the likelihood of two rare somatic mutations occurring in more than one fetal retinal cell is infinitely small. Therefore offspring of a bilaterally affected parent have a 0.5 (1 : 2) chance of inheriting the retinoblastoma mutation. Since only 0.15 of unilaterally affected retinoblastoma cases have the germ line retinoblastoma mutation, the risk that their offspring also carry the mutation is 0.15 × 0.5, or 0.075.

The risk for a sibling, offspring of unaffected sibling, or first cousin of a retinoblastoma patient depends on the number of intervening apparently unaffected individuals, each of whom has a 0.1 risk of carrying retinoblastoma mutation. Thus with each unaffected intervening individual, the risk that the next relative carries the mutation decreases by a factor of 0.1. Therefore, for example, first cousins of bilaterally affected retinoblastoma patients have a risk of 0.0005 (1 : 2,000) and of patients with unilateral retinoblastoma, 0.000075 (1 : 13,000). The monozygotic twin of a bilaterally affected individual must also have the mutation (risk = 1.0). The monozygotic twin of a unilaterally affected patient has the same risk of having the retinoblastoma mutation as the affected patient (0.15). Dizygotic twins of patients with either bilateral or unilateral cases have the same risk as siblings.

When a family history of retinoblastoma exists, risk calculations can be made as described above, considering the proband to be the nearest relative known to have the retinoblastoma mutation.

Since the likelihood that retinoblastoma mutation carriers will develop retinoblastoma tumors varies in different families [9, 62], the risk of actually developing the tumors can be obtained by multiplying the risk of the retinoblastoma mutation by a factor based on expression of the retinoblastoma mutation in the parent. If the parent is bilaterally affected, expression in the offspring with the mutation is 0.9; if the parent is unilaterally affected, expression in the offspring with the mutation is 0.76; if the parent is unaffected, expression in the offspring with the mutation is 0.54.

Recommendations for treatment of newborn relatives of retinoblastoma patients can be made

Table 16-1. *Risk of Retinoblastoma*

Retinoblastoma in Proband	Relationship to Proband	Risk of Carrying Retinoblastoma Mutation*	Risk of Developing Retinoblastoma Tumor†
Bilateral	Offspring	0.5 (0.5 × 1.0)	0.45 (0.90 × 0.5)
Bilateral	Sibling	0.05 (0.5 × 0.1)	0.027 (0.54 × 0.05)
Bilateral	Offspring of unaffected sibling	0.005 (0.5 × 0.1 × 0.1)	0.0027 (0.54 × 0.005)
Bilateral	First cousin	0.0005 (0.5 × 0.1 × 0.1 × 0.1)	0.00027 (0.54 × 0.0005)
Bilateral	Monozygotic twin	1.0	0.9 (0.9 × 1.0)
Bilateral	Dizygotic twin	0.05 (0.5 × 0.1)	0.027 (0.54 × 0.05)
Unilateral	Offspring	0.075 (0.5 × 0.15)	0.057 (0.76 × 0.075)
Unilateral	Sibling	0.008 (0.5 × 0.1 × 0.15)	0.004 (0.54 × 0.008)
Unilateral	Offspring of unaffected sibling	0.0008 (0.5 × 0.1 × 0.1 × 0.15)	0.0004 (0.54 × 0.0008)
Unilateral	First cousin	0.00008 (0.5 × 0.1 × 0.1 × 0.1 × 0.15)	0.00004 (0.54 × 0.00008)
Unilateral	Monozygotic twin	0.1 (1.0 × 0.1)	0.054 (0.54 × 0.1)
Unilateral	Dizygotic twin	0.008 (0.5 × 0.1 × 0.15)	0.004 (0.54 × 0.008)

*The retinoblastoma mutation will be inherited by 0.5 of the offspring of patients with heritable retinoblastoma. No retinoblastoma tumors will develop in 0.1 of the individuals with the mutation. Of all unilateral retinoblastoma cases 0.15 are heritable.
†Risk for retinoblastoma tumor development was obtained by multiplying the risk of carrying the retinoblastoma mutation by a factor based on expression of the retinoblastoma mutation in the carrier parent: 0.9 if the parent is affected bilaterally, 0.76 if the parent is affected unilaterally, and 0.54 if the parent is unaffected [62].

based on the calculated risk of retinoblastoma tumor involvement (Table 16-1). The frequency of retinoblastoma in the general population is approximately 0.00005 (1 in 20,000 live births). Therefore, first cousins of unilaterally affected retinoblastoma patients do not have an increased risk of retinoblastoma tumor development, since the calculated risk of their being affected is 0.00004 (1 : 25,000). Clinical examination of these babies may be recommended, but examination under anesthetic is not warranted. Offspring, twins, and siblings of retinoblastoma patients have a risk ranging from 0.45 to 0.004 (1 : 2–1 : 250) and therefore require complete retinal examination at birth and monthly without anesthetic until 3 months of age, examination under anesthetic every 2 months to age 7 months, every 3 months to age

18 months, and every 6 months to age 3 years. Subsequently annual clinical examination is advisable.

Because of the close linkage between the locus for hereditary retinoblastoma and that for the polymorphic enzyme esterase D on chromosome 13, retinoblastoma kindreds with an informative set of ESD alleles may benefit from improved genetic counseling. A retinoblastoma family is informative for a set of ESD alleles when the affected parent is heterozygous (usually ESD-1,2), the unaffected parent is homozygous, and there are normal and affected children. Unfortunately less than 20 percent of the population is heterozygous for ESD, so informative families are very rare. Also, the ESD locus is separable from the retinoblastoma locus, making meiotic recombination between these loci possible. Meiotic recombination has not yet been observed in the available informative families but potentially could lead to an error in counseling.

The patients with the deletional form of retinoblastoma have been shown to have half-normal levels of ESD and might be detected by ESD quantitative analysis. However, screening by quantitative assays of esterase D in children without other malformations of retinoblastoma has not usually detected any small deletions [23]. In summary, the usefulness of esterase D as a marker to identify carriers of the retinoblastoma mutation or deletion cases to improve genetic counseling is limited.

The detection of linked DNA marker loci or restriction fragment length polymorphisms by single-copy DNA probes has made it possible to examine genotypes at both the constitutional (germ line) and somatic cell level, has allowed identification of the chromosome 13 that carries the retinoblastoma mutation [15], and should be valuable in the genetic counseling of patients with hereditary retinoblastoma. However, the present DNA probes that identify restriction fragment length polymorphisms on the long arm of chromosome 13 can detect only a limited number of polymorphisms in the somatic cells tested and are located at variable distances from the retinoblastoma locus. Since mitotic recombination is frequent in tumors and meiotic recombination is frequent on chromosome 13 [50, 70, 82], probes very close to the retinoblastoma locus must be found. In order for prenatal diagnosis by restriction fragment length polymorphism analysis to be useful in retinoblastoma or any other genetic disorder, a large number of RFLPs must be available to allow some to be informative in a given family [27]. As more chromosome 13 probes are made in the 13q14 region and more polymorphisms are identified with new restriction enzymes, these limitations will be overcome. However, definitive genetic counseling for the presence of retinoblastoma mutation will await molecular detection of the mutation itself.

REFERENCES

1. Abramovsky-Kaplan, I., and Jones, I. S. Sister chromatid exchange induced by X-irradiation of retinoblastoma lymphocytes. *Invest. Ophthalmol. Vis. Sci.* 25:698, 1984.
2. Abramson, D. H. Retinoma, retinocytoma, and the retinoblastoma gene. *Arch. Ophthalmol.* 101:1517, 1983.
3. Abramson, D. H., et al. Second tumors and the retinoblastoma gene. *Ophthalmology (Rochester).* 91:1351, 1984.
4. Atkin, N. B., and Baker, M. C. Chromosome 1 in 26 carcinomas of the cervix uteri. *Cancer* 44:606, 1979.
5. Balaban, G., et al. Abnormalities of chromosome #13 in retinoblastomas from individuals with normal constitutional karyotypes. *Cancer Genet. Cytogenet.* 6:213, 1982.
6. Benedict, W. F., et al. Nonrandom chromosomal changes in untreated retinoblastoma. *Cancer Genet. Cytogenet.* 10:311, 1983.
7. Benedict, W. F., et al. Patient with 13 chromosome deletion: Evidence that the retinoblastoma gene is a recessive cancer gene. *Science* 219:973, 1983.
8. Bentley, D. A case of Down's syndrome complicated by retinoblastoma and celiac disease. *Pediatrics* 56:131, 1975.
9. Bonaiti-Pellie, C., and Briard-Guillemot, M. L. Segregation analysis in hereditary retinoblastoma. *Hum. Genet.* 57:411, 1981.
10. Botstein, D., et al. Construction of a genetic linkage map in man using restriction fragment length polymorphisms. *Am. J. Hum. Genet.* 32:314, 1980.
11. Carlson, E. A., and Desnick, R. J. Mutational mosaicism and genetic counseling in retinoblastoma. *Am. J. Med. Genet.* 4:356, 1979.
12. Carlson, E. A., et al. Factors for improved genetic counseling for retinoblastoma based on a survey of 55 families. *Am. J. Ophthalmol.* 87:449, 1979.
13. Cavenee, W. K., et al. Expression of recessive alleles by chromosomal mechanisms in retinoblastoma. *Nature* 305:779, 1983.
14. Cavenee, W., et al. Isolation and regional localization of DNA segments revealing polymorphic loci from human chromosome 13. *Am. J. Hum. Genet.* 36:10, 1984.
15. Cavenee, W. K., et al. Genetic origins of mutations predisposing to retinoblastoma. *Science* 228:501, 1985.
16. Cernea, P., Teodorescu, F., and Angheloni, T. Rétinoblastome: Un mosaïcisme chromosomien 46XX/47XX, G +. *Ann. Ocul. (Paris)* 206:607, 1973.
17. Chaganti, R. S. K., Schoenberg, S., and German, J. A manyfold increase in sister chromatid exchanges in Bloom's syndrome lymphocytes. *Proc. Natl. Acad. Sci. U.S.A.* 71:4508, 1974.
18. Cleaver, J. E., et al. Repair and replication of DNA in hereditary (bilateral) retinoblastoma cells after X-irradiation. *Cancer Res.* 42:1343, 1982.
19. Connolly, M. J., et al. Familial, ESD-linked retinoblastoma with reduced penetrance and variable expressivity. *Hum. Genet.* 65:122, 1983.
20. Cross, H. E., et al. Retinoblastoma in a patient with 13q×p translocation. *Am. J. Ophthalmol.* 84:548, 1977.

21. Day, R. W., et al. XXX,21-trisomy and retinoblastoma. *Lancet* 2:154, 1963.

22. Dollfus, M. A., and Aubert, B. Le gliome de le rétine et les pseudogliomes. Paris: Masson, 1953.

23. Dryja, T. P., et al. Low incidence of deletion of esterase D locus in retinoblastoma patients. *Hum. Genet.* 64:151, 1983.

24. Dryja, T. P., et al. Homozygosity of chromosome 13 in retinoblastoma. *N. Engl. J. Med.* 310:550, 1984.

25. Dryja, T. P., et al. Chromosome 13 restriction fragment length polymorphisms. *Hum. Genet.* 65:320, 1984.

26. Ejima, Y., et al. Radiosensitivity of fibroblasts from patients with retinoblastoma and chromosome 13 anomalies. *Mutat. Res.* 103:177, 1982.

27. Epstein, C. J., et al. Recent developments in the prenatal diagnosis of genetic diseases and birth defects. *Annu. Rev. Genet.* 17:49, 1983.

28. Fearon, E. R., Vogelstein, B., and Feinberg, A. P. Somatic deletion and duplication of genes on chromosome 11 in Wilms' tumors. *Nature* 309:176, 1984.

29. Fitzgerald, P. H., Stewart, J., and Suckling, R. D. Retinoblastoma mutation rate in New Zealand and support for the two-hit model. *Hum. Genet.* 64:128, 1983.

30. François, J., Berger, R., and Saraux, H. *Les Aberrations Chromosomiques en Ophtalmologie.* Paris: Masson, 1972.

31. François, J., DeBie, S., and Malton-Van Leuven, M. T. Genesis and genetics of retinoblastoma. *J. Pediatr. Ophthalmol. Strabismus* 16:85, 1979.

32. Gallie, B. L. Gene carrier detection in retinoblastoma. *Ophthalmology (Rochester)* 87:591, 1980.

33. Gallie, B. L., et al. Retinoma: Spontaneous regression of retinoblastoma or benign manifestation of the mutation? *Br. J. Cancer* 45:513, 1982.

34. Gallie, B. L., and Phillips, R. A. Multiple manifestations of the retinoblastoma gene. *Birth Defects* 18(6):689, 1982.

35. Gallie, B. L., et al. Significance of retinoma and phthisis bulbi for retinoblastoma. *Ophthalmology (Rochester)* 89:1393, 1982.

36. Gallie, B. L., Musarella, M. A., and Chan, H. Ocular Oncology. In J. S. Crawford and J. D. Morin (Eds.), *The Eye in Childhood.* New York: Grune & Stratton, 1983. Pp. 307–330.

37. Gallie, B. L., and Phillips, R. A. Retinoblastoma: A model of oncogenesis. *Ophthalmology (Rochester)* 91:666, 1984.

38. Gardner, H. A., et al. Multiple karyotypic changes in retinoblastoma tumor cells: Presence of normal chromosome no. 13 in most tumors. *Cancer Genet. Cytogenet.* 6:201, 1982.

39. Godbout, R., et al. Somatic inactivation of genes on chromosome 13 is a common event in retinoblastoma. *Nature* 304:451, 1983.

40. Grace, E., et al. The 13q$^-$ deletion syndrome. *J. Med. Genet.* 8:351, 1971.

41. Hashem, N., and Khalifa, S. H. Retinoblastoma: A model of hereditary fragile chromosomal regions. *Hum. Hered.* 25:35, 1975.

42. Hermann, J. Delayed mutation model: Carotid body tumors and retinoblastoma. In J. J. Mulvihill, R. W. Miller, and J. F. Fraumeni (Eds.), *Genetics of Human Cancer.* New York: Raven, 1977. Pp. 417–438.

43. Hida, T., et al. Bilateral retinoblastoma with 13q × p translocation. *J. Pediatr. Ophthalmol. Strabismus* 17:144, 1980.

44. Howard, R. O. Origin of retinoblastoma. *Lancet* 2:490, 1982.

45. Jackson, E. W., et al. Down's syndrome. *J. Chronic. Dis.* 21:247, 1968.

46. Judisch, G. F., and Patil, S. R. Concurrent heritable retinoblastoma, pinealoma and trisomy X. *Arch. Ophthalmol.* 99:1767, 1981.

47. Kaelin, A. Statistische Pruf-und Schatzverfaren fur die relative Haugfighert von Merkmals-tragern in Geschwislerriken vei einem der Auslese unterworfen Material mit Anwendung auf da Retinoblastom. *Arch. Julius-Klaus Stift. Vererbungsforch. Sozialanthropol. Rassenhygiene* 30(3/4), 1955.

48. Klein, G. The role of gene dosage and genetic transpositions in carcinogenesis. *Nature* 294:313, 1981.

49. Knight, L. A., Gardner, H. A., and Gallie, B. L. Absence of chromosome breakage in patients with retinoblastoma. *Hum. Genet.* 51:73, 1979.

50. Knight, L. A., Gardner, H. A., and Gallie, B. L. Familial retinoblastoma: Segregation of chromosome 13 in four families. *Am. J. Hum. Genet.* 32:194, 1980.

51. Knudson, A. G. Mutation and cancer: Statistical study of retinoblastoma. *Proc. Natl. Acad. Sci. U.S.A.* 68:820, 1971.

52. Knudson, A. G., Jr., and Strong, L. C. Mutation and cancer: A model for Wilms' tumor of the kidney. *JNCI.* 48:313, 1972.

53. Knudson, A. G., Hethcote, H. W., and Brown, B. W. Mutation and childhood cancer: A probabilistic model for the incidence of retinoblastoma. *Proc. Natl. Acad. Sci. U.S.A.* 72:5116, 1975.

54. Knudson, A. G. Model hereditary cancers of man. *Prog. Nucleic Acid Res. Mol. Biol.* 29:17, 1983.

55. Kossakowska, A. E., Gallie, B. L., and Phillips, R. A. Fibroblasts from retinoblastoma patients: Enhanced growth in fetal calf serum and a normal response to ionizing radiation. *J. Cell Physiol.* 111:5, 1982.

56. Koufous, A., et al. Loss of allele at loci on human chromosome 11 during genesis of Wilms' tumor. *Nature* 309:170, 1984.

57. Kusnetsova, L., et al. Similar chromosomal abnormalities in several retinoblastomas. *Hum. Genet.* 61:201, 1982.

58. Lele, K. P., Penrose, L. S., and Stallard, H. B. Chromosome deletion in a case of retinoblastoma. *Ann. Hum. Genet.* 27:171, 1963.

59. Lerche, W. Merkwiiridge Entartung des linken Augapfels bei allen mannlicken Kindern einer Familie (1821). Cited in Vogel [106].

60. Margo, C., et al. Retinocytoma: A benign variant of retinoblastoma. *Arch. Ophthalmol.* 101:1519, 1983.
61. Matsunaga, E. Parental age and sporadic retinoblastoma. *Annu. Rep. Jpn. Inst. Genet.* 16:121, 1965.
62. Matsunaga, E. Hereditary retinoblastoma: Penetrance, expressivity and age of onset. *Hum. Genet.* 33:1, 1976.
63. Matsunaga, E. Hereditary retinoblastoma: Delayed mutation or host resistance? *Am. J. Hum. Genet.* 30:406, 1978.
64. Matsunaga, E. Hereditary retinoblastoma: Host resistance and age at onset. *JNCI* 63:933, 1979.
65. Matsunaga, E. On estimating penetrance of the retinoblastoma gene. *Hum. Genet.* 56:127, 1980.
66. Matsunaga, E. Retinoblastoma: Host resistance and 13q− chromosomal deletion. *Hum. Genet.* 56:53, 1980.
67. Matsunaga, E. Retinoblastoma: Mutational mosaicism or host resistance? *Am. J. Med. Genet.* 8:375, 1981.
68. Migdal, C. Retinoblastoma occurring in four successive generations. *Br. J. Ophthalmol.* 60:151, 1976.
69. Miller, R. W. Neoplasia and Down syndrome. *Ann. N.Y. Acad. Sci.* 171:637, 1970.
70. Morten, J. E. N., Harnden, D. G., and Bundley, S. Family studies on the chromosomal location of the retinoblastoma gene (Rb-1). *J. Med. Genet.* 19:120, 1982.
71. Morten, J. E. N., Harnden, D. G., and Taylor, A. M. R. Chromosome damage in G_0 X-irradiated lymphocytes from patients with hereditary retinoblastoma. *Cancer Res.* 41:3635, 1981.
72. Motegi, T. Lymphocyte chromosome survey in 42 patients with retinoblastoma: Effort to detect 13q14 deletion mosaicism. *Hum. Genet.* 58:168, 1981.
73. Motegi, T. High rate of detection of 13q14 deletion mosaicism among retinoblastoma patients (using more extensive methods). *Hum. Genet.* 61:95, 1982.
74. Motegi, T., et al. A recognizable pattern of the midface of retinoblastoma patients with interstitial deletion of 13q. *Hum. Genet.* 64:160, 1983.
75. Motegi, T., Kosmastu, M., and Minoda, K. Is the interstitial deletion in 13q in retinoblastoma patients not transmissible? *Hum. Genet.* 64:205, 1983.
76. Motegi, T., and Minoda, K. A decreasing tendency for cytogenetic abnormality in peripheral lymphocytes of retinoblastoma patients with 13q14 deletion mosaicism. *Hum. Genet.* 66:186, 1984.
77. Mukai, S., et al. Linkage of gene for human esterase D and hereditary retinoblastoma. *Am. J. Ophthalmol.* 97:681, 1984.
78. Nichol, W. W., et al. Further observations on 13q×q translocation associated with retinoblastoma. *Am. J. Ophthalmol.* 89:621, 1980.
79. Nove, J., et al. Retinoblastoma, chromosome 13 and in vitro cellular radiosensitivity. *Cytogenet. Cell Genet.* 24:176, 1979.
80. O'Brady, R. B., Rothstein, T. B., and Romano, P. D-group deletion syndromes and retinoblastoma. *Am. J. Ophthalmol.* 77:40, 1974.
81. Orkin, S. H., Goldmann, D. S., and Sallan, S. E. Development of homozygosity for chromosome 11p markers in Wilms' tumor. *Nature* 309:172, 1984.
82. Palmer, R. W., and Hulten, M. A. Chiasma derived genetic maps and recombination fractions: Chromosome 13 with reference to the proposed 13q14 retinoblastoma locus. *J. Med. Genet.* 19:125, 1982.
83. Pellie, C., and Briard, M. L. Risque de récurrence et malformations associées dans le rétinoblastome. *J. Genet. Hum.* 22:257, 1974.
84. Penrose, L. S. Parental age and mutation. *Lancet* 2:312, 1955.
85. Reeve, A. E., et al. Loss of a Harney ras allele in sporadic Wilms' tumor. *Nature* 309:174, 1984.
86. Rethmore, M. D., et al. Syndrome 48,XXY, +21, et retinoblastoma. *Arch. Fr. Pediatr.* 29:533, 1972.
87. Rivera, H., et al. Report of two patients, one with a trisomic sib due to maternal insertion. Gene-dosage effect for Esterase D. *Hum. Genet.* 59:211, 1981.
88. Smith, J. L. S. Histology and spontaneous regression of retinoblastoma. *Trans. Ophthalmol. Soc. U.K.* 94:953, 1974.
89. Southern, E. M. Detection of specific sequences among DNA fragments separated by gel electrophoresis. *J. Mol. Biol.* 98:503, 1975.
90. Sparkes, R. S., et al. Gene for hereditary retinoblastoma assigned to human chromosome 13 by linkage to esterase D. *Science* 219:971, 1983.
91. Sparkes, R. S., and Sparkes, M. C. Esterase D studies in human retinoblastoma. *Isozymes Curr. Top. Biol. Med. Res. Isozymes* 11:173, 1983.
92. Sparkes, R. S., et al. Separation of retinoblastoma and esterase D loci in a patient with sporadic retinoblastoma and del(13) (q14.1q22.3). *Hum. Genet.* In press, 1985.
93. Sparkes, R. S., et al. Regional assignment of genes for human esterase D and retinoblastoma to chromosome band 13q14. *Science* 208:1042, 1980.
94. Squire, J., Gallie, B. L., and Phillips, R. A. Specific chromosomal abnormalities in retinoblastoma. *Cancer Res.* 25:143, 1984.
95. Squire, J., et al. Isochromosome 6p, a unique chromosomal abnormality in retinoblastoma: Verification by standard staining techniques, new densitometric methods, and somatic cell hybridization. *Hum. Genet.* 66:46, 1984.
96. Strong, L. C., et al. Familial retinoblastoma and chromosome 13 deletion transmitted via an insertional translocation. *Science* 213:1501, 1981.
97. Suckling, R. D., and Fitzgerald, P. H. An epidemiological study of retinoblastoma in New Zealand. *Trans. Opthalmol. Soc. N.Z.* 24:17, 1972.
98. Sugahara, T., and Uyama, M. A possible population monitoring system on environmental mutagens: Statistical studies on retinoblastoma in Japan. *Mutat. Res.* 30:137, 1975.

99. Taktikas, A. Association of retinoblastoma with mental defect and other pathological manifestations. *Br. J. Ophthalmol.* 48:495, 1964.

100. Tan, K. E. W. P., van Biervliet, J. P. G. M., and van Hemel, J. O. Retinoblastoma combined with severe chromosomal disorders. *Ophthalmologica* 176:280, 1978.

101. Taylor, A. I. Dq⁻, Dr, and retinoblastoma. *Humangenetik* 10:209, 1970.

102. Thompson, H., and Lyons, R. B. Retinoblastoma and multiple congenital anomalies associated with complex mosaicism with deletion of D-chromosome and probably D/C translocation. *Hum. Chromosome Newsletter* 15:21, 1965.

103. Turleau, C., et al. Two cases of del(13q)-retinoblastoma and two cases of partial trisomy due to a familial insertion. *Ann. Genet.* 26:158, 1983.

104. van Heyningen, V., et al. Chromosome assignment of some human enzyme loci: Mitochondrial malate dehydrogenase to 7, mannosephosphate isomerase and pyruvate kinase to 15 and probably esterase D to 13. *Ann. Hum. Genet.* 38:295, 1975.

105. van Kempen, C. A case of retinoblastoma combined with severe mental retardation and a few other congenital anomalies associated with more complex aberrations of the karyotype. *Maandschr. Kindergenesk.* 34:92, 1966.

106. Vogel, F. Genetics of retinoblastoma. *Hum. Genet.* 52:1, 1979.

107. Ward, P., et al. Location of the retinoblastoma susceptibility gene(s) and the human esterase D locus. *J. Med. Genet.* 21:9295, 1984.

108. Weichselbaum, R. R. Skin fibroblasts from a D-deletion type retinoblastoma patient are abnormally X-ray sensitive. *Nature* 266:726, 1977.

109. Weichselbaum, R. R., Nove, J., and Little, J. B. X-ray sensitivity of diploid fibroblasts from patients with hereditary or sporadic retinoblastoma. *Proc. Natl. Acad. Sci. U.S.A.* 75:3962, 1978.

110. Welch, S., and Lee, J. The population distribution of genetic variants of human esterase D. *Humangenetik* 24:329, 1974.

111. Wilson, M. G., et al. Chromosomal anomalies in patients with retinoblastoma. *Clin. Genet.* 12:1, 1977.

112. Woods, W. G., et al. Normal repair of gamma radiation-induced single-strand and double-strand DNA breaks in retinoblastoma fibroblasts. *Biochim. Biophys. Acta* 698:40, 1982.

113. Yunis, J. J., and Ramsay, N. Retinoblastoma and subband deletion of chromosome 13. *Am. J. Dis. Child.* 132:161, 1978.

17

Hereditary Macular Dystrophies

Kenneth G. Noble

There are three situations in which the macula may be involved with a hereditary disease (Table 17-1). The first is the numerous inherited systemic diseases that have as part of the constellation of abnormalities retinal and macular involvement. An awareness of the systemic disorder usually precedes the discovery of ocular findings. The cherry-red spot in the macula of infants with the lipid storage of generalized GM_1 gangliosidosis type 1 (Tay-Sachs disease) is a systemic disorder that may have a macular abnormality.

Second, there are generalized chorioretinal dystrophies in which the symptoms and fundus appearance suggest solely a macular dystrophy but visual function tests reveal diffuse retinal dysfunction. An example of this would be "inverse" retinitis pigmentosa, a generalized tapetoretinal dystrophy that presents with diminished central vision and central pigmentary alterations.

Finally, there are inherited dystrophies of the macula unassociated either with a generalized retinal dystrophy or with a systemic disorder. These may be considered truly to represent the hereditary macular dystrophies, and as such, will constitute the major portion of this chapter.

GENETICS

The inheritance of macular dystrophies may follow any of the three mendelian modes, namely, autosomal dominant, autosomal recessive, or X-linked recessive (Table 17-1). Autosomal dom-

inant disorders affect successive generations with an individual at risk having a 50 percent chance of inheriting the disorder. Dominantly inherited dystrophies are more variable in their expression and milder in their course than the recessively inherited dystrophies. Indeed, some individuals with Best's vitelliform macular dystrophy have such a mild form that the fundus appearance is entirely normal and vision 20/20 in each eye.

Autosomal recessive disorders affect individuals in the same generation, with these individuals having a 25 percent chance of inheriting the disease from their parents, both of whom are heterozygote carriers. Parental consanguinity is frequently found in autosomal recessive disorders, and this information should be routinely sought. Recessive disorders have an earlier onset, a more severe expression, and a more rapid progression than do dominant disorders.

The inheritance pattern in the X-linked recessive disorders is modified from the autosomal recessive disorders in that the affected female is essentially a heterozygote and unaffected, while the affected male is homozygous for the disease and exhibits its full manifestations. Therefore, females are carriers of the disease and will transmit it to 50 percent of their male offspring, while 50 percent of their female offspring will be carriers. Affected males cannot transmit the disease to their sons, but all of their daughters will be carriers.

The carrier female in some X-linked recessive chorioretinal dystrophies (e.g., retinitis pigmentosa, choroideremia, albinism) may show a characteristic fundus appearance that aids in the diagnosis and establishes individuals at risk. Unfortunately, there are no consistent female carrier signs in juvenile retinoschisis. The fundus appearance and visual function tests in the female

Gratitude is expressed to August F. Deutman, M.D., author of Macular Dystrophies in the first edition of this book, from which several illustrations have been utilized in the present chapter.

Table 17-1. *Hereditary Macular Dystrophies*

I. Primary hereditary macular dystrophies
  A. Stargardt's disease (AR)
  B. Variants of Stargardt's disease
    1. Fundus flavimaculatus (AR)
    2. Progressive atrophic macular dystrophy (AR)
    3. Dominant Stargardt's disease (AD)
  C. Best's vitelliform macular dystrophy (AD)
  D. Dominant drusen of Bruch's membrane (AD)
  E. Pigment pattern dystrophies (AD)
  F. Central areolar choroidal dystrophy (AD)
  G. Peripapillary (pericentral) choroidal dystrophy (AR)
  H. Hereditary hemorrhagic macular dystrophy (AD)
  I. Rare dystrophies
    1. Dominantly inherited cystoid macular edema (AD)
    2. Benign concentric annular macular dystrophy (AD)
    3. Central areolar pigment epithelial dystrophy (AD)
    4. Progressive foveal dystrophy (AD)
    5. Slowly progressive macular dystrophy (AD)
    6. Familial foveal retinoschisis (AR)
    7. Fenestrated sheen macular dystrophy (AD)
    8. Adult foveomacular dystrophy
    9. Central pigmentary dystrophy
II. Macular abnormalities with generalized chorioretinal dystrophies
  A. Cone-rod dystrophy (AR)
  B. Progressive cone dystrophy (AD)
  C. Leber's congenital amaurosis (AR)
  D. Idiopathic juvenile X-linked retinoschisis (XLR)
  E. Goldmann-Favre syndrome (AR)
III. Macular abnormalities with systemic diseases

AD = autosomal dominant; AR = autosomal recessive; XLR = X-linked recessive. If a clearly established mode of inheritance has not been established, none is listed.

carrier may range from completely normal to as severely affected as her male counterpart. This phenomenon may be understood in light of Lyon's hypothesis of random inactivation of the X chromosome.

Finally, it should be emphasized that in caring for patients with hereditary macular dystrophies, it is the ophthalmologist who very often assumes the additional role of genetic counselor. The key to proper counseling is making the correct diagnosis. Only then can the physician intelligently discuss with the parents and the patient the course and prognosis of the disease, therapy, and the like-lihood that additional children or generations will inherit the disease.

CHARACTERISTICS

A number of features help distinguish the inherited macular dystrophies from the acquired macular degenerations. Evidence of genetic inheritance may come from a history of affected family members or, in autosomal recessive diseases, of parental consanguinity. In addition, affected family members may be first diagnosed by eye examination. Since children are often accompanied by their parents, routine examination of the parents may yield helpful clues in reaching the correct diagnosis.

Hereditary macular dystrophies have an early age of onset, with the signs and symptoms usually occurring in the first or second decade. In contradistinction, acquired macular degenerations are usually age related and present from the fifth decade onward. Finally, the dystrophies, unlike the degenerations, are usually bilateral, often with a symmetrical fundus appearance.

CLASSIFICATION

In the introduction to this chapter the inherited diseases affecting the macula were divided into three groups: (1) primary hereditary macular dystrophies, (2) macular dystrophies that are part of generalized chorioretinal dystrophies, and (3) macular dystrophies associated with systemic disorders (Table 17-1). Attempts have been made to subdivide these groups further according to (1) mode of inheritance (e.g. dominant, recessive, X-linked recessive), (2) age at onset (e.g. infantile, juvenile, adult), and (3) anatomic site of primary pathology (e.g. choroid, Bruch's membrane, retinal pigment epithelium [RPE], photoreceptors, inner retinal layers). Until our scientific probes identify the basic biochemical abnormality (presumably a missing or deficient enzyme), the preferred classification would appear to be according to the presumed anatomic site of primary pathology since this classification is the most logical and most helpful in understanding the pathogenesis (Table 17-2).

PRIMARY HEREDITARY MACULAR DYSTROPHIES

The typical presentation of an individual with an hereditary macular dystrophy is a progressive cen-

Table 17-2. *Anatomic Classification of Hereditary Macular Dystrophies*

1. Choriocapillaris
   a. Central areolar choroidal dystrophy
   b. Peripapillary choroidal dystrophy
2. Bruch's membrane
   a. Drusen
   b. Hereditary hemorrhagic macular dystrophy (Sorsby's pseudoinflammatory macular dystrophy)
3. Retinal Pigment Epithelium–photoreceptor complex
   a. Stargardt's disease, fundus flavimaculatus
   b. Best's vitelliform macular dystrophy
   c. Pigment pattern dystrophies
   d. Benign concentric annular macular dystrophy
   e. Central areolar pigment epithelial dystrophy
   f. Progressive foveal dystrophy
   g. Slowly progressive macular dystrophy
   h. Fenestrated sheen macular dystrophy
   i. Adult foveomacular dystrophy
   j. Central pigmentary dystrophy
4. Inner retinal layers
   a. Familial foveal retinoschisis
   b. Dominant cystoid macular edema

Table 17-3. *Characteristics of Primary Hereditary Macular Dystrophies*

1. Evidence of genetic inheritance
2. Early age of onset
3. Presenting symptom: diminished central vision
4. Bilateral, usually symmetrical, fundus appearance
5. Abnormal ophthalmoscopic appearance and abnormal visual function confined to macula or posterior pole

eases permits a proper perspective. For example, Stargardt's disease–fundus flavimaculatus is the most common hereditary macular dystrophy, and Best's vitelliform dystrophy is the second most common. These two diseases account for nearly 90 percent of the hereditary macular dystrophies I have seen. Dystrophies such as dominant drusen, central areolar choroidal dystrophy, and pattern dystrophies of the retinal pigment epithelium, are decidedly less common, while the remaining dystrophies are limited to a few case reports in the literature.

Stargardt's Disease (Juvenile Macular Degeneration)

Stargardt's disease (juvenile macular degeneration) is the most common hereditary macular dystrophy and, by virtue of this fact, the most important. Since its description by Stargardt in 1909 [67] there have been numerous reports and several large studies [40, 56].

In its classic form this recessively inherited disorder may be considered the prototype of hereditary macular dystrophies. The symptoms of central visual loss occur in the first or second decade, and the presenting maculopathy is bilateral and symmetrical in appearance. Results of tests of general retinal function (ERG, EOG) are usually normal and remain so throughout the course. The electro-oculogram is abnormal in a few patients [56].

While visual acuity at the time of presentation may be quite variable (as good as 20/20), and in some cases quite asymmetric, the natural course is progressive in each eye with final visual acuity in most cases in the range of 20/200 to 20/400. Vision less than 20/400 is distinctly uncommon.

The macular morphology may be quite varied, and an unusual appearance, by itself, should not dissuade one from entertaining the diagnosis. In the classic example (seen in some of Stargardt's

tral visual loss in one or both eyes with the onset frequently in the first or second decade of life (Table 17-3). The ophthalmoscopic abnormalities are usually bilateral and symmetrical and are confined to the macula and macular region.

Since the dystrophy is confined to the central retina, visual function (as measured by psychophysical and electrophysiologic tests) is abnormal in the affected retina but normal in the retinal periphery. Psychophysical tests that measure visual function at various loci (e.g., perimetry, final retinal thresholds, dark adaptation) clearly indicate the dichotomy between the normal and abnormal retina. Results of electrophysiologic tests that measure general retinal function (e.g., the electroretinogram [ERG] and the electro-oculogram [EOG]) are only minimally affected in most macular dystrophies. However, results of electrophysiologic tests that measure a local retinal area (focal electroretinogram) or that are heavily macular dependent (visual-evoked response) are dramatically abnormal.

The age of onset, visual symptoms, and visual function test results are similar in most of these dystrophies. Therefore, very often the most useful method of diagnosis is an appreciation of the various macular morphologies. In addition, an appreciation of the relative frequency of these dis-

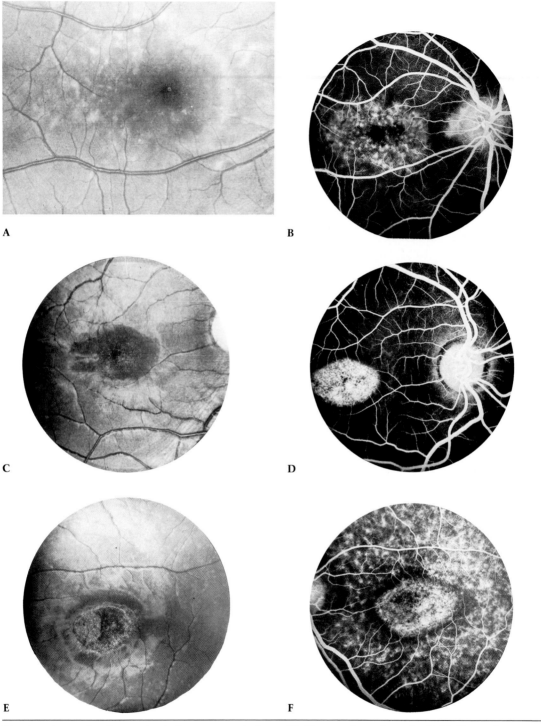

Fig. 17-1. *Stargardt's disease. Typical appearance in 3 cases. The typical appearance of the macula is a mild pigment granularity surrounded by irregular yellowish white deep flecks (A). Occasionally the pigmentary abnormalities are mild and are unassociated with these flecks (C). When the pigmentary changes are pronounced the tapetum-like reflex is referred to as a beaten-bronze appearance (E). Fluorescein angiography (B, D, F) may be revealing in demonstrating more pigmentary disturbances than are seen funduscopically in the macula (e.g., B and D) or in the posterior pole (F). A good example of the "dark" or "silent" choroid is seen in D, where the decrease in the background choroidal fluorescence allows for the visualization of the retinal capillary circulation.*

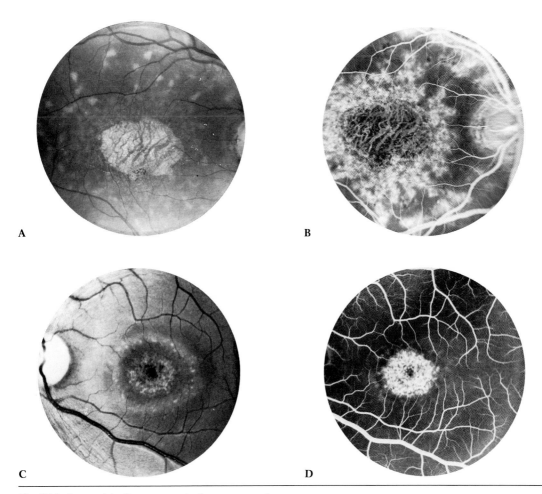

Fig. 17-2. *Stargardt's disease, atypical appearance. In these 2 cases (A and B; C and D), the typical flecks of Stargardt's disease surround an atypical maculopathy—in 1 case (A) a well-circumscribed area of choroidal atrophy; in the other (C) a "bull's-eye" ring. Fluorescein angiography shows the choriocapillaris atrophy surrounded by focal areas of transmitted hyperfluorescence (B) and the pronounced retinal capillary circulation seen in the dark, silent choroid (D).*

original patients) there is a pigmentary maculopathy surrounded by a few irregularly shaped yellow to white spots or flecks. The pigmentary alterations may include a mild tapetal sheen reflex, a marked tapetal reflex ("beaten-bronze" appearance), mottling, atrophy, and clumping (Fig. 17-1). Occasionally, the fundus appearance may be so atypical (e.g. choroidal sclerosis, bull's eye, bone spicule pigmentation) that it suggests an alternative diagnosis (respectively, central areolar

choroidal dystrophy, cone dystrophy, "central retinitis pigmentosa") (Fig. 17-2, Table 17-4). Recently Stargardt's disease has been associated with subretinal neovascularization [46].

Fluorescein angiography has proved helpful in diagnoses on certain occasions. When a subtle maculopathy is suspected, the pigmentary changes may be confirmed by noting a transmitted hyperfluorescence. Macular abnormalities without surrounding flecks may show, on angiography, the surrounding areas of patchy hyperfluorescence so typical of this disease (see Fig. 17-1F).

In a number of situations the diagnosis is not readily apparent. First, there may be a marked dissociation between vision and macular appearance. Children who complain of visual difficulties have been labeled as malingerers or hysterics or, worse yet, suspected of harboring a brain tumor because the macula appeared normal. In my experience all individuals with Stargardt's disease

Table 17-4. Differential Diagnosis of Stargardt's Disease

1. Central areolar choroidal dystrophy
2. Vitelliform macular dystrophy
3. Progressive cone dystrophy
4. X-linked retinoschisis (late atrophic stages)
5. Bull's-eye maculopathy (see Table 17-6)
6. Acquired macular degenerations

will show some slight macular pigmentary alterations, which are more obvious on fluorescein angiography. Second, although Stargardt's disease is referred to as juvenile macular dystrophy, some individuals become symptomatic later in life; the onset of symptoms in the fourth or fifth decade does not exclude this diagnosis. Third, there may be a marked asymmetry in vision despite a similar maculopathy. Unfortunately, the vision in the better eye soon catches up to the worse eye.

The differential diagnosis of Stargardt's disease is shown in Table 17-4. Stated simply, children and young adults who present with progressive central visual loss and a bilateral maculopathy, whose histories suggest an autosomal recessive inheritance, and who have a normal ERG and EOG have Stargardt's disease (juvenile macular dystrophy) until proven otherwise.

Variants of Stargardt's Disease

Several diseases bear a relationship to the previously described macular dystrophy but are different enough for some investigators to classify them into separate categories. Thus, the following disorders, and their relationship with Stargardt's disease, will now be discussed: (1) fundus flavimaculatus, (2) progressive atrophic macular dystrophy, and (3) dominant Stargardt's disease.

FUNDUS FLAVIMACULATUS

In 1963 the fundus appearance of irregularly shaped yellowish white spots (flecks) scattered throughout the posterior pole of each eye was reported, and the somewhat descriptive term of fundus flavimaculatus was coined [30]. In subsequent publications, when the features were described in some 36 patients [31], half of whom had a macular degeneration, it became apparent that many individuals with this "new" disease were funduscopically similar if not identical to some patients originally described by Stargardt. In present day parlance the term *fundus flavimaculatus* is reserved for patients with the disseminated flecks throughout the posterior pole with or without macular degenerations (Fig. 17-3).

There have been two histopathologic reports of fundus flavimaculatus. The initial report in 1967 concluded that the basic defect resided in the pigment epithelium [45]. These cells showed an altered morphology consisting of (1) great variations in size, (2) nuclear displacement from the base inwardly, (3) an acid mucopolysaccharide material in the inner half of the cell, and (4) multiple granules that stained with periodic acid–Schiff (PAS). The second report agreed with the light microscopic findings of the first case and emphasized the importance of the PAS-positive granules [20]. With additional histochemical techniques, ultraviolet fluorescent microscopy, and transmission electron microscopy, a massive intracellular accumulation of a lipofuscin-like substance in both the peripheral and posterior RPE was demonstrated.

The clinical and angiographic appearance in this disease may be explained by the large accumulation of the lipofuscin-like material. In the posterior polar RPE where the accumulation is greatest, these cells have a decreased melanin content and appear lighter (the yellow-white flecks). Since lipofuscin absorbs the blue excitatory wavelengths used in fluorescein angiography these flecks would appear hypofluorescent. Similarly, the presence of the lipofuscin-like material throughout the retina would explain the generalized relative hypofluorescence and decrease in normal background choroidal fluorescence referred to as the silent or dark choroid [6, 24]. Finally, as these cells degenerate they lose their lipofuscin-like material and melanin, resulting in the hyperfluorescence of older flecks (Fig. 17-3C).

These histologic findings documented abnormalities in the RPE throughout the entire retina although the posterior pole exhibited the most striking features. This correlates with a clinical concept that some cases of the Stargardt's disease–fundus flavimaculatus group may progress, in a centrifugal fashion, from a central to a more generalized degeneration in which reabsorption of flecks leads to chorioretinal atrophy, and, in the most advanced stages, to electrophysiologic evidence of cone and rod dysfunction [25]. However, this progression is distinctly rare.

The yellowish white flecks may be confused with features of a number of other disorders, in-

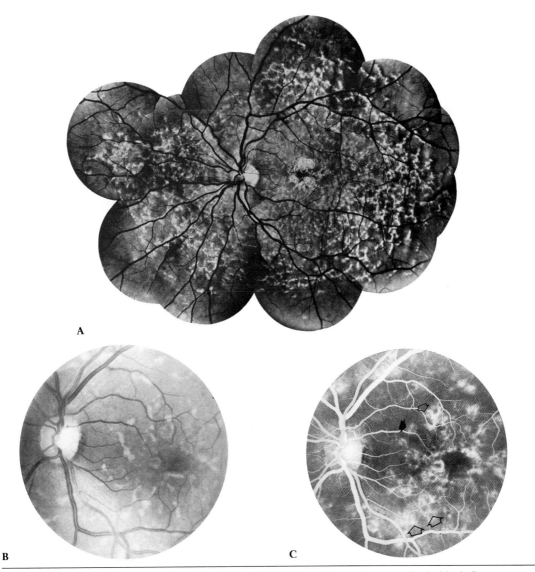

Fig. 17-3. *Fundus flavimaculatus. The typical yellowish white flecks are seen throughout the posterior pole, nasal to the optic disc, and peripheral to the temporal vessel arcades (A). A comparison of the fundus appearance (B) with the angiogram (C) demonstrates that some flecks block fluorescence (single open arrow), some transmit fluorescence (closed arrow), and some fluorescein abnormalities cannot be correlated with obvious fundus flecks (open arrows at bottom).*

Table 17-5. *Differential Diagnosis of Fundus Flavimaculatus*

1. Dominant drusen of Bruch's membrane
2. Fundus albipunctatus
3. Retinitis punctata albescens
4. Multiple vitelliform cysts
5. Flecked retina (of Kandori)

cluding dominant drusen of Bruch's membrane, fundus albipunctatus, retinitis punctata albescens, multiple vitelliform cysts, and flecked retina (of Kandori) (Table 17-5).

PROGRESSIVE ATROPHIC MACULAR DYSTROPHY

The term *progressive atrophic macular dystrophy* has been used to describe the maculopathy of Stargardt's disease without any evidence of perifoveal flecks (see Fig. 17-1C and E) [14]. Some individuals do develop flecks later in life, and they undoubtedly have Stargardt's disease. In those who do not, it is arguable whether they indeed have a distinct macular dystrophy that deserves this new name.

In 1979 the fundus morphology of 67 diagnosed cases of Stargardt's disease and fundus flavimaculatus was reviewed [56]. The cases were separated into four groups:

1. Macular degeneration without flecks (progressive atrophic macular dystrophy) (14 cases)
2. Macular degeneration with flecks (Stargardt's disease) (25 cases)
3. Macular degeneration with diffuse flecks (fundus flavimaculatus with macular degeneration) (24 cases)
4. Diffuse flecks without macular degeneration ("pure" fundus flavimaculatus) (4 cases)

It has been well documented that individuals in group 1 may progress to group 2 or 3 and that those in group 4 may develop macular degeneration (Fig. 17-4). On the basis of sex, race, age of onset, visual acuity, visual function tests, and prognosis, it is not possible to distinguish among these four morphologic groups. Thus one may conclude that these different morphologies represent the phenotypic variability of the same disease process.

DOMINANT STARGARDT'S DISEASE

Most cases previously described as dominant Stargardt's disease were in reality progressive cone dystrophies [14]. There are a few dominant pedigrees with an atrophic macular degeneration (without flecks) but without generalized cone dysfunction, and this may represent a distinct entity.

Only one well-documented dominant pedigree of a macular dystrophy with posterior polar flecks has been reported [8]. This clearly indicates that at least two distinct genetic entities may result in the similar morphology of macular degeneration and flecks.

Best's Vitelliform Macular Dystrophy

Best's vitelliform macular dystrophy is the second most common hereditary macular dystrophy. For a variety of reasons it remains the most enigmatic of all these dystrophies. Like an unruly child it obeys none of the "rules." For example, Best's dystrophy has the following features:

1. Variable onset. (The typical vitelliform lesion has been seen shortly after birth [3, 13], and a typical lesion has newly arisen in a 51-year-old man [71].)
2. Polymorphous presentations [55]. (Typically the lesion is atypical.)
3. Not uncommonly "unilateral."
4. Vision varies considerably and may improve dramatically.
5. Mildly affected individuals appear unaffected ("carrier" state) [10].
6. Invariably a dichotomy between a normal ERG and an abnormal EOG.

The intact egg yolk is one of the most striking pictures in all of ophthalmology. Unfortunately, the location and nature of this yellowish material remains a mystery. It lies in front of the choroid since it may block background choroidal fluorescence, and it has little if any effect on photoreceptor function since typically vision is normal. When the egg yolk "ruptures," resulting in the appearances of the "scrambled egg," "pseudohypopyon," or nonspecific pigmentary maculopathy, then the visual acuity diminishes (Fig. 17-5).

The classical vitelline lesion is actually encountered infrequently, and the presenting fundus morphology is often deceptive, mimicking that in other macular diseases. Pigmentary atrophy and clumping, drusen, subretinal hemorrhage, choroidal neovascularization, choroidal atrophy, and fibrosis have all been seen. When one considers

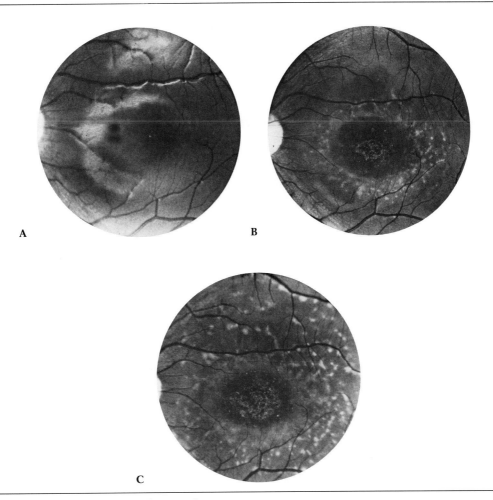

A

B

C

Fig. 17-4. *Stargardt's disease–fundus flavimaculatus spectrum. Fundus photographs from this 16-year-old girl document the transition of fundus appearances. A. Initially, the macula had an atrophic appearance without flecks. B. Six years later the maculopathy was more prominent and surrounded by flecks. C. Three years later there was a beaten-bronze maculopathy surrounded by diffuse posterior polar flecks.*

that these lesions may be multifocal, extramacular, asymmetric, and uniocular, one can see that establishing the diagnosis of vitelliform macular dystrophy can be quite frustrating.

There are two helpful guides in this regard. The first is establishing an autosomal dominant mode of inheritance. All family members should be examined since asymptomatic affected members may have normal or near normal visual acuity and yet show macular abnormalities. Some affected individuals may have 20/20 vision and a normal fundus. While these individuals have been called carriers [10], the notion of a heterozygote state is incompatible with dominant inheritance.

The second is performing an electro-oculogram. Since the first reports of an abnormal electro-oculogram in this disease [33], studies of large pedigrees have indicated the following [9, 68]:

1. The EOG is invariably abnormal (L/D* less than 1.40) in *all* affected members.
2. The EOG is abnormal in both eyes in cases of unilateral macular pathology.
3. The EOG is abnormal in "carriers."

*L = amplitude in light; D = amplitude in darkness.

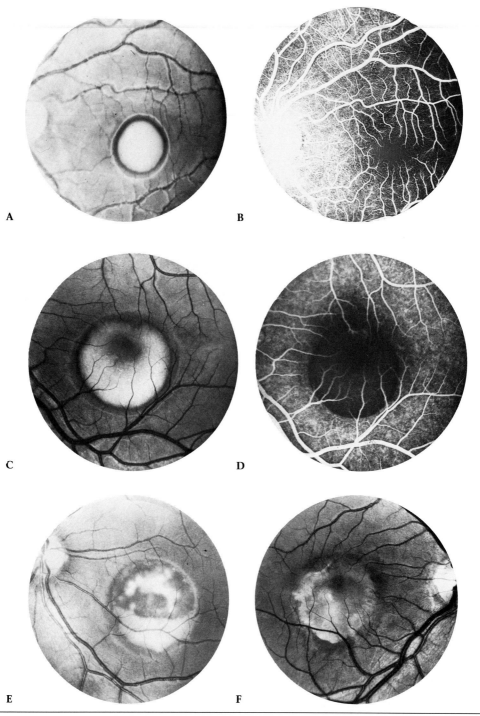

Fig. 17-5. Best's vitelliform macular dystrophy. The intact egg yolk stage has a dramatic appearance, made even more so in view of normal vision (20/20) (A and C). The angiogram at this stage may be normal (B) or show a blocked transmission corresponding to the lesion (D). Other appearances include the pseudohypopyon (E), scrambled egg (F), subretinal choroidal neovascularization (G and H), and multiple vitelliform lesions (I).

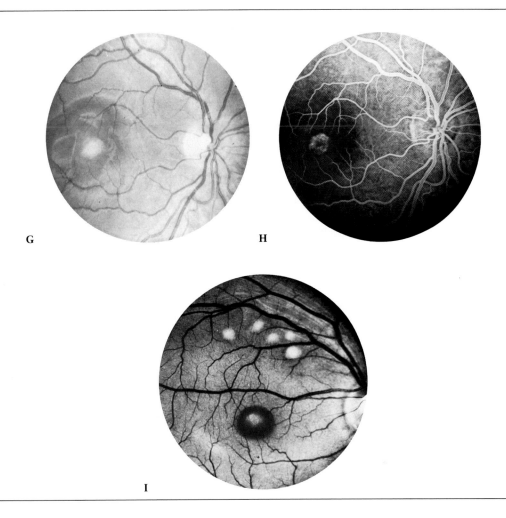

G

H

I

The conclusion to be drawn from these findings is that an abnormal EOG is a very sensitive indicator of vitelliform dystrophy and that it may be the only evidence of the inheritance of the abnormal gene. While the sensitivity approaches 100 percent, the specificity of an abnormal EOG with a normal ERG is somewhat lower, since on rare occasion other macular dystrophies (Stargardt's disease–fundus flavimaculatus, dominant drusen, pattern pigment dystrophies) can result in these findings.

The intact egg yolk is neither a common finding in vitelliform macular dystrophy nor is it pathognomonic for this disorder. Since the first report in 1973 of a normal EOG in a patient with typical bilateral vitelliform macular lesions [5], numerous examples have occurred of individuals with vitelliform lesions with a normal EOG and without evidence of a dominant maculopathy. These pseudovitelliform lesions occur in adults and have been associated with perifoveal retinal capillary leakage [29], RPE [63] and neurosensory detachments, or nonspecific pigmentary changes [21, 43, 69]. It is my feeling that these lesions are manifestations of an acquired macular degeneration.

Most previous histopathologic reports of vitelliform macular dystrophy were in elderly individuals in whom, it could be argued, age-related degenerative abnormalities may have distorted the primary pathology. Recently, however, both eyes of a 28-year-old member of a family with vitelliform dystrophy (whose macula had a scrambled egg appearance) showed an abnormal accumulation of lipofuscin granules within the retinal pig-

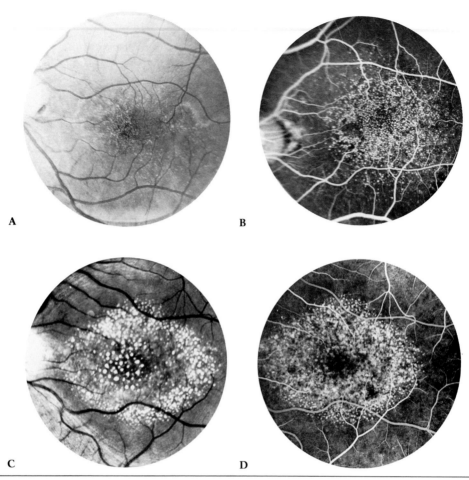

A   B

C   D

Fig. 17-6. *Dominant drusen. The fundus appearance and topographic distribution of dominant drusen of Bruch's membrane may vary from being confined to the macula (A and C) to involving the entire posterior pole (E), sparing the macula (F), and being nasal to the disk (G). The fluorescein angiogram (B and D) indicates focal areas of hyperfluorescence more widespread than seen on funduscopy.*

ment epithelium, which led the authors to conclude this is a generalized retinal pigment epithelial abnormality [70]. Another recent report of the histology of the eyes of an 80-year-old woman from a well-documented pedigree of vitelliform dystrophy showed a PAS-positive, acid-mucopolysaccharide-negative, electron-dense, finely granular material in the inner segments of the degenerating photoreceptors and the Müller cells [34]. These authors felt it most likely that the sensory retinal changes are primary and the retinal pigment epithelial changes are secondary.

Dominant Drusen of Bruch's Membrane

Dominant drusen of Bruch's membrane is usually an asymptomatic disorder noticed fortuitously on ocular examination. For this reason its true fre-

quency is undoubtedly much higher than the frequency with which it is diagnosed.

As with many dominant disorders there is a variable expressivity, which accounts for the different shapes, sizes, color, and topography of these basal laminar deposits. It is now generally agreed that the disorders referred to as Hutchinson-Tay choroiditis, Holthouse-Batten chorioretinitis, Doyne's honeycomb dystrophy, and mallatia Leventinese are different clinical manifestations of this same hereditary dystrophy.

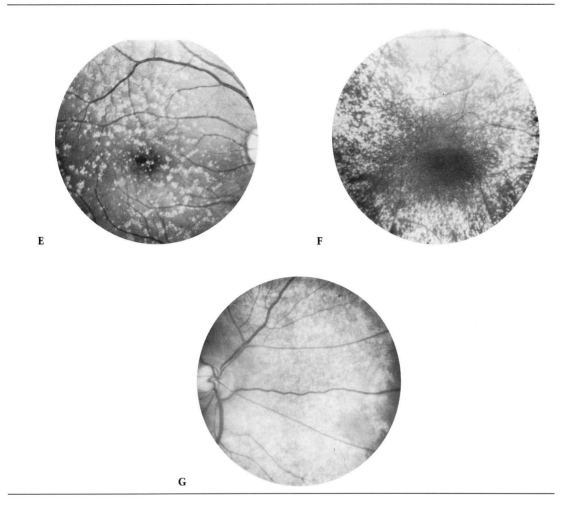

E

F

G

The drusen are round (unlike the flecks of fundus flavimaculatus), yellowish to white, discrete or confluent, and associated with various pigmentary changes. They may be focal, confined to the macula or the peripapillary region, or they may be diffuse, involving the entire posterior pole, sometimes sparing the macula. The appearance is virtually always symmetrical and similar within affected family members (Fig. 17-6).

These individuals become symptomatic from an associated exudative or nonexudative macular degeneration. The relationship between acquired drusen and macular degeneration has been well documented, and presumably a similar process is occurring in these patients.

The relationship between familial and acquired drusen is not well understood. Some claim ready methods of distinguishing these two [12, 22]; others suspect all drusens are familial [36]. While the senile or acquired drusen may have a polygenic inheritance, dominant drusen is probably a distinct entity that may be diagnosed by (1) evidence of dominant inheritance, (2) early age of onset, (3) bilateralness and symmetry, and (4) intrafamilial similarity.

Pigment Pattern Dystrophies

The term *pigment pattern dystrophies* is an attempt to group together a number of individual disease entities that share similar characteristics. Previously referred to as reticular dystrophy [62], macroreticular dystrophy [50], and butterfly dystrophy [11], these inherited diseases all have a particular bilateral, symmetrical pigmentary ap-

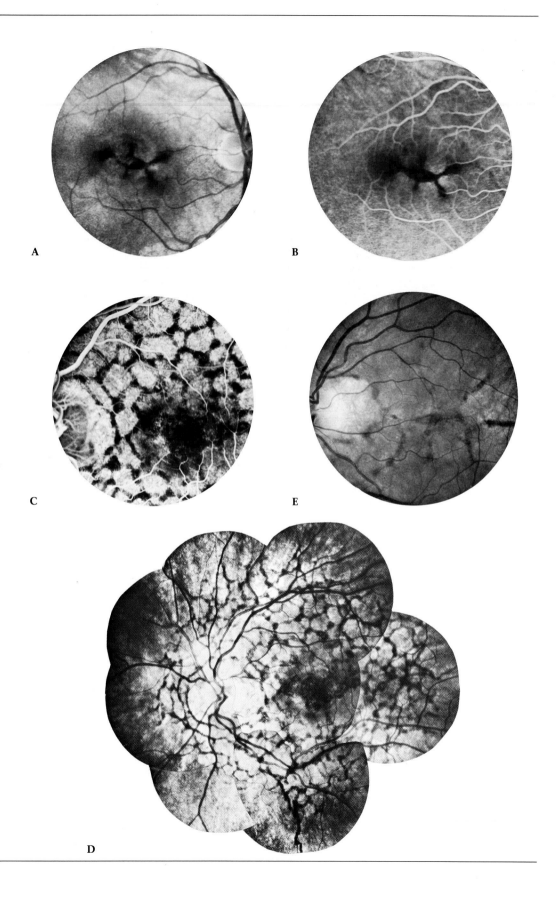

pearance of the posterior pole associated with normal or near-normal visual acuity, a normal ERG, and a variable EOG that is not diagnostic (Fig. 17-7).

The impetus for lumping these various diseases together has been the finding in different family members of dominant pedigrees each of the particular pigmentary abnormalities [42, 44, 49, 57]. Studies of large pedigrees with this disorder would be helpful in determining whether these various pigmentary configurations are indeed different phenotypic manifestations of a single genetic disorder.

One report has suggested that some of these pattern dystrophies may progress with reduced visual acuity and an abnormal ERG [28]. However, long-term studies on these patients have not yet been done.

Central Areolar Choroidal Dystrophy

Central areolar choroidal dystrophy (CACD) is an autosomal dominant maculopathy [60, 66] in which the primary abnormality is probably an abiotrophy of the choriocapillaris. While the earliest fundus changes—macular pigment granularity, transparency of the RPE, or tapetal sheen reflex—may mimic a variety of macular disorders, a fluorescein angiogram will indicate atrophy of the choriocapillaris with a diminished background choroidal fluorescence and persistent visualization of the larger choroidal vessels (Fig. 17-8) [51, 52].

With progression of the disease the underlying choroid is more easily seen, and the vessels may appear normal or sclerotic (yellowish white) (Fig. 17-8D). However, histopathology has clearly shown no evidence of vessel wall sclerosis, but rather a well-circumscribed macular zone of atrophy of the choriocapillaris, RPE, and neurosensory retina [2].

The early findings in CACD of a nonspecific macular pigmentary abnormality can mimic a wide variety of macular diseases (e.g., Stargardt's disease, vitelliform dystrophy, progressive cone dystrophies, acquired macular degeneration), while the later typical stage of circumscribed choroidal atrophy can be mimicked by many other diseases (e.g., atrophic nonexudative macular degeneration, retinochoroiditis, and the advanced stages of various hereditary dystrophies) [52]. In this regard the diagnosis of CACD is best made when the following information is available:

1. Dominant inheritance with family members demonstrating the various morphologic stages
2. Bilateral and symmetrical macular lesions
3. Evidence of choriocapillaris atrophy on fluorescein angiography

Peripapillary (Pericentral) Choroidal Dystrophy

Peripapillary choroidal dystrophy, an autosomal recessive disorder, demonstrates atrophy of the choriocapillaris surrounding the optic nerve with radiation along the temporal vessel arcades [64]. It is only in the fifth to seventh decade, when the macula becomes involved, that the patient becomes symptomatic. Fluorescein angiography clearly demonstrates choriocapillaris atrophy in the involved area (Fig. 17-9).

Hereditary Hemorrhagic Macular Dystrophy (Sorsby's Pseudoinflammatory Macular Dystrophy)

In 1949 Sorsby and colleagues described "a fundus dystrophy with unusual features" [65]. Since the late stages of this disorder resembled a postinflammatory process the term *pseudoinflammatory macular dystrophy* has been used [18]. The presence of macular subretinal choroidal neovascularization in the early stages prompted the more accurate descriptive name of *hereditary hemorrhagic macular dystrophy* (Fig. 17-10) [7].

Unlike most hereditary diseases the onset of symptoms is usually later in life. The pathophysiology is similar to the hemorrhagic and exudative maculopathy seen in acquired disciform macular degeneration except that hereditary hemorrhagic macular dystrophy (1) is inherited as an autosomal dominant trait, (2) has an earlier onset

Fig. 17-7. *Pigment pattern dystrophies. A, B. The unusual pigmentary appearance in the maculae of this patient prompted the term* butterfly-shaped pigment dystrophy. *C, D. In reticular dystrophy the network of hyperpigmentation has a mosaic pattern and involves the entire posterior pole. E. Macroreticular or spider dystrophy is an intermediate form between butterfly and reticular dystrophy. Fluorescein angiography vividly demonstrates the pigmentary abnormalities in all these cases of pigment pattern dystrophy. The finding of these pigment abnormalities in different family members of dominant pedigrees has prompted the term* pigment pattern dystrophy *to encompass these three disorders.*

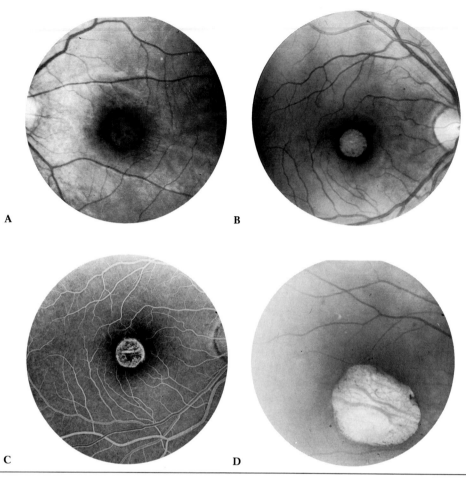

Fig. 17-8. *Central areolar choroidal dystrophy. The early pigmentary changes include atrophy (A) or a tapetal reflex (B) well circumscribed in the macula. The atrophy of the choriocapillaris is nicely seen on fluorescein angiography (C). In the later stages there is loss of the retina and choroid, and the remaining choroidal vessels are seen overlying the sclera (D).*

(in the fourth decade), (3) is unassociated with drusen, and (4) extends into the more peripheral retina in the late stages.

Because of the paucity of case reports there is some controversy as to whether this is indeed a distinct dystrophy or rather another inherited dystrophy that itself predisposes to an exudative maculopathy. For example, drusen and angioid streaks have been seen in family pedigrees with this dystrophy [41]. Histopathologic studies in two older affected individuals demonstrated findings typical of acquired macular degeneration [1]. However, other family pedigrees have shown no evidence of a hereditary disease that is associated with subretinal choroidal neovascularization [2]. Additional case reports will be necessary to clarify the nature of this disease.

Rare Dystrophies

The following hereditary dystrophies are extremely rare, having been noted in a single pedigree or a few family pedigrees, and they will be dealt with briefly.

DOMINANTLY INHERITED CYSTOID
MACULAR EDEMA

Cystoid macular edema owing to leakage from perifoveal retinal capillaries has been docu-

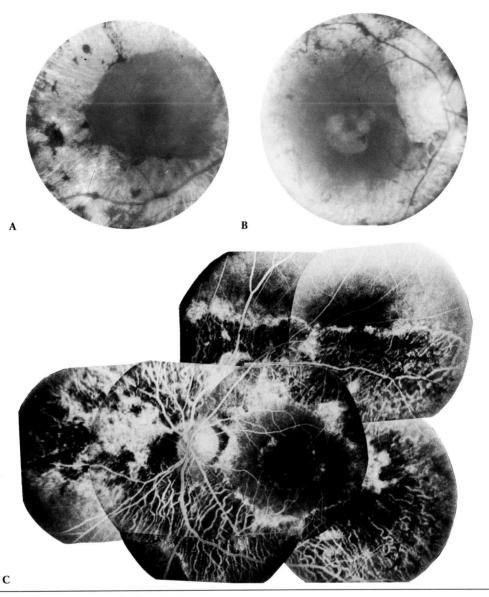

Fig. 17-9. *Peripapillary (pericentral) choroidal dystrophy. A. Unlike central areolar choroidal dystrophy, which remains localized in the macula, this dystrophy initially surrounds the optic nerve and radiates along the temporal vessel arcades, sparing the macula. B. Later in the course the macula may become involved. C. Angiography demonstrates atrophy of the choriocapillaris in the affected area and shows normal results elsewhere.*

mented in a number of dominant pedigrees [16, 59]. Other findings include hyperopia, punctate vitreous opacities, and an abnormal EOG in some.

BENIGN CONCENTRIC ANNULAR MACULAR DYSTROPHY (BULL'S-EYE MACULOPATHY)

Bull's-eye maculopathy, a disorder confined to four members of three generations in one family [15], is manifested by a bull's-eye pigmentary maculopathy with normal or near-normal vision. Since

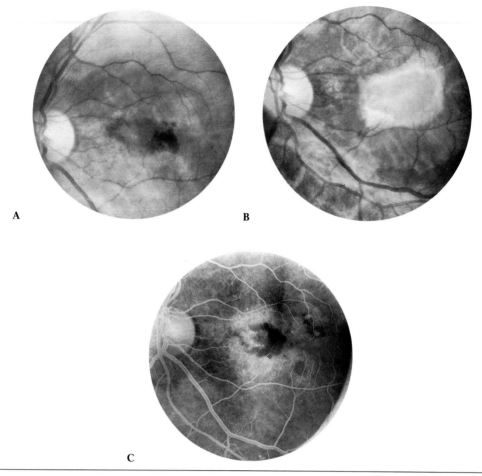

Fig. 17-10. *Hereditary hemorrhagic macular dystrophy (Sorsby's pseudoinflammatory macular dystrophy). This 30-year-old man from a family with this disorder had hemorrhagic maculopathy (A) associated with a subretinal choroidal neovascular net (B). This progressed to a dense glial scar in the macula (C) and similar changes in the periphery. (From R. E. Carr, K. G. Noble, and I. Nasaduke, Hereditary hemorrhagic macular dystrophy. Am. J. Ophthalmol. 85:318, 1978. Reprinted by permission.)*

one of the four affected individuals had tiny drusen surrounding the macular lesions, dominant drusen cannot be entirely ruled out. The normal or slightly diminished photopic ERG makes a cone dystrophy (in which occasionally there is a bull's-eye maculopathy) unlikely. The differential diagnosis of bull's-eye maculopathy is listed in Table 17-6.

CENTRAL AREOLAR PIGMENT EPITHELIAL DYSTROPHY

Central areolar pigment epithelial (CAPE) dystrophy has been reported in four members of three generations in one pedigree [23]. It is a benign, nonprogressive disorder in which the macular lesions were "central, depigmented, sharply demarcated and involved primarily the pigment epi-

thelium" [23]. Visual acuity was 20/20 except in one eye with hemorrhagic maculopathy.

PROGRESSIVE FOVEAL DYSTROPHY

The findings of progressive foveal dystrophy are confined to 50 affected members of a single pedigree [35, 47]. The early changes of drusen and pigmentary alterations are nonspecific, but the

Table 17-6. *Differential Diagnosis of Bull's-Eye Maculopathy*

1. Progressive cone dystrophy
2. Benign concentric annular macular dystrophy
3. Stargardt's disease
4. Acquired macular degeneration
5. Chloroquine-induced maculopathy
6. Trauma

early age of onset (less than 1 year of age in one case) and a rapid progression to central chorioretinal changes by late puberty are unique. An aminoaciduria has been seen in some family members, but this gene segregates independently from the gene for macular dystrophy.

SLOWLY PROGRESSIVE MACULAR DYSTROPHY

Slowly progressive macular dystrophy was described in 18 members in two generations of a single pedigree [61]. The macular changes included "perifoveal pigment epithelial atrophy, posterior pole flecks, and . . . an atrophic form of senile macular degeneration" [61].

FAMILIAL FOVEAL RETINOSCHISIS

Three young sisters (including monozygotic twins) with a mild visual loss demonstrated a foveal retinoschisis that funduscopically resembled X-linked foveal retinoschisis [48]. Unlike the X-linked disease, the ERG in familial foveal retinoschisis was normal, and the periphery was normal.

FENESTRATED SHEEN MACULAR DYSTROPHY

Fenestrated sheen macular dystrophy, a slowly progressive dystrophy, was described in 5 patients in three generations of a single family [58]. The earliest manifestations (in a 4-year-old) consisted of "a yellowish refractile sheen with red fenestrations within the sensory retina" that eventually progressed to include RPE changes, some resembling a bull's-eye lesion.

ADULT FOVEOMACULAR DYSTROPHY

The appearance of small, yellow, slightly elevated subretinal macular lesions in adults has prompted the terms *foveomacular vitelliform dystrophy* and *adult-type* or *adult-onset foveomacular pigment*

epithelial dystrophy [37, 38, 69]. The EOG results are variable and in some cases are markedly abnormal.

The presence of small paracentral drusen with occasional serous and hemorrhagic detachments in some adults suggests either an acquired exudative macular degeneration or dominant drusen. The findings in a few family members indicate this may be inherited as an autosomal dominant trait. However, studies of larger family pedigrees will be necessary to further clarify and classify this disorder. The relationship with pseudovitelliform macular dystrophy is not clear.

CENTRAL PIGMENTARY DYSTROPHY

When the posterior pole develops the typical bone spicule pigmentation seen in classic retinitis pigmentosa, the descriptive term *central retinitis pigmentosa* has been used (Fig. 17-11). While the term *central pigmentary dystrophy* avoids the comparison with the generalized tapetoretinal dystrophy retinitis pigmentosa, to which it bears little relationship, it is not clear whether this distinctive fundus appearance is a separate disease entity or represents the morphologic mimicking of many different macular dystrophies.

Most of these cases are sporadic, with occasional evidence of an autosomal recessive mode of inheritance [19, 32]. Both the visual acuity and the prognosis are quite variable. However, the disease process should never involve the retinal pe-

Fig. 17-11. *Central pigmentary dystrophy. The typical bone spicule pigmentation and grayish metallic sheen is confined to the posterior pole.*

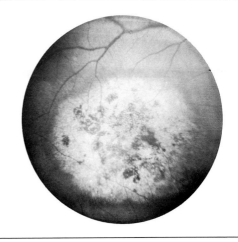

riphery, and this, in part, distinguishes it from the disorder called cone-rod dystrophy (inverse retinitis pigmentosa), which is a generalized tapeto-retinal dystrophy.

MACULAR ABNORMALITIES WITH GENERALIZED CHORIORETINAL DYSTROPHIES

On occasion, the visual symptoms or the fundus appearance may suggest a primary macular disease when in fact the macular abnormalities are part of a more generalized retinal dysfunction. The distinction between these two is made by visual function testing, including electroretinography, electro-oculography, visual fields, dark adaptation, and retinal sensitivity profiles. With generalized diseases all retinal areas tested will indicate visual dysfunction, whereas in the primary hereditary dystrophies areas outside the affected retina will be normal. It is important to make this distinction since the prognosis in the generalized chorioretinal dystrophies is invariably worse.

Cone-Rod Dystrophy (Inverse Retinitis Pigmentosa)

In the typical case of retinitis pigmentosa (rod-cone dystrophy), the symptoms of poor night vision and peripheral vision are related to the fact that the midperipheral rods are affected earliest and most severely in this disease. This has been confirmed by psychophysical, electrophysiologic, and histopathologic studies. The central retina is the most resistant to the dystrophic process, and characteristically central vision remains normal until late in the course.

In the cone-rod dystrophies the earliest manifestations of disease symptomatically, funduscopically, and functionally are in the central retina. This accounts for the early symptoms of visual loss, the preponderant pigmentary alterations occurring in the posterior pole, and an ERG that indicates predominantly cone photoreceptor dysfunction. During the course of the disease the remainder of the retina will become more involved, and these two forms of retinitis pigmentosa (rod-cone and cone-rod) merge.

Cone-rod dystrophy should be distinguished from central retinitis pigmentosa (see Central Pigmentary Dystrophy above). In the former the entire retina shows both cone and rod dysfunction, while in the latter the retinal function is normal beyond

the affected central retina. Cone-rod dystrophy must also be distinguished from the progressive cone dystrophies. In the former the rods are affected early in the course of the disease (though less so than the cones) and show progressive visual dysfunction. In the latter the rods are only minimally affected and show little inclination toward progression, while the cone function continues to worsen.

There has been a recent emphasis on the macular abnormalities that may occur in the course of otherwise typical retinitis pigmentosa (rod-cone dystrophy) [26, 27]. These abnormalities, all of which may lead to diminished vision, include cystoid macular edema (with or without perifoveal retinal capillary leakage), macular holes or cysts (possibly as a consequence of the edema), preretinal gliosis, pigmentary atrophy or accumulation, and choroidal atrophy. These macular changes in retinitis pigmentosa should not be confused with the macular abnormalities of the cone-rod dystrophies nor with features of the primary macular dystrophies.

Progressive Cone Dystrophy

There are a number of inherited dystrophies in which the cone photoreceptors are primarily, if not exclusively, affected. While the rods may show mild visual dysfunction, they do not worsen to the severe state of the cones.

The congenital stationary form of cone dysfunction known as achromatopsia (rod monochromatism) presents with poor vision, photophobia, nystagmus, and lack of color discrimination. As such it is rarely confused with the hereditary macular dystrophies even though macular changes may be seen.

A less common type of cone dystrophy has an onset in the first or second decade of life with the predominant symptom of diminished central vision and a progressive course [4, 39]. A bull's-eye maculopathy occasionally occurs in this disease, but more often the macula pigmentary abnormalities are variable (Fig. 17-12). A bull's-eye maculopathy, as already noted, is a very nonspecific change that may be seen in numerous disorders (see Table 17-6). The key to making the diagnosis of a progressive cone dystrophy is not the macular appearance but the ERG, which shows a reduced photopic single-flash response, an absent photopic flicker response, and a normal scotopic response (Fig. 17-12E). Unlike the cone-rod dystro-

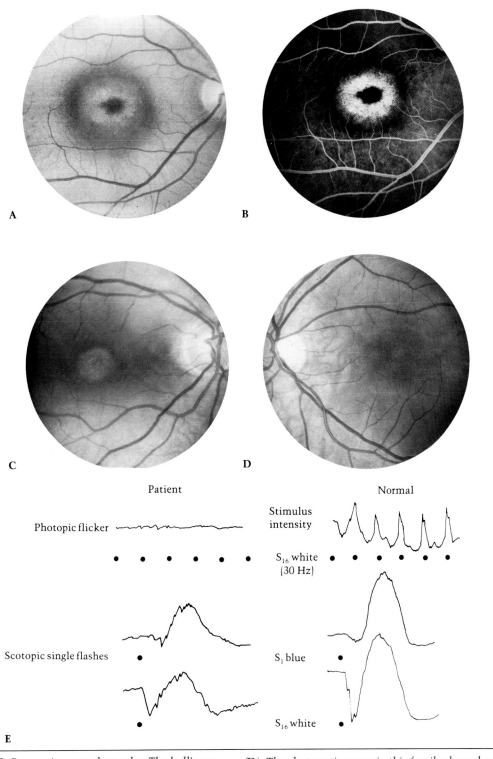

Patient

Normal

Photopic flicker

Stimulus
intensity

S_{16} white
(30 Hz)

Scotopic single flashes

S_1 blue

S_{16} white

A

B

C

D

E

Fig. 17-12. *Progressive cone dystrophy. The bull's-eye appearance of the macula is uncommon in this disease but striking when it occurs (A and B). The more likely appearance is nonspecific pigmentary changes, as are seen in this mother (C) and daughter (D). The electroretinogram in this family showed an absent photopic flicker response with a normal or near-normal scotopic response (E). (Time and amplitude calibration is 40 msec and 200 μv, respectively).*

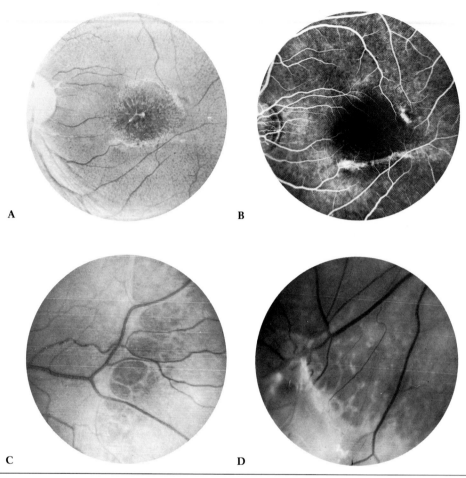

A

B

C

D

phies previously discussed, in progressive cone dystrophy the rod function remains essentially normal.

Leber's Congenital Amaurosis

Leber's congenital amaurosis usually presents with poor vision (20/200 or worse) and nystagmus. The fundus findings are extremely variable, in the early stages appearing quite normal but in the late stages exhibiting diffuse chorioretinal atrophy with heavy pigment proliferation. On rare occasions the fundus changes appear localized to the posterior pole. However, the markedly abnormal or extinguished ERG clearly differentiates this from a localized macular dystrophy [53].

Fig. 17-13. *Idiopathic juvenile X-linked retinoschisis. The macula has the characteristic spoke-wheel appearance (A), which is not apparent in the angiogram (B) since the pathology is in the superficial retina. Peripheral retinoschisis with superficial retinal holes and white dendritic figures are seen in another patient (C and D). When the macular retinoschisis flattens, a nonspecific maculopathy usually results (E). The fluorescein angiogram reveals a transmitted hyperfluorescence indicating pigmentary abnormalities (F). However, it is the electroretinogram (G) in this man that establishes the diagnosis since it shows the deep a wave with a b wave that does not return to the baseline (electronegative response) that is so characteristic of this disorder. (Time and amplitude calibration is 40 msec and 200 μv, respectively.)*

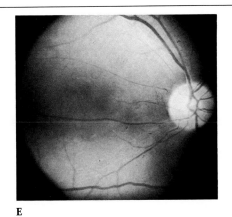

E

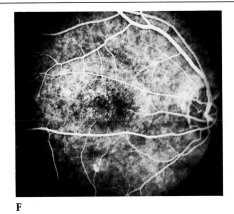

F

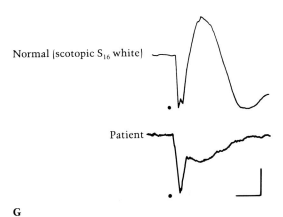

Normal (scotopic S_{16} white)

Patient

G

Idiopathic Juvenile X-Linked Retinoschisis

Juvenile retinoschisis does not readily fit into one of the neat classifications. Some would place it with the primary hereditary macular dystrophies since the macula is invariably involved. Others, in view of the ERG abnormalities, would consider it a generalized vitreotapetoretinal dystrophy along with Goldmann-Favre and Wagner's syndromes.

In this X-linked recessive disorder only males are affected and there is no reliable female carrier sign. The macula is said to be affected in 100 percent of cases with a retinoschisis of that portion of the retina [14]. The superficial retinal layer is elevated and thin and shows folds that radiate from the center of the fovea in a spoke-wheel fashion (Fig. 17-13A). While this appearance is encountered in other rare diseases [48, 54], foveal retinoschisis is virtually pathognomonic for juvenile X-linked retinoschisis.

In approximately half the cases the fovea will show the only fundus abnormality. Other patients will show peripheral changes including retinoschisis (most often in the inferotemporal quadrant), perivascular sheathing, white dendritic figures, veils in the vitreous (with or without attached retinal vessels), and pigmentary atrophy and migration (Fig. 17-13C and D).

Interestingly, whether or not the periphery is involved, the scotopic ERG is invariably abnormal, showing a deep a wave and a b wave that does not return to the baseline (electronegative response) (Fig. 17-13G). This ERG finding places the anatomic abnormality in the bipolar cell region. However, histopathologic studies demonstrate a splitting superficially in the nerve fiber layer and not in the midretinal layers, as is seen in senile retinoschisis [72].

Visual symptoms are due to the macular lesion

or to vitreous hemorrhage secondary to traction from the peripheral retinoschisis on a retinal blood vessel. When the macular retinoschisis flattens, it may be difficult to distinguish the nonspecific pigmentary changes from those in the other macular dystrophies (Fig. 17-13E). The X-linked mode of inheritance, peripheral retinoschisis (if present), and, most important, the electronegative ERG are methods of establishing the diagnosis.

GOLDMANN-FAVRE SYNDROME

Like the preceding disorder, Goldmann-Favre syndrome is classified as one of the vitreotapetoretinal dystrophies. While there are certainly some differences among this group, they do share a number of characteristics including vitreous degeneration (optically empty vitreous; fibrillar strands, veils, and sheets), retinoschisis (peripheral and central), pigmentary abnormalities, and an abnormal ERG (electronegative, moderately to markedly reduced, absent).

The cystic macular elevation that occurs in this recessive disease is coarser than the delicate radial folds of juvenile retinoschisis. The ERG resembles that in the generalized retinal dystrophies with the a and b waves markedly reduced or absent.

MACULAR ABNORMALITIES WITH SYSTEMIC DISEASES

There are a number of inherited systemic diseases that have as part of their syndrome an associated retinal dystrophy. In some of these the prominent retinal finding will be exhibited as macular abnormalities.

These syndromes are rarely confused with a primary macular dystrophy since it is unusual for the presenting symptom to be related solely to the eye. The more common of these diseases include Laurence-Moon and Bardet-Biedl syndromes, the ceroid lipofuscinoses, albinism and its various syndromes, angioid streaks associated with various diseases (pseudoxanthoma elasticum, Ehlers-Danlos syndrome, Paget's myotonic dystrophy), abetalipoproteinemia, and the mucopolysaccharidoses. In addition, several metabolic storage disorders may show a characteristic macular cherry-red spot.

A more detailed discussion of these diseases may be found in Chapters 2 and 5 and elsewhere [17].

REFERENCES

1. Ashton, N., and Sorsby, A. Fundus dystrophy with unusual features: A histological study. *Br. J. Ophthalmol.* 35:751, 1951.
2. Ashton, N. Central areolar choroidal sclerosis: A histopathological study. *Br. J. Ophthalmol.* 37:140, 1953.
3. Barkman, Y. A clinical study of a central tapetoretinal degeneration. *Acta Ophthalmol. (Copenh.)* 39:663, 1961.
4. Berson, E. L., Gouras, P., and Gunkel, R. D. Progressive cone degeneration, dominantly inherited. *Arch. Ophthalmol.* 80:77, 1968.
5. Birndorf, L. A., and Dawson, N. W. A normal electrooculogram in a patient with a typical vitelliform macular lesion. *Invest. Ophthalmol.* 12:830, 1973.
6. Bonnin, P., Passot, M., and Trilaire, M. T. Le Signe du Silence Choroidien dans les Dégénérescences tapeto-rétiennes posterieures. *Doc. Ophthalmol.* 9:461, 1976.
7. Carr, R. E., Noble, K. G., and Nasaduke, I. Hereditary hemorrhagic macular dystrophy. *Am. J. Ophthalmol.* 85:318, 1978.
8. Cibis, G. N., Morey, M., and Harris, D. J. Dominantly inherited macular dystrophy with flecks (Stargardt). *Arch. Ophthalmol.* 98:1785, 1980.
9. Cross, H. E., and Bard, L. Electro-oculography in Best's macular dystrophy. *Am. J. Ophthalmol.* 77:46, 1974.
10. Deutman, A. F. Electro-oculography in families with vitelliform dystrophy of the fovea: Detection of the carrier state. *Arch. Ophthalmol.* 81:305, 1969.
11. Deutman, A. F., et al. Butterfly-shaped pigment dystrophy of the fovea. *Arch. Ophthalmol.* 83:558, 1970.
12. Deutman, A. F., and Jansen, M. A. Dominantly inherited drusen of Bruch's membrane. *Br. J. Ophthalmol.* 54:373, 1970.
13. Deutman, A. F. *The Hereditary Dystrophies of the Posterior Pole of the Eye.* Assen, Netherlands: 1971. P. 210 (citing a personal communication of A. E. Braley, 1968).
14. Deutman, A. F. Macular Dystrophies. In M. F. Goldberg (Ed.), *Genetic and Metabolic Eye Disease* (1st ed.). Boston: Little, Brown and Co., 1974.
15. Deutman, A. F. Benign concentric annular macular dystrophy. *Am. J. Ophthalmol.* 78:384, 1974.
16. Deutman, A. F., Pinckers, A. J. L. G., and aan de Kerk, A. L. Dominantly inherited cystoid macular edema. *Am. J. Ophthalmol.* 82:540, 1976.
17. Deutman, A. F. Hereditary Diseases and Syndromes with Retinal, Choroidal, or Optic Nerve Abnormalities. In *Krill's Hereditary Retinal and Choroidal Diseases.* Hagerstown, Md.: Harper & Row, 1977. P. 1299.
18. Duke-Elder, S., and Perkins, E. S. *System of Ophthalmology, Vol. 9: Diseases of the Uveal Tract.* St. Louis: Mosby, 1966. P. 715.
19. Duke-Elder, S. *System of Ophthalmology, Vol. 10: Diseases of the Retina.* St. Louis: Mosby, 1967. P. 591.

20. Eagle, R. C., et al. Retinal pigment epithelial abnormalities in fundus flavimaculatus. *Ophthalmology (Rochester)* 87:1189, 1980.

21. Epstein, G. A., and Raab, M. F. Adult vitelliform macular degeneration: Diagnosis and natural history. *Br. J. Ophthalmol.* 64:733, 1980.

22. Farkas, T. G., Krill, A. E., and Sylvester, V. M. Familial and secondary drusen: Histologic and functional correlations. *Trans. Am. Acad. Ophthalmol. Otolaryngol.* 75:33, 1971.

23. Fetkenhour, C. L., et al. Central areolar pigment epithelial dystrophy. *Am. J. Ophthalmol.* 81:745, 1976.

24. Fish, G., et al. The dark choroid in posterior retinal dystrophies. *Br. J. Ophthalmol.* 65:359, 1981.

25. Fishman, G. A. Fundus flavimaculatus: A clinical classification. *Arch. Ophthalmol.* 94:2061, 1976.

26. Fishman, G. A., Fishman, M., and Maggiano, J. Macular lesions associated with retinitis pigmentosa. *Arch. Ophthalmol.* 95:798, 1977.

27. Fishman, G. A., Maggiano, J. M., and Fishman, M. Foveal lesions seen in retinitis pigmentosa. *Arch. Ophthalmol.* 95:1993, 1977.

28. Fishman, G. A., et al. Reticular tapeto-retinal dystrophy: As a possible late stage of Sjögren's reticular dystrophy. *Br. J. Ophthalmol.* 60:35, 1976.

29. Fishman, G. A., et al. Pseudovitelliform macular degeneration. *Arch. Ophthalmol.* 95:73, 1977.

30. Franceschetti, A. Über tapeto-retinale Degenerationen im Kindesalter. In *Entwidklung und Fortschritt in der Augenheilkunde.* Stuttgart: Ferdinand Enke, 1963.

31. Franceschetti, A., and François, J. Fundus flavimaculatus. *Arch. Ophthalmol.* 25:505, 1965.

32. Franceschetti, A., François, J., and Babel, J. *Chorioretinal Heredodegenerations.* Springfield, Ill.: Thomas, 1974. P. 275.

33. François, J., DeRouck, A. and Ferandez-Sasso, D. Electro-oculography in vitelliform degeneration of the macula. *Arch. Ophthalmol.* 77:726, 1967.

34. Frangieh, G. T., Green, W. R., and Fine, S. L. A histopathologic study of Best's macular dystrophy. *Arch. Ophthalmol.* 100:1115, 1982.

35. Frank, H. R., et al. A new dominant progressive foveal dystrophy. *Am. J. Ophthalmol.* 78:903, 1974.

36. Gass, J. D. M. Drusen and disciform macular detachment and degeneration. *Arch. Ophthalmol.* 90:206, 1973.

37. Gass, J. D. M. A clinicopathologic study of a peculiar foveomacular dystrophy. *Trans. Am. Ophthalmol. Soc.* 72:139, 1974.

38. Gass, J. D. M. *Stereoscopic Atlas of Macular Diseases: Diagnosis and Treatment* (2nd ed.). St. Louis: Mosby, 1977. P. 170.

39. Goodman, G., Ripps, H., and Siegel, I. M. Progressive Cone Degeneration. In *Clinical Electroretinography: Proceedings of the 3rd International Symposium, 1964.* Oxford, England: Pergamon, 1966. P. 363.

40. Hadden, O. B., and Gass, J. D. M. Fundus flavimaculatus and Stargardt's disease. *Am. J. Ophthalmol.* 82:527, 1976.

41. Hoskin, A., Sehmi, K., and Bird, A. R. Sorsby's pseudoinflammatory macular dystrophy. *Br. J. Ophthalmol.* 65:859, 1981.

42. Hsieh, R. C., Fine, B. S., and Lyons, J. S. Patterned dystrophies of the retinal pigment epithelium. *Arch. Ophthalmol.* 95:429, 1977.

43. Kingham, J. D., and Lochen, G. P. Vitelliform macular degeneration. *Am. J. Ophthalmol.* 84:526, 1977.

44. Kingham, J. D., et al. Reticular dystrophy of the retinal pigment epithelium. *Arch. Ophthalmol.* 96:1177, 1978.

45. Klein, B. A., and Krill, A. E. Fundus flavimaculatus: Clinical, functional and histopathologic observations. *Am. J. Ophthalmol.* 864:3, 1967.

46. Klein, R., et al. Subretinal neovascularization associated with fundus flavimaculatus. *Arch. Ophthalmol.* 96:2054, 1978.

47. Lefler, W. H., Wadsworth, J. A. C., and Sidbury, J. B. Hereditary macular degeneration and aminoaciduria. *Am. J. Ophthalmol.* 71:224, 1971.

48. Lewis, R. A., et al. Familial foveal retinoschisis. *Arch. Ophthalmol.* 95:1190, 1977.

49. Marmor, M. F., and Byers, B. Pattern dystrophy of the pigment epithelium. *Am. J. Ophthalmol.* 84:32, 1977.

50. Mesker, R. P., Oosterhuis, J. A., and Delleman, J. W. A Retinal Lesion Resembling Sjögren's Dystrophia Reticularis Laminae Pigmentosae Retinae. In J. E. Winkelman and R. A. Crone (Eds.), *Perspectives in Ophthalmology.* Amsterdam: Excerpta Medica, 1970. Vol. 2, p. 40.

51. Noble, K. G., Carr, R. E., and Siegel, I. M. Fluorescein angiography of the hereditary choroidal dystrophies. *Br. J. Ophthalmol.* 61:43, 1977.

52. Noble, K. G. Central areolar choroidal dystrophy. *Am. J. Ophthalmol.* 84:310, 1977.

53. Noble, K. G., and Carr, R. E. Leber's congenital amaurosis: A retrospective study of 33 cases and a histopathological study of one case. *Arch. Ophthalmol.* 96:818, 1978.

54. Noble, K. G., Carr, R. E., and Siegel, I. M. Familial foveal retinoschisis associated with a rod-cone dystrophy. *Am. J. Ophthalmol.* 85:551, 1978.

55. Noble, K. G., Scher, B. M., and Carr, R. E. Polymorphous presentations in vitelliform macular dystrophy: Subretinal neovascularization and central choroidal atrophy. *Br. J. Ophthalmol.* 62:561, 1978.

56. Noble, K. G., and Carr, R. E. Stargardt's disease and fundus flavimaculatus. *Arch. Ophthalmol.* 97:1281, 1979.

57. O'Donnell, F. E., et al. Autosomal dominant dystrophy of the retinal pigment epithelium. *Arch. Ophthalmol.* 97:680, 1979.

58. O'Donnell, F. E., and Welch, R. B. Fenestrated sheen macular dystrophy. *Arch. Ophthalmol.* 97:1292, 1979.

59. Pinckers, A. J. L. C., Deutman, A. F., and Notting, J. G. A. Retinal functions in dominant cystoid macular dystrophy. *Acta Ophthalmol. (Copenh.)* 54:579, 1976.

60. Sandvig, K. Familial central areolar choroidal atrophy of autosomal dominant inheritance. *Acta Ophthalmol. (Copenh.)* 33:71, 1955.

61. Singerman, L. J., Berkow, J. W., and Patz, A. Dominant slowly progressive macular dystrophy. *Am. J. Ophthalmol.* 83:680, 1977.

62. Sjögren, H. Dystrophia reticularis laminae pigmentosae retinae. *Acta Ophthalmol. (Copenh.)* 28:279, 1950.

63. Snyder, D. A., et al. Vitelliform lesions associated with retinal pigment epithelial detachments. *Ann. Ophthalmol.* 10:1711, 1978.

64. Sorsby, A. Choroidal angio-sclerosis with special reference to its hereditary character. *Br. J. Ophthalmol.* 23:433, 1939.

65. Sorsby, A., Joll-Mason, M. E., and Gardener, N. A fundus dystrophy with unusual features. *Br. J. Ophthalmol.* 33:67, 1949.

66. Sorsby, A., and Crick, R. P. Central areolar choroidal sclerosis. *Br. J. Ophthalmol.* 37:129, 1953.

67. Stargardt, K. Über familiare progressive Degeneration in der Makulagegend des Auges. *Albrecht von Graefes Arch. Klin. Ophthalmol.* 71:534, 1909.

68. Thorburn, W., and Nordstrom, S. EOG in a large family with hereditary macular degeneration. *Acta Ophthalmol. (Copenh.)* 56:455, 1978.

69. Vine, A. K., and Schatz, H. Adult-onset foveomacular pigment epithelial dystrophy. *Am. J. Ophthalmol.* 89:680, 1980.

70. Weingeist, T. A., Kobrin, J. L., and Watzke, R. C. Histopathology of Best's macular dystrophy. *Arch. Ophthalmol.* 100:1108, 1982.

71. Wiznia, R. A., Perina, B., and Noble, K. G. Vitelliform macular dystrophy of late onset. *Br. J. Ophthalmol.* 65:866, 1981.

72. Yanoff, M., Rahn, E. K., and Zimmerman, L. E. Histopathology of juvenile retinoschisis. *Arch. Ophthalmol.* 79:49, 1968.

18

Heredofamilial Disorders of the Optic Nerve

Joel S. Glaser

DEVELOPMENTAL ANOMALIES

The number of genetically determined developmental malformations of the eye, with and without associated major and minor defects of other organ systems, is legion. The majority of such embryologic dysplasias are linked to autosomal aberrations including trisomy, translocation, and deletion (see Chap. 8). The discussion here, however, will be limited to those anomalies of the optic nerve that reflect genetic patterns conforming mostly to concepts of mendelian heredity.

Isolated Defects of the Optic Disc

Waardenburg and associates have commented that the polymorphic appearance of the optic disc is so great and varied that it is difficult to assess the precise role of heredity [129]. Bonamour and coauthors of the admirable *La Papille Optique* devote less than three pages in five hundred to the question of heredity of disc malformations [11]. In a subsequent essay Bonamour again alludes to the unknown role of heredity in variations of the arterial pattern on the nerve head, with the possible exception of arterial trifurcations, which he observed in three members of a family [10]. The incidence of retinal vessel trifurcation is not known. However, this finding is not infrequently encountered with various congenital anomalies of the optic nerve head (Fig. 18-1). In fact, in monozygotic twins vessel patterns may show marked differences [128]. Collier reported a family with the following findings: maternal grandmother with congenital dilated superior retinal veins in one eye; mother with a flat venous loop of one disc; daughter with epipapillary membrane in one eye

and mild microphthalmos of the other; and three other daughters with "blurred disc margins," two of whom had cilioretinal arteries [21].

Armaly in 1967 concluded that the cup-disc ratio of the optic nerve head is genetically determined and that an individual's cup size varies directly with those of the parents and siblings [3]. Armaly suggested that the mode of inheritance is polygenic and multifactorial. Bengtsson also has concluded that disc diameter and cup diameter resemblance among first-degree relatives (father-son, mother-daughter, father-daughter, mother-son, brother-brother, and sister-sister pairs) is highly significant [7]. Since absence of excavation is a factor contributing to the ophthalmoscopic picture of pseudoneuritis and pseudopapilledema (Fig. 18-2), examination of family members is helpful when this diagnostic dilemma presents itself. Witusik provides the following figures in regard to disc excavation: without physiologic excavation, 21 percent; with excavation, 79 percent [143].

ANOMALIES OF SIZE AND SHAPE

Considerable variation in disc size exists, influenced at least partially by refractive error. In 1950 Franceschetti and Bock measured disc diameters in 100 normal eyes, taking into account refractive error, and found an ideal gaussian curve between 1.23 and 1.99 mm (averages of vertical and horizontal diameters) [36]. In their patient with "megalopapilla," disc diameters measured 2.11 and 2.45 mm, statistically well beyond the normal distribution curve, and the father of that patient also had an asymmetric large disc. Megalopapilla must be considered exceedingly rare [119], and insuf-

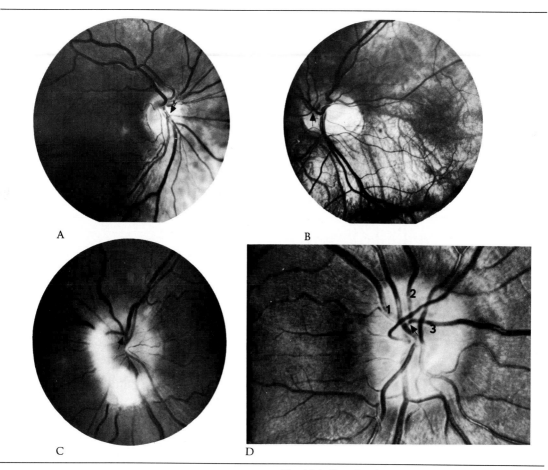

Fig. 18-1. *Vessel trifurcations associated with congenital anomalies of the optic disc. A, B. Arterial trifurcations (arrows) occurring with inferior crescents of the nerve head. C. Venous trifurcation (arrow) on anomalously elevated disc with medullated nerve fibers. D. Venous trifurcation (arrow), partially obscured by overlying artery, occurring on anomalously elevated disc.*

ficient data exist for hereditary analysis. Mikuni and co-workers found the following disc diameters in Japanese cadaver eyes, corrected for shrinkage: males 1.66 × 1.84 mm; females 1.5 × 1.74 mm [91]. However, Abe, using photographic techniques, calculated mean horizontal diameters of 1.74 mm in males and 1.76 mm in females [1]. Abe also provided a figure for heritability of disc size, namely, 0.92.

While colobomatous malformations of the optic nerve often occur in association with uveal colobomas, the disc defect may be isolated. Most colobomas of the optic disc occur either in overt association with choroidal and iris defects or accompany gross ocular dysplasias (microphthalmos) or congenital malformations of the forebrain (sphenoidal encephalocele, arhinencephalia, holoprosencephaly) or cerebral hemispheres (hydranencephaly). Waardenburg and associates suggest that, unlike typical iridochoroidal colobomas, optic colobomas often behave as recessive traits

[130], although Weyert's original family demonstrated dominant inheritance of optic colobomas in three generations [138].

Savell and Cook have reported on 15 members of a family with bilateral optic nerve colobomas characterized by variable amounts of glial tissue within the disc cavities, and macular or extramacular serous detachments in 21 of 30 affected eyes [110]. No skull or endocrine abnormalities were obvious. Disc coloboma may also be observed in Aicardi's syndrome, the essential features of which are infantile spasms, lacunar (geographic) pigmentary chorioretinopathy, scleral ectasia, and agenesis of the corpus callosum. This

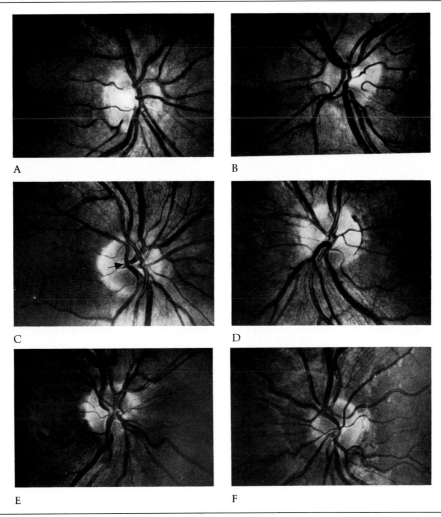

Fig. 18-2. *Optic discs in family consisting of 34-year-old mother (A and B), 12-year-old daughter (C and D), and 14-year-old son (E and F), demonstrating role of heredity in disc appearance. A diagnosis of papilledema had been made in the boy. There is absence of any real central cup in all discs. Note the "engorged" veins (B, D, E, and F) and prominent nerve pattern. A central venous trifurcation is seen in C (arrow), and multiple arterial branching is seen on the discs (especially in C, E, and F).*

syndrome occurs only in female infants, but is not familial, which suggests a sex-mediated embryopathy, possibly infectious [53].

Optic pits, although possibly related to colobomas, have not been reported with familial occurrence [72, 120, 131], except in a father and daughter [4]. Hoffmann described a family of five children with the following optic nerve anomalies: (1) right eye, inferior crescent, left eye, temporal crescent; (2) bilateral inferior crescents; (3) unilateral optic pit; (4) unilateral inferior crescent; (5) right eye, persistent hyaloid artery, left eye, temporal crescent [49].

Hypoplasia of the optic disc may be unilateral or bilateral, marked or minimal, and associated with good or poor visual function; it may occur in isolation or accompany ocular or forebrain malformations. The condition has alternately been termed micropapilla, partial aplasia, and, incorrectly, aplasia. Literature related to optic disc hypoplasia has for years almost exclusively consisted of isolated case reports with only occasional reviews [113, 116]. Walton and Robb [136] and Edwards and Layden [28] have reported an additional 45 cases, with no evidence of heredofamilial tendency. It is interesting that in the Walton-Robb series the patients described enjoyed normal growth and development, while in the Edwards-Layden series about one-third of the patients had major concomitant central nervous system (CNS) anomalies. Ellenberger and Runyan have admirably reviewed optic nerve dysplasia accompanying congenital cerebral anomalies and have recorded a case of optic nerve hypoplasia, dwarfism, and agenesis of the septum pellucidum [29]; this constellation comprises the septo-optic dysplasia syndrome of DeMorsier [25]. Skarf and C. Hoyt have reviewed the incidence of endocrine and CNS anomalies in 93 children with disc hypoplasia and found that 78 percent of cases with bilateral disc smallness, poor vision, and nystagmus had non-ocular developmental abnormalities, including absent septum pellucidum, absent corpus callosum, porencephalic cyst, transethmoidal encephalocele, hypothyroidism, growth hormone insufficiency, diabetes insipidus, neonatal hypoglycemia, and ventriculoseptal defect. There was no instance of familial occurrence [114a].

Sporadic occurrence of bilateral disc hypoplasia has led to the concept of autosomal recessive inheritance. However, since the hypoplasias cannot be considered a homogeneous group, such conclusions regarding hereditary patterns are unfounded. Misseroli reported a sibship of one brother and two sisters, otherwise well developed and with normal eyes, all with bilateral hypoplastic discs and binasal hemianopia [92]. Kytilä and Miettinen examined two blind brothers with hypoplastic discs, normal intellect, and no neurologic deficits [74]. Hackenbruch and colleagues described a third familial instance of bilateral optic nerve hypoplasia affecting five individuals in four generations, which suggests an autosomal dominant trait. None of these patients was subjected to neuroradiologic procedures [47].

While optic nerve hypoplasia not infrequently accompanies a variety of malformations of the globe, the association with aniridia is of special interest. Bonamour and associates presented such

Fig. 18-3. *Hypoplastic optic discs in mother (B) and daughter (A) with familial aniridia. In fundi of mother (B), arrows indicate actual disc margins. (Courtesy of Paul Layman, M.D.)*

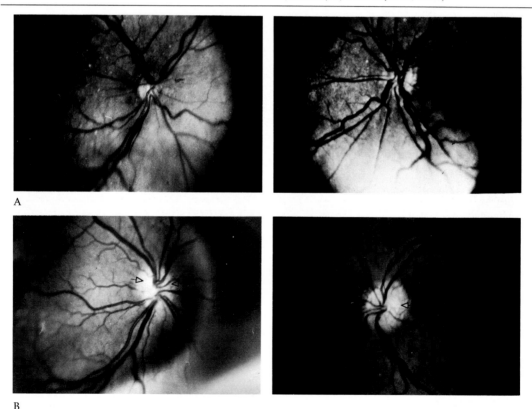

a case [12], as did Collier and Adais [23]. At the Bascom Palmer Eye Institute, Miami, a number of patients with aniridia and disc hypoplasia have been seen, including a mother and daughter with bilateral involvement (Fig. 18-3). Collier has reported a family with hypoplastic discs and mandibulofacial dysostosis [22].

Inferior crescents of the nerve head (see Fig. 18-1A and B) rarely occur in a familial grouping, but Riise is of the opinion that conclusions may not be drawn regarding the mode of inheritance [99]. Fishman and coauthors have recorded familial dextrocardia, divergent strabismus, and situs inversus of the optic disc [33], and Hittner and colleagues have reported tilted discs in association with X-linked recessive congenital stationary night blindness [48]. Anomalous vessel entrance, situs inversus, disc crescents, large cups, and pigment epithelial hypopigmentation have been documented in association with craniofacial syndromes including hypertelorism, Crouzon's disease, and Apert's disease [87]; these craniofacial dysostoses are transmitted as autosomal dominant traits.

ANOMALOUS ELEVATIONS OF THE OPTIC DISC: PSEUDOPAPILLEDEMA, PSEUDONEURITIS, AND HYALINE BODIES

Anomalous elevation of the optic nerve head, with or without ophthalmoscopically detectable hyaline bodies, is a major cause of unnecessary alarm and misdirected diagnostic procedures. Because the funduscopic appearance resembles that of papilledema, patients have been subjected to cerebral arteriography, pneumoencephalography, computerized tomography, and even craniotomy for innocent headaches, vertigo, or more trivial symptoms! The fact that these conditions are not infrequently familial makes examination of family members mandatory when the distinction between true papilledema and pseudopapilledema is in doubt (see Fig. 18-2).

Congenitally elevated discs have been called pseudopapilledema or pseudoneuritis, but the suggestion by Walsh and Hoyt that, when possible, more specific funduscopic characteristics should be described (e.g., intrapapillary drusen, hyperopia, persistent hyaloid tissue) seems reasonable [134]. It is very likely that the majority of cases of anomalous elevation are associated with nerve head drusen, alternately termed colloid or hyaline bodies (rarely, concretions). Not uncommonly, drusen progressively become visible as they enlarge toward the disc surface and margins. The occurrence of overt disc drusen in parents of patients with anomalously elevated discs, but without apparent drusen, attests to both the progressive and the heredofamilial nature of disc drusen. Some family members may be observed to have visible drusen, while others have only elevated discs without ophthalmoscopically distinct drusen.

According to the genetic analysis of Lorentzen, disc drusen are inherited as an autosomal irregular dominant trait [82]. However, in addition, there would appear to be a distinct tendency for occurrence of drusen in fair Caucasians [134]. I am personally aware of the case recorded in a black by Sanders and co-workers [107, case 7], and of the 5 black patients in the series with Rosenberg et al. [103].

From a study of 142 cases (250 eyes) the clinical features of pseudopapilledema may be summarized [103, 111]. Patients were classified into two groups: those with ophthalmoscopically visible hyaline bodies (HB), and those with disc elevation without visible HB. Although one disc may have been more elevated than the other, both with or without apparent HB, there was a tendency toward bilaterality. However, one-third of HB were strictly unilateral (compare with Lorentzen's estimate of 27% unilaterality [82] and Mustonen's of 26% [93]), and 14 percent of all anomalous elevation was unilateral. On only extremely rare occasions do HB account for diminished visual acuity [70, 93, 103]. Although HB were previously thought to be especially common in hyperopia, analysis shows a distribution of refractive errors that parallels that in the general population. Anomalous vascular patterns are common (see Fig. 18-2). Except for the tapetoretinal degenerations and X-linked retinoschisis, there apparently is no statistically significant association of HB with the numerous and diverse ocular and neurologic disorders (including tuberous sclerosis) with which HB have been described [82, 93, 103, 111].

Defects Associated with Ocular and Cerebral Malformations

Hypoplasia and colobomatous malformations of the optic nerve not infrequently accompany gross defects of the eye, including microphthalmos and cystic globe. Similarly, optic nerve dysplasias may be associated with congenital malformations of the forebrain such as the following: arrhinencephalia (DeMyer and associates include an instance of familial alobar holoprosencephaly with optic colobomas [26]), agenesis of the corpus callosum, agenesis of the septum pellucidum [29], and transsphenoidal encephalocele [96]. The majority of such cases occur sporadically, but chromosome analysis may demonstrate aneuploidy or aberration, including deletion and translocation (see Chap. 8). In the absence of arhinencephalia there is no documented instance of genetically determined septo-optic dysplasia [75].

DEGENERATIONS AND ABIOTROPHIES; HEREDITARY OPTIC ATROPHIES

Heredofamilial degeneration or abiotrophy of the optic nerves may occur as a primary event, either as a monosymptomatic lesion or accompanying other nervous system lesions. Optic atrophy may also occur secondarily in heritable neurolipid storage disorders (e.g., Tay-Sachs disease), in which accumulation of abnormal material in retinal ganglion cells results in consecutive atrophy. Retinal dystrophies, including Leber's congenital amaurosis, and tapetoretinal abiotrophies show variable degrees of optic atrophy, but the primary disorder is retinal. In addition, the optic nerves may be compromised in familial cranioskeletal anomalies and the craniosynostoses, such as oxycephaly and Crouzon's disease. (See Cranial Dysplasia, below, and Chap. 9).

Simple or complicated optic atrophy occurs with various patterns of transmission and graded symptoms, such that a vast and heterogeneous literature has accrued. Lodberg and Lund [81] and Kjer [65] point out that preoccupation with Leber's optic atrophy resulted in much confusion in case reports and retarded adequate classification of other forms of hereditary optic atrophy. These authors have provided useful classifications of other patterns of genetically determined optic atrophy. Table 18-1 is an attempt at pragmatic classification and by no means should be considered complete. Texts by François [37] and Waardenburg and coauthors [129] contain numerous genealogical studies and bibliographic material that cannot be duplicated here.

Recessive Optic Atrophies

SIMPLE OPTIC ATROPHY

Optic atrophy of recessive inheritance is a relatively rare entity, noted occasionally in the neonate and therefore termed congenital, but more frequently discovered at some point before the patient is 3 to 4 years of age. Severe visual impairment is the rule, and nystagmus is variably present. The optic disc is quite pale, and attenuation of arteries may suggest a tapetoretinal degeneration. However, electroretinography will distinguish between the two conditions, the electroretinogram (ERG) being normal in optic atrophy. According to François, consanguineous parentage is uncovered in more than half of the cases [37].

COMPLICTED OPTIC ATROPHY (INFANTILE, RECESSIVE; BEHR'S SYNDROME)

In 1909 Behr described six male children in whom optic atrophy was associated with mild mental deficiency, spasticity, hypertonia, and ataxia [6]. Subsequent study by Saleeby indicated no sex predilection, although all of Behr's original patients were boys [106]. The disorder has its onset in childhood (range, 1–9 years) and stabilizes after a variable period of progression. Pallor of the disc tends to be temporal. Nystagmus is present in half of the patients, and strabismus in two-thirds [37]. It is generally thought that Behr's infantile complicated optic atrophy may represent a transitional form between simple hereditary optic atrophy and the hereditary cerebellar ataxias of the Marie type (Fig. 18-4). Autopsy in a case of Behr's syndrome with only moderately atrophic optic nerves revealed extensive degenerative changes in the lateral geniculate bodies, characterized by axonal spheroids consistent with the neuropathologic changes of infantile neuroaxonal dystrophy [51].

RECESSIVE OPTIC ATROPHY AND JUVENILE DIABETES (WOLFRAM SYNDROME)

Rose and colleagues in 1966 reviewed the association of optic atrophy and juvenile diabetes [102], and Rorsman and Söderström in 1967 added a family of four involved siblings [100]. The latter authors discussed the frequency of bilateral nerve deafness and the lesser occurrence of Friedreich's ataxia. According to Thorén, there is a 20 percent incidence of diabetes in Friedreich's ataxia [122]. Bretz and associates call attention to the further association of diabetes insipidus to juvenile diabetes mellitus and optic atrophy [13]. Lessell and Rosman have reviewed the literature on this form of genetically determined optic atrophy and reported their experience with 9 additional cases

Table 18-1 *Heredofamilial Optic Atrophies*

Feature	Dominant	Recessive			Undetermined
	Juvenile (Infantile)	Early Infantile (Congenital); Simple	Behr's Syndrome; Complicated*	With Diabetes Mellitus ± Deafness	Leber's Disease
Age of onset	Childhood (4–8 yr)	Early childhood† (3–4 yr)	Childhood (1–9 yr)	Childhood (6–14 yr)	Early adulthood (18–30 yr; up to sixth decade)
Visual impairment	Mild to moderate (20/40–20/200)	Severe (20/200–HM)	Moderate (20/200)	Severe (20/400–FC)	Moderate to severe (20/200–FC)
Nystagmus	Rare‡	Usual	In 50%	Absent	Absent
Optic disc	Mild temporal pallor ± temporal excavation	Marked diffuse pallor (± arteriolar attenuation)§	Mild temporal pallor	Marked diffuse pallor	Moderate diffuse pallor; disc swelling in acute phase
Color vision	Blue-yellow dyschromatopsia	Severe dyschromatopsia, achromatopsia	Moderate to severe dyschromatopsia	Severe dyschromatopsia	Dense central scotoma for colors
Course	Variable, slight progression	Stable	Stable	Progressive	Acute visual loss, then usually stable; may improve or worsen

*See Optic Atrophy and Heredodegenerative Neurologic Syndromes, in text.
†Difficult to assess in infancy, but visual impairment usually manifest by age 4 years.
‡Presence of nystagmus with poor vision and early onset suggests separate congenital or infantile form.
§Distinguished from tapetoretinal degenerations by normal electroretinogram.
HM = hand motions; FC = finger counting.

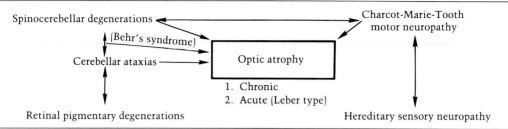

Fig. 18-4. *Continuum of heredodegenerative syndromes associated with optic atrophy. Behr's syndrome may represent a transitional form between simple (monosymptomatic) hereditary optic atrophy and heredoataxias. Acoustic nerve degeneration is another frequent concomitant.*

[79]. A variety of associated manifestations were recorded, including sensorineural hearing loss, ptosis, ataxia, nystagmus, seizures, mental retardation, abnormal ERG, elevated spinal fluid protein and cells, and small stature. It has also been pointed out that optic atrophy may precede diabetes mellitus by several years and that diabetes insipidus may precede optic atrophy [139].

Brief mention should be made of an acquired form of transient ischemic optic neuropathy characterized by florid disc swelling in relatively young juvenile diabetics, with minimal visual disturbance [5].

In essence, autosomal recessive optic atrophy is quite rare, and, in fact, several authors have pointed out that cases previously categorized as autosomal recessive congenital or infantile optic atrophy may indeed be examples of retinal dysplasias.

Dominant Heredofamilial Optic Atrophies

The monograph on dominant optic atrophy by Paul Kjer in 1959 [65] was an important milestone in nosologic analysis of the heritable optic atrophies. Kjer's study defined the clinical features of dominant optic atrophy and provided further evidence for distinction from Leber's disease, with which it had previously been confused. Kjer distinguished two dominant forms, separated primarily by the presence of nystagmus, but Waardenburg and coauthors take exception, commenting that "nystagmus is too unspecific a symptom to be used as a reliable criterion for differential diagnosis" [129]. They mention the possibility of separate genotypes for a form of dominant infantile optic atrophy with severe visual loss, versus that more benign form with mod-

erate visual dysfunction. However, since there is considerable intra- and interfamilial variability as regards vision, this point remains unsettled. Kivlin and co-workers have also commented on the variable expressivity of dominant optic atrophy, and their linkage analysis suggests that the locus for this disorder is on chromosome 2 [64].

Smith has provided an admirable review of dominant optic atrophy and has defined diagnostic criteria and clinical variants [115]. Smith's analysis reveals eight major clinical manifestations: (1) dominant autosomal inheritance, (2) insidious onset between the ages of 4 and 8 years, (3) moderately reduced visual acuity about 20/40–20/200, (4) temporal pallor of optic discs, (5) centrocecal enlargement of the blind spot, (6) full peripheral fields to white targets, (7) inverted peripheral fields to color, and (8) acquired blue-yellow dyschromatopsia.

Kjer noted that many of his patients were ignorant of the familial nature of their disease and that many had noticed no symptoms [65]. These phenomena attest to the insidious onset in childhood, mildly progressive course, and usual mild degree of visual dysfunction. There is some evidence for progression, since patients less than 15 years of age did not show vision below 20/200, while 10 percent of patients 15 to 44 years old and 25 percent of patients 45 years old and older had visual function below 20/200. No patient had vision reduced to hand motion or light perception levels. Kline and Glaser noted that acuity could be strikingly asymmetric in any individual case, for example, 20/30 in one eye and 20/200 in the other, and that pattern-reversal visual-evoked cortical potentials were characterized by diminished amplitude and prolonged latency [67].

Optic disc changes may take the form of temporal pallor (Fig. 18-5) or a peculiar pie-shaped excavation of the temporal sector. Still other discs demonstrate diffuse pallor with sharp margins. Atrophy may be difficult to establish by ophthalmoscopic criteria alone. In fact, the diagnosis of optic atrophy is probably best never made solely

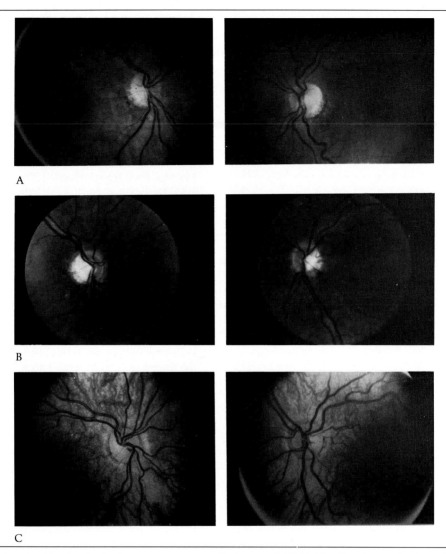

Fig. 18-5. *Dominant optic atrophy in three generations. Disc pallor is primarily confined to the temporal sector. A. Paternal grandmother, aged 60. B. Father, aged 32. C. Daughter (propositus), aged 5. (Courtesy of John T. Flynn, M.D.)*

on fundus appearance. That is, whether or not a disc is pale, *optic atrophy* implies a loss of function (visual acuity, visual field, color perception, sluggish pupil, and so on), which must be demonstrable before such a diagnosis is made.

Regarding visual fields, Kjer states that the characteristic defect is a centrocecal scotoma, which may be quite minimal [65]. Subtle scotomata can enlarge the blind spot vertically and superficially resemble depression of the temporal field. With colored targets especially, a pseudotemporal hemianopic defect may be simulated (Fig.

18-6) [85]. The field for blue may fall within that for red, a phenomenon called *inverted* color fields by both Kjer [65] and Smith [115], simply reflecting preferential diminution of blue perception. The central field defect for colored targets is greater and easier to plot than for white, a finding commonly seen in optic nerve lesions. The peculiar acquired tritanopia of this disorder has been adequately documented [73] and, although at times subtle, should be considered a characteristic and relatively constant finding. Eventually, achromatopsia may ensue. Kline and Glaser reported

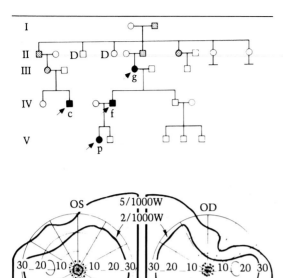

Fig. 18-6. *A. Pedigree of family in Fig. 18-5. Propositus (p) with 20/70–20/100 acuity and tritanopia. Father (f) with 20/40–20/50 acuity and mild unclassified dyschromatopsia. Grandmother (g) with 20/30–20/40 acuity and tritanopia. Cousin (c) with 20/70–20/100 acuity and undetermined color defect. Arrows indicate family members examined. Other family members (stippling) reportedly have poor vision. B. Visual field in patient with dominant optic atrophy. Note indefinite central scotomata with slightly ectopic blind spots owing to poor fixation. There is relative depression of the superior temporal fields, which superficially simulates the bitemporal depression of chiasmal interference. These defects were actually somewhat less distinct than illustrated.*

the results of the Farnsworth-Munsell 100-hue color test in 22 eyes with dominant optic atrophy [67]. In 15 eyes a tritan confusion axis was identified, and in 5 of these a deutan or protan axis was also present. The remaining 7 eyes showed a generalized dyschromatopsia with no discernible confusion axis. Moreover, there was no correlation between the severity of the dyschromatopsia and the level of visual acuity.

Regarding nystagmus, interestingly, none of Kjer's patients was unequivocally demonstrated to have the combination of optic atrophy and nystagmus [65]. Therefore the presence of nystagmus with early severe visual loss may constitute either

a separate nosologic type of congenital dominant optic atrophy or may represent the extreme degree of a single genetic disorder with great symptomatic variability. According to Smith, few patients with "congenital" optic atrophy have been observed at birth or shortly thereafter, the age of onset usually being inferred from the history or presence of nystagmus [115]. There is no authoritative consensus on this point. Hoyt has described 4 patients with severe visual loss, pendular nystagmoid eye movements, and neural hearing loss, from among 31 individuals in six pedigrees of dominant optic atrophy [52]. Also, there was 1 case each of mild retardation, ataxia, seizures, and ulnar neuropathy. Kjer included 9 patients with mild "presenile" dementia in his original monograph [65].

Kjer and colleagues had the opportunity to examine the visual system and vestibulocochlear nerves in an 86-year-old man with well-established dominant optic atrophy but without nystagmus or hearing loss [66]. Findings included normal retinal photoreceptors but reduced ganglion cells and thickened internal limiting membrane; decreased myelin sheaths and axon cylinders of the optic nerves, chiasm, and tracts; massive loss of ganglion cells and fibrillar gliosis in the lateral geniculate bodies; normal calcarine cortex; and a decreased number of neurofibrils and myelin sheaths of the vestibulocochlear nerves. Kjer and coauthors concluded that dominant optic atrophy is a primary degeneration of the ganglion cell layer of the retina, with ascending optic atrophy.

Sufficient case material has accrued to indicate that dominant (juvenile-onset) optic atrophy is the most common heredofamilial simple (monosymptomatic) optic atrophy. Visual dysfunction in this disorder is considerably milder than in either Leber's optic neuropathy or recessive optic atrophy. As a rule, progression is minimal and prognosis good. Grützner adds one cautious note: In rare cases relatively rapid deterioration may occur, even after years of stable visual function [46].

There is no known medical relief for this common form of hereditary optic atrophy, but Imachi and Mimura have reported finding round-cell infiltrations of perichiasmal arachnoid, with thickening of connective tissue and hyalinization of capillary walls [59]. The authors stated that, after craniotomies for "perichiasmal arachnoiditis" with "removal of thickened membranes from the chiasm," visual acuity improved in 8 eyes of 6 patients (e.g., from 20/200 and 20/100 to 20/50

OU in 1 case, and from 20/400 OU to 20/100 and 20/200 in another).

Leber's Disease

In 1871 Theodore Leber described a nosologically distinct hereditary form of optic neuropathy that now bears his name [76]. This entity is characterized by sudden loss of central vision occurring in the second and third decades of life and nondirect transmission with male preponderance. Subsequently, other heredofamilial optic atrophies have emerged as distinct clinical entities, but only after a confusing period in which the literature was preoccupied with "Leber's disease."

Although the disorder has been classically considered X-linked recessive, pedigrees of indisputable Leber's disease do not conform to rigid mendelian rules. For example, there is absence of transmission through males, and passage occurs from the female to most of her offspring. According to van Senus [126] and Wallace [132], the pattern of female-line inheritance argues strongly in favor of vertical transmission of an infective agent. Transmitted maternal mitochondrial DNA may be defective. Leber's disease complicated by neurologic disorders suggests the possibility of a slow virus mechanism (as in the kindred with encephalitis reported by Wallace [133]), in which the expression of disease may be dependent on genetically determined resistance.

The hereditary pattern of Leber's disease may be summarized as follows:

1. Males are predominantly affected (males and females are equally affected in Japan).
2. There is no transmission in the male line; that is, an affected male does not transmit to his issue, unlike transmission in X-linked disorders, in which an affected male transmits through his daughters (see Lundsgaard [83], Waardenburg et al. [129], and Seedorff [114]).
3. The heterozygous female can transmit the trait to sons and the carrier state to daughters.
4. There is no genotypic difference between a female carrier and a manifestly affected woman.
5. According to Lundsgaard, 50 percent of sons and about 10 percent (expected, 50%) of daughters are manifestly affected [83].
6. According to Seedorff, all women born in pedigrees with only females affected are carriers; that is, the carrier rate is 100 percent [114].

Combined data indicate an age of onset usually in the second or third decade, typically in the late teens to midtwenties, with a range from 5 to 65 years of age. Lundsgaard feels that there are insufficient data to support a different age-of-onset incidence in females, but she points out the remarkably constant age of onset for members of the same sibship [83]. The interval between onset in one eye and onset in the other is difficult to assess because of patient subjectivity, but some interval of days to weeks would appear to be the rule. Entirely unilateral cases are distinctly rare and, at the time of Lundsgaard's review, had been found only in females.

Loss of central visual function progresses rapidly to levels of 20/200 or finger counting, although more benign and more severe loss is not infrequent. Although relative stability of visual function is anticipated after initial loss, gradual decline or sudden improvement after years of stationary vision has been reported [83]. Such spontaneous variation after stationary intervals makes objective studies of treatment difficult, and ultimate visual outcome cannot be forecast with certainty. The family described by Brunette and Bernier, in which there was spontaneous recovery to normal vision in 6 of 51 affected members, is of great interest [14, 15]. Four other members recovered vision of 20/50 in at least one eye. Lessell et al. [78] have suggested that spontaneous recovery in Leber's disease may be related to absence of the usual microvascular anomalies observed around the nerve head. Certainly, this high recovery rate must be kept in mind in evaluating suggested forms of therapy, including neurosurgical intervention, which will be discussed below.

During the acute neuritic phase (Fig. 18-7) the fundus findings are characterized by a somewhat small, usually cupless disc elevated slightly above the retinal plane. The nerve fiber layer appears thick and swollen, especially on the disc and in the arcuate temporal nerve fiber bundles, but fluorescein angiography shows no leakage or staining. Large vessels are tortuous, and smaller circumpapillary capillaries appear telangiectatic; hemorrhages are extremely rare. Of great interest is the observation that asymptomatic family members in the female line may have premorbid peripapillary telangiectatic microangiopathy, very much resembling the fundus findings during visual loss of the acute neuritic phase [94]. Three asymptomatic boys with such angiopathy subsequently developed classic symptomatic Leber's disease.

Carroll and Mastaglia have demonstrated mildly

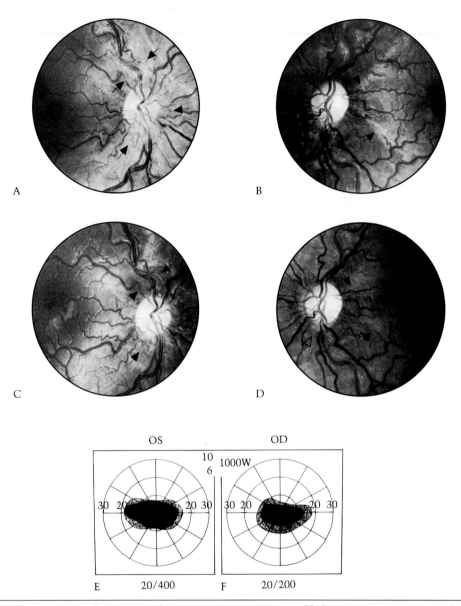

Fig. 18-7. *Leber's optic atrophy. A–D. In the acute stage the disc appears hyperemic, the nerve fiber layer is swollen and opacified (compare arrows in A and C), and the retinal internal limiting membrane appears wrinkled (compare arrows in B and D). As swelling of the disc and retina recedes, a flat, pale disc remains. E. Visual fields show dense central scotomata including the blind spots.*

impaired color vision in asymptomatic (presymptomatic?) family members, even in the male line [16]. Also, Livingstone and colleagues found Farnsworth-Munsell 100-hue color vision anomalies and evoked potential latency delays in asymptomatic family members in the female, but not the male, lineage. In another series of 72 individuals at risk

and 14 proven carriers, it was concluded that numerous presymptomatic signs of Leber's disease were present, including tortuosity of peripapillary capillaries, hyperemia and indistinct disc borders, relative central and paracentral scotomata, abnormal evoked potentials, and increased error scores on Farnsworth-Munsell 100-hue color testing [117]. The genetic or therapeutic significance of these findings is yet to be fully appreciated.

Headaches may accompany the onset of visual loss and are construed as meningeal signs by advocates of an arachnoidal causation. Atrophy ensues, often progressing slowly over many months, leaving a flat pale disc. The visual fields show large, dense central scotomata at the fixational area. Lundsgaard discussed pericentral annular scotomata with relative sparing of function in the central fenestration and suggested that this form of defect is relatively frequent and prognostically favorable [83].

Although the hereditary nature and cause of Leber's disease remain obscure, therapeutic measures have been suggested. Wilson and colleagues feel that failure to detoxify cyanide may be the basic heritable defect in Leber's disease [140–142] and suggest the therapeutic use of hydroxocobalamin [35]. This theory of cyanide toxicity in Leber's disease, as well as in tobacco and nutritional amblyopias, is very much unconfirmed, despite enthusiastic advocates. David Knox (personal communication) has seen a patient with Leber's disease in whom optic neuritis developed in the second eye while the patient was taking large doses of hydroxocobalamin for visual loss in the first eye, and Nikoskelainen and co-workers unsuccessfully treated two affected brothers in the early stages of the disease, employing both hydroxocobalamin and prednisone [95].

Imachi and associates [57, 58] and others have advocated craniotomy with lysis of opticochiasmal arachnoidal adhesions. The success rate reported at Kobe University has not been duplicated elsewhere, but this form of therapy for Leber's disease is rarely attempted outside of Japan. (See discussion above regarding spontaneous recovery above.)

Lees and coauthors [77] and de Weerdt and Went [27] have pointed out the association of typical Leber's disease with signs and symptoms indistinguishable from those of disseminated sclerosis, including involvement of cerebellar and pyramidal systems. It is important to note that the failure to remit and the degree of symmetry serve to distinguish most cases of Leber's disease from the retrobulbar neuritis of multiple sclerosis. The work of de Weerdt and Went suggests the following declining order of incidence of neurologic abnormalities in Leber's disease kindreds: Leber patient, brothers of patient, sisters of patient, individuals in the "female line" [27]. Those authors

concluded that patients with Leber's disease are likely to have minor neurologic abnormalities, as are direct relatives who potentially carry the gene and may be at risk of developing optic atrophy. Schapira and co-workers noted that, in the family of a patient with multiple sclerosis, the chances that multiple sclerosis will develop are three times greater for a female member than for a male member [112]. McLeod and colleagues have documented a family with visual failure typical of Leber's disease, associated with hypertrophic Charcot-Marie-Tooth disease, but they concluded that the two conditions were inherited independently [90] (see Optic Atrophy and Heredodegenerative Neurologic Syndromes, below). Rose and associates cite the occurrence of electrocardiographic abnormalities in 2 patients with Leber's optic atrophy but properly draw no firm conclusions other than to point out the association of cardiac disorders with other heredofamilial neurologic diseases [101].

Dominant Pseudoglaucoma

In 1961 Sandvig reported three Norwegian families with a peculiar hereditary abnormality characterized by deeply excavated optic discs and slowly progressive glaucomatous visual field defects, but with normal intraocular pressure and outflow facility [108]. In this condition visual symptoms start when patients are 20 to 35 years of age and progress to severe depression of visual function. Unlike some patients with early dominant optic atrophy, these patients do not have nystagmus. Although dominant juvenile atrophy may show isolated temporal excavation, patients with that condition do not have marked visual deficits or glaucoma-type field defects. Wium also had previously called attention to this rare form of familial optic atrophy, recording details of 5 cases in a single family [144].

Optic Atrophy and Heredodegenerative Neurologic Syndromes

There is considerable overlapping of syndromes variously combining progressive degeneration of cerebellar and pyramidal systems, deafness, and optic atrophy. To add to the nosologic confusion, familial progressive polyneuropathies of the Charcot-Marie-Tooth type have occasionally been associated with optic atrophy [54], and their association with spinocerebellar degenerations is well established [44]. Visual evoked occipital potentials have shown abnormalities in a number of

Table 18-2. Syndromes with Hereditary Association of Optic Atrophy and Deafness

Syndrome	Inheritance	Vision	Hearing	Associated Findings
Progressive optic atrophy and congenital sensorineural deafness	Autosomal dominant	Progressive optic atrophy with visual loss in middle to late life	Congenital severe sensorineural deafness	None
Optic atrophy with diabetes mellitus and sensorineural hearing loss	Autosomal recessive	Progressive visual loss; bilateral optic atrophy before age 16 yr	Onset in childhood; progressive hearing loss	Diabetes mellitus with onset in the first or second decade
Optic atrophy, ataxia, and progressive hearing loss (Sylvester's syndrome)	Autosomal dominant	Progressive visual loss secondary to optic atrophy onset 2½–9 yr of age	Moderate to severe progressive sensorineural deafness	Ataxia particularly involving the legs, weakness and muscle wasting particularly involving the shoulder girdle and hands
Opticocochleodentate degeneration	Autosomal recessive	Optic atrophy with onset of visual loss in infancy	Progressive hearing loss resulting in severe deafness	Onset in infancy of progressive spastic quadriplegia, progressive mental deterioration, and death in childhood
Optic atrophy, polyneuropathy, and sensorineural deafness (Rosenberg-Chutorran syndrome)	X-chromosome linked or autosomal recessive	Visual loss with optic atrophy beginning at age 20 yr	Progressive sensorineural hearing loss with deafness by age 6 yr	Progressive peripheral polyneuropathy beginning in early childhood

Source: From C. R. Kollarits et al. [71].

genetic neurologic disorders, including hereditary spastic paraplegia, Friedreich's ataxia, and olivopontocerebellar atrophy [9]. This frequent intermingling of spinocerebellar degenerations, heredoataxias, motor and sensory neuropathies, deafness, and optic atrophy strongly suggests a complex genetic continuum in which discrete distinctions are not possible (see Fig. 18-4). Transmission may be dominant, as in Charcot-Marie-Tooth polyneuropathy and some cases of Friedreich's ataxia, or recessive, as in Behr's syndrome and the majority of cases of Marie's disease, or may not conform to strict mendelian rules.

A detailed discussion of these syndrome variations is beyond the scope of the present work. As previously noted, optic atrophy associated with neurologic signs may take the form of an acute optic neuritis, at least superficially resembling Leber's disease, or may occur as a recessive optic atrophy in childhood, associated with ataxia (Behr's syndrome). Weiner and coauthors [137] and, earlier, Jampel and colleagues [60] have reviewed other ocular findings associated with cerebellar ataxia, including ophthalmoplegia and retinal pigmentary degenerations with optic atrophy. Gillespie [39] and Sarsfield [109] have reported cases of cerebellar ataxia associated with aniridia. It is of great interest that the optic discs in these patients were described as small and round and undoubtedly were hypoplastic. (See Anomalies of Size and Shape, above). Rosenberg and Chutorian discuss (and provide a bibliography related to) the concurrence of optic atrophy and heredodegenerative neurologic syndromes [104].

With reference to the special association of sensorineural hearing loss and optic atrophy, Kollarits and associates have provided a useful summary (Table 18-2) [71].

HERITABLE NEOPLASMS AND HAMARTOMAS: NEUROCUTANEOUS SYNDROMES

Several of the heredofamilial neurocutaneous disorders grouped as phakomatoses may involve the optic nerve and anterior visual pathways, but only neurofibromatosis and tuberous sclerosis do so with any consistency. A detailed discussion of the phakomatoses is beyond the scope of this chapter; the reader is referred to the well-illustrated review by Gass [38], the very complete section in the text of Walsh and Hoyt [135], and Chapter 19.

Tuberous sclerosis often shows the stigmata of retinal astrocytic hamartomas in epipapillary and parapapillary locations as well as in the retinal periphery (Fig. 18-8). These characteristic lesions appear as elevated semitransparent domes in the nerve fiber layer of the retina and may undergo calcification as the patient ages. The calcified hamartomas, when on or near the optic disc, have been termed giant drusen but should not be confused with common drusen (hyaline bodies) within the substance of the nerve head, nonhamartomatous lesions that are not characterized by astrocytic hyperplasia. There is little evidence [50, 82] to support Reese's suggestion [98] that hyaline bodies of the optic disc are minor manifestations of tuberous sclerosis. The retinal hamartomas of tuberous sclerosis are rarely symptomatic but are of great help in establishing the diagnosis.

Gliomas of the optic nerves and chiasm are distinctly associated with neurofibromatosis, the patients either having other characteristic stigmata or having affected relatives (Fig. 18-9). The frequency of this association cannot be established with accuracy, and, as pointed out by Davis, it is far more common than generally recognized [24]. A review by Hoyt and Baghdassarian includes 36 cases of anterior visual pathway gliomas, of which 21 were associated with neurofibromatosis; in one family, two siblings had optic gliomas, and in a second family, a mother and child had gliomas [55]. Manshot has described a kindred with optic glioma and neurofibromatosis in two children and stigmata of neurofibromatosis in their mother and a third sibling [86], and Cartwright has described monozygotic twins with identical chiasmal gliomas and neurofibromatosis [17].

Stern and co-workers suggest that the clinical presentation and morphology of optic gliomas differ in patients with and without neurofibromatosis [118]: Gliomas associated with neurofibromatosis tend to be multicentric or occupy a single optic nerve; chiasmal gliomas are less likely to be associated with neurofibromatosis. Of 84 patients with chiasmal glioma, only 6 were considered to have neurofibromatosis, while 21 of 30 patients with a single optic nerve glioma, and 6 of 8 patients with multicentric gliomas, had neurofibromatosis. In another series of 38 patients with optic gliomas, 22 showed stigmata of neurofibromatosis, including 13 of 14 with diffuse thickening of both nerves and chiasm; only 1 of 13 with primarily chiasmal glioma had neurofibromatosis [69]. On the other hand, Rush and associates found a high incidence of chiasmal tumors among their patients with optic glioma and neurofibromatosis [105].

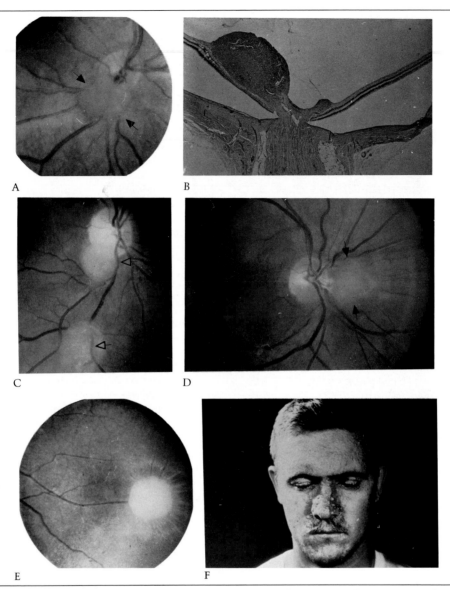

Fig. 18-8. *Retinal astrocytic hamartomas in tuberous sclerosis. Lesion may occur in epipapillary location (A–C), parapapillary location (D), or retinal periphery (E). Note glial hamartoma of nerve fiber layer (B).* *Retinal vessels may be seen passing beneath the hamartoma (C). Note "adenoma sebaceum" (F). (A, B, and F courtesy of Donald Gass, M.D.)*

Considerable controversy exists regarding the natural course, growth potential, and efficacy of therapy in optic gliomas. In 1922 Verhoeff remarked that, since the great majority of optic gliomas become manifest in early childhood, it is highly likely that these tumors "are really congenital in origin and due to some more or less localized abnormality in the embryonic development of the neuroglia of the nerve" [127]. Fur-

thermore, Verhoeff felt that a glioma "does not increase in size by invading or destroying . . . . but by causing preexisting neuroglia in the vicinity of the growth to proliferate."

Hoyt and Baghdassarian in 1969 [55] and Glaser, Hoyt, and Corbett in 1971 [41] stressed the indolent nature of these tumors and the monotonously stable clinical course. In that series of patients, 80 percent of tumors were diagnosed in

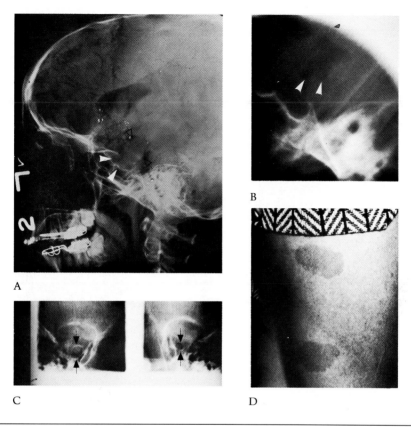

A

B

C

D

Fig. 18-9. *Neurofibromatosis. A. Pneumoencephalogram demonstrates massive enlargement of optic nerves and chiasm (*open arrows*). Note also dysplastic sella turcica with absence of tuberculum and undercutting of anterior clinoids (*white arrowheads*). The posterior clinoid is blunted.*

B. Arrows indicate elevation and blunting of anteroinferior aspect of third ventricle because of suprasellar mass, compatible with chiasmal glioma. C. Regular, enlarged optic foramina with typical sclerotic rims. D. Café au lait spots of neurofibromatosis.

infancy and preschool years. Ocular signs were chronic when first observed. Over long follow-up periods, patients not subjected to radiotherapy fared as well as patients who were irradiated, and the efficacy of irradiation was, therefore, questioned. A review by Wong and Lubow reaffirms these concepts [146]. Other authors attribute stability to the effects of radiotherapy [18, 121, 123, 124]. Accumulation of carefully scrutitnized data will, it is hoped, provide further information on the natural course of optic gliomas and the efficacy of therapy.

Childhood optic gliomas should not be confused with malignant glioblastomas, which are rare tumors of the optic nerves and chiasm that occur in adults [56].

Anderson and Spencer investigated in detail the histopathology of optic glioma and reported that (1) microcystic areas of tumor are neither necrotic nor degenerated, but made up of highly differentiated glial cells; (2) the "microcysts" are extracellular accumulations of mucosubstance that stains with periodic acid–Schiff (PAS), mucosubstance presumably synthesized by tumor cells; (3) the space around axons is distended by mucosubstance, which has a tendency to collect in central areas of the glioma; and (4) the hydrophilic property of mucosubstance may contribute to rapid expansion of the glioma (simulating "growth"), with concurrent loss of visual function or increase in proptosis [2].

Taking into account their occurrence in infancy

and early childhood, their natural course, growth characteristics, histopathologic picture, and association with neurofibromatosis, it is not unreasonable to consider gliomas of the anterior visual pathways as hereditary congenital hamartomas. Indeed, Gass suggests the term *hereditary hamartomatosis* as a more accurate description of the nosologically related entities grouped as phacomatoses [38]. By definition, a hamartoma is a tumor of anomalous origin, composed of elements normally present in the tissue in which it originates, and with a limited capacity for proliferation. The following tumors may be classified as hamartomas: (1) in neurofibromatosis: optic gliomas, neurofibromas, and ganglioneuromas; (2) in tuberous sclerosis: retinal and cerebral astrocytomas, cutaneous angiofibromas ("adenoma sebaceum"), rhabdomyomas, and leiomyomas; (3) in von Hippel-Lindau disease: hemangioblastomas of the cerebellum and retina (including optic nerve head) and renal hypernephromas or cysts; and (4) in Sturge-Weber disease: facial and choroidal cavernous hemangioma and meningeal angiomatous malformations.

Neurofibromatosis, tuberous sclerosis, and von Hippel-Lindau disease are transmitted as irregular dominants with considerable variation in penetrance. No hereditary tendency in Sturge-Weber disease has been recorded.

METABOLIC STORAGE DISEASES

The Neurolipidoses

In recent years biochemical assays have considerably clarified the nosologic status of a group of storage diseases previously classified as the "cerebromacular degenerations," of which Tay-Sachs disease is the eponymous prototype. Although these disorders share a superficial resemblance, showing a progressive neurodegenerative course with variable fundus findings, they are now best classified by abnormal storage products (sphingolipidoses, mucopolysaccharidoses, mucolipidoses) and lysosomal enzyme deficiencies (see Chap. 2).

The optic nerve may be involved via several mechanisms. Optic atrophy results when abnormal glycolipids are stored in retinal ganglion cells, as occurs in Tay-Sachs disease (GM_2 gangliosidosis), with subsequent neuronal death and nerve pallor. However, ophthalmoscopic evidence of optic atrophy is not invariable. Similarly, GM_1 gangliosidosis (generalized gangliosidosis, "Tay-Sachs disease with visceral involvement") also deposits an abnormal ganglioside in the retina, with subsequent atrophy of the nerve [31]; however, an abnormal mucopolysaccharide is deposited in the viscera. Metachromatic leukodystrophy (sulfatide lipidosis) demonstrates an abnormal ceramidegalactose sulfate in retinal ganglion cells and glial cells, and macrophages of the optic nerve [20]. The optic atrophy that occurs with Krabbe's disease (formally considered one of the familial diffuse scleroses) is due to extensive demyelination associated with the accumulation of globoid bodies containing ceramide galactose [19].

In late infantile amaurotic idiocy (Bielschowsky-Jansky disease) ganglioside is deposited in ganglion cells with a decrease in their number, thinning of the nerve fiber layer, and optic atrophy. In addition, there is invovement of the outer segments [145], with degeneration of the rods and cones and pigmentary clumping in the outer retinal layers. Juvenile amaurotic idiocy (Batten-Mayou, Spielmeyer-Vogt) is, briefly, characterized by retinal pigmentary changes predominantly at the macula, with late and minimal pallor of the discs. There is evidence that excessive amounts of lipofuscin are deposited in neurons [147], and therefore the juvenile form of amaurotic idiocy is not technically a lipidosis.

The late form of amaurotic idiocy ascribed to Kufs paradoxically is associated neither with amaurosis nor retardation to the degree of "idiocy." According to van Bogaert, in the true chronic form the ocular fundus is normal [125].

The Mucopolysaccharidoses

Optic nerve involvement may occur in the mucopolysaccharidoses taking the form of optic atrophy or papilledema. While true papilledema doubtless occurs in association with hydrocephalus seen in these disorders [43], there are other instances of "papilledema" in which fundus descriptions or photographs are not convincing. Goldberg and Duke reported the ocular histopathologic findings in a case of Hunter's syndrome (mucopolysaccharidosis II; MPS II), in which examination ante mortem included the observation of "bilateral chronic papilledema" [42]. On microscopic examination, the optic nerve was normal, despite marked retinal pigmentary degeneration, showing neither atrophy nor changes compatible with chronic papilledema. Similarly, Kenyon and associates have reviewed the systemic mucopolysaccharidoses and included an instance (case 2) of a 26-year-old man with Hunter's syndrome (MPS II), whose ophthalmoscopic examination revealed "blurred disc margins in both fundi (without venous congestion, hemorrhages or exudates), compatible with mild chronic papilledema" [62]. No further comment was made in elucidation of this finding, and one wonders if this is not an example of pseudopapilledema owing to congenital anomalous elevation of the optic nerve head.

Mailer reviewed 16 cases of optic atrophy in gargoylism and concluded that communicating hydrocephalus was the most frequent cause [84]. Although hydrocephalus has long been recognized to occur in MPS [88], it is uncovered more frequently at the autopsy table than clinically. Goldberg and colleagues have reported a case of Maroteaux-Lamy syndrome (MPS VI) with hydrocephalus and papilledema, treated with a ventriculojugular shunt [43]. These authors discussed the following possible pathogenetic mechanisms of visual dysfunction caused by optic nerve involvement in MPS: optic atrophy secondary to glaucoma, retinal pigmentary degeneration, or mucopolysaccharide deposition in the retinal elements; infiltration of the nerve substance or meninges; narrowing of the optic canals; and hydrocephalus, with or without papilledema [40].

Kenyon [63] lists the heritable lysosomal disorders that may variably be associated with optic nerve atrophy (see Tables 5-1 and 5-2).

CRANIAL DYSPLASIA

The Craniostenoses

Congenital cranial malformations produced by premature synostoses of sutures are not infrequently associated with optic nerve atrophy. Craniofacial dysostosis (Crouzon's disease) is an autosomal dominant disorder that occasionally occurs sporadically. Acrocephalosyndactyly (Apert's disease) is a less regular dominant (see Chap. 9), and the simple cranial synostoses are infrequently heritable. However, there is a greatly increased incidence of monozygotic twins in the simple craniosynostoses—some 10 times greater than in the normal population. Table 18-3 is modified from the monograph of Bertelsen, in which data from 219 cases were collected [8].

Optic nerve involvement in the craniostenoses may take the form of optic atrophy or papilledema. It should be noted that, according to Bertelsen, patients with oxycephaly and Crouzon's disease show considerably more hypermetropia than do normal subjects (21% above +1.5 D). This leads to an interesting problem, that of distinguishing true chronic papilledema from pseudopapilledema occurring in hyperopia, which has a high incidence among these patients, as do tortuous retinal veins!

Optic atrophy in craniostenosis would appear to be due to one of three mechanisms: narrowed optic canals, chronic increased intracranial pressure with papilledema, or angulation of the optic nerves. Optic nerve involvement is best correlated with the number of fused sutures and their location, with subsequent elevation of cerebrospinal fluid pressure. However, Bertelsen pointed out that papilledema had never been observed in his 33 patients with optic atrophy [8]. There was also a high concurrence rate of optic nerve involvement in oxycephalic patients with exophthalmos.

Fishman and colleagues pointed out that the mechanisms responsible for hydrocephalus in the

Table 18-3. *Optic Nerve Involvement in Hereditary and Nonhereditary Cranial Synostoses*

Disorder (219 cases)	Frequency (%)	Inheritance	Optic Nerve Involvement (%)
Simple cranial synostoses			
Oxycephaly	79.9	—*	36
Scaphocephaly	5.5	—	—
Trigonocephaly	3.7	—	—
Plagiocephaly	1.8	—	—
Craniofacial dysostosis (Crouzon)	6.8	Dominant	80
Acrocephalosyndactyly (Apert)	2.3	Dominant	(1 of 4)

*In the simple craniosynostoses (199 cases), there was a male to female ratio of about 2 : 1.
Source: Modified from T. I. Bertelsen [8].

craniostenoses are not clear and that hydrocephalus appears to be associated with premature synostosis rather than a direct consequence of it [34]. Communicating or noncommunicating hydrocephalus can be present, and ventricular enlargement may progress even after surgical treatment of the cranial defect.

As noted by Bertelsen, chronically elevated intracranial pressure may result in sellar enlargement, but primary dysplastic deepening of the middle fossa may also cause sellar abnormalities without increased pressure [8]. It has been suggested that short anterior fossae result in posterior displacement of the frontal lobes, with subsequent pushing backward of the third ventricle and distortion of the optic nerves [45]. Foreshortening of the anterior fossae would thus result both in exophthalmos and in retropulsion of the chiasm, with subsequent stretching of the optic nerve.

Osteopetrosis

First described by Albers-Schönberg in 1907, osteopetrosis is a rare disorder of bone formation, occurring in two major forms: (1) an autosomal recessive ("malignant") form, resulting in early death from pancytopenia and intercurrent infections; and (2) a relatively benign autosomal dominant form characterized by spontaneous fractures and osteomyelitis.

Ophthalmologic interest arises over the incidence of optic nerve complications, usually attributed to bony sclerosis with narrowing of the optic canal. Ellis and Jackson pointed out the high incidence of optic atrophy in severe involvement and suggested early unroofing of canals to prevent optic atrophy [30]. However, Keith has reported a case with central retina atrophy not associated with narrowing of the optic canals [61]. Keith's review of the literature indicates that many patients had optic pallor with no definite evidence of bony pressure. Klintworth has reviewed other neurologic manifestations, including papilledema, facial palsies, and deafness [68].

Paget's Disease

McKusick considers Paget's disease a heritable abiotrophy of the collagen matrix of bone, transmitted as a simple autosomal dominant gene [89]. Optic atrophy may occur as a result of progressive narrowing of the optic canals, and deafness is also frequent (Fig. 18-10). Exophthalmos, papilledema, angioid streaks, and cranial nerve palsies are also observed.

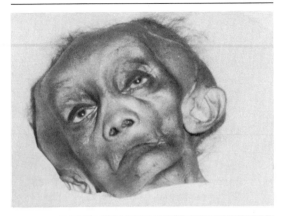

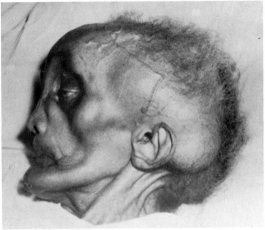

Fig. 18-10. *Severe Paget's disease with complete blindness and deafness. Pupils are dilated and nonreactive to light. The fundi demonstrated profound optic atrophy. Note the position of the ears caused by grotesque dysplasia of temporal bones. It is presumed that deafness is the result of closure of the acoustic canals.*

Eretto and coauthors provide a useful review of the optic neuropathy that variably occurs in Paget's disease [32]. Of 22 patients (18 men, 4 women) with radiographic and clinical evidence of Paget's disease, only 3 cases had visual acuity depression associated with optic atrophy, although 3 others showed optic atrophy with good acuity. Arcuate scotomata were common field defects, but only 2 of 9 patients with visual field defects had pagetic optic canal encroachment. The authors conclude that optic neuropathy in Paget's disease is not always due simply to bony mechanical impingement, and that calcitonin therapy does not reverse optic neuropathy.

Craniometaphyseal Dysplasia

Craniometaphyseal dysplasia is usually inherited as an autosomal dominant disorder characterized by facial abnormalities that may be apparent even in the first year of life, including broad nasal root and hypertelorism. Bone development shows typically marked sclerosis and hyperostosis of the skull, and abnormal modeling of the long bones. New bone formation leads to progressive encroachment on cranial foramina with dysfunction especially of the facial and acoustic nerves. Optic atrophy evolves when the optic canals are narrowed. Puliafito and co-workers have recorded optic atrophy in two of four members of a family with craniometaphyseal dysplasia, with visual acuity ranging from 20/30 to severe impairment [97].

REFERENCES

1. Abe, K. Dimensions de la papille. *Jpn. J. Clin. Ophthalmol.* 19:1227, 1965.
2. Anderson, D. R., and Spencer, W. H. Ultrastructural and histochemical observations of optic nerve gliomas. *Arch. Ophthalmol.* 83:324, 1970.
3. Armaly, M. F. Genetic determination of cup/disc ratio of the optic nerve. *Arch. Ophthalmol.* 78:35, 1967.
4. Babel, J., and Farpour, H. L'origine génétique des fossettes colobomateuses de nerf optique. *J. Genet. Hum.* 16:187, 1967.
5. Barr, C. C., Glaser, J. S., and Blankenship, G. Acute disc swelling in juvenile diabetes: Clinical profile and natural history of 12 cases. *Arch. Ophthalmol.* 98:2185, 1980.
6. Behr, C. Die komplizierte, heredität-familiäl Optikusatrophie des Kindesalters. *Klin. Monatsbl. Augenheilkd.* 47:138, 1909.
7. Bengtsson, B. The inheritance and development of cup and disc diameters. *Acta Ophthalmol. (Copenh.)* 58:733, 1980.
8. Bertelsen, T. I. The premature synostosis of the cranial sutures. *Acta Ophthalmol. [Suppl.] (Copenh.)* 51, 1958.
9. Bird, T. D., and Crill, W. E. Pattern-reversal visual evoked potentials in the hereditary ataxias and spinal degeneration. *Ann. Neurol.* 9:243, 1981.
10. Bonamour, G. Émergénces et divisions anormales de l'artère centrale de la rétine sur la papille. *Ann. Ocul. (Paris)* 203:639, 1970.
11. Bonamour, G., et al. *La Papille Optique.* Paris: Masson, 1968. Pp. 161–164.
12. Bonamour, G., et al. *La Papille Optique.* Paris: Masson, 1968. P. 59.
13. Bretz, G. W., et al. Coexistence of diabetes mellitus and insipidus and optic atrophy in two male siblings: Studies and review of literature. *Am. J. Med.* 48:398, 1970.
14. Brunette, J.-R., and Bernier, G. Study of a Family of Leber's Optic Atrophy with Recuperation. In J. R. Brunette and A. Barbeau (Eds.), *Progress in Neuro-Ophthalmology.* Amsterdam: Excerpta Medica, 1969. Pp. 91–98.
15. Brunette, J.-R., and Bernier, R. G. Diagnostic et pronostic de la maladie de Leber: Incidence de la récupération totale spontanée. *Union Med. Can.* 99:643, 1970.
16. Carroll, W. M., and Mastaglia, F. L. Leber's optic neuropathy. *Brain* 102:559, 1979.
17. Cartwright, S. C. Concordant optic glioma in a pair of monozygotic twins with neurofibromatosis. *Clin. Pediatr. (Phila.)* 21:236, 1982.
18. Chutorran, A. M., et al. Optic gliomas in children. *Neurology (Minneapolis)* 14:83, 1964.
19. Cogan, D. G., and Kuwabar, T. The sphingolipidoses and the eye. *Arch. Ophthalmol.* 79:437, 1968.
20. Cogan, D. G., et al. Histochemistry of the eye in metachromatic leucoencephalopathy. *A.M.A. Arch. Ophthalmol.* 60:397, 1958.
21. Collier, M. Anomalies papillaires dans trois générations successives. *Ann. Ocul. (Paris)* 193:881, 1960.
22. Collier, M. Dysostose mandibulo-faciale et hypoplasia papillarie. *Bull. Soc. Ophtalmol. Fr.* 61:873, 1961.
23. Collier, M., and Adais, L. Les anomalies congénitales des dimensions papillaires. *Clin. Ophthalmol.* 2:1, 1960.
24. Davis, F. A. Primary tumors of the optic nerve (a phenomenon of Recklinghausen's disease): A clinical and pathologic study with a report of five cases and a review of the literature. *Arch. Ophthalmol.* 23:735, 1940.
25. DeMorsier, G. Études sur les dysgraphies cranio encephaliques: Agénésie de septum lucidum avec malformation du tractus optique. La dysplasie septooptique. *Schweiz. Arch. Neurol. Psychiatr.* 77:267, 1956.
26. DeMyer, W., Zeman, W., and Palmer, C. G. Familial alobar holoprosencephaly (arhinencephaly) with median cleft lip and palate: Report of patient with 46 chromosomes. *Neurology (Minneapolis)* 13:913, 1963.
27. de Weerdt, C. J., and Went, L. N. Neurological studies in families with Leber's optic atrophy. *Acta Neurol. Scand.* 47:541, 1971.
28. Edwards, W. C., and Layden, W. E. Optic nerve hypoplasia. *Am. J. Ophthalmol.* 70:950, 1970.
29. Ellenberger, C., Jr., and Runyan, T. E. Holoprosencephaly with hypoplasia of the optic nerves, dwarfism and agenesis of the septum pellucidum. *Am. J. Ophthalmol.* 70:960, 1970.
30. Ellis, P. P., and Jackson, W. E. Osteopetrosis: A clinical study of optic nerve involvement. *Am. J. Ophthalmol.* 53:943, 1962.
31. Emery, J. M., et al. GM_1-gangliosidosis: Ocular and pathological manifestations. *Arch. Ophthalmol.* 85:177, 1971.

32. Eretto, P., et al. Optic neuropathy in Paget's disease. *Am. J. Ophthalmol.* 97:505, 1984.

33. Fishman, J., Spaier, A. H., and Cohen, M. M. Familial dextrocardia, divergent strabismus, and situs inversus of the optic disc. *Am. J. Med. Sci.* 271:225, 1976.

34. Fishman, M. A., Hogan, G. R., and Dodge, P. R. The concurrence of hydrocephalus and craniosynostosis. *J. Neurosurg.* 34:621, 1971.

35. Foulds, W. S., et al. Hydroxocobalamin in the treatment of Leber's hereditary optic atrophy. *Lancet* 1:896, 1968.

36. Franceschetti, A., and Bock, R. H. Megalopapilla: A new congenital anomaly. *Am. J. Ophthalmol.* 33:227, 1950.

37. François, J. *Heredity in Ophthalmology.* St. Louis: Mosby, 1961.

38. Gass, J. D. M. The Phakomatoses. In J. L. Smith (Ed.), *Neuro-Ophthalmology.* St. Louis: Mosby, 1965. Vol. 2, pp. 223–268.

39. Gillespie, F. D. Aniridia, cerebellar ataxia, and oligophrenia in siblings. *Arch. Ophthalmol.* 73:338, 1965.

40. Gills, J. P., et al. Electroretinography and fundus oculi findings in Hurler's disease and allied mucopolysaccharidoses. *Arch. Ophthalmol.* 74:596, 1965.

41. Glaser, J. S., Hoyt, W. F., and Corbett, J. Visual morbidity with chiasmal glioma: Long-term studies of visual fields in untreated and irradiated cases. *Arch. Ophthalmol.* 85:3, 1971.

42. Goldberg, M. F., and Duke, J. R. Ocular histopathology in Hunter's syndrome: Systemic mucopolysaccharidosis type II. *Arch. Ophthalmol.* 77:503, 1967.

43. Goldberg, M. F., Scott, C. I., and McKusick, V. A. Hydrocephalus and papilledema in the Maroteaux-Lamy syndrome (mucopolysaccharidosis type VI). *Am. J. Ophthalmol.* 69:969, 1970.

44. Greenfield, J. G. *The Spino-cerebellar Degenerations.* Oxford: Blackwell, 1954. P. 82.

45. Grundy, L., Goree, J. A., and Jimenez, J. P. Oxycephaly in the adult simulating pituitary tumor: Clinical and roentgenologic manifestations. *Am. J. Roentgenol. Radium Ther. Nucl. Med.* 108:762, 1970.

46. Grützner, P. Über Diagnose und Funktionsstörungen bei der infantilen, dominant vererbten opticus-Atrophie. *Ber. Dtsch. Ophthalmol. Ges.* 65:268, 1964.

47. Hackenbruch, Y., et al. Familial bilateral optic nerve hypoplasia. *Am. J. Ophthalmol.* 79:314, 1975.

48. Hittner, H. M., Borda, R. P., and Justice, J. X-linked recessive congenital stationary night blindness, myopia and tilted discs. *J. Pediatr. Ophthalmol. Strabismus* 18:15, 1981.

49. Hoffmann, H. Über eine seltene Strangbildung in Augenhinterngrund (Arteria hyaloidea persistens). *Klin. Monatsbl. Augenheilkd.* 77:370, 1926.

50. Hogan, M. J., and Zimmerman, L. E. *Ophthalmic Pathology* (2nd ed.). Philadelphia: Saunders, 1962. P. 580.

51. Horoupian, D. S., et al. Behr syndrome: A clinicopathologic report. *Neurology (N.Y.)* 29:323, 1979.

52. Hoyt, C. Autosomal dominant optic atrophy: A spectrum of disability. *Ophthalmology (Rochester)* 87:245, 1980.

53. Hoyt, C., and Billson, F. Ocular features of Aicardi's syndrome. *Arch. Ophthalmol.* 96:291, 1978.

54. Hoyt, W. F. Charcot-Marie-Tooth disease with primary optic atrophy: Report of a case. *Arch. Ophthalmol.* 64:925, 1960.

55. Hoyt, W. F., and Baghdassarian, S. B. Optic glioma of childhood: Natural history and rationale for conservative management. *Br. J. Ophthalmol.* 53:793, 1969.

56. Hoyt, W. F., et al. Malignant optic glioma of adulthood. *Brain* 96:121, 1973.

57. Imachi, J. Neuro-surgical Treatment of Leber's Optic Atrophy and Its Pathogenetic Relationship to Arachnoiditis. In J.-R. Brunette and A. Barbeau (Eds.), *Progress in Neuro-Ophthalmology.* Amsterdam: Excerpta Medica, 1969. Pp. 121–127.

58. Imachi, J., Yaso, I., and Matsumoto, S. On thirty-two craniotomized cases of Leber's disease with reference to its genetic problems. *Jpn. J. Ophthalmol.* 1:236, 1957.

59. Imachi, J., and Mimura, O. Infantile dominant optic atrophy. *Doc. Ophthalmol.* 17:127, 1978.

60. Jampel, R. S., Okazaki, H., and Bernstein, H. Ophthalmoplegia and retinal degeneration associated with spinocerebellar ataxia. *Arch. Ophthalmol.* 66:123, 1961.

61. Keither, C. G. Retinal atrophy in osteopetrosis. *Arch. Ophthalmol.* 79:234, 1968.

62. Kenyon, K. R., et al. The systemic mucopolysaccharidoses: Ultrastructural and histochemical studies of conjunctiva and skin. *Am. J. Ophthalmol.* 73:811, 1972.

63. Kenyon, K. R. Lysosomal Disorders Affecting the Ocular Anterior Segment. In D. H. Nicholson (Ed.), *Ocular Pathology Update.* New York: Masson, 1980. Pp. 1–22.

64. Kivlin, J. D., et al. Linkage analysis in dominant optic atrophy. *Am. J. Hum. Genet.* 35:1190, 1983.

65. Kjer, P. Infantile optic atrophy with dominant mode of inheritance: A clinical and genetic study of 19 Danish families. *Acta Ophthalmol.* [Suppl.] (Copenh.) 54, 1959.

66. Kjer, P., Jensen, O. A., and Klinken, L. Histopathology of eye, optic nerve and brain in a case of dominant optic atrophy. *Acta Ophthalmol. (Copenh.)* 61:300, 1983.

67. Kline, L. B., and Glaser, J. S. Dominant optic atrophy: The clinical profile. *Arch. Ophthalmol.* 97:1680, 1979.

68. Klintworth, G. K. The neurologic manifestations of osteopetrosis (Albers-Schönberg's disease). *Neurology (Minneapolis)* 13:512, 1963.

69. Klug, G. L. Gliomas of the optic nerve and chiasm in children. *Neuro-Ophthalmology* 2:217, 1981.

70. Knight, C. L., and Hoyt, W. F. Monocular blindness from drusen of the optic disc. *Am. J. Ophthalmol.* 73:890, 1972.

71. Kollarits, C. R., et al. The autosomal dominant syndrome of progressive optic atrophy and congenital deafness. *Am. J. Ophthalmol.* 87:789, 1979.

72. Kranenburg, E. W. Crater-like holes in the optic disc and central serous retinopathy. *Arch. Ophthalmol.* 64:912, 1960.

73. Krill, A. E., Smith, V. C., and Pokorny, J. Similarities between congenital tritan defects and dominant optic nerve atrophy: Coincidence or identity? *J. Opt. Soc. Am.* 60:1132, 1970.

74. Kytilä, J., and Mitettinen, P. On bilateral aplasia of the optic nerve. *Acta Ophthalmol.(Copenh.)* 39:416, 1961.

75. Landrieu, P., and Eurard, P. La dysplasia septo-optique: Étude clinique et éléments d'un conseil génétique. *J. Genet. Hum.* 27:329, 1979.

76. Leber, T. Über hereditäre und congenitalangelegte Sehnervenleiden. *Albrecht von Graefes Arch. Ophthalmol.* 17(Abst. 2):249, 1871.

77. Lees, F., MacDonald, A. M. E., and Turner, J. W. A. Leber's disease with symptoms resembling disseminated sclerosis. *J. Neurol. Neurosurg. Psychiatry* 27:415, 1964.

78. Lessell, S., Gise, R. L., and Krohel, G. B. Bilateral optic neuropathy with remission in young men: Variation on a theme by Leber? *Arch. Neurol.* 40:2, 1983.

79. Lessell, S., and Rosman, N. P. Juvenile diabetes mellitus and optic atrophy. *Arch. Neurol.* 34:759, 1977.

80. Livingstone, I. R., et al. Leber's optic neuropathy: Clinical and visual evoked response studies in asymptomatic and symptomatic members of a 4-generation family. *Br. J. Ophthalmol.* 64:751, 1980.

81. Lodberg, C. V., and Lund, A. Hereditary optic atrophy with dominant transmission: Three Danish families. *Acta Ophthalmol. (Copenh.)* 28:437, 1950.

82. Lorentzen, S. E. Drusen of the optic disc, a clinical and genetic study. *Acta Ophthalmol. [Suppl.] (Copenh.)* 90, 1966.

83. Lundsgaard, R. Leber's disease: A genealogic, genetic and clinical study of 101 cases of retrobulbar optic neuritis in 20 Danish families. *Acta Ophthalmol. [Suppl.] (Copenh.)* 21, 1944.

84. Mailer, C. Gargoylism associated with optic atrophy. *Can. J. Ophthalmol.* 4:266, 1969.

85. Manchester, P. T., and Calhoun, F. P., Jr. Dominant hereditary optic atrophy with bitemporal field defects. *A.M.A. Arch. Ophthalmol.* 60:479, 1958.

86. Manshot, W. A. Primary tumours of the optic nerve in von Recklinghausen's disease. *Br. J. Ophthalmol.* 38:285, 1954.

87. Margolis, S., and Siegel, I. M. The Tilted Disc Syndrome in Craniofacial Diseases. In J. L. Smith (Ed.), *Neuro-Ophthalmology Focus 1980.* New York: Masson, 1979. Pp. 97–116.

88. McKusick, V. A. *Heritable Disorders of Connective Tissue* (3rd ed.). St. Louis: Mosby, 1966. P. 421.

89. McKusick, V. A. *Heritable Disorders of Connective Tissue* (3rd ed.). St. Louis: Mosby, 1966. Pp. 325–399.

90. McLeod, J. G., Low, P. A., and Morgan, J. A. Charcot-Marie-Tooth disease with Leber's optic atrophy. *Neurology (N.Y.)* 28:179, 1978.

91. Mikuni, M., Ishii, K., and Makabe, R. Zum Durchmesser der Sehnervenpapille bei Japanern. *Klin. Monatsbl. Augenheilkd.* 136:544, 1960.

92. Misseroli, G. Una nuova sindrome congenita a carattere famigliare: Ipoplasia del nervoottico ed emianopsia binasale. *Boll. Ocul.* 26:683, 1947.

93. Mustonen, E. Pseudopapilloedema with and without verified optic disc drusen: A clinical analysis I. *Acta Ophthalmol. (Copenh.)* 61:1037, 1983.

94. Nikoskelainen, E., Hoyt, W. F., and Nummelin, K. Ophthalmoscopic findings in Leber's hereditary optic neuropathy: I. Fundus findings in asymptomatic family members. *Arch. Ophthalmol.* 100:1597, 1982.

95. Nikoskelainen, E., et al. The early phase of Leber's hereditary optic atrophy. *Arch. Ophthalmol.* 95:969, 1977.

96. Pollock, J. A., Newton, T. H., and Hoyt, W. F. Transsphenoidal and transethmoidal encephaloceles: A review of clinical and roentgen features in 8 cases. *Radiology* 90:442, 1968.

97. Puliafito, C. A., et al. Optic atrophy and visual loss in craniometaphyseal dysplasia. *Am. J. Ophthalmol.* 92:292, 1981.

98. Reese, A. B. Relation of drusen of the optic nerve to tuberous sclerosis. *Arch. Ophthalmol.* 24:187, 1940.

99. Riise, D. The nasal fundus ectasia. *Acta Ophthalmol. [Suppl.] (Copenh.)* 126, 1975.

100. Rorsman, G., and Söderström, N. Optic atrophy and juvenile diabetes mellitus with familial occurrence. *Acta Med. Scand.* 182:419, 1967.

101. Rose, F. C., Bowden, A. N., and Bowden, P. M. A. The heart in Leber's optic atrophy. *Br. J. Ophthalmol.* 54:388, 1970.

102. Rose, F. C., et al. The association of juvenile diabetes mellitus and optic atrophy: Clinical and genetic aspects. *Q. J. Med.* 35:385, 1966.

103. Rosenberg, M. A., Savino, P. J., and Glaser, J. S. A clinical analysis of pseudopapilledema: I. Population, laterality, acuity, refractive error, ophthalmoscopic characteristics, and coincident disease. *Arch. Ophthalmol.* 97:65, 1979.

104. Rosenberg, R. N., and Chutorran, A. Familial optico-acoustic nerve degeneration and polyneuropathy. *Neurology (Minneapolis)* 17:827, 1967.

105. Rush, J. A., et al. Optic glioma: Long-term follow-up of 85 histopathologically verified cases. *Ophthalmology (Rochester)* 89:1213, 1982.

106. Saleeby, S. S. Maladie de Behr ou atrophie optique infantile compliquée hérédo-familiale: Étude de 19 cas (thesis). Geneva, 1960. Cited by J. François: Genetic aspects of ophthalmology. *Int. Ophthalmol. Clin.* 8(4):1043, 1968.

107. Sanders, T. E., Gay, A. J., and Newman, M. Hemorrhagic complications of drusen of the optic disc. *Am. J. Ophthalmol.* 71:204, 1971.

108. Sandvig, K. Pseudoglaucoma of autosomal domi-

nant inheritance: A report on three families. *Acta Ophthalmol. (Copenh.)* 39:33, 1961.

109. Sarsfield, J. K. The syndrome of congenital cerebellar ataxia, aniridia and mental retardation. *Dev. Med. Child Neurol.* 13:508, 1971.

110. Savell, J., and Cook, J. R. Optic nerve colobomas of autosomal-dominant heredity. *Arch. Ophthalmol.* 94:395, 1976.

111. Savino, P. J., Glaser, J. S., and Rosenberg, M. A. A clinical analysis of pseudopapilledema: II. Visual field defects. *Ophthalmology (Rochester)* 97:71, 1979.

112. Schapira, K., Poskanzer, D. C., and Miller, H. Familial and conjugal multiple sclerosis. *Brain* 86:315, 1963.

113. Scheie, H. G., and Adler, F. H. Aplasia of the optic nerve. *Arch. Ophthalmol.* 26:61, 1941.

114. Seedorff, T. Leber's disease, V. *Acta Ophthalmol. (Copenh.)* 48:186, 1970.

114a. Skarf, B., and Hoyt, C. S. Optic nerve hypoplasia in children. Association with anomalies of the endocrine and CNS. *Arch. Ophthalmol.* 102:62, 1984.

115. Smith, D. P. Diagnostic criteria in dominantly inherited juvenile optic atrophy: A report of 3 new families. *Am. J. Optom.* 49:183, 1972.

116. Smith, H. E. Aplasia of the optic nerve: Report of three cases. *Am. J. Ophthalmol.* 37:498, 1954.

117. Stehauwer, A., and Went, L. N. Leber's optic neuropathy: I. Clinical studies. *Doc. Ophthalmol.* 53:97, 1982.

118. Stern, J., DiGiacinto, G. V., and Housepian, E. M. Neurofibromatosis and optic glioma: Clinical and morphologic correlations. *Neurosurgery* 4:524, 1979.

119. Streiff, B. Über Megalopapille. *Klin. Monatsbl. Augenheilkd.* 139:824, 1961.

120. Sugar, H. S. Congenital pits in the optic disc and their equivalents (congenital colobomas and colobomalike excavations) associated with submacular fluid. *Am. J. Ophthalmol.* 63:298, 1967.

121. Taveras, J. M., Mount, L. A., and Wood, E. H. The value of radiation therapy in the management of glioma of the optic nerves and chiasm. *Radiology* 66:518, 1956.

122. Thorén, C. Diabetes mellitus in Friedreich's ataxia. *Acta Paediatr. Scand. [Suppl.]* 135:239, 1962.

123. Throuvalas, N., Bataini, P., and Ennuyer, A. Les gliomes du chiasma et du nerf optique: L'apport de la radiothérapie transcutanée dans leur traitement. *Bull. Cancer (Paris)* 56:231, 1969.

124. Tym, R. Piloid gliomas of the anterior optic pathways. *Br. J. Surg.* 49:322, 1961.

125. van Bogaert, L. Chronic amaurotic idiocy without amaurosis. *World Neurol.* 3:512, 1962.

126. van Senus, A. H. C. Leber's disease in the Netherlands. *Doc. Ophthalmol.* 17:1, 1963.

127. Verhoeff, F. H. Primary intraneural tumors (gliomas) of the optic nerve. *Arch. Ophthalmol.* 51:120, 239, 1922.

128. Waardenburg, P. J. Twin research in ophthalmology. *Doc. Ophthalmol.* 4:154, 1950.

129. Waardenburg, P. J. Franceschetti, A., and Klein, D. *Genetics and Ophthalmology*, Vol. 2. Assen, Netherlands: van Gorcum, 1963.

130. Waardenburg, P. J., Franceschetti, A., and Klein, D. *Genetics and Ophthalmology*, Vol. 2. Assen, Netherlands: van Gorcum, 1963. P. 1607.

131. Waardenburg, P. J., Franceschetti, A., and Klein, D. *Genetics and Ophthalmology*, Vol. 2. Assen, Netherlands: van Gorcum, 1963. P. 1600.

132. Wallace, D. C. Leber's optic atrophy: A possible example of vertical transmission of a slow virus in man. *Australas. Ann. Med.* 19:1, 1970.

133. Wallace, D. C. A new manifestation of Leber's disease and a new explanation for the agency responsible for its unusual pattern of inheritance. *Brain* 93:121, 1970.

134. Walsh, F. B., and Hoyt, W. F. *Clinical Neuro-Ophthalmology* (3rd ed.). Baltimore: Williams & Wilkins, 1969. Vol. 1, pp. 673–680.

135. Walsh, F. B., and Hoyt, W. F. *Clinical Neuro-Ophthalmology* (3rd ed.). Baltimore: Williams & Wilkins, 1969. Vol. 3, pp. 1939–1989.

136. Walton, D. S., and Robb, R. M. Optic nerve hypoplasia: A report of 20 cases. *Arch. Ophthalmol.* 84:572, 1970.

137. Weiner, L. P., Konigsmark, B. W., and Stoll, J., Jr. Hereditary olivopontocerebellar atrophy with retinal degeneration: Report of a family through six generations. *Arch. Neurol.* 16:364, 1967.

138. Weyert, F. Zur Heredität der Opticuskolobome. *Klin. Monatsbl. Augenheilkd.* 28:325, 1890.

139. Wijngaarde, R., Blaauw, G., and Bosman, H. Optic atrophy and non-tumoral hypothalamic disorders. *Doc. Ophthalmol.* 17:139, 1978.

140. Wilson, J. Leber's hereditary optic atrophy: Some clinical and aetiological considerations. *Brain* 86:347, 1963.

141. Wilson, J. Leber's hereditary optic atrophy: A possible defect of cyanide metabolism. *Clin. Sci.* 29:505, 1965.

142. Wilson, J., Linnell, J. C., and Matthews, D. M. Plasma-cobalamins in neuro-ophthalmological diseases. *Lancet* 1:259, 1971.

143. Witusik, W. Types of physiologic excavation of the optic nerve head. *Ophthalmologica* 152:57, 1966.

144. Wium, E. Hereditary opticusatrophy with excavation of the papilla. *Acta Ophthalmol. (Copenh.)* 26:195, 1948.

145. Wolter, J. R., and Allen, R. J. Retinal neuropathology of the late infantile amaurotic idiocy. *Br. J. Ophthalmol.* 48:277, 1964.

146. Wong, I. G., and Lubow, M. Management of Optic Glioma of Childhood: A Review of 42 Cases. In J. L. Smith (Ed.), *Neuro-Ophthalmology.* St. Louis: Mosby, 1972. Vol. 6, pp. 51–60.

147. Zeman, W., and Hoffman, J. Juvenile and late forms of amaurotic idiocy in one family. *J. Neurol. Neurosurg. Psychiatry* 25:352, 1962.

Oculocutaneous Genetic Diseases

Sophie Marie Worobec-Victor
Michelle Ann Bené Bain

The eye and skin share prominently exposed positions, and, since both have ectodermal and mesodermal components, numerous hereditary, inflammatory, and infectious diseases affect both of these organs. An adequate examination of both organs is necessary in evaluating and treating these oculocutaneous disorders [19]. In this chapter we will confine our considerations to genetic diseases involving both the skin and eye.

PIGMENTARY DISORDERS

A number of hereditary disorders involve a disturbance in melanin metabolism; the resultant effects may be a loss or increase of pigment in the skin and eye.

Human Melanogenesis

During the first 8 to 10 weeks of human embryonic development, melanoblasts differentiate in the neural crest and then migrate to the developing central and peripheral nervous systems, the epidermis, eyes, ears, gastrointestinal tract, ovaries, and adrenal systems. In the eye dendritic melanocytes derived from the neural crest form the choroid, and cuboidal melanocytes derived from the neuroectoderm form the retinal pigment epithelium, which also extends to the iris and ciliary body structures. Similarly, in the developing ear, pigment cells are involved in the development of

the following inner ear structures: the cochlea, stria vascularis, and organ of Corti. Because of this wide distribution of melanocytes, it is not surprising to find that a number of pigment disorders are associated with multisystemic effects such as deafness and neurologic disorders. The function of melanocytes in all the organ systems to which they are dispersed is not completely understood; however, it is known that melanin acts as a free-radical receptor, and in this role it may exert a protective effect in a number of tissues.

Melanocytes contain membrane-bound organelles, the melanosomes, within which melanin formation occurs. The primary melanogenic enzyme is tyrosinase, which catalyzes the hydroxylation of tyrosine to dopa and the oxidation of dopa to dopaquinone. Tyrosine hydroxylation to dopa is also catalyzed by peroxidase enzyme. Dopa serves as both substrate and cofactor in the conversion of tyrosine to melanin with both enzyme systems. Tyrosinase is a copper-containing enzyme, and dopa reduces the copper, enabling the tyrosinase to function as a catalyst in melanogenesis. Dopaquinone then undergoes nonenzymatic oxidation resulting in its polymerization into melanin.

There are two types of melanin: eumelanin, which is a brown to black polymer, and phaeomelanin, which is a yellow to brown polymer. The formation of phaeomelanin requires the covalent bonding of cysteine and other thiol compounds to dopaquinone in the melanin synthesis pathway. This divergence to either eumelanin or phaeomelanin formation is believed to be under genetic control, as evidenced by familial patterns of red hair and the autosomal recessive inheri-

We thank our mentors, Drs. Lawrence M. Solomon and Nancy B. Esterly, authors of The Skin and the Eye, in the first edition of this book, from which sections and illustrations are utilized in the present chapter.

tance pattern of yellow mutant oculocutaneous albinism. A lesser degree of cysteine binding to dopa intermediates also occurs in eumelanin synthesis, and this is probably the mechanism of reddish hair tints in brunettes and blonds.

Based on electron microscopic appearance, cutaneous melanosomes are classified into four developmental stages: Stage I melanosomes are round organelles containing filaments with intense melanogenic enzyme activity but containing no melanin. Melanin deposition is first seen in stage II melanosomes. As the melanin content increases in individual melanosomes, the amount of melanogenic enzyme decreases. Stage III melanosomes show very little enzyme activity, and stage IV melanosomes show no enzyme activity. Continued melanin formation occurs largely in stage III (and completely in stage IV) melanosomes through nonenzymatic polymerization. The internal structure of stage IV melanosomes is completely obscured on electron micrographs by melanin.

Transfer of melanosomes to surrounding keratinocytes and hair cortex cells from cutaneous melanocytes occurs by way of phagocytosis of melanocytic dendrites, but in the uveal tract the melanocytes contain no dendrites and melanosomes remain within melanocytes. In the skin one melanocyte serves approximately 36 keratinocytes. When melanosomes are engulfed within keratinocytes, the melanin is then slowly degraded and fragmented into small, dense particles that localize to a position covering and protecting the basal cell nucleus from the noxious effects of ultraviolet light. The known diseases of hypopigmentation have been classified according to the following defects [175]:

1. Failure of melanoblast migration to the skin (piebaldism)
2. Failure of melanoblast differentiation into melanocytes (piebaldism)
3. Failure of mitotic devision of melanocytes (?vitiligo)
4. Defect of synthesis of functional tyrosinase (albinism)
5. Failure of synthesis of melanosome matrix
6. Defect of tyrosinase transport
7. Failure of melanosome formation
8. Failure of melanosome melanization (albinism)
9. Defect of melanosome transfer
10. Alteration in degradation of melanosomes
11. Melanin removal with loss of stratum corneaum (trauma)

The exact genic control of pigmentation in humans is unknown. However, in laboratory mice more than 147 genes at 62 different loci have been found to influence hair and skin color, and often different genes controlling different steps in the melanization process produce phenotypically similar effects. These findings suggest that human disorders of pigmentation are under very complex genic control.

Hypopigmentation Disorders

The number of described human genetic syndromes of which pigment loss is a part increases every year. Doubtlessly many more will be entered into the medical literature. The hereditary syndromes resulting in oculocutaneous hypomelanization have been classified by Witkop as shown in Table 19-1 [280].

ALBINISM

All forms of albinism, both oculocutaneous and ocular, are distinguished by foveal hypoplasia, photophobia, nystagmus, and decreased visual acuity. In oculocutaneous albinism (OCA), pigmentation is decreased or absent in the skin, hair, and eyes. In ocular albinism (OA) primarily the eyes are affected with normal or slightly altered skin and hair pigmentation. (Albinoidism differs from albinism in that nystagmus and photophobia are not manifested by albinoid individuals.)

Albino individuals have normal visual fields; however, they lack well-developed binocular vision. This is believed to be due to the development of abnormal optic pathways in two areas: (1) the cross-over of most temporal retinal neurons to the contralateral side of the brain, and (2) the rearrangement of geniculocortical tracts. In normally pigmented individuals, the temporal retinal neurons pass instead to the same side of the brain as the eye of origin. Ida Mann in 1937 postulated that the pigmentation of the optic cup was a prerequisite for the direction of optic neurons toward normal brain targets and also for normal foveal development [28]. In albinos, however, fundal pigmentation is lacking at birth and also during the postnatal period during which final

Table 19-1. *Types of Albinism and Albinoidism Classified by Response to Hair Bulb Tyrosine Incubation Test*

I. Albinism: hypopigmentation with nystagmus, photophobia, and decreased visual acuity
   A. Oculocutaneous albinism (OCA)
      1. Hair bulb tyrosine test negative
         a. Tyrosinase-negative (ty-neg) OCA (AR)
      2. Hair bulb tyrosine test positive
         a. Tyrosinase-positive (ty-pos) OCA (AR)
         b. OCA–hemorrhagic diathesis, Hermansky-Pudlak syndrome (AR)
         c. Béguez César disease, Chédiak-Higashi syndrome (AR)
         d. Hypopigmentation-microphthalmos, Cross-McKusick-Breen syndrome (AR)
         e. Brown OCA (AR)
         f. Rufous OCA (AR)
         g. Autosomal dominant OCA (AD)
         h. Black locks, deafness of the sensorineural type (BADS syndrome) (AR)
      3. Hair bulb tyrosine test variable
         a. Yellow mutant albinism (AR)
   B. Ocular albinism (OA)
      1. X-linked (Nettleship)
      2. X-linked (Forsius-Eriksson)
      3. Autosomal recessive
      4. OA, lentigines, deafness (AD)
II. Albinoidism: hypopigmentation without nystagmus, photophobia, and decreased visual acuity
   A. Hair bulb tyrosine test positive
      1. Autosomal dominant albinoidism (AD)
      2. Punctate ocular albinoidism (AD)
      3. Brachymetapody, anodontia, hypotrichosis, albinoid trait (AR)
      4. Ocular hypopigmentation and Apert's disease (AD, sporadic)
      5. Phenylketonuria (AR)
   B. Hair bulb tyrosine test negative
      1. Menkes' syndrome (X-linked)

AD = autosomal dominant; AR = autosomal recessive.
Source: Adapted from C. J. Witkop, Jr. [280].

optic neuronal development is completed. These neural abnormalities are found in albino individuals and are absent in albinoid patients.

At birth albino infants respond little, if at all, to visual stimuli. Their lack of skin and hair pigmentation can be difficult to discern in infancy. Early diagnosis is best made on the basis of the following ocular findings: transillumination of the iris, a blond fundus with clearly visible choroidal vasculature, absence of macular pigmentation, and a poor macular reflex. At 2 to 3 months of age albino infants start to show visual responsiveness and develop nystagmus [81]. It is estimated that 9 percent of all visually handicapped children have some form of oculocutaneous albinism, and about 1 percent have ocular albinism [281]. The various forms of albinism are distinguished on the basis of clinical, biochemical, and genetic criteria.

Oculocutaneous Albinism. Serum tyrosinase levels are normal in all forms of oculocutaneous albinism, but in vitro incubation of freshly epilated hair bulbs from albino individuals in tyrosine solutions can distinguish between tyrosinase-negative (ty-neg) OCA (incubation shows no pigmentation of the bulbs), yellow mutant (ym) OCA (no or questionable pigmentation), and tyrosinase-positive (ty-pos) OCA (definite pigmentation). In the other forms of oculocutaneous albinism, results on tyrosine hair bulb tests are positive. The tyrosine hair bulb test is a test of the ability to form melanin, and, since this ability may be delayed until 1 to 2 years of age in tyrosinase-positive OCA, tyrosinase-positive and tyrosinase-negative albinos may be indistinguishable at birth.

Tyrosinase-negative OCA (classic or Garrod type) is the most severe form of albinism. It occurs in about 1 in 34,000 births. The phenotypic expression does not vary with the patient's ethnic origin. Tyrosinase-negative albinos have snow-white hair, pink-white skin, blue to gray irides, prominent red reflexes, severe nystagmus, photophobia, and visual acuity of 20/400 or less. Myopic astigmatism and strabismus are frequent findings. Electron microscopy of hair bulbs shows only stage I and II melanosomes, which lack melanin. Skin or hair bulbs incubated in tyrosine or dopa are negative for melanogenesis. There is a marked risk of skin neoplasms, especially squamous cell carcinomas. Photoprotection is essential.

Yellow mutant oculocutaneous albinism (Amish albinism, xanthous albinism) is indistinguishable at birth from ty-neg OCA, but at age 3 transillumination of the iris shows a cartwheel effect in ym OCA. Phenotypic expression varies with the patient's ethnic origin. Retinal pigment is visible in black patients. Nystagmus and photophobia are present. Visual acuity is in the 20/90 to 20/400 range. The hair is white at birth, then turns a yellow shade by 6 weeks to 6 months of age. The skin is fair with slight tanning ability, and in blacks pigmented nevi are found. Incubation of the hair bulbs in a tyrosine-cystine solution causes increased red-yellow pigmentation because of phaeomelanin production. Stage III melanosomes are seen on electron microscopy. Ym OCA is allelic with ty-neg albinism. It is common in the Amish community and also occurs among American blacks and Americans of Polish and German extraction as well as among Ceylonese and African blacks.

Tyrosinase-positive oculocutaneous albinism (complete, imperfect albinism; albinism II) is distinguished from ty-neg OCA by the presence of some pigment in the skin, hair, and eyes. The appearance of this pigment formation is delayed until 1 to 2 years of age, and the amount of pigment formed depends on the patient's ethnic origin. Ty-pos albinos can tan slightly by age 2 years and may even develop yellow, brown, or red hair color. The eyes may develop yellow, hazel, or even brown coloration. A ty-pos albino of black parentage may even be darker than some fair-skinned Caucasians. The red reflex is a constant finding only in ty-pos albinos of Caucasian origin. Ocular findings resemble those in ty-neg albinos but are less severe. Visual acuity in adults varies from 20/90 to 20/400. There is a cartwheel effect at the pupil and limbus on transillumination. Risk of skin neoplasia is less severe than in ty-neg OCA. Freckles and nevi may be present. Numerous stage III and even rare stage IV melanosomes are seen on electron microscopy of skin and hair tissue. The biochemical defect of this condition is unknown. Ty-pos OCA is not allelic with ty-neg

OCA. Ty-pos OCA has a prevalence of 1 in 15,000 among blacks and 1 in 40,000 among Caucasians.

Hermansky-Pudlak syndrome is a form of ty-pos OCA with hemorrhagic episodes caused by a platelet storage pool defect and interstitial pulmonary fibrosis caused by deposition of a ceroid-like material. This material is also found throughout the reticuloendothelial system, oral and gastrointestinal mucosa, and urine. There are cytoplasmic inclusions in circulating leukocytes. Eye color is blue-gray to brown. There is no variation of pigmentation of the uveal tract and retina [241]. On electron microscopy melanosomes in Stage III, and rarely in stage IV, maturation are present, and there are numerous irregular phaeomelanosomes, resembling those seen in normal redheads. About 50 cases of this disorder have been reported. Because all its features are present in affected patients, its genetic basis is believed to be a pleiotrophic effect of a single gene rather than the effect of two or more closely linked genes.

Chédiak-Higashi syndrome (CHS, Béguez César disease, Steinbrink syndrome) is a rare imperfect form of oculocutaneous albinism with a fatal outcome usually in the teen years because of infection or lymphoreticular malignancy. Its laboratory characterization is based on the finding of giant granules within granulocytes and monocytes. These giant granules form by the fusion of primary lysosomes with one another and with incorporation of cytoplasmic material, thereby leading to the creation of secondary lysosomes or phagolysosomes. In this disease microorganisms are phagocytized in a normal fashion by white blood cells; however, their destruction is impeded because of the inability of giant phagolysosomes to discharge bactericidal enzymes [274].

Melanocytes in CHS contain a few stage IV melanosomes and numerous giant melanosomes. The giant melanosomes are formed by a fusion process similar to that observed in lysosomes, and the giant melanosomes even fuse with each other, followed by degenerative changes. The normal melanosomes, upon transfer to keratinocytes and hair cortex cells, are packaged into abnormally large phagolysosomes. It is likely that this segregation of melanosomes within giant phagolysosomes, instead of their fine dispersion, causes the hypopigmentation seen in this syndrome [286]. Similar changes occur in the retina, choroid plexus, limbal area, and pia-arachnoid membrane [175]. The pigment dilution present in this syndrome depends on ethnic origin and presents the following phenotypic expressions: light cream to slate gray skin, blond-brunette to metallic gray hair, and blue-violet to brown irides. Ocular examination reveals normal to cartwheel-type iris pigmentation, a red reflex that diminishes after 5 years of age, and diminished uveal and retinal pigmentation. Nystagmus and photophobia are variably present. Childhood vaccinations are well tolerated by affected individuals, but recurrent staphylococcal and streptococcal infections are common presenting problems. Convulsions and neuropathy start around 5 years of age, followed by an "accelerated phase" of pancytopenia, splenomegaly, and lymphadenopathy, which portend malignancy and early death. In the late stages of this disease, papilledema is present, because of lymphocytic infiltration of the optic nerve.

Cross-McKusick-Breen syndrome was first described in one Amish family with multiple consanguineous marriages. It is a form of oculocutaneous albinism characterized by microphthalmos and ill-defined corneas. In two affected individuals the cornea was cloudy and vascularized, and it was impossible to visualize the fundi. No response to bright light was seen, and blindness was assumed. Ectropion with conjunctival injection and a severe jerky nystagmus were present. Other findings included gingival fibromatosis, ichthyosis, and severe physical and mental retardation. Hair was white to blond, and skin was pink to white. Scanty clustered stage III melanosomes were seen in skin biopsies.

Brown oculocutaneous albinism has been seen among natives of Nigeria and New Guinea. It differs from ty-pos OCA in showing only slight pigment formation with aging, and the incubation of hair bulbs in tyrosine produces only slightly positive pigmentation. Brown albinos have darker constitutional pigmentation than do ty-pos albinos of similar ethnic origin; however, they sunburn easily and have a high rate of squamous cell carcinomas. They are brunette with olive to light brown skin. Irides are diaphanous with blue to hazel to light brown pigmentation. Nystagmus, strabismus, and slight photophobia are present in a majority of studied patients. Visual acuity is in the 20/30 to 20/100 range. Numerous stage III melanosomes and moderate numbers of stage IV melanosomes are seen on electron micrographs. The biochemical defect is unknown.

Rufous oculocutaneous albinism has been seen among Africans, American blacks, and the natives of New Guinea. Both skin and hair coloration is reddish brown. The tyrosine hair bulb test is positive. The irides show slight transillumination and

are reddish brown. The fundus background too appears reddish brown. Mild nystagmus and photophobia are present. Visual acuity ranges from normal to 20/100.

Autosomal dominant OCA has been observed in two families (Swiss and American), and its phenotypic presentation includes completely white to reddish-tinted cream-colored hair, white to creamy skin, gray to blue irides, moderate to severe nystagmus, and photophobia. Irides are translucent or show a cartwheel effect on transillumination. Visual acuity is in the 20/70 to 20/200 range. There is little or no detectable fundal pigment. Melanocytes are structurally normal, present in normal numbers, and reach early stage III maturation.

Black locks, oculocutaneous albinism, and deafness of the sensorineural type (BADS syndrome) has been seen in two kindred groups and is assumed to be autosomal recessive. Skin and hair are white with scattered locks of black hair and scattered round brown skin macules. The deafness is congenital and is believed to be due to failure of embryonic migration of neural elements from the neural tube to the ear. In one patient with a black hair lock above one ear, that ear had a 50-dB hearing loss, with complete deafness of the opposite ear, which was surrounded by white hair. One heterozygote had a white hair lock in the midscalp associated with an unusual pigmentary lesion of the fundus. The entire posterior pole was covered by circles and lines of hyperpigmentation and hypopigmentation. The diameter of these zones approximated one-half the diameter of the optic disc. The retinal vasculature was not visible. In affected homozygotes eye findings include foveal hypoplasia, marked nystagmus, photophobia, translucent gray irides, a prominent red reflex, and visual acuity ranging from 20/250 and 20/400. This condition differs from other forms of OCA in that melanocytes are absent, either through a migration defect or failure to survive, in the nonpigmented areas and present in normal numbers with normal structure and function in the pigmented areas.

Ocular Albinism. Patients classified as having ocular albinism have hypomelanosis primarily of the retinal and uveal tracts, with either focal cutaneous hypopigmentary defects or normal to near-normal skin coloration. Four types of ocular albinism have been described:

Ocular albinism of the X-linked Nettleship type (XOAN) is mainly manifested in affected males by reduced ocular pigmentation. The irides may vary from pale blue to pale green with the presence of some brown pigment at the pupillary border. The irides are diaphanous, and eye color usually darkens with age. Photophobia, refraction errors, strabismus, exotropia, esotropia, and nystagmus (rotary or horizontal or both) are common problems. Head nodding or tilting is present in about one-half of affected males. Visual acuity ranges from 20/50 to 20/300 in affected Caucasians but is near normal in blacks.

In black patients with XOAN the most characteristic ocular feature has been foveal hypoplasia, as the irides and fundi can be moderately pigmented. Hypomelanotic macules were also found on the torsos of 7 of 9 affected males in the first reported black kindred. Females who are heterozygous for XOAN show a mosaic pigment pattern in the fundus and have translucent irides; however, some female carriers are as severely affected as male patients. These findings are in accord with Mary Lyon's hypothesis of random X chromosome inactivation in females, which in the more severely affected females is explained by chance selection of the X chromosome bearing the mutant gene by progenitor optic nerve cells.

Microscopic examination of both retinal epithelium and skin from affected males and heterozygous females has revealed macromelanosomes (giant pigment granules) within melanocytes. This is a nonspecific finding since macromelanosomes have also been described in several other disorders, including Hermansky-Pudlak syndrome and the ocular albinism–lentigines–deafness syndrome. Nonalbino conditions in which macromelanosomes occur include nevus spilus, generalized lentigines, xeroderma pigmentosum, and neurofibromatosis.

Autosomal recessive ocular albinism (AROA) has now been established in over 18 kinship systems. Eye findings include a prominent red reflex, photophobia, nystagmus, strabismus, diaphanous irides, light yellow fundi, and foveal hypoplasia. Visual acuity ranges from 20/100 to 20/400. Skin and hair color is slightly lighter than that of unaffected siblings. Macromelanosomes do not occur in this disorder, and the hair bulb tyrosine incubation test result is positive. The nature of the pigmentary defect is unknown.

X-linked ocular albinism of the Forsius-Eriksson type (Aland eye disease, Forsius-Eriksson syndrome) differs from the XOAN type in that males affected with the former frequently have protanomalous color blindness and a high degree of axial myopia. Female carriers do not show a mosaic pigmented pattern in the fundus; however, they may show slight color discrimination defects and latent nystagmus. Foveal hypoplasia and nystagmus are constant features. O'Donnell and colleagues have hypothesized that in this condition there is either defective induction of retinal pigment or that retinal hypopigmentation results from retinal stretching because of the high degree of axial myopia [186]. No macromelanosomes are found in this condition.

Ocular albinism–lentigines–deafness syndrome is an autosomal dominant syndrome described in three generations of one Caucasian family. Ocular albinism is accompanied by congenital nystagmus, strabismus, and hypermetropic refractive error. Systemic features are congenital deafness, vestibular abnormalities, and multiple cutaneous lentigines containing macromelanosomes [159].

ALBINOIDISM

Albinoidism differs from albinism in that albinoidism shows milder ocular involvement: Usually there is no nystagmus nor photophobia present, and the fovea is normally developed. Visual acuity is usually normal. There are several different forms, which, on the basis of tyrosine test results, have been divided into two groupings.

Hair Bulb Tyrosine-Test-Positive Albinoidism. Autosomal dominant oculocutaneous albinoidism has been described in several families. The irides are blue with a diffuse pattern of pigment distribution on transillumination. Diffuse punctate pigmentation is seen in the retina. Hair color ranges from white to yellow to strawberry blond. Skin is pink-white and easily reddens with ultraviolet B (UVB) light or sun exposure, with very slight tanning in a few patients.

Autosomal dominant albinoidism and deafness was described by Tietz in a six-generation kinship in which the patients were reported to have cutaneous hypomelanosis, blond hair, blue irides, and deaf mutism [262]. However, reexamination of several members of the same family by Reed and associates cast doubt on the existence of albinoidism, as unaffected and affected siblings had similar coloring [212]. The reported family probably had dominantly transmitted deafness but no albinoidism.

Punctate ocular albinoidism has been reported by Bergsma and Kaiser-Kupfer as an autosomal dominant trait observed in one kindred [25]. Affected patients were blond. The pupils were dilated and anisocoric. The irides showed a punctate type of transillumination, and retinal fluorescein angiography revealed a punctate window pattern in the retinal pigment epithelium.

Brachymetapody, anodontia, hypotrichosis, and albinoid trait were reported by Toumaala and Haapanen in three siblings in an inheritance pattern consistent with autosomal recessive transmission [263]. Affected patients had white hair, pale skin, generalized hypotrichosis, hypoplastic breasts, hypoplastic maxilla, anodontia, and shortened digits. Eye findings included nystagmus, cataracts, and myopia.

Ocular hypopigmentation in Apert's disease was observed by Margolis and co-workers on examination of 9 patients with Apert's disease. In this group 7 patients had mild loss of visual acuity (20/25–20/50), 5 had localized fundal hypopigmentation, 4 had mild photophobia, and 1 had nystagmus.

Phenylketonuria (PKU, phenylpyruvic oligophrenia) is an autosomal recessive metabolic disorder in which most untreated patients show hypopigmentation of the skin, hair, and irides in comparison with unaffected family members. The estimated prevalence rate of PKU is 1 in 20,000 births [96]. Affected patients have the normal means by which to synthesize melanin from tyrosine and structurally normal melanosomes, but they have a block in the conversion of phenylalanine to tyrosine, usually caused by a deficiency of the enzyme L-phenylalanine hydroxylase. However, the exact relationship of the clinical features to the biochemical defect remains a source of lively controversy. The inability to convert phenylalanine to tyrosine may lead to (1) an inadequate store of melanin precursor; (2) an accumulation of phenylalanine and some of its catabolites, as well as a deficiency of other metabolities that depend on the tyrosine-to-melanin sequence; and (3) inhibition of other metabolic processes by the abnormal accumulation of phenylalanine and its residues. It seems reasonably certain, however, that the cutaneous and ocular hypopigmentation results from competitive inhibition of tyrosinase activity by excessive phenylalanine, thus compounding the lack of melanin substrate. Phenylketonuria is usually diagnosed soon after birth, since it has been routine pediatric practice since the 1960s in the United States to study the urine or capillary blood of newborn infants for the presence of phenylketones.

Any abnormal test result must be followed up by a plasma phenylalanine assay after there has been normal protein ingestion for several days. In untreated PKU patients this level is always greater than 16mg/100ml. Dietary restriction of phenylalanine has been successful in preventing the clinical manifestations of this disease in most patients. When the mother is affected, in utero exposure to phenylalanine levels equal to or greater than 20mg/100ml results in a 92 percent incidence of mental retardation, a 73 percent incidence of microcephaly, and a 10 percent incidence of cardiac defects [242, 245]. Therefore, affected women who wish to bear children must follow a strict low-phenylalanine diet [245, 283].

In untreated symptomatic patients PKU results in neurologic abnormalities including mental retardation, epilepsy, agitated behavior, hyperkinesia, tremors, muscular hypertonia, hyperactive tendon reflexes, inability to talk and walk, and microcephaly. There is decreased pigmentation in the brain, locus ceruleus, and substantia nigra [55]. Eczema is found in about 25 to 50 percent of the cases [248]. High myopia with choroidosis was observed in one case [85]. The irides are blue in about 70 percent of the cases. Cutaneous and hair pigmentation are normal at birth, but lighten in the first few weeks of life in two-thirds of untreated cases.

About 1 to 3 percent of infants with PKU fail to respond clinically to dietary restriction of phenylalanine. These infants lack the enzyme dihydropteridine reductase, which is needed for the regeneration of the tetrahydrobiopterin cofactor of phenylalanine hydroxylase. This cofactor is also essential in the hydroxylation of tryptophan to 5-hydroxytryptophan and of tyrosine to L-dopa. These biochemical deficits are believed to be responsible for the progressive and severe neurologic deficits and seizures seen in this PKU variant, which has been termed malignant hyperphenylalaninemia since most children die within the first few years of life. Dietary treatment has been attempted with tetrahydrobiopterin and the neurotransmitters hydroxytryptophan and levodopa [59].

Hair Bulb Tyrosine-Test-Negative Albinoidism. *Menkes' kinky-hair syndrome* is an X-linked recessive disease that is believed to occur in 1 in 35,000 live births [58]. It is characterized by failure to gain weight, myoclonic seizures, and opisthotonos, which develop within the first 2 months of life. Hair color and texture are usually normal at birth, but the hair soon becomes "metallic" white with a twisted kinky configuration termed pili torti. Rarely, the hair abnormality is present at birth. Blindness owing to optic nerve atrophy with tortuosity of the retinal blood vessels develops along with neurologic signs of neuronal degeneration and demyelination [52]. Histopathologic examination reveals decreased numbers of retinal ganglion cells and nerve fibers in the optic tract and microcysts in the iris pigment epithelium [252]. The exact biochemical defect is unknown: Affected patients have low serum copper and ceruloplasmin levels, increased copper uptake and intracellular copper levels in cultured fibroblasts, but decreased copper content in liver, basal ganglia, and cerebral cortex tissues. Prenatal diagnosis is possible by studying copper incorporation in cultured fibroblasts. Copper serves as a coenzyme in a number of enzyme systems including tyrosinase and lysyl oxidase, which are essential for proper cross-link formation in elastin and collagen tissues [117]. Resulting malformation of collagen and elastin is believed to result in a cascade of multisystemic effects including impaired internal elastic laminae of blood vessels, osteoporosis because of impaired bone collagen formation, optic atrophy, and cerebral and cerebellar degeneration. Death occurs within the first 3 years of life. Attempts at copper replacement therapy have been unsuccessful in the treatment of this disease.

CUTANEOUS HYPOPIGMENTARY DISORDERS
WITHOUT DEAFNESS

Various disorders involving pigment defects of the skin and its appendages are generally free of ocular defects; however, sporadic cases include ocular abnormalities.

Incontinentia pigmenti achromians (hypomelanosis of Ito) is a rare disorder of uncertain inheritance in which jagged swirls of hypopigmentation develop in the trunk and extremities soon after birth or during childhood. In late childhood there is a tendency towards repigmentation. In the few familial cases reported, autosomal dominant inheritance seems probable. Of the initial 36 reported cases, females had been affected four times as frequently as males, but this ratio is decreasing with increased recognition of cases. Histologic study of the hypopigmented skin shows a decreased number of melanocytes. Multisystem abnormalities of the eyes, central nervous system, hair, and teeth are present in 43 percent of cases [137, 231].

Ocular findings have included strabismus, tessellated fundus [113], exotropia [67], hypertelorism, corneal opacification, equivocal optic atrophy, myopia, choroidal atrophy, ptosis, papillary dislocation [137], and heterochromia iridis [231].

Hypopigmentation-immunodeficiency disease is an autosomal recessive disorder in which generalized pigment dilution is associated with multiple deficiencies of immune function [29, 112, 239]. Affected individuals have pale gray skin and silver gray hair. Cutaneous melanocytes contain numerous melanin granules but lack normal dendrites, and only a few isolated melanosomes can be identified in adjacent keratinocytes. One patient was reported to have depigmented spots on the retina, but there are no reports of photophobia or nystagmus.

Piebaldism (partial albinism) is an autosomal dominant trait in which melanocytes are missing in localized hypopigmented patches. Eye involvement is rare but has been reported in the form of heterochromia iridis [50]. The underlying mechanism of this disease is either a failure of melanocyte migration to target organs or a failure of melanocyte survival in the hypopigmented areas.

Vitiligo is a condition in which there is an acquired patchy destruction of the cutaneous, ocular, otic, and leptomeningeal melanocytes. Vitiligo occurs in about 1 percent of the general population [155]. Both sporadic and familial cases have occurred, and several authors believe that vitiligo is inherited as an autosomal dominant trait [154, 168] in which either precipitating stress factors are necessary for phenotypic expression or a mutant gene controlling melanocyte function in discrete clones of cells is activated [110]. Manifestations include halo nevi and early graying of hair (poliosis). Depigmentation may be localized or generalized or rarely may even become universal. Symmetrical loss of pigment is frequently seen in generalized involvement, and similar patterns of pigment loss have been seen in identical twins. Spontaneous repigmentation occurs in a small percentage of patients. Therapy consisting of oral or topical psoralen together with exposure to ultraviolet light has been followed by repigmentation in 30 percent of treated patients. However, often treatment causes hyperpigmentation of the surrounding normal skin with a worse appearance than seen before therapy. Vitiligo has been associated in a minority of affected patients with several autoimmune diseases including pernicious anemia, alopecia areata, and the complex of Addison's disease, idiopathic hypoparathyroidism, and thyroid disease. It is seen in association with malignant melanoma [3] or, rarely, other malignancies.

Periocular involvement consists of external eyelid, eyebrow, and eyelash depigmentation or, more rarely, alopecia areata of the eyebrows and eyelashes. Vitiligo can include depigmentation of the fundus and sometimes the irides as well. Ocular involvement is usually seen in patients with cutaneous involvement, but in some cases the changes are confined to the eyes [3, 4].

Vogt-Koyanagi-Harada syndrome is a rare complex consisting of uveitis, alopecia, vitiligo, poliosis, tinnitus, and deafness. It often presents with a febrile episode, headache, and other neurologic symptoms suggesting meningoencephalitis. Spinal fluid examination has shown increased mononuclear cells and elevated protein levels. Initial eye findings include iridocyclitis, which usually quickly subsides, and choroiditis, which tends to be patchy and recurrent. The optic disc may become hyperemic and the veins engorged. The choroiditis has been associated with serous exudative retinal detachment and formation of a coarse irregular retinal pigment epithelial pattern. The uveitis clears in about 50 percent of patients, and then the retinal detachment subsides. Complications can include glaucoma, cataract, and phthisis bulbi. If only posterior eye disease is present, this disease is termed Harada's syndrome; this pattern is more frequent among Hispanic populations, while the complete syndrome is most frequent in Orientals and Filipinos. An immunogenetic mechanism with uveal pigment sensitivity is believed responsible for this syndrome complex [77, 148]. The meningeal irritation present in Harada's and Vogt-Koyanagi syndromes may result from destruction of melanocytes in the leptomeninges. Destruction of pigment cells with release of those cells' products may evoke an immunologic response in which antibodies are produced against pigment cells. When ocular pigment cells are involved, this immune mechanism could account for uveitis or sympathetic ophthalmia [156, 162, 181].

Neuroectodermal melanosomal disease is a rare congenital condition seen in three families in which consanguineous marriages had occurred. The disease consists of severe hypotonia, seizures, mental retardation, failure to thrive, and death in early childhood. Affected children have blue irides, silver gray hair, and general skin hypopigmentation. One of the three affected children had severe myopia. Electron microscope studies re-

veal abnormal hypomelanized and clumped melanosomes, which are not transferred to keratinocytes [72], and abnormal inclusion bodies in fibroblasts, bone marrow histiocytes, and lymphocytes. Familial patterns suggest that the disease is due to a single autosomal recessive gene with pleiotropic effects on neuroectodermal and mesodermal structures.

CUTANEOUS HYPOPIGMENTATION
WITH DEAFNESS

Several syndromes exist in which cutaneous hypopigmentation, either patchy or generalized, is associated with hearing loss. This is to be expected since melanocytes migrate to the inner ear during embryologic development and are essential for the proper development of inner ear structures. These syndromes have been reviewed by Witkop [280], and several of them have been associated with ocular abnormalities.

Waardenburg's syndrome exists in two genetic variants, type I and type II, both of which show an autosomal dominant inheritance pattern. These syndromes are a special form of piebaldism. Both type I and type II show a highly variable expressivity and incomplete penetrance. Type I includes dystopia canthorum, which is absent in type II. Unilateral or bilateral deafness occurs in 20 percent of affected persons and is more frequent in type II. Eyebrows are confluent in 50 percent of cases. A white forelock occurs in 20 to 40 percent of cases, depigmented skin patches in 15 percent, and heterochromia iridis or blue eyes in 25 percent. Albinotic fundi are occasionally seen. The variation in fundus pigment in most of these patients follows the pigmentary pattern in the iris. When the iris is hypopigmented, the ipsilateral fundus is usually also hypopigmented. When a sector of the iris is light, the corresponding sector in the fundus is often found to be similarly light. In an area of retinal hypopigmentation the choroidal vessels stand out sharply. The decrease in retinal pigment apparently does not reduce visual acuity or cause changes in the electroretinogram [101].

In four families Hirschsprung aganglionic megacolon has been seen in association with Waardenburg's syndrome [187]. A failure of migration or survival of neural crest cells during embryonic development is the probable cause of the pleiotropism seen in this syndrome.

Pseudo-Waardenburg syndrome is a name given to a tetrad of findings suggestive of a cervical sympathetic lesion: ptosis, meiosis, heterochromia, and unilateral facial atrophy associated with deafness [280]. The deafness in one reported case could have been congenital or due to a 5-day course of streptomycin at the age of 5 months. There was no family history of deafness, dystopia, heterochromia, or a white forelock in the affected patient [193].

Waardenburg ocular albinoidism [280] was described by Bard in one family [13]. The 4 affected patients had findings of Waardenburg's syndrome type II associated with fundal pigmented defects, foveal hypoplasia, and transilluminable irides. All had amblyopia and either esophoria or esotropia. None had photophobia or nystagmus.

Ziprowski-Margolis syndrome is an X-linked disease described in a Moroccan Jewish family [287]. Affected individuals had congenital sensorineural deafness and were albinotic at birth except for slight pigmentation of the gluteal and scrotal areas. These areas darkened during childhood, and new pigmented spots appeared, giving the patients a leopardlike appearance. Within the hypopigmented areas, melanocytes were weakly dopa positive; they were strongly positive in the pigmented areas. Ocular findings included heterochromia iridis and one patient with blue eyes. The fundi were normally pigmented; there was no dystopia canthorum or hyperplasia of the nasal base [287].

MISCELLANEOUS CUTANEOUS DISORDERS WITH HAIR HYPOPIGMENTATION

Hypomelanosis affecting the hair in the form of premature canities (graying) or poliosis (focal hypomelanosis) can occur in various syndromes of disparate causation. The syndromes that also manifest ocular involvement are listed in Table 19-2.

Hyperpigmentation Disorders

Cutaneous disorders with primary hyperpigmentation, either localized or generalized, are often associated with extracutaneous malformations [93]. The disorders reviewed here are limited to those with ocular involvement.

INCONTINENTIA PIGMENTI

Incontinentia pigmenti is a hereditary disorder that affects the eye, skin, teeth, hair, nails, skeletal system, heart, and central nervous system.

Its mode of inheritance is probably that of an X-linked trait, lethal in the majority of males [38, 276]. As a result, the disease is extremely uncommon among living males, and female carriers tend to have a 25 percent incidence of aborted pregnancies.

The cutaneous lesions are usually present at birth or shortly afterward and undergo three identifiable morphologic stages. The initial lesions are linearly arranged inflammatory blisters that usually are succeeded in the second to sixth week of life by dark, warty outgrowths. The verrucous lesions then resolve, forming flat, hyperpigmented lines arranged in a strange whorled or feathered pattern. The hyperpigmentation appears generally between the twelfth and twenty-sixth week of life and may remain for many years. Histologic examination reveals intraepidermal eosinophilic vesicles and dermal eosinophilic perivascular infiltrates in the first stage; acanthosis, papillomatosis, dyskeratosis, and hyperkeratosis in the second stage; and extensive deposits of melanin within melanophages in the upper dermis in the third stage. In all three stages macrophages can be found containing dystrophic cells, melanosome complexes, or both within their cytoplasm. Numerous Schwann's cells phagocytosing melanosomes are found at the basal lamina in both the second and third stages [228]. These linear skin lesions are mostly on the trunk and limbs. Localized alopecia, hair hypoplasia, and nail abnormalities may also be present.

The cutaneous lesions of incontinentia pigmenti are self-limiting and require only symptomatic treatment during the bullous and warty phases of the disease. During the vesicular stage concomitant leukocytosis (as high as 43,000 cells) and eosinophilia (as high as 65%) are found in seventy-five percent of patients [38].

Incontinentia pigmenti is complicated by faulty dentition in 65 percent of patients and abnormalities of the central nervous system in 31 percent of patients.

Affected patients require regular ophthalmologic examinations.

Ocular abnormalities occur in about 35 percent of affected patients and are severe enough in 8 percent to result in blindness of one or both eyes [84]. Another 10 percent of patients have considerable loss of vision because of cataracts, retinitis proliferans, retrolental fibroplasia (without neonatal oxygen therapy), metastatic ophthalmia, chorioretinitis, uveitis, pseudoglioma, retinal detachment, optic nerve atrophy, or a combination

Table 19-2. *Miscellaneous Dermatologic Syndromes with Hair Pigment Loss and Ocular Manifestations*

Syndrome	Epidemiology	Eye Involvement	General Involvement
Fanconi's syndrome	Idiopathic or associated with cystinosis, Lowe's syndrome, tyrosinemia, Wilson's disease, galactosemia, and hereditary fructose intolerance	With cystinosis: deposits of soluble cystine crystals in the conjunctiva, cornea, sclera, and choroid; cornea is cloudy owing to crystal deposition, especially at periphery; with Lowe's syndrome: glaucoma	Renal tubular dysfunction with hypophosphatemic rickets; glucosuria; aminoaciduria; fair hair and skin
Rothmund-Thomson syndrome	Recessive	Cataracts	Poikiloderma; alopecia; photosensitivity; hypogonadism
Myotonia dystrophica	Dominant	Cataracts; retinal degenerative changes	Myotonia; muscle wasting; premature frontal balding
Werner's syndrome	Recessive	Cataracts; retinal degenerative changes	Premature aging; sclerodermatous skin changes; atherosclerosis
Progeria	Sporadic	Prominent eyes; infrequent: cataracts	Premature aging; sparse hair
Seckel's syndrome	Recessive	Prominent eyes; possible strabismus	Bird-headed dwarfism; baldness; hypopigmented skin macules
Treacher Collins (Franceschetti's) syndrome	Dominant	Lower lid coloboma; microphthalmos; antimongoloid slanting of lids with downward collapse of lateral orbital tissue	Micrognathia; small jaw; malformed ears and conduction deafness
Pierre Robin syndrome	Sporadic	Congenital glaucoma; cataracts; myopia; esotropia, retinal detachment; microphthalmos	Micrognathia; glossoptosis; isolated cleft palate
Hallermann-Streiff syndrome	Sporadic	Microphthalmos; cataracts; nystagmus; strabismus; blue	Mandibulofacial dysostosis
Tyrosinuria	Recessive	Corneal lesions and thickening of conjunctival epithelium	Erosive hyperkeratotic lesions of the palms and soles
Down's syndrome	1 : 1000 live births, mosaicism for trisomy 21 common; trisomy 21 or translocation of a D or G group chromosome to chromosome 21	Brushfield's spots; strabismus; keratoconus; cataract; epicanthus; mongoloid slant to palpebral fissures; hypoplasia of iris; esotropia; ectropion	Normal to typical Down's syndrome phenotype

of these problems. It is postulated that retinal vascular changes and abnormalities of the retinal pigment epithelium lead to the above changes with resultant loss of vision. The vascular abnormalities follow a pattern of ectasia, microhemorrhage, avascularity, hypoxia, retinitis, and atrophy [38]. In one case histologic study of an enucleated blind eye with retinal detachment showed alternate areas of depigmentation and hyperpigmentation in the retinal pigment epithelium and a placoid, multilayered, occasionally nodular proliferation of the retinal pigment cells. Pigment granules were present among the sheets of the pigment epithelium. Nevoid patches or pigmentary mottling of the retina have also been reported in cases without retinal detachment. These findings indicate that the same inflammatory process that affects the cutaneous melanocytes also affects the retinal melanocytes [23].

Strabismus occurs in 18 percent and nystagmus in 5 percent of affected patients. Rare associations include glaucoma and blue sclera.

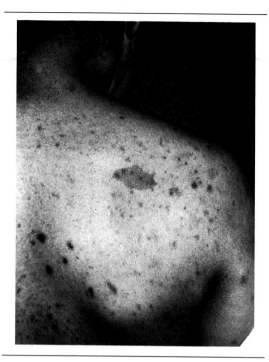

Fig. 19-1. *Multiple café au lait spots in neurofibromatosis.*

CAFÉ AU LAIT SPOTS

A flat localized area of cutaneous hyperpigmentation, usually light brown (like coffee with milk, or café au lait), may become the focus of attention in a given patient. These lesions are generally uniform in color (although much darker in blacks than in whites). Their significance varies with the family history, associated findings, size, shape, and number. The incidence of these café au lait spots (CLS) in the general population is about 10 percent. In individuals with peripheral neurofibromatosis the incidence of CLS is 90 to 100 percent; CLS numbering more than six or those greater than 3 cm are found in neurofibromatosis (Fig. 19-1). CLS may occur also in tuberous sclerosis, Albright's syndrome (35% of patients), Watson's syndrome (60%), Russell-Silver dwarfism (45%), leopard syndrome (see below under Lentiginoses) (38%), Westerhof's syndrome, Lescke's disease, Cowden's disease, basal cell nevus syndrome, Gaucher's disease, Hunter's syndrome, Bloom's syndrome, ataxia-telangiectasia, and the epidermal nevus syndrome.

There is *no specific* histologic nor ultrastructural marker differentiating CLS of normal individuals from those found in individuals with diseases such as Albright's syndrome or neurofibromatosis [189]. All CLS reveal increased numbers of melanocytes and basal layer melanization.

Giant pigment granules can frequently be found in CLS of adult neurofibromatosis patients but may be absent, especially in affected children. These giant pigment granules are nonspecific, being sometimes found in normal human epidermis, Albright's syndrome, leopard syndrome, speckled lentiginous nevus, and melanocytic nevi [174].

ALKAPTONURIA (OCHRONOSIS)

Alkaptonuria, inherited as an autosomal recessive trait, is a disorder in the metabolism of phenylalanine and tyrosine caused by a lack of the enzyme homogentisic acid oxidase, with the result that homogentisic acid accumulates. The oxidation and polymerization of homogentisic acid produces a dark ochronotic pigment. After a number of decades, deep black pigmentary changes develop in the cartilage, skin, tendons, and sclerae. The brown pigment is deposited in those areas of the skin that are richest in sweat gland ducts. The sweat may stain the clothes. Arthropathic changes are prominent. Prostatic and renal calculi are frequent complications.

Alkaptonuria, a rare disease, is more common

among Slovaks, in whom the incidence is estimated at 1 in 25,000, than in other groups [251].

Ocular deposition of pigment occurs in the sclera, conjunctiva, and limbic cornea. On electron microscopic examination the pigment granules are extracellular, attaching to collagen fibers and fibrinocytes [142]. For the ophthalmologist the pigmented sclerae may present a diagnostic challenge, since they so much resemble dermal oculomelanocytosis (nevus of Ota) and, sometimes, senile hyaline plaques of the sclera. In Srsen's series of 126 patients, the earliest sign of scleral pigmentation was seen in a 14-year-old girl [250]. The ocular findings have been reviewed by François [85]. In ochronosis the sclerae and conjunctivae may have black bilateral pigmentation. Well-circumscribed golden brown to black deposits can occur at the periphery of Bowman's membrane and in the superficial layers of the cornea near the limbus [65]. The diagnosis is made by finding the pigment elsewhere (in cartilaginous areas of the body), and by the late onset of the disease, a family history of ochronosis, and the coexistence of arthritis. Alkalized urine from these individuals will turn brown after exposure to air for 5 minutes [250].

B-K MOLE SYNDROME (FAMILIAL ATYPICAL MULTIPLE MOLE MELANOMA; FAMM'S SYNDROME)

The B-K mole syndrome is inherited as an autosomal dominant trait. Affected patients develop many dysplastic melanocytic nevi, predominantly on the upper trunk and extremities, during their teens or early adulthood. New lesions continue to appear throughout adult life, and these dysplastic nevi are at a very high risk of transformation into malignant melanomas. On clinical examination, these nevi are 5- to 15-mm macular lesions of various shades of tan, brown, red, and black, with irregular borders, and sometimes a red halo. Often, part of a dysplastic nevus is papular. Histologically these lesions resemble compound melanocytic nevi, but the nevus cells are atypical, and a heavy lymphocytic infiltrate with capillary proliferation is found in the surrounding tissue [43]. When there is no familial history of these lesions, the condition is termed dysplastic nevus syndrome. Cutaneous melanomas in affected patients can also arise de novo in addition to developing within dysplastic nevi. For ophthalmologists the importance of this syndrome lies in

these patients' probable increased propensity for development of ocular melanomas [1].

NEVUS OF OTA (OCULODERMAL MELANOCYTOSIS; NEVUS FUSCOCERULEUS OPHTHALMOMAXILLARIS)

Nevus of Ota is a congenital pigmentary disorder presenting as an ill-defined brown to blue-gray to blue-black hyperpigmentation in the distribution of the maxillary and ophthalmic branches of the fifth cranial nerve. The cutaneous hyperpigmentation is clinically apparent in the first year of life in about 60 percent of cases and has a delayed onset during adolescence or rarely in the twenties in the remainder of affected individuals. The pigmentation persists throughout life, and individuals with neonatal onset tend to have a darkening of their lesions during puberty. Histologic examination reveals that this hyperpigmentation is due to the presence of melanocytes in the upper dermis with rare hypermelanization of the epidermal basal layer. Melanosis oculi occurs in two-thirds of patients with cutaneous involvement [122], and it has been proposed that the finding of melanosis oculi without cutaneous involvement be considered a variant of nevus of Ota [192]. The ocular hyperpigmentation most commonly affects the sclera but can extend to the conjunctiva, subconjunctival connective tissue, Tenon's capsule, iris, choroid, retina, optic nerve, and the muscles and connective and fatty tissue of the orbit. Central nervous system involvement can include the pineal gland and the leptomeninges. The hyperpigmentation is bilateral in about 5 percent of cases; occasionally, the hyperpigmentation extends to the palate, tongue, gums, buccal mucosa, pharynx, nasal mucosa, concha auriculae, external ear canal, and tympanic membrane [122, 171, 213]. Ipsilateral sensorineural deafness has been reported with an extensive unilateral lesion, and bilateral hearing loss with a bilateral lesion [94]. Glaucoma is commonly associated with the melanosis oculi [122, 171], and malignant melanoma of the skin, eye, or brain is a rare association [213]. Several case reports exist of neurologic and vascular disorders being associated with nevus of Ota: Sturge-Weber syndrome [183], Sturge-Weber syndrome with multiple gastrointestinal hemangiomas [215], Sturge-Weber syndrome with Klippel-Trenaunay syndrome [94], spinocerebellar degeneration [205], and familial cerebellar degeneration with slow eye movement [275] and Takayasu arteritis [144].

A hereditary influence is suggested by the increased frequency of this lesion among Orientals. This disorder has been variously presumed to be due to either faulty migration of melanocytes from the neural crest or to a persistence of fetal dermal melanocytes. The incidence of this disorder in Orientals varies from 2 to 8 in 1,000. The rate of consanguinity among parents of affected Japanese individuals is about the same as seen in the general Japanese population, so that autosomal recessive inheritance is unlikely [122]. Familial cases have been reported. In Hidano and colleagues' series, affected children in two families had lesions symmetrical to those seen in their parents [122].

LENTIGINOSES

Lentiginoses are dermatologic syndromes characterized by lentigines (well-defined hyperpigmented macules). Histologically lentigines are characterized by elongated rete ridges, increased numbers of basal melanocytes, and basal melanization.

Generalized lentigines with concomitant nystagmus and strabismus is an autosomal dominant syndrome described in 8 individuals belonging to three generations of a Maltese-Lebanese family. The lentigines were present on the entire body including the ears, eyelids, lips, and palms, and their onset varied from 4 to 10 years of age. There was no hyperpigmentation of the conjunctivae, sclerae, or fundi. Six affected individuals had nystagmus, and three exhibited strabismus. Neither ocular problem was found in unaffected family members [200].

Peutz-Jeghers syndrome is an autosomal dominant syndrome consisting of hamartomatous gastrointestinal polyps associated with lentiginosis. Fewer than 50 percent of affected patients have relatives with both features, and *formes frustes* may exist with lentigines or polyps alone [14]. The incidence is estimated at 1 in 200,000 population. The lentigines are present in periorificial areas (lips and buccal mucosa in 96% of affected patients) and also frequently on the palms, soles, and conjunctivae. The lentigines appear in infancy and early childhood and precede the onset of gastrointestinal symptoms. The polyps undergo malignant degeneration in 13 percent of affected patients [266], but pain, bleeding, intussusception, and obstruction are common complications. About 10 percent of affected women have ovarian tumors, and polyps are sometimes present in other organs, for example, nose and bladder.

Leopard syndrome (multiple lentigines syndrome) is a rare autosomal dominant syndrome of variable expressivity whose acronym stands for its cardinal features: multiple lentigines (*l*), electrocardiographic abnormalities (*e*), ocular hypertelorism (*o*), pulmonary stenosis (*p*), genital abnormalities (*a*), growth retardation (*r*), and neurosensory deafness (*d*). One or two café au lait macules and axillary freckling may be present. The distribution of lentigines is densest on the face, neck, and upper chest, although the entire skin surface is involved. The lentigines vary from pinpoint to several centimeters in size and spare the mucous membranes [182]. Lentigines are not a constant finding, and severe deafness is present in 15 percent of affected patients. Leopard syndrome in the absence of lentigines has to be differentiated from Noonan's syndrome, which includes ocular hypertelorism, ptosis, short stature, pulmonary stenosis, cryptorchidism, and delayed sexual maturation.

Ocular examination of some patients affected by leopard syndrome has revealed multiple small white punctate and comma-shaped lenticular opacities. These usually appear in the third decade and do not impair visual acuity for at least 20 years [129].

EPIDERMAL (KERATINOCYTIC) NEVI AND TUMORS

Basal Cell Nevus Syndrome

Ocular changes in the basal cell nevus syndrome are not so frequent as those found in the skin, skeleton, and central nervous system [109], but they may be serious enough to be chronic, requiring an ophthalmologist's continual care. The syndrome is transmitted as an autosomal dominant trait, which is usually fully penetrant. Affected individuals may show mental retardation and have a broad face. About 40 percent of affected patients have ocular hypertelorism. The development of the teeth may be complicated by odontogenic cysts. The hands are short and flat, with shortening of the fourth metacarpals. There are frequently asymptomatic bifid or missing ribs. The falx cerebri is calcified in nearly all patients. Medulloblastomas have been observed in a few patients within the first 2 years of life.

The cutaneous findings are most striking and are the greatest source of distress for the patient. At about adolescence in affected individuals, papillomas and small nodules begin to develop on the

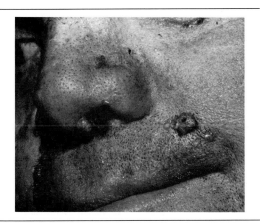

Fig. 19-2. *Basal cell nevus syndrome.*

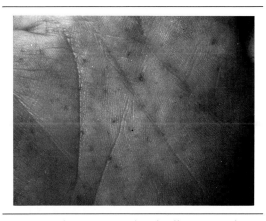

Fig. 19-3. *Palmar "pits" in basal cell nevus syndrome.*

face, neck, ears, scalp, arms, chest, and back (Fig. 19-2). These lesions may vary in shape and size, from a small pearly excrescence to a large cauliflower-like tumor. Histologically, the lesions are basal cell epitheliomas. These are aggressive tumors; affected individuals even in their thirties have been known to develop more than 300 basal cell epitheliomas. Exposure to ultraviolet light or ionizing radiation results in an increased number of these tumors.

Frequently, the eyelids and periorbital skin are studded with tumors. Milia are also present around the eyes. Punctate depressions ("pits") may be found on the palms (Fig. 19-3). Multicentric basal cell carcinomas can arise within the palmar pits [128].

Ocular complications including direct involvement of the orbit by tumor [78] and congenital blindness or partial loss of vision caused by corneal dystrophy, cataracts, strabismus, glaucoma, and colobomas of the choroid and optic nerve occur in about one-third of patients. Deformities of the sella turcica and vertebral column, genital infantilism, and ovarian fibromas and cysts have also been described in the basal cell nevus syndrome.

The following extracutaneous malignant tumors have been reported in affected patients: medulloblastomas, fibrosarcomas of the palate or maxilla, malignant melanomas of the iris, congenital rhabdomyosarcomas, and adenocarcinoma of the colon.

Cytogenetic studies of cultured fibroblasts have revealed an increased number of spontaneous chromosomal breaks [115].

Cowden's Disease (Multiple Hamartoma and Neoplasia Syndrome)

Cowden's disease is a rare multisystem disease transmitted in an autosomal dominant fashion with incomplete penetrance and variable expressivity [227]. Characteristic mucocutaneous lesions include

1. Facial 1- to 5-mm papules with a predilection for the centrofacial and periorificial area (83% of patients). On histologic examination these lesions are trichilemmomas.
2. Oral mucosal papillomatosis (83% of patients), which histologically are benign fibromas.
3. Acral keratosis (63% of patients).
4. Palmar and plantar keratosis (42% of patients).

Histologically, examination of the keratoses shows nonspecific or thokeratosis, hypergranulosis, and acanthosis. The multiple extracutaneous hamartomas that have been reported include fibrocystic breast disease, thyroid goiters and adenomas, multiple polyposis of the gastrointestinal tract, and ovarian cysts. High-arched palate occurs in 15 percent of patients and adenoid facies in 11 percent. In a series of 46 patients, 52 percent of the women and 23.8 percent of the men developed malignancies. Breast carcinoma was reported in 36 percent and thyroid carcinoma in 12 percent of affected women. Three patients had primary malignant neoplasms in more than one organ system.

Ocular findings have included cataracts, glaucoma, retinal gliomas, drusen, and, in one case, bilateral angioid streaks [6].

Epidermal Nevus Syndrome

Epidermal nevi are a group of tumors consisting primarily of the keratin-producing cells (keratinocytes) of the epidermis. Most of these leions are present at birth or appear soon thereafter. They may take several forms: small warty papules arranged in a stringlike distribution; large, linear, scaly, streaky plaques involving 50 percent or more of the body surface (also called ichthyosis hystrix); long, unilateral, pigmented, warty streaks involving a limb or two (nevus unius lateris); and a large cerebriform verrucous lesion involving the scalp and extending onto the face and bulbar conjunctiva (sebaceous nevus of Jadassohn). In a highly significant number of these cases there are associated skeletal and central nervous system anomalies. These associations with epidermal nevi have recently been reviewed [247], and the constellation of these findings has been called the epidermal nevus syndrome.

A variety of ocular changes have been seen in approximately one-third of patients with this condition. The most common ocular involvement consists of extension of the epidermal nevus to the eyelid, lid margin, and conjunctiva. On the conjunctival surface, the nevus becomes vascular and proliferative and can interfere with lid closure. Other ocular abnormalities found are as follows:

Periorbital and orbital tissue hypertrophy (but no exophthalmos) associated with hemihypertrophy of the rest of the body.

Dermoid tumors of the bulbar conjunctiva. The tumors examined histologically contained elements of lacrimal glands, vascular tissue, nerves, cartilage, smooth muscle, bone, epidermis, sebaceous glands, hair, collagen, and apocrine ductal tissue.

Ectopic lacrimal glands; colobomas of lids, iris, choroid, and retina; corneal opacity and pannus formation; oculomotor dysfunction; nystagmus and cortical blindness; and coexistent portwine hemangioma of the face, including the upper lid.

The means of genetic transmission is not clear. In a few cases a similar process may have existed in other family members, which suggests an autosomal dominant form of transmission [247].

DYSPLASTIC DISEASES

A number of genetically transmitted diseases result in poorly developed skin and ocular defects as well as in other ectodermal and mesodermal malformations. The causes or mechanisms of these processes are unknown, but they have enough in common for them to be grouped together for purposes of discussion.

Rothmund-Thomson Syndrome (Congenital Poikiloderma)

Rothmund-Thomson syndrome is a very rare congenital multisystem disorder [109]. Genetic heterogeneity is suggested by the available case reports. The syndrome is sometimes inherited in an autosomal recessive fashion; several of the reported 65 patients have been the product of a consanguineous marriage. However, in one Canadian family with three affected children and no unaffected children, the parents were of Swiss-Italian and of German, Scottish, and Canadian Indian ancestry, with no history of consanguineous marriages. Two boys and one girl showed the complete syndrome, and no ancestors were affected, which suggests autosomal dominant transmission of a mutant gene. A preponderance of affected females (70% of affected patients) has been noted, but the reason for this is unknown.

The cutaneous lesions are the most constant feature of the syndrome. The initial changes, usually observed between the third and sixth month of life, consist of plaques of erythema and edema that are most prominent on the face but may also appear on the ears, buttocks, and extremities. This eruption is superseded by a macular and reticular erythema, atrophic lesions, scarring, linear telangiectases, and hyper- and hypopigmentation. Photosensitivity, although not a universal finding, may cause exacerbation of existing lesions and result in the formation of bullae during early childhood. Scalp hair, eyebrows, and eyelashes may be sparse or absent. The nails are often dystrophic and the dentition faulty. Bony defects include abnormalities of the skull, shortening of the long bones, body asymmetry, absence of bones, and roentgenographic changes resembling those of chondrodystrophy. Short stature, hypogonadism, and mental retardation have also been noted occasionally.

Developmental cataracts are present in 75 percent of the patients. The usual age at onset is 3 to 7 years; however, lenticular opacities have been detected in the first few months of life. Cataracts are bilateral, complete, and semisolid and evolve rapidly over a period of weeks. When observed, the cataracts initially are posterior or anterior subcapsular opacities that soon involve the nucleus and proceed to total opacity. Band-shaped degenerative lesions of the cornea, at times preceding surgical intervention for cataracts, have been reported in a few cases [240]. Keratoconus, iris anomalies, amblyopia with tilted optic disks, strabismus, and microcornea have also been reported [145]. Aneurysmal dilatations of the retinal veins have been described in one patient with probable Rothmund-Thomson syndrome [258].

Werner's Syndrome (Adult Progeria)

Werner's syndrome is a rare heritable disorder of which about 50 cases have been reported [198]. It is clinically similar to the Rothmund-Thomson syndrome but has its onset after adolescence. There is no sexual predilection, and the high incidence of consanguineous marriage in families of affected individuals suggests an autosomal recessive mode of inheritance.

Patients with the Werner's syndrome usually experience the first manifestations of their disease during the second decade. Short stature resulting from early cessation of growth and atrophy of the muscles and subcutaneous tissue, and graying and loss of scalp, body, and pubic hair contribute to an impression of premature senility. In addition to sclerodermatous fibrosis of the subcutaneous tissue, progressive changes consisting of atrophy, telangiectasia, and hyperkeratosis cause the skin to appear stretched and adherent to underlying structures; indolent, painful ulcers occur over pressure points, particularly on the distal extremities. Tautness of the facial skin, combined with recession of the chin, beaking of the nose, and microstomia, results in a birdlike facies.

Other prominent findings include hypogonadism (representing regression of sexual maturation after a relatively normal puberty) and infertility, diabetes (which is usually mild and nonketotic), a high-pitched voice, generalized atherosclerosis, osteoporosis, calcification of the aorta and coronary arteries, and osteoarthritis of the peripheral joints. An increased incidence of neoplasia, particularly of the sarcomatous type, has also been noted.

Diabetes mellitus occurs in 45 percent of patients; however, neither the vascular disease nor the cataracts seen in this syndrome are explained by the diabetes. Senile cataracts, the most frequent ocular manifestations, initially appear as homogeneous or striate posterior cortical and subcapsular opacities. They have a sudden onset during the third or fourth decade. Cataract surgery

may be complicated by bullous keratopathy and degenerative corneal changes with loss of vision. Blue sclera, retinal lesions, and telangiectatic irides have been observed in a small number of patients. The retinal lesions have consisted of retinitis pigmentosa, senile macular degeneration, and chorioretinitis.

The life span of patients with the Werner's syndrome is decreased. Sister chromatid exchanges in cultured lymphocytes from an affected patient have been normal. Cultured fibroblasts from these patients have shown a reduced capacity for mitotic division [184].

Hallermann-Streiff Syndrome (Oculomandibulofacial Dyscephaly)

The salient features of the Hallermann-Streiff syndrome are (1) malformations of the skull and face, (2) dental abnormalities, (3) hypotrichosis, (4) anomalies of the eye, (5) dwarfism, and (6) motor, and occasional mental, retardation. The head is brachycephalic, the fontanelles may remain patent for long periods, and the facial skeleton is underdeveloped, with a pinched, hooked nose, a small jaw, microstomia, and a high-arched palate. The skin over the scalp, face, and particularly the nose exhibits striking atrophic changes, permitting increased visibility of the dermal vasculature. Thin, sparse hair, with frontal balding or patchy alopecia along the coronal and lambdoid sutures, and absence of the eyebrows and lashes are characteristic of this syndrome. Hypodontia, malformed teeth, and limited mobility of the temporomandibular joint are also frequently noted.

The anomalous changes encountered in the eyes are cataracts, microphthalmos, nystagmus, strabismus, and optic disc colobomas [88]. Rare findings include blue sclera, cloudy media, poor reactivity to light, underdeveloped irides, posterior synechiae of irides, and spontaneous rupture of cataract [76].

Degenerative retinal diseases, such as chorioretinal atrophy or peripapillary choroidal atrophy, have been reported in several cases [126].

A genetic causation has not been well established for this syndrome; however, a single mutant gene (dominant) has been postulated as the cause.

Dyskeratosis Congenita (Zinsser-Engman-Cole Syndrome)

Dyskeratosis congenita (DKC), a very rare syndrome reported almost exclusively in males, involves both ectodermal and mesodermal derivatives and has its onset in early childhood [109, 243]. It is clearly familial, since affected siblings have been described, and the few available pedigrees suggest genetic heterogeneity with X-linked recessive and autosomal recessive forms of this disorder. An autosomal dominant form has also been reported, but only in an abstract [232].

The initial manifestation is a severe nail dystrophy, which may result in complete destruction of the nail plate. Cutaneous changes, which appear simultaneously or later, consist of brownish gray reticulated hyperpigmentation, atrophy, and telangiectasia, most prominently on the neck, thorax, and arms. The dorsal skin on the hands and feet becomes atrophic, and, although the palms and soles may be thickened, there is often striking hyperhidrosis. Acrocyanosis develops in half of the affected patients. In almost 90 percent, blisters, erosions, and patches of leukoplakia occur on the mucous membranes of the mouth and may also affect the urogenital and anorectal tissues. The incidence of squamous cell carcinoma developing in areas of leukoplakia is high.

Similar lesions of the conjunctiva may obliterate the lacrimal puncta. Repeated blepharitis (causing ectropion, epiphora, and loss of cilia) and bullous conjunctivitis have also been noted. One affected individual had retinal atrophy with infarctions and hemorrhages. Another patient had pallor of the optic disc [243].

Of the numerous other associated defects that have been reported, the most common are retarded physical and mental development, dystrophic teeth, blood dyscrasias because of aplasia of the bone marrow, and a heightened susceptibility to infection. Affected individuals must be followed closely because of the possibility of a complicating malignancy. Two reported patients had multiple primary malignancies. This predisposition is presently unexplained. Cytologic studies of one affected patient have shown a sister chromatid exchange (SCE) rate (12.2 per mitosis) twice as high as that seen in 33 normal controls, which indicates chromosomal instability. However, several studies have shown no increase in chromosome breakage rates over those seen in normal controls [34]. The significance of increased SCE rate is not clearly understood. One theory is that SCE represents poorly repaired DNA damage. Experimental work with fibroblast cultures from two unrelated DKC patients has indicated slow repair of DNA cross-links formed by exposure of the cell cultures to ultraviolet light and psoralens [41].

Focal Dermal Hypoplasia (Goltz's Syndrome)

Goltz's syndrome, a rare disorder, is also one of combined ectodermal and mesodermal anomalies. The cutaneous lesions, probably the most outstanding identifying feature, are the result of defective development of the dermal tissue, a finding readily demonstrable on skin biopsy. Apparent at birth are asymmetric, irregular, linear streaks of hyperpigmentation, atrophy, and telangiectasia that may resemble scars. Also common are groups of soft, reddish yellow nodules, which represent herniation of the subcutaneous fat through an attenuated dermis; these lesions occur most frequently over the posterior thigh, groin, and iliac crest. Occasionally, there may be total absence of skin in localized areas. Multiple papillomas occur on the oral mucosa, lips, perianal skin, and genital mucosa. Hypotrichosis and dystrophic nails are usual manifestations.

Associated defects in this syndrome are manifold [109, 202] and will be mentioned only briefly. Physical and mental development are retarded, and asymmetry of the face, trunk, and limbs may be present. Skeletal anomalies include syndactyly, polydactyly, hemimelia, absent digits, microcrania, and spinal and pelvic deformities. Longitudinal striations in the metaphyseal areas of the long bones (osteopathic striae) on radiologic examination have been reported in 80 percent of cases. Microdontia, dysplastic or absent teeth, enamel defects, malocculusion, and a high-arched palate are the most frequent oral anomalies. A number of abnormalities of the soft tissues, such as protruding ears, hernias, and hypoplasia of the thenar and hypothenar eminences, may occur.

Ocular abnormalities, reported in 40 percent of affected patients [133, 261], include colobomas of the iris, retina, choroid, and optic nerve; microphthalmos; unilateral anophthalmia; aniridia; pupillary irregularities; subluxation of the lens; pigmentary changes of the retina; clouding of the vitreous and cornea; strabismus; nystagmus; ptosis; blue sclera; thickening of the conjunctiva; ectropion; and blockage of the lacrimal ducts. Photophobia is a common symptom. Many of the defects reflect abnormal ocular development during early gestation.

Of approximately 60 patients reported, all but 8 were girls. Unfortunately, there is little pedigree information available to substantiate a genetic causation. However, a few patients have had relatives with anomalies such as ocular defects, syndactyly, and skin lesions. Goltz and his colleagues have postulated that the condition may be caused by a single mutant gene transmitted as an X-linked dominant or by a sex-limited autosomal dominant gene with variable expressivity [107]. Linkage studies may clarify the genetics and provide further support for an X-linked type of inheritance. Happle and Lenz have theorized that the striate nature of both the skin and radiologic lesions is due to chromosomal mosaicism [116].

Ectodermal Dysplasias

Ectodermal dysplasia (ED) is frequently used as a descriptive term for a heterogeneous group of disorders with a constellation of defects affecting the skin and its appendages. *Ectodermal dysplasia* has been used traditionally to connote one of two specific disease entities, anhidrotic and hidrotic ED. It should not be applied indiscriminately to any symptom complex that includes ectodermal defects. Solomon and Keuer have proposed that the term *ectodermal dysplasia* be limited to generalized, congenital, nonprogressive progeria-like disorders that involve the epidermis and at least one of the appendages [249]. In a number of congenital and hereditary diseases there is abnormal development of one or several of the appendages, and such conditions may superficially resemble the phenotype of anhidrotic ectodermal dysplasia. Whenever possible, these rare syndromes, which do not conform to the classic types of ectodermal dysplasia, should be defined in terms of the dysplastic changes of the specific tissues involved.

Anhidrotic (hypohidrotic) ectodermal dysplasia (Christ-Siemens-Touraine syndrome) is characterized by a triad of absence of sweating, hypotrichosis, and defective dentition (Fig. 19-4) [47]. The facies is distinctive because of frontal bossing, a flattened nasal bridge, and depression of the central portion owing to hypoplasia of the maxillary alveolar processes ("dish face" profile). The eyebrows are absent or sparse, and the eyelashes are absent or fine and set in double rows. The skin around the eyes is wrinkled and frequently hyperpigmented. The ears and chin are prominent; the lips, thick and everted.

The skin over the remainder of the body is thin, dry, and hypopigmented, with prominent cutaneous vessels. A variable degree of alopecia is present; the scalp hair is sparse, blond, fine, and has an unruly appearance. Dental anomalies range from total anodontia to hypodontia, with defective teeth that are discolored, peg shaped, or conical.

The most striking physiologic abnormality is

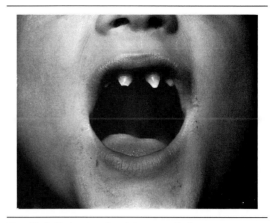

Fig. 19-4. *Defective dentition in anhidrotic ectodermal dysplasia.*

the absence of sweating, which can be demonstrated by a variety of techniques. Absence or severe hypoplasia of the eccrine sweat glands can be confirmed by skin biopsy, which should be obtained from the palm, an area normally replete with these structures. Abnormal dermatoglyphics and absent or diminished sweat pores on the fingertips are additional findings. Sweat pore counting can be useful for genetic counseling when a patient from an affected family is a questionable carrier. Heterozygote carriers have a reduced to high number of sweat pores in a patchy distribution because of the Lyon effect and interfamily variability. Therefore, sweat pore counting should be done on several fingertips of as many family members, affected and nonaffected, as possible in deciding whether a given individual is a carrier [146]. The glandular structures in the nasal mucosa, pharynx, larynx, bronchi, esophagus, duodenum, and colon may also be atrophic or absent. Atrophic rhinitis, recurrent pneumonia and bronchitis, hoarseness, and intermittent aphonia may occur. The incidence of atopic diseases, asthma, allergic rhinitis, and atopic dermatitis is increased in these patients.

In addition to changes in the periorbital skin and hair, photophobia may be a disturbing ocular symptom. Injection of the conjunctiva is common because of dryness and lack of protection by eyelashes. Keratitis, as evidenced by diffuse punctate staining with fluorescein, may be a prominent feature. Lacrimation may be diminished or absent, as is demonstrable by Schirmer's test. The lacrimal puncta may be stenotic. Congenital glaucoma is occasionally found [138]. Other reported ocular problems have included corneal opacities, congenital cataracts [47], absence of the iris, luxation of the lens, and inability of the iris to respond to mechanical and chemical stimuli [211].

In most kindreds the disorder is inherited as an X-linked recessive trait. Affected males show full phenotypic expression of the syndrome, whereas carrier females may have minor stigmata. The phenotypic variability in carrier females has been attributed to the Lyon hypothesis, namely, random inactivation of one X chromosome in each somatic cell of the female early in embryogenesis. However, 35 cases of the complete syndrome in females have been documented, and in their families an autosomal recessive gene appears to be operating [109].

The most serious effect of anhidrotic ectodermal dysplasia is marked heat intolerance because of an inability to regulate the body temperature adequately by sweating. In caring for these children, every effort should be made to moderate environmental temperatures by air conditioning. Deficient lacrimation can be palliated by regular use of artificial tears. The nasal mucosa can be protected by intermittent saline irrigations and application of petrolatum. Dental prostheses should be provided when necessary, and reconstructive procedures can be performed to improve facial contours.

Kline and his colleagues reported on a single family with both anhidrotic ectodermal dysplasia and a corneal dystrophy [147]. Of 56 members studied, 10 had ectodermal dysplasia, 4 had corneal dystrophy, and 9 had both disorders. The corneal lesions were of the granular type, began in the first decade, and involved the central portion of the cornea. Visual acuity was decreased only in adulthood, if at all. The corneal dysplasia was present in both sexes and was clearly inherited as an autosomal dominant trait. Although the authors suggest that the ectodermal dysplasia is also inherited in this fashion, the available data do not support this contention, since the affected females in this pedigree do not show full expression of the syndrome. In the absence of male-to-male transmission, it is difficult to argue against X-linked inheritance with partial expression of the gene in carrier females. Thus in this kindred the two conditions (corneal dystrophy and ectodermal dysplasia) appear to have been inherited independently.

Another family, described by Marshall, showed ocular anomalies in association with mild hypohidrosis, partial deafness, depressed nasal bridge, hypoplasia of the maxilla, and thickened lips [165].

The patients were myopic and had congenital or juvenile cataracts (some of which resorbed spontaneously) associated with glaucoma, dislocation of the lens, or both. Inheritance was thought to be autosomal.

Hidrotic ectodermal dysplasia (Clouston's syndrome) is a dominantly inherited disorder that has been described in a few kinships. It is characterized by nail dystrophy, palmar and plantar hyperkeratosis, alopecia, and dental anomalies. Less frequent findings are mental deficiency, hyperpigmentation, polydactyly, syndactyly, and hearing loss. Associated ocular abnormalities are uncommon. Strabismus is a rare finding. Conjunctivitis and pterygium are thought to result from mechanical irritation owing to absence of lashes. In one kindred 2 of 7 affected patients had pointlike lenticular opacities, and in another kindred 4 of 5 affected members had bilateral premature cataracts [119].

EEC syndrome (ectrodactyly, ectodermal dysplasia, and cleft lip and palate) is a rare constellation of defects that to date has been described in only 30 patients. Dominant inheritance with variable expressivity and incomplete penetrance has been proposed on the basis of existing data [109]. The cutaneous features consist of a thick, dry, poorly pigmented skin; mild hyperkeratosis over the elbows; dystrophic and deformed nails; sparse scalp hair and eyebrows; and absent lashes. Other findings include bilateral cleft lip, median cleft of the palate, granulomatous perlèche, and lobster-claw deformity of the hands and feet. Six patients with EEC were found to have normal sweat gland function and histology but either absent or extremely sparse sebaceous glands.

Ocular findings in reported cases involve the ocular adnexal and anterior segments: chronic blepharitis, photophobia, decreased tear formation, scarring of the lacrimal puncta, cicatricial narrowing of palpebral fissures, and absence of meibomian gland orifices. Superficial corneal vascularization or scarring or both are present in most patients. One patient had esotropia, and one patient had central corneal opacification, causing decreased visual acuity [204].

ELASTIC AND CONNECTIVE TISSUE DEFECTS

Pseudoxanthoma Elasticum

Pseudoxanthoma elasticum (PXE) is an uncommon, generalized, genetically heterogeneous group

Table 19-3. *Clinical Features of Autosomal Dominant and Recessive Forms of Pseudoxanthoma Elasticum*

Characteristics	Dominant I	Dominant II	Recessive I	Recessive II
Number of patients examined	12	54	54	3
Classical peau d'orange and flexural pseudoxanthomas	12 (100%)	12 (24%)	40 (77%)	—
Macular rash	—	35 (70%)	7 (13%)	—
General increase of extensibility	1 (58%)	33 (66%)	2 (4%)	—
General cutaneous PXE	—	—	—	3 (100%)
Vascular disease				
Angina	7 (58%)	—	—	—
Claudication	7 (58%)	—	—	—
Hypertension	9 (75%)	4 (8%)	10 (19%)	—
Hematemesis	1 (8%)	2 (4%)	8 (15%)	—
Ophthalmic features				
Severe choroiditis	9 (75%)	4 (8%)	18 (33%)	—
Angioid streaks	4 (34%)	24 (47%)	24 (44%)	—
Washed-out pattern		6 (12%)	1 (2%)	—
Peau d'orange		4 (8%)	—	—
Prominent choroidal vessels		9 (18%)	—	—
Myopia	3 (25%)	24 (48%)	3 (6%)	—
High-arched palate	—	27 (54%)	3 (6%)	—
Blue sclera	1 (8%)	21 (41%)	5 (9%)	—
Loose jointedness	—	18 (35%)	3 (6%)	

PXE = pseudoxanthoma elasticum.
Source: Adapted from F. M. Pope [201].

of disorders that involve the skin, eyes, and vasculature. Although the cause remains unknown, the most widely held concept is that the disorders result from a molecular defect or defects in elastic tissue. Genetic studies have indicated the existence of four clinical types: dominant type I and type II, and recessive type I and type II (Table 19-3) [201].

The age of onset is extremely variable, perhaps in part because the cutaneous lesions, which are often the presenting complaint, may be minimal or may go unnoticed for long periods. In 50 percent of affected patients lesions are noticed by 10 years of age; however, some patients are not diagnosed until their fourth decade. The classic lesions in the dominant and recessive type I forms consist of small, yellow papules, approximately 1 to 3 mm in diameter, which may coalesce to form plaques and give the involved skin a pebbly appearance resembling that of a plucked chicken. The sides of the neck, axillae, inguinal folds, and the periumbilical, antecubital, and popliteal areas are the sites of predilection. The involved skin has a velvety feel and, in more advanced stages, may hang in lax folds. Similar plaques of infiltrated, yellow papules may be found on the inner

surface of the lip, palate, buccal mucosa, oral mucosa, tonsillar area, vagina, and rectum. Less commonly, the serpiginous lesions of a perforating elastoma may occur.

A canary yellow macular rash is found in 70 percent of dominant type II individuals and 13 percent of recessive type I individuals. The recessive type II form has been observed in only three British families and shows only skin involvement manifesting as a yellowish generalized cutaneous laxity.

While the cutaneous lesions are a valuable clue to the diagnosis of PXE, they represent mainly a cosmetic problem, in contrast to the ocular lesions, which can cause severe disability. Angioid streaks are the most characteristic ocular finding and occur in a high percentage of patients with PXE. These lesions, which appear as broad, irregular gray or red lines that radiate from the peripapillary area, are due to breaks in the elastic tissue to Bruch's membrane. Fluorescein angiography is useful in detecting streaks not detectable on funduscopy and in recognizing the extent of any subretinal choroidal neovascularization [39]. In advanced disease, or, more rarely, after strenuous physical exercise or relatively minor ocular contusion, chorioretinal rupture, hemorrhage, scarring, and retinal pigment proliferation in the macular area may be accompanied by marked diminution in visual acuity. Severe choroidoretinitis occurs in 75 percent of individuals with dominant type I PXE and in 33 percent of recessive type I individuals. Myopia, blue sclera, and prominent choroidal vessels are the most frequent ocular findings in the dominant type II form. Less common findings include peau d'orange (diffuse mottling of the retinal pigment epithelium), salmon spots (yellowish deposits at the fundal periphery), and "punched-out lesions" (peripheral dehiscences of Bruch's membrane) [44].

Gastrointestinal hemorrhage is another of the more serious complications of PXE. Rarely, the bleeding results from aggravation of a preexisting and unrelated lesion, but the usual cause is primary disease in the wall of the gastric vessels. Yellow cobblestone lesions in the gastric mucosa similar to those of the skin have been visualized by gastroscopy. Bleeding from the urinary tract has also been observed.

Diminished peripheral pulses and calcification of the peripheral arteries, most commonly the femoral arteries, are present in a large proportion of PXE patients over 33 years of age. Despite impairment of blood flow in all extremities, ischemic and atrophic symptoms are usually confined to the legs. The arterial media are the predominant site of calcification, although intimal lesions do occur; the changes are slowly progressive and usually allow ample time for an adequate collateral circulation to develop.

The earliest detectable histologic abnormality in PXE is the deposition of calcium on the elastic fibers. When altered skin is examined with appropriate histochemical stains, the elastic fibers in the middle and lower dermis appear distorted, fragmented, and granular. What mechanism renders the elastic fibers susceptible to calcification is unknown. Fibroblasts from PXE patients when grown in tissue cultures have proteolytic activity not found in fibroblasts from normal individuals. It is possible that a proteolytic process affects elastin's affinity for calcium. High calcium levels are also found to a lesser degree in clinically unaffected skin of PXE patients [214].

Marfan's Syndrome

Marfan's syndrome is a connective tissue disorder characterized by a triad of skeletal anomalies, ocular defects, and cardiovascular defects. Its U.S. prevalence has been estimated at 1.5 in 100,000. Marfan's syndrome until very recently was considered a single autosomal dominant disease of variable expressivity. However, current thought is that it represents a genetically heterogeneous group of disorders that share similar phenotypic expressivity and that quite probably a number of molecular defects will be uncovered in Marfan's syndrome. In some, but not all, affected patients, levels of urinary hydroxyproline are increased, indicating increased collagen turnover. In one study of collagen types and cross-linking, skin samples from 3 patients with Marfan's syndrome had markedly decreased numbers of stable intermolecular collagen cross-links, compared to 3 control skin samples taken post mortem from previously healthy accident victims. The same finding held in comparing aortic tissue from a Marfan patient and an unaffected control patient. Since the basic molecular defect or defects in Marfan's patients are still unknown, no specific biochemical test exists. The diagnosis has to be based on clinical criteria.

In Marfan's syndrome the cutaneous findings are minimal and consist only of diminished subcutaneous tissue and striae in the pectoral, deltoid, and buttock areas. Occasional skin abnormalities include elastosis perforans and anetoderma. The more characteristic features are tall stature, long limbs with arachnodactyly, dolichocephaly, pectus excavatum or carinatum, muscle hypotonia, laxity of the joints, kyphoscoliosis, hernias, incompetence of the aortic or mitral valves or both, and dilatation of the ascending aorta with or without dissecting aneurysm.

Ocular findings have been reviewed by Cross and Jensen [56]. Lens dislocation occurs in at least 79 percent of patients, is usually bilateral, and is generally in a superior or superotemporal direction. In some patients it is congenital. It occurs in 50 percent of patients by 5 years of age, but in 5 percent it is not detected until the fourth decade or even later. Glaucoma occurs in 8 percent, and retinal detachment occurs in 9 percent of eyes with dislocated lenses. Glaucoma can result from lens subluxation into the anterior chamber. Chronic simple glaucoma occurs as well.

Retinal detachment has been diagnosed at an average age of 26 years in the presence of ectopia lentis and at an average age of 22 years among aphakic patients. The detachment seen after lens surgery follows the surgery by an average of 7.6 years, indicating that the aphakic individuals have more severe eye disease and are operated on at an early age. Cross and Jensen advise educating patients to avoid contact sports in order to minimize chances of a retinal detachment or an anterior lens dislocation [56]. Goldberg and Ryan have described a 5-year-old girl who developed a rapidly progressive intercalary staphyloma after being hit in the eye by a stone [103].

Abnormalities of the iridocorneal angle including abnormal iris insertions with bridging pectinate strands, inconspicuous Schwalbe's line, wide iris processes, and a broad trabecular meshwork are common. Strabismus occurs in approximately 20 percent of patients. Other ocular abnormalities seen less frequently in Marfan's syndrome include elongated suspensory ligaments, blue sclera, aplasia of the pupillary dilator muscle, high axial myopia, buphthalmos, microphthalmos, keratoconus, megalocornea, microcornea, and colobomas of the lens, fundus, macula, and optic nerve [167].

Ehlers-Danlos Syndrome

Ehlers-Danlos syndrome (EDS) is a group of hereditary disorders of connective tissue characterized by hyperelasticity of the skin, joint hypermobility, fragility of the tissues, and a hemorrhagic diathesis. Phenotypic variability is considerable, but the severity of the manifestations tends to be constant within families. To date, at least 11 different types of EDS have been classified (Table 19-4):

I. *EDS gravis type.* Skin hyperextensibility and fragility are prominent; bruising tendency, moderate; molluscoid pseudotumors, subcutaneous spheroids, varicose veins, common. Generalized joint hypermobility with gross musculoskeletal deformity are often present, and there is an increased incidence of premature births.
II. *EDS mitis type.* All stigmata are of minor degree. Prematurity is not usual.
III. *EDS benign hypermobile type.* Joint hypermobility is prominent, skin hyperextensibility is variable, and other stigmata are less severe.
IV. *EDS Sack's ecchymotic type.* Joint hypermobility is limited to the digits. The skin is thin and pale, but hyperextensibility is minimal. There are extensive ecchymoses secondary to minor trauma, and systemic complications are frequent and serious. Both autosomal dominant and autosomal recessive forms exist.
V. *EDS X-linked type.* Skin hyperextensibility is marked; fragility, bruising, spheroids, and pseu-

dotumors are usual; joint hypermobility is unimpressive.
VI. *EDS ocular type (fragilitas oculi).* The ocular fragility is characterized by blue sclera, keratoglobus or keratoconus, and rupture of the globe, especially the cornea, after minor trauma. Other features include marked skin hyperextensibility, scoliosis, dolichostenomelia, arachnodactyly, hyperextensible joints, sensorineural hearing defects, microcornea, retinal detachment, myopia, and fragilitas ossium. Protective eye wear is essential for these patients. Two variants have been reported: one with normal [141] and the second with defective [199] lysyl hydroxylase enzyme activity in cultured skin fibroblast assays. Heterozygotes of the latter variant have intermediate lysyl activity [199]. Large-dose ascorbate therapy was effective in one reported case [73].
VII. *EDS arthrochalasis multiplex congenita type.* Congenital hip dislocation; hypermobile joints; stretchable, velvety skin; and short stature are present.
VIII. *EDS periodontal type.* Cutaneous fragility, especially of lower extremities; pretibial, tender, yellow-brown atrophic scarring; and periodontitis are features. There is no skin hyperextensibility, and joint hypermobility is minimal.
Three different syndromes have been proposed for the title of EDS type IX:

a. *EDS mental retardation type.* Findings include severe mental deficiency, hypermobile joints, fragile skin with poor healing, inguinal hernias, and protuberant ears [18, 120, 199]. Inheritance is autosomal recessive.
b. *EDS occipital horns type (originally classified as X-linked cutis laxa).* Mild hypermobility of small joints; skeletal dysplasia of the wrists and elbows; soft, velvety skin with mild hyperelasticity but no laxity; easy bruising and atrophic scarring; bladder diverticula; inguinal hernias; pectus excavatum; and short broad clavicles are present. The so-called occipital horns are bony spurs seen projecting inferiorly from the occiput on radiologic examination [31, 127, 153].
c. *EDS fibronectin type.* Striae (usually not seen even in parous EDS patients), moderate skin extensibility, marked joint hypermobility, and platelet aggregation defect are features. On the basis of limited pedigree data inheritance is thought to be autosomal recessive [7].

The cutaneous manifestations described may vary in severity in different kindreds, but basi-

Table 19-4. *Types of Ehlers-Danlos Syndrome*

Type	Inheritance	Ultrastructural defect	Biochemical defect
I. Gravis	Autosomal dominant	Increased collagen fibril diameter	Unknown
II. Mitis	Autosomal dominant	Increased collagen fibril diameter	Unknown
III. Benign hypermobile	Autosomal dominant	Increased collagen fibril diameter	Unknown
IV. Ecchymotic	A. Autosomal dominant	Not determined	Unknown
	B. Autosomal recessive	Not determined	Diminished type III collagen synthesis
	C. Unknown	Small collagen fibril diameter; massive dilatation of rough endoplasmic reticulum	Intracellular accumulation of collagen (? type III)
V. X-linked	A. X-linked recessive	Not determined	Lysyl oxidase deficiency
	B. X-linked recessive	Increased collagen fibril diameter	Unknown
VI. Ocular	A. Autosomal recessive	Small collagen fibril diameter	Lysyl hydroxylase deficiency
	B. Not determined	Not determined	Normal lysyl hydroxylase activity
VII. Arthrochalasis multiplex congenita	A. Autosomal recessive	Not determined	Procollagen aminoprotease deficiency
	B. Probable sporadic heterozygote	Not determined	Probably structural mutation of procollagen α_2 (I)
VII. Periodontal	Autosomal dominant	Not determined	Unknown
IX. Mental retardation type	Autosomal recessive	Not determined	Unknown
Fibronectin type	Autosomal recessive	Not determined	?Functional abnormality of fibronectin
Occipital horns type	X-linked	Increased collagen fiber diameter; defective collagen cross-link formation	Diminished lysyl oxidase activity; low serum copper and ceruloplasm

cally the changes are similar. Skin hyperextensibility may vary in degree at different sites, but the skin can often be pulled out several inches without discomfort to the patient, snapping back into place when released. This last feature, in combination with joint hypermobility, has permitted many affected individuals to exhibit themselves as contortionists or "elastic men" in circuses and sideshows. Cutaneous fragility may be extreme, with minor trauma leading to extensive tearing. Lacerations occur most frequently on exposed surfaces and bony prominences. The resultant scars are irregular, thin, and often referred to as having a papyraceous or "cigarette-paper" appearance. If a hemorrhagic diathesis is present, the scars may become deeply pigmented, and bruising and hematomas are common. Heaped-up nodular lesions known as molluscoid pseudotumors may form at sites of trauma.

Multiple, hard, mobile bodies that feel like grains of rice may be palpable in the subcutaneous tissue, particularly over the forearms and anterior lower legs. These calcified bodies have a characteristic appearance and can be demonstrated roentgenographically.

Joint hypermobility may be associated with a

hypotonic musculature, the combination of which leads to joint dislocations and other skeletal deformities, including spinal abnormalities and thoracic asymmetry. Thoracic deformity may cause secondary cardiac disability. Gastrointestinal complications, most frequently hematemesis and melena, may occur because of the fragility of the tissues of the gastrointestinal tract. Hernias are also common findings. Of the variety of neurologic complications that have been observed, intracranial vascular lesions, although unusual, probably pose the most life-threatening hazard. Sudden death from rupture of the larger arteries has been reported.

Ophthalmologic abnormalities include laxity of the eyelids, epicanthal folds, strabismus, subluxation of the lens, posterior staphyloma, keratoconus, strabismus, high myopia, and blue sclera resulting from a relative thinning of the sclera. Metenier's sign (easy eversion of the eyelids) may be present. Fundal findings include angioid streaks, choroidal hemorrhages rupturing into the vitreous, and disciform macular degeneration. Rarely, progressive retinal lesions and retinal detachment may eventuate in blindness [197].

Cutis Laxa

Cutis laxa refers to a specific dermatologic sign: skin that is loose and pendulous but does *not* have increased elasticity. Light microscopic examination of involved skin reveals reduced numbers of elastic fibers. Electron microscopy reveals short, fragmented, clumped fibers that appear to be undergoing granular degeneration.

A heterogeneous group of heritable disorders featuring cutis laxa have been described: an autosomal dominant form and two autosomal recessive forms. An X-linked form described by Lazoff more properly belongs to the Ehler-Danlos group of connective tissue disorders [31, 127] and has also been dubbed Ehler-Danlos type IX and occipital horn syndrome.

Rarely, neonatal cutis laxa is due to maternal D-penicillamine treatment. Cutis laxa can also occur as a manifestation of autosomal recessive pseudoxanthoma elasticum or an autosomal dominant form of amyloidosis [163]. The pathogenesis of acquired cutis laxa diagnosed in later life is unclear. It may be acquired after inflammatory skin disease or gradually appear with no preceding skin inflammation. Most acquired forms are nonmendelian and are limited to skin involvement.

In the autosomal dominant form of cutis laxa, skin involvement can appear at infancy or as late as middle age. Systemic involvement is much less severe than in the recessive forms. Bronchiectasis, premature cardiac death in adulthood, mitral valve prolapse, and dilatation of the sinuses of Valsalva on echocardiography have been reported in several patients [31]. Ultrastructural studies of skin tissue have revealed regions of atypical globular elastic fibers with loose association of microfibrils on the surface of elastic fibers. The abnormal elastic fibers were associated with atypical collagen fibers, which showed irregular diameters and contour. Therefore, the underlying defect of this disorder affects both collagen and elastic tissue. Only a few kinship systems have been reported with this disorder.

The two autosomal recessive forms both show congenital skin involvement and postnatal growth retardation. In one form the infants have joint laxity and hip dislocation, large fontanelles with delayed closure, and retarded development. In the second and more common form, severe respiratory problems develop with progressive emphysema and cor pulmonale. Death from pulmonary problems frequently occurs within the first 3 years of life. Other systemic findings include multiple hernias, diverticula of the gastrointestinal and genitourinary tracts, and vaginal and rectal prolapse. Ultrastructural studies of skin biopsies from two affected siblings have shown abnormal collagen cross-linking, as well as the elastic tissue changes described previously.

The most frequent ocular abnormality is distortion of the lids (blepharochalasis) because of laxity of the skin. Surgery may be indicated because of the ocular complications of ectropion or entropion, as well as for cosmetic reasons. Rarely, one may find coloboma of the macula and severe myopia.

METABOLIC AND IMMUNE DEFICIENCY DISEASES

Xeroderma Pigmentosum

Xeroderma pigmentosum is a serious, life-limiting disorder occurring in approximately 1 in 250,000 births. It is inherited as an autosomal recessive trait with the exception of one reported dominant kindred.

Extensive studies [79] have uncovered various abnormalities in nucleic acid metabolism in xeroderma pigmentosum that result in photosensitivity, pigmentary changes, and a propensity for continuous formation of a variety of cutaneous and mucosal malignant tumors that can be mutilating and fatal.

There are now eight known genetic forms of xeroderma pigmentosum [95]. In nine groups, there is diminished DNA repair in cells that have been exposed to light in the sunburn wavelengths (290–310 nm). Affected individuals have impaired removal of pyrimidine dimers because of deficient endonuclease activity. These patients, who have defective DNA excision repair, may be assigned to one of the nine complementation groups, A, B, C, D, E, F, or G, based on in vitro cell fusion studies. However, no specific enzyme defect has been determined for any individual complementation group. A group of individuals with "variant xeroderma pigmentosum" has a normal excision repair mechanism but has a defect in S-phase DNA synthesis after ultraviolet irradiation. Sister chromatid exchanges are normal in xeroderma pigmentosum before irradiation but increase much more than in controls after ultraviolet irradiation [105].

During the first few months of life, affected infants develop photophobia and chronic conjunctivitis. These changes are soon followed by severe sunburnlike reactions accompanied by scaling and limited mostly to the light-exposed areas of the body. The erythema subsides, leaving freckling interspersed with areas of hypopigmentation. In 75 percent of patients between 6 months and 3 years of age, blepharitis, symblepharon, and crusts develop on the lid margins. The skin of the face may become atrophic and the superficial blood vessels visible and permanently dilated. Blisters, crusts, actinic keratoses, and scars supervene. Considerable distortion of the mouth, eye, and nose may result from progressive dermal sclerosis and contractures.

At about 6 years of age, basal cell epitheliomas, squamous cell carcinomas, and malignant melanomas (in decreasing order of frequency) cause considerable tissue destruction. Less common tumors include keratoacanthomas, sarcomas, fibromas, and angiomas [253]. Rarely, internal malignancies including medulloblastomas and neuromas develop [105]. Ultimately, metastatic disease presages the demise of the patient, usually before 20 years of age.

Ophthalmic findings in xeroderma pigmentosum occur in up to 80 percent of cases and have been excellently reviewed by Stenson [253]. She reports that pathology is virtually confined to the anterior segment of the globe, although postmortem findings of choroidal melanomas have been reported. The lids (especially the lower) are often involved with progressive madarosis, scarring, entropion or ectropion, trichiasis, lagophthalmos, symblepharon, ankyloblepharon, and frequent eventual loss of the entire lower lid substance. Basal cell and squamous cell cancer occur frequently on lid margins. Conjunctival and corneal involvement occur either primarily or as a complication of infection and exposure owing to lid defects. Conjunctival findings may include hyperemia, xerosis, edema, tenacious mucoid exudates, keratinization, hyperpigmentation, atrophy, pinguecular and pseudopterygial changes, or frank malignancy. The limbus is preferentially involved, especially in the exposed interpalpebral zone. The cornea is frequently affected with vascularization, opacification, recurrent ulceration, exposure, and band-shaped nodular growths; corneal neoplasms may occur. According to Robbins, benign and malignant tumors commonly develop at the corneal-scleral junction [222]. Inflammation of the iris may result in atrophy, abnormal pigmentation, and synechiae. No characteristic alterations of the lens or fundus are seen [79]. Any of the malignancies that invade the orbit and spread to the base of the brain may lead to third, fourth, sixth, and seventh cranial nerve palsies.

Overall, xeroderma pigmentosum occurs more commonly in whites, but in blacks the disease displays more severe ocular pathology and less severe skin involvement [21, 90].

Goldsmith reports that 20 to 60 percent of patients in various series have the disease with severe nervous system involvement (De Sanctis-Cacchione syndrome) [105]. In addition to skin findings, there may be microcephaly, choreoathetosis, cerebellar ataxia, sensorineural deafness, mental retardation, testicular hypoplasia, seizures, and quadriparesis [253]. Emotional lability, electroencephalographic changes, and hyporeflexia may be partial manifestations.

Xeroderma pigmentosum may be accompanied by metabolic and biochemical abnormalities, including renal impairment, aminoaciduria, and adrenal hypofunction, or by skeletal or other developmental abnormalities.

It has been possible to diagnose xeroderma pigmentosum prenatally by showing a decrease in DNA repair. Treatment, then, should include genetic counseling; rigorous protection against ultraviolet light with sunscreens of the highest possible sun protection factor; early removal of small cutaneous and ocular malignant tumors by excision, chemosurgery, or cryosurgery; and the use of topical antimitotic agents such as fluorouracil on the skin.

Familial Dysautonomia (Riley-Day Syndrome)

Familial dysautonomia is transmitted by an autosomal recessive gene, and consanguineous marriage is a relatively frequent finding in the affected individual's family history. The disease occurs most frequently among Ashkenazic Jews originating in eastern Europe. It was reviewed by Pearson in 1979 [196] and Brunt and McKusick in 1970 [33]. In summary, these investigators report that most of the patients suffer from episodic hypertension, profuse sweating, and blotching of the skin; impaired swallowing reflexes (which may lead to life-threatening regurgitation, aspiration, and pneumonia); locomotor incoordination with diminished or absent tendon reflexes; poor postural muscle control leading to marked scoliosis early in life; episodic bouts of fever with hypothermia of the extremities; recurrent infections; dry eyes; and poor general somatic growth.

The cutaneous findings, besides excessive sweating and vasomotor lability, include an absence of lingual fungiform papillae and a truncated cutaneous response to histamine (the erythematous flare component of the triple response of Lewis is absent). Temporary erythematous eruptions may occur, particularly after eating. Pustules, vesicles, and erythematous patches may appear after excitement or anxiety, which may leave hyperpigmented patches on resolution [86].

The ocular findings, studied by François [86] and Goldberg and associates [102], include corneal hypoesthesia and reduction or absence of tears leading to recurrent superficial punctate keratitis, epithelial erosions (mostly in the center or lower third of the cornea), or true ulcerations, which may lead to perforation and may be recurrent. Corneas may become keratinized, thin, and vascularized. All of these changes occur without pain, photophobia, or hyperemia. The application of 2.5% methacholine to the eye results in prompt miosis. This response is not pathognomonic of familial dysautonomia (it may be found in patients with Adie's pupil and in some normal people), but it has been used as a screening test for dysautonomia. Myopia and exodeviations are also common in the syndrome. Inconstant features include anisocoria, anisometropia, ptosis, corneal

leukoma, dry conjunctivitis, swelling of periorbital tissues, several rows of eyelashes, lateral ankyloblepharon, partial symblepharon, cataract, and increase of ocular pressure. Besides lubrication, tarsorrhaphy, and scleral contact lenses, corneal transplantation may be of use in therapy for the eye in familial dysautonomia [143].

Other findings of the disease include drooling, facial grimacing, tongue thrusting, rhythmic body movements, gastrointestinal motility dysfunction, emotional lability, postural hypotension, and indifference to pain. Breath-holding spells may cause seizures to occur. Hypercapnia and hypoxia do not cause compensatory increases in respiratory effort; thus comas or rapid deaths have occurred in tunnels, at high altitudes, and under water. Spontaneous fractures and osteochondritis may be present. Diminished renal function frequently occurs secondary to glomerulosclerosis with arterial hypertension and subnormal renin excretion [196].

The clinical and pathologic features of familial dysautonomia suggest that neuronal deficits are present at birth and worsen with age. Sympathetic ganglia are hypoplastic, averaging 34 percent of normal volume and 12 percent of normal neuronal counts. Parasympathetic sphenopalatine ganglia and lingual mucosa have severely depleted neuronal populations. Sensory neurons in spinal ganglia, dorsal root entry zones, and Lissauer's tracts are hypoplastic. A report of increased circulating nerve growth factor suggests that there may be abnormalities in nerve growth factor function. Norepinephrine and epinephrine catabolite excretion is diminished, but dopamine metabolism is normal. A 60 percent decrease in norepinephrine synthesis may result from a block in the synthesis of epinephrine and norepinephrine from dopamine, but this block has not been documented. During emotional crises in familial dysautonomia, norepinephrine, epinephrine, and dopamine levels rise markedly, which usually correlates with vomiting and hypertension [196].

Fabry's Disease (Angiokeratoma Corporis Diffusum, Anderson-Fabry Disease)

Fabry's disease is an incompletely recessive (intermediate) X-linked disorder of glycosphingolipid catabolism resulting from deficiency of α-galactosidase A, a lysosomal hydrolase. Consequently, ceramide trihexoside accumulates in the lysosomes of a variety of organ systems, which may produce serious complications [61, 87]. Eventually enough glycosphingolipid accumulates that lysosomal function is totaly disrupted; lysosomes become secondary lysosomes and functionally inert. Thus cell metabolism is interrupted and tissue dysfunction ensues. For unknown reasons, individuals with blood types B and AB appear to accumulate more of the ceramide trihexoside. The locus for the α-galactosidase A gene resides in the region of bands Xq22–q23 on the long arm of the X chromosome and is not linked to the Xg blood group locus [208].

Symptoms usually begin in late childhood or early adolescence with episodes of fever, painful burning extremities, irregular sweating, and skin and eye lesions. Deposition of the glycosphingolipid in endothelial, perithelial, and smooth muscle cells of the cardiovascular, renal, and cerebrovascular systems leads to progressive impairment [219]. Cerebrovascular accidents may result in hemiplegia, aphasia, vertigo, or collapse. Cardiac disease may manifest with congestive failure or arrhythmias. Renal vascular hypertension, renal failure, and anemia often lead to death by the fifth decade. Heterozygous females are variably affected.

In the skin characteristic angiokeratomas begin to develop as punctate dark blue, red, or black macules that do not blanch and are often first called petechiae. They are distributed in the bathing trunk area, most densely around the umbilicus and pressure points. Individual lesions then enlarge to become 1- to 2-mm papules that may blanch. A few angiomas may appear in the mouth. Rare patients have otherwise typical Fabry's disease with no angiokeratomas [208].

Pathologically, the angiokeratomas are subepidermal ectasias with thin vascular walls accompanied by epidermal hyperplasia and minimal hyperkeratosis of the stratum corneum. Moderate dilatation of deeper dermal vessels may also occur. In the dilated vessels, fibrinous thrombi with partial organization may be seen. Though the glycosphingolipid accumulation in the skin is sparse, it concentrates in the endothelial cells and pericytes of the dilated capillaries, fibroblasts, and muscles of hair, leading to damage and dilatation of the vessels. The lipid in the skin and other affected organs is demonstrable with Sudan black B and periodic acid–Schiff (PAS) (diastase resistant) and by polariscopy [157]. Ultrastructural examination of the angiokeratomas reveals myelinlike intralysosomal accumulations of ceramide trihexoside in the endothelial cells [264]. In uninvolved skin, glycosphingolipid also accumu-

lates in endothelial cells, pericytes, vascular smooth muscle, interstitial and perineural fibroblasts, and, rarely, axons of unmyelinated nerves (which degenerate and fibrose). The lipid may be membrane-bound in lysosomes or free in the cytoplasm, vascular lumina, and interstitial spaces. It has been postulated that the painful paresthesias are related to the accumulations in vascular and nerve cells [69].

The ophthalmologic findings in Fabry's disease are often unique and diagnostic; they have been excellently reviewed by many authors [27, 61, 68, 83, 87, 124, 208, 236, 237]. Usually vision is not affected in Fabry's disease, though many patients are myopic. Eyelids may be edematous. Aneurysmal dilatation and corkscrew tortuosity of conjunctival vessels are seen in about three-fourths of hemizygotes and one-half of heterozygotes. Veins of the inferior bulbar conjunctivae are preferentially involved.

Corneal involvement is highly specific and is present in virtually every hemizygote over the age of 4 years, and in heterozygotes over 10 years. Whorl-like corneal opacities radiating from a nodal point near the center of the cornea against a red reflex are seen in the subepithelial layers of the cornea at or near the level of Bowman's membrane. They are usually inferior and cream colored, though they range from very faint to white to golden brown. Corneal dystrophy (cornea verticillata) appears in a variety of patterns and may involve the upper cornea as well. The corneal lesions may appear as a diffuse epithelial haze in younger patients.

Two types of lens changes may be seen in Fabry's disease. Granular anterior or subcapsular lens deposits of various densities are present bilaterally in about one-third of hemizygotes but no heterozygotes. They typically are inferior in location, wedge shaped near the lenticular equator, and radially aligned with apices near the center of the anterior capsule in a "propeller" fashion. In addition, an unusual type of posterior lens opacity in about 37 percent of hemizygotes and 14 percent of heterozygotes has been named the Fabry cataract because of its specificity for this disease. These opacities are characteristically linear, whitish to translucent, spokelike deposits of fine granular material on or near the posterior lens capsule. They radiate from the central part of the posterior cortex, frequently along the posterior sutures. These cataracts are best viewed by retroillumination and can be easily missed by an unsuspecting examiner.

Retinal involvement clinically is much more frequent and severe in hemizygotes than in heterozygotes. Retinal vessels, especially veins, are variably tortuous or corkscrewlike; these changes may be primary or secondary to the arterial hypertension and renal disease. Segmented dilatations of veins may be seen at arteriovenous crossings. Central retinal artery and inferior temporal branch vein occlusion have also been observed.

Less consistent eye findings include myelinated nerve fibers radiating from the optic disc, mild optic atrophy, chorioretinal scarring, papilledema, nevi, iris cysts, nystagmus, and internuclear ophthalmoplegia.

Pathologically, glycosphingolipid deposits or osmophilic inclusion bodies or both are found throughout the ocular vasculature, preferentially in the endothelial, perithelial, and smooth muscle cells [219]. Ultrastructurally, in the corneal epithelium small osmiophilic inclusions are seen that correspond to lysosomes, which are more numerous than normal, and to lamellar bodies. These inclusions are responsible for the diffuse corneal haze. Punctiform gray opacities could be due to giant inclusions (unusually large secondary lysosomes) in the corneal epithelium. Subepidermal ridges in the cornea composed of thin strands of reduplicated basement membrane and an amorphous material may be responsible for the whorl-like opacities [68, 87, 264].

The diagnosis of Fabry's disease is confirmed by measuring ceramide trihexoside in plasma or urine [61] or by demonstrating a deficiency of α-galactosidase A activity in plasma, leukocytes, or tears [236].

General medical management is nonspecific and directed at individual complications. Transient decreases in plasma ceramide trihexoside occur after intravenous infusion of α-galactosidase A or plasmapheresis, but the long-term efficacy of these treatments has not been established.

Fucosidosis

Fucosidosis is an autosomal recessive lysosomal enzyme deficiency (defective α-L-fucosidase) in which fucose-containing glycolipids accumulate in many locations. The activity of the enzyme is less than 10 percent of normal.

A typical patient manifests psychomotor regressions, spasticity, and seizures first at age 12 to 18 months. Only type III disease is associated with cutaneous lesions consisting of angiokeratomas, primarily on the tunk and thighs. These lesions are indistinguishable from angiokeratoma corporis diffusum of Fabry but develop between age 6 months and 8 years, earlier than in Fabry's disease. Ophthalmologic manifestations include diffuse and lobulated corneal opacities and conjunctival and retinal vessel tortuosity [91, 157, 236].

On electron microscopy, many greatly distended vacuolated lysosomes with finely granular content are seen in endothelial cells, fibroblasts, histiocytes, keratinocytes, and secretory cells of eccrine glands [157].

Lipogranulomatosis (Farber's Disease)

Lipogranulomatosis is a rare autosomal recessive sphingolipidox's in which excess ceramide accumulates in many organs as a result of deficient ceramidase activity.

The disease manifests early in infancy with a feeble, hoarse cry and painful periarticular and tendinous swellings (which are inflammatory initially, then nodular in consistency) eventuating in flexion contractures. Cutaneous and subcutaneous nodules develop primarily over the wrists and ankles. Affected children are irritable and progressively cachectic. Involvement of cranial nerves and spinal cord leads to motor weakness, hypotonia, loss of reflexes, extreme amyotrophia, and death during the first year of life because of chronic respiratory insufficiency [17, 157, 178].

Ophthalmologic examination reveals distinctly gray maculae with mild cherry-red centers. Optic discs are slightly atrophic. The fundi have diffuse peppery pigmentation. Xanthoma-like granulomas may be evident periocularly, on the conjunctivae, or within the eye [178, 207].

Ultrastructural examination of skin lesions demonstrates highly characteristic features including curvilinear bodies (Farber bodies) in fibroblasts, histiocytes, and endothelial cells; elongated membranes in fibroblasts and endothelial cells; zebra bodies in endothelial cells; and spindle-shaped bodies in Schwann's cells [230].

Tyrosinemia Type II (Richner-Hanhart Syndrome)

Tyrosinemia type II is an autosomal recessive disorder characterized by mental retardation, keratitis, and palmar and plantar erosions and hyperkeratosis. The syndrome is caused by a deficiency of hepatic tyrosine aminotransferase with increased serum tyrosine levels and deposition of tyrosine crystals in the eye and skin. This deposition leads to corneal and skin inflammation.

Ocular symptoms have started at 2 weeks to 8 years of age and include tearing, redness, pain, and photophobia. Eye findings include corneal clouding, central or paracentral opacities progressing to erosions, dendritic ulcers, and deep ulcers. Chronic effects include scarring, nystagmus and exodeviation, and conjunctival plaques with neovascularization. Examination of a conjunctival plaque biopsy specimen by light microscopy has revealed eosinophilic inclusions in the superficial epithelial cells and endothelial cells of blood vessels within the plaque. On electron microscopy these were membrane-bound inclusions. Increased keratofibrillar bundles and alcian blue inclusions have also been seen in conjunctivae.

The skin lesions, which have their onset weeks to months later than the eye lesions, are limited to the palms and soles and consist of hyperhidrosis, blisters, painful erosions that become crusted and hyperkeratotic, and occasional hyperkeratotic subungual lesions. Electron microscopy of skin lesions may show lipidlike granules and filaments and myelin figures intermixed with the granules. Increased tonofibrils and keratohyalin and very tightly packed microtubular and tonofibrillar masses have been seen.

Renal and hepatic test results are normal in tyrosinemia type II, in contrast to tyrosinemia type I, which is an autosomal recessive disease with severe liver and renal involvement. Treatment with a low-tyrosine, low-phenylalanine diet has resulted in resolution of eye and skin lesions as well as normal growth and development [106].

Hereditary Hyperlipoproteinemias and Hypolipoproteinemias

Xanthomas of the skin, small and large, localized and disseminated, may be manifestations of hyperlipemia. Most of the blood lipids (with the exception of free fatty acids) are transported by proteins to which they are attached, so that hyperlipoproteinemia is a more accurate term. Excess serum lipoproteins may result from secondary causes such as obstructive liver disease and myxedema but are primary (i.e., genetically determined) in origin in most cases. Several rare disorders of hypolipoproteinemia may likewise be inherited.

The hyperlipoproteinemias were originally divided into five types by Fredrickson based on the paper electrophoretic separation of the plasma lipoproteins. Presently six, rather than five, types of

hyperlipoproteinemias are recognized since type II has been separated into types IIa and IIb. Types I, III, and V are rare, whereas types IIa, IIb, and IV are quite common [157]. There is a remarkable association between each type of xanthoma and the elevation of a characteristic lipoprotein fraction. Trauma predisposes to xanthoma formation but does not alter the type of xanthoma to appear [118]. Each major type of hyperlipoproteinemia with its characteristic eye findings, and several hypolipoproteinemic disorders, will be discussed.

HYPERLIPOPROTEINEMEA TYPE I: HYPERCHYLOMICRONEMIA (BÜRGER-GRÜTZ SYNDROME)

Hyperchylomicronemia is an autosomal recessive disease that begins in infancy and is caused by a deficiency of lipoprotein lipase, which results in the accumulation of chylomicrons without an excess of other lipoprotein fractions [279]. Cutaneous lesions are characterized by an acute disseminated eruption of small yellow or reddish brown papules (eruptive xanthomas). Ophthalmologic manifestations include lipemia retinalis (in which the contents of retinal vessels appear milky), synchysis scintillans "asteroid bodies," and dot-type exudates [28]. Abdominal pain owing to pancreatitis and hepatosplenomegaly are always present.

HYPERLIPOPROTEINEMIA TYPE IIA: HYPERBETALIPOPROTEINEMIA

Also termed familial hypercholesterolemia, hyperbetalipoproteinemia, a disorder of elevated low-density lipoproteins (LDL) has an autosomal dominant pattern of inheritance. In the homozygote the disease may be severe with the development of periocular xanthelasmas, tuberous xanthomas (large and slowly growing lesions localized over bony prominences and joints), and tendinous xanthomas (especially of Achilles tendons and digital extensor tendons) in childhood. These cholesterol-laden yellowish plaques and nodules reflect the high serum cholesterol level that characterizes the underlying disorder; triglycerides may be normal or only slightly elevated. (It is noteworthy that 50% of individuals with xanthelasmas alone are normolipemic, though some of this group are obese [279].) Death from coronary occlusion occurs at a young age in homozygous familial hypercholesterolemia. Symptoms in the heterozygote do not usually develop until the third to sixth decade [157]. Characteristic eye findings include premature arcus senilis, flame- or line-shaped hemorrhages, and plaque-type exudates [28]. Xanthomatous deposits may rarely affect other ocular sites including the iris and possibly the retina and choroid [279].

HYPERLIPOPROTEINEMIA TYPE IIB:
COMBINED HYPERLIPOPROTEINEMIA

Combined hyperlipoproteinemia, a newly recognized type also inherited as an autosomal dominant trait, manifests in adulthood with moderately elevated LDL (β-lipoproteins) and very-low-density (pre-β-) lipoprotein (VLDL) fractions. These patients may show eruptive xanthomas or, less commonly, tuberous and tendinous xanthomas. Ophthalmologic findings are similar to those in type IIa. Atherosclerotic coronary disease and diabetes mellitus may be associated [157].

HYPERLIPOPROTEINEMIA TYPE III: BROAD-
BETA LIPOPROTEINEMIA

Impaired interconversion of VLDL to LDL forms the basis of excess intermediate-density lipoprotein accumulation in broad-beta disease, an autosomal recessive disorder. Apolipoprotein E peptides are also associated. Clinical expression begins in adulthood and may require precipitating factors such as obesity, alcoholism, or glucose intolerance [279]. Linear palmar and digital crease xanthomas (plane xanthomas) are the highly characteristic skin lesion [118, 267]. Xanthelasmas and eruptive, tendinous, and tuberous xanthomas may also be present. Associated ophthalmologic signs include arcus senilis, synchysis scintillans asteroid bodies, lipemia retinalis, dot-type hemorrhages, and dot- or plaque-type exudates [28]. Atherosclerotic coronary heart disease and occlusive peripheral vascular disease, especially of the lower extremities, are common complications.

HYPERLIPOPROTEINEMIA TYPE IV:
HYPERPREBETALIPOPROTEINEMIA

Type IV disease, a common autosomal dominant disorder, may begin with elevated triglyceride levels in childhood, but clinical symptoms do not develop until adult life. These consist of eruptive and rarely tuberous xanthomas, as well as diabetes mellitus; generalized atherosclerosis, hepatosplenomegaly, and pancreatitis are less common.

Type IV fundal changes can be dominated by exudates, hemorrhages, lipemia retinalis, extravasations, and other vascular changes and papillary abnormalities that are usually mistaken for diabetic retinopathy. Thus it is important that patients with these eye findings be tested for aberrant fat metabolism even if the diagnosis of diabetes mellitus has been made [28]. Fat may be demonstrated in retinal vessel walls as well as the lumen. It appears that lipid reaches the perivascular retinal tissue by transport through the endothelial cells, intramural pericytes, and basement membranes rather than through spaces between endothelial cells. The presence of fibrin and blood cells in the vicinity of lipid deposition suggests that some of the lipid is accounted for by rupture of vessels and hemorrhage [151]. Retinal arterial, central vein, and branch vein occlusion may occur because of the intravascular lipid deposits. These may be heralded by visual field defects, diplopia, or episodes of aphasia thought to result from recurrent emboli in the distribution of the vertebral and internal carotid arteries [63, 64, 151, 279]. Several months of hypolipidemic therapy may result in re-perfusion and reduced leakage of the peripheral retinal circulation [64].

HYPERLIPOPROTEINEMIA TYPE V: MIXED
HYPERPREBETALIPOPROTEINEMIA AND
HYPERCHYLOMICRONEMIA

Biochemically, type V disease is a combination of types I and IV resulting in unusually severe hyperlipidemia in affected individuals and many first-degree relatives (autosomal dominant inheritance). Triglyceride concentrations may exceed 2000 mg/dl, and cholesterol levels may likewise be quite elevated [89]. Occasionally there is a deficiency of lipoprotein lipase activity. Eruptive xanthomas are the most common skin manifestation. Eye findings resemble those in type IV hyperlipoproteinemia, though asymptomatic opaque milky white fluid (lipids) in the anterior chamber may be the initial manifestation of type V hyperlipoproteinemia [2]. Caloric and alcohol excess, nonketotic diabetes mellitus, hepatosplenomegaly, pancreatitis, and hyperuricemia are very commonly associated with type V disease and usually do not manifest themselves before the fourth or fifth decade [89, 157].

MISCELLANEOUS LIPOPROTEIN DISORDERS

Corneal opacities occur in two rare familial conditions in which there are low serum levels of high-density lipoproteins (HDL), namely Tangier disease (familial HDL deficiency) and lecithin-cholesterol acyltransferase (LCAT) deficiency. In Tangier disease, opacities are evident only on slit-lamp examination and do not cause visual impairment. Usually, the skin is free of lesions, but numerous scattered papules have been seen in Tangier disease. In LCAT deficiency, the corneal opacities are clearly visible to the naked eye, but visual acuity is not reduced.

In 1979 a new entity termed fish-eye disease was described in a man and his three daughters (among five children), all of whom demonstrated massive corneal opacities (resembling the eyes of boiled fish) and dyslipoproteinemia [37]. The small dotlike gray, white, or yellow opacities formed a mosaic pattern in all layers of the cornea except the epithelium. Most of the cornea was uniformly turbid. Corneal sensation was normal. Conjunctivae were slightly yellow. Visual acuity diminished with age. Laboratory analysis revealed normal serum cholesterol levels, but elevated serum triglycerides. LDL were strikingly elevated, while VLDL were moderately raised. The LDL contained normal-sized as well as abnormally large particles, and there was a 90 percent reduction in the level of HDL. LCAT activity and the percentage of plasma cholesterol esters were normal, which excluded LCAT deficiency.

A variant of fish-eye disease in which several corneal opacities were associated with high total cholesterol, HDL, and LDL values, but normal serum triglycerides and total serum lipids, has also been seen [49]. LCAT activity was likewise normal. Thus it has been suggested that fish-eye disease must be a heterogeneous entity.

ATAXIA-TELANGIECTASIA (LOUIS-BAR SYNDROME)

Ataxia-telangiectasia is an autosomal recessive disease manifested by oculocutaneous telangiectasias, cerebellar ataxia, choreic movements and dystonic posturing, recurrent sinopulmonary infections, persistent α-fetoprotein production (a chemical marker for the disease), ovarian agenesis or testicular hypoplasia, and a high incidence of reticuloendothelial neoplasia (10% of patients, usually before age 15 years). Affected individuals have a defect in DNA repair associated with increased sensitivity to ionizing radiation and to bleomycin [172, 269, 271]. Twenty-five percent of patients demonstrate chromosomal breakage, especially of chromosome 14. Endoreduplication and polyploidy are frequent, but there is no increased rate of sister chromatid exchanges [157, 285].

Individuals affected with ataxia-telangiectasia demonstrate variable abnormalities of both cellular and humoral immune systems including an abnormal or absent thymus gland, defective delayed hypersensitivity to skin test antigens, delayed rejection of histoincompatible skin grafts, decreased T-cell proliferative responses to mitogens and antigens, decreased generation of virus-specific immune cytotoxic T lymphocytes, and impaired helper T-cell function, which contributes to the humoral abnormalities. Seventy to eighty percent of patients synthesize low molecular weight IgM and have IgA and IgE deficiencies either alone or conjointly. There may be selective IgA2, IgG2, or IgG4 deficiencies, at times associated with compensatory increases in IgG1, IgG3, or both. Patients with very low or absent IgG2 tend to have chronic lung disease, chronic sinusitis, or both. Frequently a defect in antibody responsiveness to viral immunization is observed. There appears to be an intrinsic B-cell maturation defect contributing to the immunoglobin abnormalities. Occasionally, circulating anti-IgA antibodies contribute to a high rate of IgA catabolism [172, 190, 221, 269]. Defective neutrophil chemotaxis has also been documented [97].

Telangiectasias are the primary skin manifestation of this disease. Large, tortuous vessels initially appear after age 3 on the bulbar conjunctivae between the limbus and canthi in a symmetrical pattern. Telangiectasias are subsequently seen on the cheeks, eyelids, "butterfly" areas of the face, external ears, and neck. They may also appear in the antecubital or popliteal fossae, on the buttocks or extremities, and occasionally on mucous membranes. These telangiectasias seldom bleed. Histopathologically, markedly dilated vessels that belong to the subpapillary venous plexus may be seen in the dermis [157, 179]. A number of patients may likewise manifest atopic dermatitis, areas of hypopigmentation, café au lait spots, premature graying of hair, early loss of subcutaneous fat, and generalized skin atrophy [269]. Cutaneous and conjunctival infections are rare.

Oculomotor signs include nystagmus, strabismus, and failure of purposeful eye movements [285]. In young patients with ataxia-telangiectasia, increased saccadic reaction time may be the initial eye movement abnormality. Later, progressively longer saccadic reaction times and marked hypometria of all voluntary saccades (horizontal and vertical) are noted. Affected individuals have difficulty initiating voluntary saccades. During optokinetic and vestibular stimulation (involuntary saccades), the eyes deviate toward the slow component, rather than toward the fast component as in normal persons. The eye movement abnormalities in ataxia-telangiectasia are quite similar to those of congenital oculomotor apraxia but may be distinguished by normal vertical saccades in the latter [12]. Additional observations include contraversive eye movements without reflex saccades in the direction of the target and head thrusts when making horizontal refixations.

The normal amplitude–maximum velocity relationship for both voluntary and involuntary saccades in the horizontal and vertical planes demonstrates that the pretectal and parapontine pulse-generating neurons and the oculomotor neurons are intact in ataxia-telangiectasia. It has been suggested that the abnormality in this disease resides in the supranuclear control of these brain stem structures, perhaps in the cerebellum, which is usually atrophic in affected individuals [12], with degeneration of Purkinje's cells, basket cells, and granular cells [179]. Defects in the basal ganglia and substantia nigra may be additional causes for abnormal eye movements.

Other systemic associations in ataxia-telangiectasia include glucose intolerance associated with hyperinsulinism, insulin resistance, and hyperglycemia in over one-half of patients. Forty to fifty percent of affected persons have mild hepatic functional abnormalities [269]. Generalized muscle weakness secondary to a peripheral neuropathy occurs later in the disease [194]. Growth and mental retardation are common [285]. Patients with ataxia-telangiectasia have a reduced life span, since chronic and repeated flare-ups of sinopulmonary disease cause death in a majority of cases by age 20. Immunoglobulin prophylaxis may be helpful against the infections in patients with IgG2 and IgA deficiency [190].

At least four different genetic complementation groups are now known to exist among individuals affected with ataxia-telangiectasia, which suggests extensive genetic heterogeneity [135].

Bloom's Syndrome

Bloom's syndrome is a rare autosomal recessive, life-limiting disorder characterized by a photosensitive telangiectatic facial erythema, dwarfism, and a high incidence of various malignancies. Ashkenazic Jews are more commonly affected than the population as a whole; males, more often than females.

The telangiectatic erythema commonly develops in the first few months of life with redness or blistering in the butterfly area of the nose and cheeks progressing to persistent erythema and telangiectasias on nose, cheeks, and ears. The forearms and the dorsal surface of the hands may be likewise affected. Sunlight, especially the UVB wavelengths, exacerbates the eruption in summer. Café au lait spots and axillary acanthosis nigricans may be present [105, 157, 229].

Ophthalmologic associations include conjunctivitis, conjunctival telangiectasias, and drusen at the posterior poles [207].

The stunted growth is intrauterine in onset and proceeds to proportionate dwarfism in individuals who survive to adulthood. Normal intelligence and sexual development are the rule [105, 229].

Respiratory and gastrointestinal infections commonly occur in Bloom's syndrome. Patients often have deficiencies of serum IgG, IgM, IgA, or a combination of these. Peripheral blood lymphocytes in these individuals are defective in both B-cell ability to produce immunoglobulins and T-cell help for B-cell differentiation. Delayed hypersensitivity reactions are sometimes absent, which suggests an arrest in functional maturation of lymphocytes early in the development of the immune system [157, 256].

Malignancies often develop in Bloom's syndrome. Acute leukemia most commonly occurs in the second and fourth decades. Tissues with high mitotic indices (bone marrow, lymphoid tissues, and gastrointestinal mucosa) are the most frequent sites of neoplasia [105, 229]. German and co-workers in 1979 reported on 77 patients with Bloom's syndrome who lived beyond the age of 3 years of whom 16 developed a total of 18 malignancies, or one cancer per 4.3 patients [100].

Multiple abnormalities in DNA repair and chromosomal structure have been found in Bloom's syndrome: a decreased rate of DNA replication; chromatid and isochromatid gaps, breaks, and rearrangements; acentric segments; dicentric chromosomes; abnormal monocentric chromosomes; ring chromosomes; and a markedly increased (6- to 12-fold) frequency of sister chromatid exchanges with increased triradial and quadriradial configurations [15, 62, 105, 229, 268].

Cockayne's Syndrome

Cockayne's syndrome is an autosomal recessive disorder with clinical onset after a normal first year of life. It is characterized by dwarfism, a prematurely senile appearance with "birdlike" facies, microcephaly, normal-pressure hydrocephalus, prognathism, moderate kyphosis, proportionately long limbs, sensorineural deafness, mental retardation, photosensitive dermatitis, and distinctive ophthalmologic aberrations. Additional features often included in the syndrome are carious teeth, nephropathy leading to hypertension, hepatomegaly, progressive upper motor neuron and cerebellar dysfunction, joint contractures, atrophy of skeletal muscles, incontinence, and intracranial calcifications in the regions of the basal ganglia, lateral ventricles, and frontal lobes. Death usually occurs between 10 and 30 years of age [30, 48, 158, 195, 246].

The dermatologic manifestations of Cockayne's syndrome often begin with a scaly erythematous dermatitis in sun-exposed areas. This eruption may resolve leaving hyperpigmentation. These changes, together with progressive subcutaneous and periorbital fat atrophy, contribute to the prematurely senile appearance. An absence of sweating has been reported [30, 48, 158].

Consistent ocular signs include a discrete "salt and pepper" pigmentary retinal degeneration, optic atrophy, and arteriolar narrowing. It is now thought that the optic atrophy occurs as a result of the retinal degeneration. Photophobia, enophthalmos, exotropia, corneal dystrophy with recurrent epithelial erosions or band-shaped keratopathy, hypoplastic irides, irregular pupils, vitreous floaters, small punctate lens opacities (which may be congenital), loss of macular reflex, nystagmus, lack of tearing, and poor response to mydriatic drugs constitute the variable eye findings. Hyperopia and narrowed visual fields may occur. Vision tends to decrease as the disease progresses [48, 158, 195, 265].

Histopathologic studies of the eye reveal hyperpigmentation and hypopigmentation of the retinal pigment epithelium, some loss of photoreceptors, and the presence of pigment-laden cells in the retina and subretinal space. Lipofuscin is deposited in the peripheral retinal pigment epithelium [158]. In the vicinity of Bowman's layer, irregular masses of vertically oriented fibrillar material accumulate with a virtual lack of true basement membrane system. It is uncertain whether these changes represent an end point of degeneration or fibrillogenesis replacing Bowman's layer after injury [30].

Neuropathologic studies demonstrate diffuse, extensive demyelination of the central and peripheral nervous systems beginning with pericapillary calcification in the cortex and basal ganglia.

Neuronal loss ensues in the cerebral cortex, cerebellum, and spinal cord along with lipofuscin accumulation in the remaining neurons. These findings are compatible with physiologic changes of aging and suggest that premature aging is a fundamental problem in Cockayne's syndrome [206].

No enzyme or chromosomal abnormalities have been found in Cockayne's syndrome [30]. However, cultured fibrocytes and lymphocytes from affected individuals have shown abnormal sensitivity to the lethal effects of ultraviolet irradiation [158, 206, 246]. While several studies suggest an aberration in the recovery of post-UV DNA synthesis [92, 209], other work demonstrates a primary defect in DNA metabolism unrelated to DNA repair [45], possibly in replication or excision repair [125].

Children with Cockayne's syndrome have a decreased or undetectable serum level of thymic hormone, reminiscent of the similar decline in thymic hormone in physiologic aging and suggestive of premature immunologic aging in this disorder. T-cell function, measured by phytohemagglutinin and concanavalin A responses in mixed lymphocyte cultures, may be normal or decreased [22].

Chronic Granulomatous Disease

Chronic granulomatous disease is an X-linked recessive disorder of neutrophil and monocyte function that is characterized by a relentless course of superficial and systemic granulomatous and suppurative lesions. An uncommon variant of the disease caused by a deficiency of leukocyte glutathione peroxidase is inherited in an autosomal recessive manner [40, 166].

The disease begins in the first year of life with chronic superficial pyodermas (impetigo, infected seborrheic dermatitis, or infectious eczematous dermatitis), particularly around the mouth. These infections often develop into granulomatous lesions accompanied by cervical and, at times, inguinal adenopathy. Despite aggressive therapy, the lesions remain purulent and necrotic. Culture of the purulent exudates may produce saprophytic nonpathogenic organisms, *Staphylococcus aureus*, or no growth [16, 166, 272].

Infections and granulomas later occur in widespread sites, manifesting as soft tissue abscesses, perianal abscesses and fistulas, ulcerative stomatitis, blepharitis, conjunctivitis, keratitis, otitis media, pneumonia, lung abscesses, granulomatous colitis, esophagitis, osteomyelitis, arthritis, myocarditis, and hepatosplenomegaly with perihepatic abscesses. While most lesions are localized, septicemia and meningitis signify dissemination, and death commonly occurs by adolescence [177, 282].

Histopathology of the infections reveals microabscesses and granulomas; the observation of pigmented histiocytes is helpful in establishing the diagnosis of chronic granulomatous disease [282].

Chorioretinal lesions are consistently present in patients affected with chronic granulomatous disease. Diffuse, well-demarcated areas of destruction and scarring may be seen in the choroid and retina without accompanying signs or symptoms of uveitis. These defects are generally distributed along the retinal vessels centrifugally, sparing the macula, a pattern consistent with metastatic infection. Peripapillary involvement and optic pallor are evident at times. Generally, vision is unimpaired, though occasionally visual fields are depressed in correspondence with specific areas of retinal damage. After early childhood the progression of chorioretinal scarring usually halts [166, 191].

While the specific molecular abnormality in chronic granulomatous disease is unknown, the defect lies in the neutrophils and monocytes, which ingest, but are unable to consume oxygen and kill, catalase-positive microorganisms. The host's leukocytes cannot produce H_2O_2, and the H_2O_2 generated by the pathogens is destroyed by their own catalase. However, catalase-negative organisms that are ingested are killed by their own H_2O_2, together with myeloperoxidase from the leukocyte. In vitro these neutrophils are unable to reduce nitroblue tetrazolium (NBT) dye. Heterozygous female carriers demonstrate only one-third to one-half of the normal neutrophil NBT reduction capability, though they are phenotypically normal with no infection tendencies [16, 177, 272, 282].

Dermatologic markers for the female carrier state include discoid lupus-erythematosus-like dermatoses or arcuate dermal erythemas that may be indistinguishable from Jessner's lymphocytic infiltration. Some female carriers have been reported to have arthritis, pleuritis, fever, Raynaud's phenomenon, photosensitivity, or recurrent aphthous stomatitis without serologic evidence of systemic lupus erythematosus [177].

Treatment of chronic granulomatous disease is usually unrewarding, though one boy was suc-cessfully treated with a bone marrow transplant from a fully compatible unrelated donor [82].

SCALING DISEASES

Disorders of keratinization logically would be expected to involve the ocular apparatus, and, indeed, a number of them may result in changes in the lids, conjunctivae, corneas, and lenses.

The ichthyosiform dermatoses, disorders of keratinization manifesting as visible scaling of skin, can be classified into four major types [75]. Two of these entities, ichthyosis vulgaris and bullous ichthyosis (also called epidermolytic hyperkeratosis, formerly called bullous congenital ichthyosiform erythroderma), are inherited as autosomal dominant traits. Lamellar ichthyosis, formerly termed nonbullous congenital ichthyosiform erythroderma, is transmitted as an autosomal recessive trait. X-linked ichthyosis, phenotypically evident only in the male, is transmitted by a gene on the X chromosome. *Collodion baby* is a descriptive term for affected infants of a particular appearance but does not represent a specific type of ichthyosis. Harlequin fetus is the most severe form of ichthyosis and is carried by an autosomal recessive gene. The remainder of the ichthyoses may be classified among several less common forms.

Several syndromes include ichthyosis as a constant or variable feature. Those with ocular abnormalities are reviewed below, after discussion of the ichthyoses.

Ichthyosis Vulgaris

Ichthyosis vulgaris, the most common (comprising 95% of all types) [10] and often the mildest form of ichthyosis, is present in about 0.3 percent of the population. It is manifested predominantly in childhood and early adulthood. The trunk, particularly the back, and the extensor surfaces of the limbs are the sites of predilection. Flexural areas are always spared, which is a helpful feature in differential diagnosis. The forehead and cheeks may be scaly in young children, but involvement in these areas diminishes with age. The scales are fine, white, and adherent but may be coarser over lower extremities. The turned-up margins of the scales feel rough to the touch and account for the "pasted-on" appearance [10]. Discrete, shiny, hyperkeratotic plaques on the elbows and knees, accentuation of palmar and plantar markings, follicular hyperkeratosis (keratosis pilaris), and chapping of the hands and feet are frequent findings. About half of affected individuals have manifestations of atopy [277]. The disease often worsens in cold, dry weather.

The fundamental defect in ichthyosis vulgaris is not known. Kinetic studies have revealed normal epidermal transit time from basal layer to stratum corneum, which suggests that the excessively thick stratum corneum is due to enhanced retention of scale rather than to hyperproliferation; however, no structural defects have been found to account for this [277].

The ocular manifestations in this form of ichthyosis are usually minimal. Rarely, affected individuals may have corneal erosions, punctate keratitis, multiple deep-gray stromal opacities over the entire cornea similar to those seen in X-linked ichthyosis, corneal fibrinoid degeneration, or band-shaped keratopathy. In mild cases involvement usually is anterior to Descemet's membrane, while more severe cases may extend to the posterior half of the stroma. Lenticular changes may consist of cuneiform, nuclear, cupuliform, coronary, or blue dot opacities, and granular pigmentation of the peripheral fundus has been observed [114, 136, 207].

X-linked Ichthyosis

X-linked ichthyosis, occurring in 1 in 6,000 male births, is, unlike ichthyosis vulgaris, often detectable at birth. A few of these infants may be enveloped in a collodion-like membrane that is subsequently shed. All of the body surfaces may be involved, but dark scaling is often heaviest over the sides of the neck and ears, giving the patient an unwashed appearance. Hyperkeratosis of the flexures is variable, with the axillae and antecubital fossae more often affected during childhood. Adults may instead display more prominent scaling in the popliteal fossae and over the anterior lower legs and abdomen. Hair, nails, palms, and soles are usually normal, and there is no associated atopy. In contrast to ichthyosis vulgaris, the scales of X-linked ichthyosis are large and dark brown and may be shed profusely in a cyclical fashion.

Corneal opacities are frequently present in patients with X-linked ichthyosis and to a lesser extent in female carriers but usually are not manifest before adolescence. The opacities are discrete and diffusely distributed; they are shaped like filaments, commas, or dots and are located on the posterior part of Descemet's membrane or in the deep corneal stroma in older patients. These lesions are detectable only by slit-lamp examination, and vision is not affected. There appears to be a wide clinical spectrum of severity, but within a given individual the changes tend to remain static [10]. Rare changes include punctate, coarse, subepithelial stromal keratopathy, lenticular cuneiform or nuclear opacities, peripheral granular pigmentation of the fundus, Marcus Gunn lid phenomenon, and buphthalmos [136].

Kinetic studies of epidermal cell renewal have normal results in X-linked ichthyosis, as in ichthyosis vulgaris. Recent studies strongly suggest that X-linked ichthyosis may result from a single genetic mutation that causes defective production of a microsomal enzyme, steroid sulfatase, in many or all tissues of the body [149, 234, 235]. One of the enzyme's substrates, cholesterol sulfate, accumulates in the pathologic scale [277], serum [74], and red blood cell membranes [24], strongly implicating the missing enzyme in the pathogenesis of X-linked ichthyosis. In fact, the increased cholesterol sulfate content of serum low-density lipoproteins confers on them increased electrophoretic mobility; thus X-linked ichthyosis may be diagnosed by routine serum lipoprotein electrophoresis without quantitation of either enzyme or substrate [74]. It has been demonstrated that epidermal cholesterol sulfate content is highest in the intercellular membrane region of the stratum granulosum and may be vital to adherence of cells [277]. It is conceivable that interference with cholesterol sulfation may produce increased cell adherence and decreased desquamation, as is probable in X-linked ichthyosis.

The X-linked ichthyosis gene locus has been assigned to the p22 to pter region of the human X chromosome [173].

Lamellar Ichthyosis

Lamellar ichthyosis is evident at birth with generalized redness and scaling in about 1 in 300,000 infants; occasionally infants may be covered with a collodion-like membrane that is shed gradually over the first days or weeks of life. Affected children usually have intense erythroderma, which decreases with age. The hyperkeratosis is generalized, with accentuation in flexural areas. The scales vary from yellow to brownish black and may form extensive, thick, horny plates. The palms and soles may show increased skin markings or a greatly thickened horny layer. Obstruction of sweat glands by scales may lead to hyperpyrexia during hot weather or exercise. Scalp hair may be matted down with scales, and recurrent infection may cause scarring alopecia [10].

Early in life, tension from the collodion membrane or excessively dry skin leads to marked ectropion and eclabium, which are important diagnostic signs. Exposed conjunctivae may become thickened and hyperemic, with punctate epithelial erosions that may be severe enough to perforate [136]. Corneal scarring, vascularization, and abnormal corneal nerves (with irregular diameters and brushlike endings) have been observed [188, 238]. Rare peripheral granular pigmentation of the fundus [136] and aggressive eyelid basaloma [255] have been reported.

Kinetic studies in lamellar ichthyosis have revealed increased mitotic activity and reduced cell transit time from basal layer to stratum corneum [210]. Recent work by Williams and Elias has demonstrated large quantities of n-alkanes in a homologous series of C_{19} to C_{35} with equal representation of odd and even chains in scales in some cases of lamellar ichthyosis but not in others [278]. These data may support biochemical heterogeneity within this disorder.

Bullous Ichthyosis

Also termed epidermolytic hyperkeratosis, bullous ichythyosis is a rare syndrome (1 in 300,000 births) that manifests at birth with generalized erythema and widespread or localized hyperkeratosis. There may be extensively denuded areas with secondary infection that may emit unpleasant odors and lead to sepsis [10]. The flexures are always involved, and wrists, ankles, elbows, and knees, commonly so. The scales are large, thick, dark, and often verrucous and are shed in large quantities over short intervals. Palms, soles, hair, and mucous membranes are usually normal. During the first few years of life, recurrent crops of bullae occur over the entire body surface; during late childhood they become localized to the lower legs, and by adulthood, only 20 percent of affected individuals continue to blister [10]. In contrast to the other types of ichthyosis, no specific eye lesions are seen in bullous ichthyosis.

The underlying defect in bullous ichthyosis is not known. Isolated reports of altered epidermal keratin patterns have recently been published but are conflicting and inconclusive [277]. The epi-

dermal transit time from basal layer to horny layer is markedly shortened, to 4 days.

Harlequin Fetus

Harlequin fetus is an extremely severe disorder of keratinization but should not be included in the spectrum of lamellar ichthyosis, as in the past, for there are no cross-overs between these groups [10, 11]. In harlequin fetus from birth skin has a hard, thick, armorlike covering with deep fissures running transversely and vertically, resembling tree bark. The ears and nose are underdeveloped, flattened, and distorted, and the lips are everted and gaping. Hands and feet have a gray-white color with necrotic-looking digits.

Rigidity of the periorbital skin results in marked ectropion. Chemosis of the palpebral conjunctiva may completely obscure the globe. Keratopathy and congenital cataracts may be present [207].

These infants are so severely affected that virtually all die within the first days or weeks of life. There are no consistent abnormalities of other organ systems [10].

Recent reports of harlequin fetus have shown diverse stratum corneum x-ray diffraction patterns and varying keratin polypeptide composition, which suggest heterogeneity in the disorder [210]. Another harlequin fetus exhibited none of these protein abnormalities but demonstrated abnormalities of lipid metabolism [36].

Sjögren-Larsson Syndrome

Sjögren-Larsson syndrome is characterized by the triad of ichthyosis, mental retardation, and spastic diplegia. The disease is transmitted as an autosomal recessive trait. Ichthyosis is present at birth, with erythema or large scales resembling those of lamellar ichthyosis. Severe acral skin involvement seems to correlate with a higher degree of mental retardation [233]. Neurologic signs appear later with marked spastic diplegia in the legs and much less severe or no involvement in the arms. Epilepsy may occur.

Fifty to one hundred percent of patients demonstrate ophthalmologic defects. Almost all patients have marked photophobia [134]. Ectropion occurs rarely. Retinal degeneration and a specific type of macular degeneration termed "glistening dots" or "snail tracts" are present in a high proportion of patients and are usually stationary [134, 259]. Glistening dots may be an early marker of

Sjögren-Larsson syndrome, though they are not always present at birth. Pathologically, glistening dots represent fatty degeneration of microglia [57]. These changes may be so slight as to be overlooked [134], but vision is impaired in some cases.

In a study of serum fatty acids in Sjögren-Larsson syndrome, Hernell and colleagues observed a decrease in certain metabolites of linoleic acid, thus implicating a specific block in fatty acid desaturation in the causation of Sjögren-Larsson syndrome [121].

Refsum's Disease

Refsum's disease consists of atypical retinitis pigmentosa; generalized, symmetrical motor and sensory peripheral neuropathy with progressive paresis of the distal extremities, ataxia, and other cerebellar signs; and an elevated cerebrospinal fluid protein without pleocytosis. Less constant findings include nerve deafness, ichthyosis (ranging from mild hyperkeratosis of palms and soles to severe ichthyosis on the trunk), anosmia, pupillary abnormalities, skeletal defects, and nonspecific electrocardiographic changes. Transmission is autosomal recessive. Initial symptoms of weakness, difficulty in walking, and failing vision, especially at night, usually begin before the age of 10 years [210].

The defect of Refsum's disease involves the metabolism and accumulation of phytanic acid. The diagnosis is confirmed by finding excess phytanic acid in the triglyceride portion of the serum lipids [210].

In the epidermis in Refsum's disease, phytanic acid becomes the predominant fatty acid, with a relative decrease in normal fatty acids [277]. Thus the ichthyotic skin in Refsum's disease has been likened to that in essential fatty acid deficiency, in which there is inability to generate arachidonic acid and its prostaglandin metabolites [277].

Rud's Syndrome

The clinical features of Rud's syndrome are ichthyosis, infantilism, hypogonadism, mental retardation, epilepsy, and oligophrenia. Specific skin manifestations include ichthyosiform erythroderma, acanthosis nigricans, hyperkeratosis and hyperhidrosis of palms and soles, and traumatic alopecia of scalp hair [210].

Other defects may include dwarfism, gigantism, arachnodactyly, polyneuritis, tetany, nerve deafness, macrocytic anemia, structural defects of hands and feet, and defective teeth [10]. Eye abnormalities include strabismus, retinitis-pigmentosa-like lesions [61], ptosis, nystagmus, and blepharospasm. The disease appears to be inherited as an autosomal recessive trait, but X-linked recessive inheritance cannot be excluded [10].

Chondrodysplasia Punctata (Conradi's Syndrome)

Chondrodysplasia punctata is a heterogeneous group of disorders including an extensive array of anomalies affecting the bones, joints, lens, skin, and occasionally the cardiovascular and central nervous systems. The sine qua non of these disorders is the roentgenographic finding of stippled epiphyses in the cartilaginous skeleton, involving at times the vertebral discs, joint capsules, larynx, trachea, and hyoid bone. Also common are shortening of the femur and humerus, flexion contractures of the large joints, and saddle nose.

Cataracts are present in many patients at birth, with or without optic atrophy [71]. Congenital heart defects, hernias, physical and mental retardation, abnormal facies, and hematologic disorders have been associated. Skin changes consisting of universal or localized erythema and thick, white, adherent scales that may have a distinctive whorled pattern appear in approximately 25 percent of affected infants. There is palmar and plantar hyperkeratosis. Skin changes usually disappear by 6 months of age but may be superseded by follicular atrophoderma, cicatricial alopecia, and blotchy hyperpigmentation [10].

The disease has been further categorized into type 1, Conradi-Hünerman syndrome, which is inherited as an autosomal dominant trait, and more severe type 2, rhizomelic dwarfism, which may be an autosomal recessive trait. Morbidity and mortality in chondrodysplasia punctata are related to the severity of the associated anomalies rather than to the basic skeletal defects.

KID Syndrome

The term *KID syndrome* names the constellation of keratitis, ichthyosis, and deafness [244]. Patients with this syndrome have a distinctive ichthyosis from birth that begins with generalized erythema and evolves into fine, dry scales with follicular hyperkeratotic spines and a reticulated hyperkeratosis on palms and soles. Occasionally, serpiginous, verrucous plaques develop. Oral lesions include lingua plicata, rugae on buccal mucosa, leukoplakia, and squamous cell carcinoma of the tongue. Fifty percent of patients have absent or scanty hair from childhood. Fifty percent likewise demonstrate severe recurrent skin infections with no demonstrable humoral or cell-mediated immune defects. Neurosensory deafness from birth is a consistent finding [244].

About three-fourths of patients are affected by a vascularizing keratitis resulting in photophobia and decreased vision, occasionally progressing to total blindness. Intelligence is usually normal.

Several patients have displayed abnormally low serum carotene, vitamin A, or zinc levels, possibly implicating gastrointestinal malabsorption. The inheritance pattern is not known.

BIDS Syndrome (Trichothiodystrophy)

The BIDS syndrome is named for the combination of brittle hair, intellectual impairment, decreased fertility, and short stature. Ichthyosis of variable severity is a regular feature, manifested by generalized erythroderma. Other abnormalities may include hypoplastic nails, punctate lenticular cataracts, abnormal dentition, and cerebellar ataxia [139, 140]. There are distinctive hair shaft abnormalities termed trichoschisis (transverse fractures) and trichorrhexis nodosa (transverse, frayed fractures); these probably result from a markedly deficient sulfur content of hair [140, 203].

Neutral Lipid Storage Disease

Neutral lipid storage disease is an autosomal recessive entity reported by Dorfman and associates in 1974 [66]. Generalized gray-white scaling of the skin is accompanied by variable erythema, mild ectropion, and low intelligence. Three of the four patients had impaired retinal function; two had nystagmus, ataxia, and neurosensory deafness. Results of blood lipid studies, including phytanic acid levels, were normal. But a systemic lipidosis was confirmed when free neutral (triglyceride) lipid droplets were seen in peripheral blood and bone marrow, granulocytes, monocytes, and megakaryocytes, with severe fatty changes in the liver.

Miscellaneous Syndromes

Another postulated error in lipid metabolism has been seen in at least 3 patients with lamellar ichthyosis, ectropion, steatorrhea, and slowly progressive proximal limb weakness. In these cases cholesterol and triglyceride storage was marked in skin and muscle cultures [170].

Cremers and colleagues reported a syndrome of early childhood deafness, lamellar ichthyosis, corneal pannus, photophobia, chronic blepharoconjunctivitis, hypotrichosis, anhidrosis, hyperkeratosis of nails, and dental dysplasia [54]. At least 8 similar patients have been described in the literature.

In 1982 Loffredo and coauthors described 3 cases of familial microphthalmos associated in 2 cases with ichthyosis and in another with deafness [161]. In 2 patients the microphthalmos was unilateral; in the third it was bilateral. The ichthyotic skin was more pronounced on the limbs than on the trunk. A fourth family member demonstrated ichthyosis and partial lagophthalmos secondary to peripheral facial nerve paralysis but had normal vision.

BLISTERING DISORDERS

Epidermolysis Bullosa

Epidermolysis bullosa (EB) is a generic term for a heterogeneous group of hereditary, chronic, blistering disorders that may represent 16 different entities. Blistering occurs as a result of incidental trauma. Severity depends on the particular variety of EB, ranging from mild blistering of the hands and feet to severe, extensive, hemorrhagic bulla formation on skin and mucous membranes in recessive dystrophic EB. Sequelae include nonhealing erosions or ulcers, infection, scarring, mitten-like deformities of the phalanges, and flexural joint contractures. Bony resorption of the digits may occur secondarily. Blood and protein are lost through denuded skin and gastrointestinal lesions; thus severely affected individuals frequently develop dysphagia, strictures, and malnourishment with anemia and growth retardation [51, 98, 99].

The various EB entities may best be understood histologically, as they may be divided into three major categories [51, 98, 99, 123]:

1. *Epidermolytic EB.* Blister cleavage occurs within the epidermis, and healing occurs without scarring. Included in this group are four autosomal dominant (D) types of EB simplex (Köbner type, localized Weber-Cockayne type, mottled pigmentation variant, and Ogna type) as well as D-EB herpetiformis Dowling-Meara, D-EB Bart, and X-linked recessive Mendes da Costa syndrome.

2. *Junctional EB*. Blister separation occurs below the epidermis but above the basal lamina. These blisters heal with mild atrophic changes. Entities in this category have autosomal recessive (R) inheritance and include EB letalis of Herlitz, EB atrophicans mitis, EB atrophicans localisata, EB atrophicans inversa, and EB progressiva.

3. *Dermolytic or dystrophic EB*. Blister formation occurs below the basal lamina in the papillary dermis, and scarring and milia inevitably occur as sequelae to blistering. Included are two dominant forms (Cockayne-Touraine and Pasini variants) and two recessive types (Hallopeau-Siemens and inversa variants).

Electron microscopy is used to differentiate junctional from dystrophic disease by assessing features such as tonofilament clumping, hemidesmosomal or anchoring fibril defects, cytolysis, collagenolysis, and junctional deposits. Immunofluorescence techniques that map the dermal-epidermal junction with specific antisera against type IV collagen (in the basal lamina), laminin, and bullous pemphigoid antigen (both in the lamina lucida) can further assess the site of blister cleavage [70].

Clinical correlation involves assessment of lesion morphology, distribution, and severity; atrophy; dystrophy; milia formation; and degree of mucosal and gastrointestinal involvement.

Ocular involvement may occur in several EB types but most characteristically occurs in patients with dystrophic EB. Bullous keratitis and subepithelial blisters may lead to erosions, ulcerations, scarring, corneal clouding or opacities in the region of Bowman's membrane and epithelium, or perforation. Sclerae may be similarly involved. Additional findings include blepharitis, conjunctivitis, conjunctival contraction, symblepharon, and pseudomembrane formation [8, 111, 152]. In R-dystrophic EB (Hallopeau-Siemens type), eye pathology is especially extensive, with more conjunctival than corneal involvement [98].

In Herlitz-type junctional EB, edema of the cornea may accompany extensive edematous changes in the trabecular meshwork, ciliary body, lens, and optic nerve. The retina may have areas of necrosis and detachment; occasional defects in Bruch's membrane may be seen [8]. Corneal blistering would be expected in Herlitz patients who survive infancy [98].

Individuals affected with R-EB atrophicans inversa characteristically develop corneal blisters or erosions after trivial trauma. Similar localized corneal involvement may occur intermittently in D-EB herpetiformis Dowling-Meara [98].

In two members of a family with EB simplex (type unspecified), an annular configuration of fine bullous lesions in the midperiphery bilaterally at the level of the deep corneal epithelium superficial to Bowman's membrane has been reported. These lesions were asymptomatic until some of the bullae ruptured through to the corneal epithelial surface [111].

Treatment in EB is primarily supportive and aimed at decreasing trauma. Phenytoin may be useful in inhibiting blister formation (up to 40% reduction in number of blisters) in R-dystrophic EB, perhaps by inhibiting the excess synthesis or secretion (or both) of collagenase by skin fibroblasts [51, 260]. Blistering may also improve with phenytoin in junctional EB, though the mechanism of action is unknown [223].

Fetoscopy has been used to diagnose R-dystrophic EB and junctional EB prenatally.

NEUROVASCULAR AND VASCULAR DISORDERS (PHAKOMATOSES)

A number of diseases that are characterized by tumors of neural and vascular tissues and involve the nervous system, eyes, and skin have been called phakomatoses. Some of them clearly have a hereditary cause; others (such as Sturge-Weber syndrome) do not.

Neurofibromatosis (von Recklinghausen's Disease)

Neurofibromatosis (NF) is a highly variable disease whose defining features include multiple café au lait spots, axillary freckling, multiple neurofibromas, and Lisch nodules (pigmented iris hamartomas) [218]. Lisch nodules are present in 95 percent of patients over 6 years of age and in 28 percent of younger patients [160]. Neurofibromatosis has a reported frequency of 1 in 3,000 individuals, and 50 percent of cases are due to fresh gene mutations. Riccardi has proposed that the disease is genetically heterogeneous and has devised a classification system of eight types [216]:

1. NF I (peripheral NF, the von Recklinghausen form, classic NF) has autosomal dominant transmission and accounts for 85 to 90 percent of cases. It is characterized by multiple café au lait spots, axillary freckling, multiple neurofibromas, and Lisch nodules.

2. In NF II (central or acoustic NF), another autosomal dominant form, patients have few café au lait spots and skin neurofibromas but almost a 100 percent incidence of bilateral acoustic neuromas. The CLS also tend to be very large and quite pale. Iris Lisch nodules are not found.

3. In NF III (mixed NF) patients tend to have fewer, larger, and paler café au lait spots than in classic NF, but they also have more numerous cutaneous neurofibromas than patients with NF I or NF II. Patients with NF III are more likely to develop central nervous system tumors, such as optic gliomas, neurilemomas, and meningiomas, than those with classic NF. The mode of transmission is autosomal dominant.

4. NF IV (variant NF) is marked by a highly variable presentation not permitting classification in the above groupings. Cutaneous, acoustic, and central nervous system lesions may be present.

5. NF V (segmental NF) is a nonhereditary form with involvement of only one body segment and is believed to be due to a postzygotic mutation in a primitive neural crest cell. Iris Lisch nodules are not found.

6. NF VI is an autosomal dominant hereditary form with café au lait spots as a primary feature and no neurofibromas.

7. In NF VII (late-onset NF) affected patients do not develop cutaneous neurofibromas until their twenties. Thus far no café au lait spots have been seen in late-onset disease. It is unknown at present whether the offspring of these patients inherit the disease.

8. The classification NF VIII ("not otherwise specified" NF) has been proposed by Riccardi for affected patients not fitting into any of the above categories.

In the matter of classification, all the hereditary forms (NF I–IV and VI) "breed true"; therefore, examination of patients' family members is helpful in assigning them to a particular type. Riccardi has suggested that examination of patients should include the following tests: complete neurologic and ophthalmologic examination; intelligence and psychological evaluations; electroencephalogram; audiogram; radiologic skeletal survey with emphasis on the skull, optic foramina, spine, and auditory canals; cranial computed tomography (CT) scan with inclusion of the orbits and optic chiasm; and measurement of 24-hour urine epinephrine and noreprinephrine levels.

Although early childhood changes may be restricted to six or more 1.5-cm café au lait spots, in about 75 percent of cases areas of hypopigmentation, axillary freckling, and tumors of neural sheaths in skin, bone, nervous system, and eyes develop around adolescence. The bony changes include short stature, scoliosis, osseous hypertrophy, pseudarthroses, and bowing of the limbs. Cutaneous lipomas or angiomas and neurofibromas of the internal organs may also develop. About 2 to 5 percent of patients are mentally retarded. Many have difficulty in schooling but function well in adulthood. Speech impediments are present in 30 to 40 percent of patients.

The cutaneous neurofibromas are most striking and may number from several to thousands. They are evident as soft, skin-colored, nipplelike lesions or pedunculated, unencapsulated masses. Diffuse involvement of an area (plexiform neuroma) may cause horrendous deformity of the region. The skin overlying a plexiform neuroma may be hyperpigmented and have a coarse, thickened texture. If this hyperpigmentation extends over the midline, the tumor may involve the spinal cord. Areolar neurofibromas appear after puberty in 85 percent of female patients. During pregnancy there tends to be a great increase in the size and numbers of both cutaneous and internal neurofibromas.

Tumors of the central nervous system, including optic gliomas, occur in 5 to 10 percent of patients and are usually present in the first decade of life. This fact underscores the need for neurologic and ophthalmologic examination when NF is suspected.

A predisposition to malignancies has been noted in affected patients, with an incidence of 3 to 13 percent reported in the literature. Excessive rates of neurofibrosarcomas, malignant schwannomas, Wilms' tumor, rhabdomyosarcoma, and several leukemias have been noted.

Pheochromocytomas are present in fewer than 1 percent of patients and almost always occur in adulthood.

The above-mentioned Lisch nodules are the most constant ocular manifestation, but NF also can affect the lids, orbit, and globe in a variety of ways. These protean manifestations have been reviewed by Woog and coauthors [284] and Tasman [257]. Eyelid involvement with a neurofibroma or plexiform neuroma tends to become evident between 2 and 5 years of age and is usually unilateral. The affected lid may be ptotic, have an S-shaped margin, and have a "bag of worms" consistency on palpation. The overlying skin may be thickened and rough textured with rostral displacement of the eyelashes.

Orbital involvement can take the form of skeletal anomalies or tumors of the extraocular soft tissue with resultant exophthalmos. Exophthalmos can also result from tumor involvement of the optic nerve. Tumors of the optic nerve and orbital soft tissues include neurofibromas, schwannomas, optic nerve gliomas, and optic nerve sheath meningioma. Rarely, congenital malformation or erosion of oribital bones causes protrusion of brain tissue through the defect.

Neurofibromas and schwannomas have also occurred in the ocular layers within the conjunctiva, episclera, sclera, cornea, uveal tract, and ciliary nerves [273]. Uveal tract involvement frequently results in obstruction of aqueous outflow at the iridocorneal angle and secondary glaucoma. Melanocytosis of the conjunctiva, episclera, and sclera; nevus of Ota; and rare, perhaps chance, associations with choroidal malignant melanomas have been noted. Prominent corneal nerves are common in NF but are nonspecific, being also found in multiple endocrine neoplasia syndrome type 2B, which is typified by mucosal neuromas, medullary carcinoma of the thyroid, and pheochromocytoma.

Retinal lesions, rare in NF, have included small, white tumors that histologically were schwannomas; astrocytic hamartomas; and café au lait spots of the fundus [53].

Involvement of the optic nerve may gradually result in blindness. Optic nerve glioma, meningioma, and, rarely, diffuse hyperplasia and neurofibromas have been reported. Visual loss may also occur if the intracranial structures around the sella are affected. Optic nerve atrophy has been reported in the absence of an associated neoplasm or glaucoma; however, in 70 percent of cases of NF it is due to an optic nerve glioma.

Between 7 and 38 percent of all optic nerve gliomas are associated with neurofibromatosis. The distribution of gliomas in NF patients is as follows: within the optic chiasm in 70 percent of cases; within a single nerve in 25 percent of cases; and multifocal (within one or both optic nerves and the chiasm) in 5 percent of cases. In 17 of 18 NF patients with optic nerve gliomas studied by Stern and colleagues, the gliomas had a perineural growth pattern in the subarachnoid space, while in 14 of 16 non-NF patients with optic nerve gliomas the tumor was exclusively intraneural [254]. The gliomas usually occur within the first decade and sometimes develop sarcomatous changes. Optic nerve meningiomas usually appear at a later age and are more likely to invade non-nerve tissue.

Tuberous Sclerosis (Bourneville's Disease, Adenoma Sebaceum, Epiloia)

Tuberous sclerosis (TS) is transmitted by an autosomal dominant gene, with 25 to 50 percent of cases representing fresh mutations [217]. Its incidence is estimated at 1 in 30,000 individuals. The affected individual may have a number of organ systems involved. Most prominent among these are the brain, eye, skin, bone, and kidney.

The basic pathologic lesion is a fibroangioma or glioma-angioma. In the brain these lesions displace the white matter and cause increased pressure on the cortex. Radiologically, the potato-like tumors ("tubers") give rise to intracranial calcifications and are manifested clinically by epileptiform seizures. These tumors can be detected by CT scan before their calcification [35]. Presentation is most frequently with seizures, which start as infantile spasms in 30 percent of cases. Developmental delay or mental retardation constitutes the second most frequent presentation. In older patients rarer features of TS may be the mode of presentation: renal angiomyolipomas, pulmonary cystic lesions, and cardiac rhabdomyomas.

Cutaneous changes are present in over 80 percent of affected patients: Linear, oval, or lance-ovate hypopigmented macules (ash-leaf spots) are present in 50 to 90 percent of affected patients either at birth or soon afterward. These differ histologically from vitiliginous macules by the presence of hypoactive melanocytes, which are missing in areas of vitiligo. The ash-leaf spots, while not pathognomonic, can assist in making the diagnosis of tuberous sclerosis. The detection of these macules is greatly aided by examining the skin surface with a Wood's light. The other cutaneous markers of TS appear later: Cutaneous angiofibromas, the "adenoma sebaceum" lesions, usually appear between 2 and 6 years of age but can also be present at birth or appear as late as the midtwenties. These lesions, reported in 70 to 90 percent of affected patients, are 1- to 10-mm, pink to red, dome-shaped papules, occurring over the nasolabial folds, cheeks, and chin. Histologic examination of these lesions reveals dermalfibrosis and capillary dilatation but no sebaceous component.

"Shagreen patches" are usually seen after the first 5 years of life in 36 to 70 percent of TS pa-

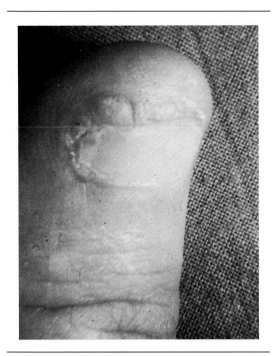

Fig. 19-5. *Periungual fibromas in tuberous sclerosis.*

tients. These are plaques of slightly thickened and raised leatherlike skin in the lumbosacral area. Histologically they differ from other connective tissue nevi by a lack of increased elastic tissue. Subungual and periungual fibromas (Fig. 19-5) are 5- to 10-mm firm, smooth papules growing out of the nail bed. These appear first at puberty and are present in about 10 to 50 percent of cases. Less common cutaneous findings include café au lait spots and large, soft, brownish fibromas on the face and scalp.

Retinal hamartomas are seen in 50 percent of affected patients [185]. The retinal hamartomas present in two forms: One is a flat, smooth-appearing semitranslucent lesion with poorly defined borders; the other is the classic elevated, multinodular tumor that has been described as resembling salmon eggs, frog's eggs, tapioca, or mulberries. The evolution of a mulberry-type lesion from a flat lesion over a 22-year period has been photographically recorded in one patient. In a study of 44 infants with infantile spasms, flat retinal hamartomas were found in 7 children, and a mulberry-type lesion was found in a single child who was 27 months old. The flat lesions are difficult to visualize unless fully dilated indirect

ophthalmoscopy is done. When a child is having frequent seizures the best way of accomplishing this is to do the exam when the child is sedated, preferably at the same time the CT scan is scheduled [130].

Ocular findings also include glial hamartomas of the optic disc, which are sometimes referred to as giant drusen; adenoma sebaceum of the lid; white pedunculated tumors of the palpebral conjunctiva; and yellow-red thickenings of the bulbar conjunctiva (see Chapter 8) [150].

Loss of visual acuity is rare and is more likely to result from intracranial lesions, which can cause papilledema and optic atrophy, than from the retinal lesions, whose effect is dependent on their size and location. Rarely, visual acuity is affected by secondary glaucoma, inflammation, or intraocular hemorrhage [257].

Hemangiomas

A number of syndromes characterized by malformations of vascular tissue give rise to hemangiomas that may involve the skin and eye: Sturge-Weber syndrome, von Hippel-Landau disease, Riley-Smith syndrome, and Osler-Weber-Rendu disease. In addition, there are several reports of retinal cavernous hemangiomas being associated with cutaneous and central nervous system vascular anomalies [104]. Whether these latter findings are chance associations owing to the frequent occurrence of cutaneous angiomas in the general population or distinct syndromes is as yet undetermined.

ENCEPHALOFACIAL ANGIOMATOSIS (STURGE-WEBER SYNDROME)

Sturge-Weber syndrome consists of a port-wine (rarely, cavernous) hemangioma, usually involving the region innervated by the ophthalmic and maxillary portion of the trigeminal nerve; unilateral cortical hemangiomas and calcifications; choroidal angiomas; and sometimes buphthalmos and glaucoma. Rarely, iris colobomas are noted [217]. When the facial hemangioma covers one or both eyelids there can be angiomatosis of the sclera and conjunctiva [9]. This disease has not been shown to have a genetically determined transmission and therefore must be considered a congenital malformation rather than a hereditary disease.

VON HIPPEL-LANDAU DISEASE

von Hippel-Landau disease involves the retina and cerebellum with hemangiomas but rarely has a similar cutaneous component. This entity has an autosomal dominant inheritance pattern with variable expressivity, and a relatively high percentage of cases are the result of a new mutation [217]. Fluorescein angiography and indirect ophthalmoscopy aid in the diagnosis of early retinal changes [270]. Four of five reported cases of optic nerve hemangioblastomas have occurred in patients with von Hippel-Landau disease [131].

RILEY-SMITH SYNDROME

A family has been reported by Riley and Smith in which multiple, widespread cutaneous and subcutaneous cavernous hemangiomas were found in association with macrocephaly and pseudopapilledema [220]. The disorder is probably due to an autosomal dominant gene.

HEREDITARY HEMORRHAGIC TELANGIECTASIA
(OSLER-WEBER-RENDU DISEASE)

Conjunctival telangiectasia may be present in association with widespread similar lesions on face, ears, mucosal surfaces, fingertips, nail beds, bladder, gastrointestinal tract, lung, and brain. Pulmonary arteriovenous fistulas also occur. This autosomal dominant disease results in postpubertal nosebleeds, occasional gastrointestinal hemorrhages, and menometrorrhagia. The cutaneous and conjunctival lesions are usually not apparent in childhood but may become visible in adolescence and troublesome during pregnancy. Rarely, the retinal vessels show telangiectasia, venous tortuosity, and segmental dilatations; retinal and disc neovascularization; vitreous hemorrhages [9, 60].

MISCELLANEOUS CONDITIONS

Lipoid Proteinosis (Hyalinosis Cutis et Mucosae, Urbach-Wiethe Disease)

Lipoid proteinosis is a rare disease of autosomal recessive inheritance, of which approximately 200 cases have been reported. It is often manifested in infancy and is characterized by hoarseness and skin and mucous membrane lesions. The hoarseness is due to infiltrative thickening of the vocal cords. Skin lesions usually start within the first 2 years of life and are more common on the ex-

posed areas of the face, neck, and extremities. Early lesions resemble impetigo but are followed by pocklike scars and infiltrated skin lesions marked by nodularity and plaque formation. The oral mucosa shows waxy or yellowish papules and plaques. Characteristic tiny gray-white papules with a "string of beads" appearance are found on the eyelid margins in most affected patients. Intracranial calcification in the hippocampal area is diagnostic but not always present.

Obstruction of Stensen's ducts can cause recurrent suppurative parotitis. Upper respiratory lesions may be so severe as to cause acute and fatal respiratory obstruction in infants and young children. Chronic, recurring cutaneous and respiratory tract infections are a common problem [108].

The papular eyelid lesions may result in loss of eyelashes. Macular degeneration, drusen, chorioretinitis, and a yellow conjunctival nodule have been reported. The microscopic appearance of the drusenlike material is similar to that reported for skin and mucous membrane lesions [176].

Microscopy of cutaneous lesions reveals deposition of a hyalin-like material that is PAS positive and diastase resistant. This material is first seen around capillaries and eccrine sweat glands but eventually accumulates throughout the dermis. Ishibashi hypothesized, on the basis of his electron microscopic studies, that this hyaline material represents an accumulation of basal lamina glycoprotein consisting of mucopolysaccharides and probably also type III or type IV collagen or both [132]. Further studies by Fleishmajer and co-workers have confirmed that the thickened basement membranes around capillaries stain intensively for laminin and type IV collagen [80]. The chemical nature of the dermal hyaline material is still unknown, but present studies point to a noncollagenous structural glycoprotein composition.

Darier-White Disease (Keratosis Follicularis)

Darier-White disease is an autosomal dominant disease. Affected individuals develop keratotic follicular papules, particularly on the face, scalp, and upper trunk, starting in late childhood or during adolescence. Individual lesions may coalesce into crusted, verrucous plaques. Secondary pyogenic infections are common. Lesions worsen with prolonged exposure to sunlight, humidity, and heat. Histologic examination of the skin lesions is diagnostic, revealing dyskeratotic corps ronds and grains, suprabasal epidermal acantholysis, and proliferation of dermal papillae lined by a single layer of basal cells [157].

In a recent series, 16 of 21 affected patients had corneal lesions consisting of both peripheral nebular and central "cobweb" opacities. Histopathologic examination revealed epithelial cell edema and decreased desmosomes [26]. Eyelid problems noted were keratotic papules on the eyelid margins and staphylococcal blepharoconjunctivitis.

Rosenthal-Kloepfer Syndrome

A Louisiana family has been reported by Rosenthal and Kloepper in which corneal leukomas were associated with acromegaly and cutis verticis gyrata [225]. The leukomas appeared in childhood and were progressive, leading eventually to blindness. Signs of cutis verticis gyrata appeared in the fourth or fifth decade. No evidence of endocrine disease was seen. X-rays of the sella turcica were normal in examined individuals. The transmission pattern observed was autosomal dominant. Of 13 affected individuals, one had no eye lesions and one had no skin lesions.

de Lange's Syndrome

de Lange's syndrome, a rare and serious disorder, has an unknown cause but may be due to an autosomal recessive gene. It results in severe mental retardation, arrested growth, phocomelia, other skeletal anomalies, a characteristic feeble cry, and an arresting facial appearance. The eyes are large and expressive, the eyebrows always meet in the midline (synophrys), the eyelashes are long, and the nostrils are anteverted. The cutaneous findings include hypertrichosis, cutaneous vasomotor lability and mottling, and cyanotic erythema around eyebrows. The inconstant ocular findings, which have been reviewed by Nicholson and Goldberg [180] and Milot and Demay [169], include antimongoloid slant of the palpebral fissures, telecanthus, ptosis, high myopia, pale optic disc, nystagmus, strabismus, and partial absence of the pupillary annulus minor with anisocoria.

Pachyonychia Congenita

Pachyonychia congenita is a localized disorder of keratinization, resulting in extensive hyperkeratosis and hyperhidrosis of the palms and soles,

marked thickening of the nails, and blister formation on the feet. The hyperkeratosis becomes most marked in the third and fourth decade and is often disabling. There may be keratotic papules on the thighs, buttocks, and shoulders. Leukoplakia frequently affects the mucous membranes of the mouth and larynx and may even proceed to malignant transformation. Ocular changes occur rarely but may include dyskeratosis of the cornea leading to blindness. Bilateral cataracts have also been seen [46]. The disease is probably heterogeneous, with both autosomal recessive and autosomal dominant transmission [42].

Atopic Dermatitis

Atopic dermatitis is a hereditarily determined chronic pruritic disorder that can be exacerbated by a number of unrelated factors, including sudden changes in environmental temperature and humidity, psychological stress, and bacterial and viral infections [224, 226]. Since the exacerbating causes are not specific, it is not, as has been suggested, an allergic disease; rather, the underlying cause appears to be an inherited abnormality in the autonomic functions of the skin and may be associated with some degree of immunodeficiency. The mode of genetic transmission at this time remains unclear, although the disease probably affects between 2 and 5 percent of the population.

Clinically, the dermatitis may start before the age of 2 years and seems to have several stages, with recurrent flare-ups throughout the adolescent and adult years. The pruritis *precedes* the lesions, which are caused by scratching. The lesions undergo four stages: redness, weeping, scaling, and lichenification. The distribution of the lesions on the body depends somewhat on the age of the patient. In the infant the disorder affects the cheeks, extensor surfaces of the limbs, and diaper area; in the adolescent it affects the flexures; and later it may affect the hands and feet. In severe cases the entire body may be involved.

Infection with herpes simplex virus or vaccinia virus can result in a disseminated eruption called Kaposi's varicelliform eruption. This eruption is accompanied by fever and a high mortality rate.

The ocular complications of atopic dermatitis are important because they are more frequent than most practitioners suspect. The orbital skin often shows distinctive findings. There is frequently an extra fold under the lower lid, which appears as a line radiating out from the inner canthus (Morgan's fold). The lids may show dermatitis and hyperpigmentation as a result of rubbing.

More serious than the cutaneous lesions around the eyes are the intraocular complications occurring in these patients. In one series cataracts were found in about 10 percent of adults with *severe* atopic dermatitis [32]. The lenticular opacities appeared most frequently between the ages of 15 and 30 years. Almost 70 percent of the cataracts were bilateral, and 10 percent of these patients developed retinal detachment as a *pre*operative complication. Keratoconus occurs occasionally. A characteristic type of cataract has been described in atopic dermatitis: The earliest changes consist of an anterior subcapsular opacification, which, as it thickens, tends to distort the anterior capsule. This polar opacification develops a shieldlike or "bearskin" character. However, nonspecific cataracts have also been noted in patients with atopic dermatitis [10]. After lens extraction, additional complications may ensue: retinal detachment, severe uveitis, hemorrhage, glaucoma, and phthisis bulbi [224].

REFERENCES

1. Abramson, D. H., Rodriguez-Sains, R. S., and Rubman, R. B-K mole syndrome: Cutaneous and ocular malignant melanoma. *Arch. Ophthalmol.* 98:1397, 1980.
2. Ursin, K. V., et al. Ocular contusion and hyperlipidaemia. *Br. J. Ophthalmol.* 56:706, 1972.
3. Albert, D. M., Nordlund, J. J., and Lerner, A. B. Ocular abnormalities occurring with vitiligo. *Ophthalmology* (Rochester) 86:1145, 1979.
4. Albert, D. M., Nordlund, J. J., and Lerner, A. B. Ocular change in vitiligo. *Pigment Cell* 5:62, 1979.
5. Albert, D. M., Sober, A. J., and Fitzpatrick, T. B. Iritis in patients with cutaneous melanoma and vitiligo. *Arch. Ophthalmol.* 96:2081, 1978.
6. Allen, B. S., Fitch, M. H., and Smith, J., Jr. Multiple hamartoma syndrome: A report of a new case with associated carcinoma of the uterine cervix and angioid streaks of the eyes. *J. Am. Acad. Dermatol.* 2:303, 1980.
7. Arneson, M. A., et al. A new form of Ehlers-Danlos syndrome: Fibronectin corrects defective platelet defect. *JAMA* 244:144, 1980.
8. Aurora, A. L., Madharan, M., and Rao, S. Ocular changes in epidermolysis bullosa letalis. *Am. J. Ophthalmol.* 79:464, 1975.
9. Ausberger, J. J., Goldberg, R. E., and Magargal, L. E. Retinal and Choroidal Vascular Abnormalities. In R.

D. Harley (Ed.), *Pediatric Ophthalmology* (2nd ed.), Vol. 1. Philadelphia: Saunders, 1983.
10. Baden, H. P., and Hooker, P. Ichthyosiform Dermatoses. In A. E. H. Emery and D. L. Rimion (Eds.), *The Principles and Practice of Medical Genetics.* London: Churchill Livingstone, 1982.
11. Baden, H. P., et al. Keratinization in the harlequin fetus. *Arch. Dermatol.* 118:14, 1982.
12. Baloh, R. W., Yee, R. D., and Boder, E. Eye movements in ataxia-telangiectasia. *Neurology (Minneapolis)* 28:1099, 1978.
13. Bard, L. A. Heterogeneity in Waardenburg's syndrome: Report of a family with ocular albinism. *Arch. Ophthalmol.* 96:1193, 1978.
14. Bartholomew, L. G., and Dahlin, D. C. Intestinal polyposis and mucocutaneous pigmentation. *Minn. Med.* 41:848, 1958.
15. Bartram, C. R., Koske-Westphal, T., and Passarge, E. Chromatid exchanges in ataxia telangiectasia, Bloom syndrome, Werner syndrome, and xeroderma pigmentosum. *Ann. Hum. Genet.* 40:79, 1976.
16. Bass, L. J., et al. Chronic granulomatous disease of childhood. *Arch. Dermatol.* 106:68, 1972.
17. Battin, J., Vital, C. L., and Azanza, X. La lipogranulomatose disséminée de Farber. *Ann. Dermatol. Syph.* 97:241, 1970.
18. Beasley, R. P., and Cohen, M. M., Jr. A new presumably autosomal recessive form of the Ehler-Danlos syndrome. *Clin. Genet.* 16:19, 1979.
19. Beerman, H., Kirshbaum, B. A., and Cowan, L. K. Oculocutaneous diseases and internal medicine: A review of some of the literature. *Am. J. Med. Sci.* 238:491, 1959.
20. Beetham, W. P. Atopic cataracts. *Arch. Ophthalmol.* 24:21, 1940.
21. Bellows, R. A., et al. Ocular manifestations of xeroderma pigmentosum in a black family. *Arch. Ophthalmol.* 92:113, 1974.
22. Bensman, A., et al. Decrease of thymic hormone serum level in Cockayne syndrome. *Pediatr. Res.* 16:92, 1982.
23. Berbich, A., Dhermy, P., and Majbar, M. Ocular findings in a case of incontinentia pigmenti (Bloch-Sulzberger syndrome). *Ophthalmologica* 182:119, 1981.
24. Bergner, E. A., and Shapiro, L. J. Increased cholesterol sulfate in plasma and red blood cell membranes of steroid sulfatase deficient patients. *J. Clin. Endocrinol. Metab.* 53:221, 1981.
25. Bergsma, D. R., and Kaiser-Kupfer, M. A new form of albinism. *Am. J. Ophthalmol.* 77:837, 1974.
26. Blackman, H. J., Rodrigues, M. M., and Peck, G. L. Corneal epithelial lesions in keratosis follicularis (Darier's disease). *Ophthalmology (Rochester)* 87:931, 1980.
27. Bloomfield, S. E., David, D. S., and Rubin, A. L. Eye findings in the diagnosis of Fabry's disease. *JAMA* 240:647, 1978.
28. Bolmers, D. M. Ocular anomalies in the types of Fredrickson. *Ophthalmologica* 171:86, 1975.

29. Brambilla, E., Dechelette, E., and Stoebner, P. Partial albinism and immunodeficiency: Ultrastructural study of haemophagocytosis and bone marrow erythroblasts in one case. *Pathol. Res. Pract.* 167:151, 1980.

30. Brodrick, J. D., and Dark, A. J. Corneal dystrophy in Cockayne's syndrome. *Br. J. Ophthalmol.* 57:391, 1973.

31. Brown, F. R., 3d, et al. Cutis laxa. *Johns Hopkins Med. J.* 150:148, 1982.

32. Brunsting, L. A., Reed, W. B., and Bair, H. L. Occurrence of cataracts and keratoconus with atopic dermatitis. *A.M.A. Arch. Dermatol.* 72:237, 1955.

33. Brunt, P. W., and McKusick, V. A. Familial dysautonomia: A report of genetic and clinical studies, with a review of the literature. *Medicine (Baltimore)* 49:343, 1970.

34. Burgdorf, W., Kurvink, K., and Cervenka, J. Sister chromatid exchange in dyskeratosis congenita lymphocytes. *J. Med. Genet.* 14:256, 1977.

35. Burkhart, C. G., and El-Shaar, A. Computerized axial tomography in the early diagnosis of tuberous sclerosis. *J. Am. Acad. Dermatol.* 4:59, 1981.

36. Buxman, M. M., et al. Harlequin ichthyosis with epidermal lipid abnormality. *Arch. Dermatol.* 115:189, 1979.

37. Carlson, L. A., and Philipson, B. Fish-eye disease: A new familial condition with massive corneal opacities and dyslipoproteinaemia. *Lancet* 2:922, 1979.

38. Carney, R. G. Incontinentia pigmenti: A world statistical analysis. *Arch. Dermatol.* 112:535, 1976.

39. Carr, R. E., and Noble, K. G. Angioid streaks. *Ophthalmology (Rochester)* 87:263, 1980.

40. Carruthers, J. A., and Greaves, M. W. Chronic granulomatous disease. *Br. J. Dermatol.* 95 (Suppl. 24):72, 1976.

41. Carter, D. M., et al. Psoralen-DNA cross-linking photoadducts in dyskeratosis congenita: Delay in excision and promotion of sister chromatid exchange. *J. Invest. Dermatol.* 73:97, 1979.

42. Chong-Hai, T., and Rajagopalan, K. Pachyonychia congenita with recessive inheritance. *Arch. Dermatol.* 113:685, 1977.

43. Clark, W. H., Jr., et al. Origin of familial malignant melanomas from heritable melanocytic lesions: The B-K mole syndrome. *Arch. Dermatol.* 114:732, 1978.

44. Clarkson, J. G., and Altman, R. D. Angioid streaks. *Surv. Ophthalmol.* 26:235, 1982.

45. Cleaver, J. E. Normal reconstruction of DNA supercoiling and chromatin structure in Cockayne syndrome cells during repair of damage from ultraviolet light. *Am. J. Hum. Genet.* 34:566, 1982.

46. Cockayne, E. A. Pachyonychia congenita. In *Inherited Abnormalities of the Skin and Its Apppendages.* London: Oxford University Press, 1933.

47. Cole, H. M., et al. Congenital cataracts in sisters with congenital ectodermal dysplasia. *JAMA* 129:723, 1945.

48. Coles, W. H. Ocular manifestations of Cockayne's syndrome. *Am. J. Ophthalmol.* 67:762, 1969.

49. Comas, A. P. Variant fish-eye disease? *Lancet* 1:881, 1980.

50. Comings, D. E., and Odland, G. F. Partial albinism. *JAMA* 195:519, 1966.

51. Cooper, T. W., and Bauer, E. A. Epidermolysis bullosa: A review. *Pediatr. Dermatol.* 1:181, 1984.

52. Cotineau, J., Rozelle, A., and Treppoz, M. Menkes' disease: A new case. *J. Fr. Ophtalmol.* 2:33, 1979.

53. Cotlier, E. Café-au-lait spots of the fundus in neurofibromatosis. *Arch. Ophthalmol.* 95:1990, 1977.

54. Cremers, C. W. R. J., Philipsen, V. M. J. G., and Mali, J. W. H. Deafness, ichthyosiform erythroderma, corneal involvement, photophobia and dental dysplasia. *J. Laryngol. Otol.* 91:585, 1977.

55. Crome, L. The association of phenylketonuria with leucodystrophy. *J. Neurol. Neurosurg. Psychiatry* 25:149, 1962.

56. Cross, H. E., and Jensen, A. D. Ocular manifestations in the Marfan syndrome and homocystinuria. *Am. J. Ophthalmol.* 75:405, 1973.

57. Daicker, B. Zur kenntnis von substrat und bedeutung der sogenannten schneckenspuren der Retina. *Ophthalmologica* 165:360, 1972.

58. Danks, D. M., et al. Menkes' kinky hair disease: Further definition of the defect in copper transport. *Science* 179:1140, 1973.

59. Danks, D. M., et al. Malignant hyperphenylalaninemia: Clinical features, biochemical findings and experience with administration of biopterins. *Pediatr. Res.* 13:1150, 1979.

60. Davis, D. G., and Smith, J. L. Retinal involvement in hereditary hemorrhagic telangiectasia. *Arch. Ophthalmol.* 85:618, 1971.

61. Delaney, W. V., Jr. *Physicians' Guide to Oculosystemic Diseases.* Oradell, N. J.: Medical Economics, 1982.

62. Dicken, C. H., Dewald, G., and Gordon, H. Sister chromatid exchanges in Bloom's syndrome. *Arch. Dermatol.* 114:755, 1978.

63. Dodson, P. M., et al. Retinal vein occlusion and the prevalence of lipoprotein abnormalities. *Br. J. Ophthalmol.* 66:161, 1982.

64. Dodson, P. M., Galton, D. J., and Winder, A. F. Retinal vascular abnormalities in the hyperlipidaemias. *Trans. Ophthalmol. Soc. U.K.* 101:17, 1981.

65. Donaldson, D. D. Ochronosis. In *Atlas of External Diseases of the Eye, Vol. 1: Congenital Anomalies and Systemic Diseases.* St. Louis: Mosby, 1966.

66. Dorfman, M. L., et al. Ichthyosiform dermatoses with systemic lipidoses. *Arch. Dermatol.* 110:261, 1974.

67. Dotson, A. D., and Raimer, S. S. Incontinentia pigmenti achromians. *Int. J. Dermatol.* 20:357, 1981.

68. Dufier, I. L., et al. La maladie de Fabry et ses manifestations ophtalmologiques. *J. Fr. Ophtalmol.* 3:625, 1980.

69. Dvorak, A. M., et al. Fabry's disease: Use of biopsies from uninvolved skin. Acute and chronic changes

involving the microvasculature and small unmyelinated nerves. *Pathol. Annu.* 16:139, 1981.

70. Eady, R. A. J., and Tidman, M. J. Diagnosing epidermolysis bullosa. *Br. J. Dermatol.* 108:621, 1983.

71. Edidnin, D. V., et al. Chondrodysplasia punctata: Conradi-Hunerman syndrome. *Arch. Dermatol.* 113:1431, 1977.

72. Elejalde, B. R., et al. Mutations affecting pigmentation in man: I. Neuroectodermal melanosomal disease. *Am. J. Med. Genet.* 3:65, 1979.

73. Elsas, L. J., Miller, R. L., and Pinnell, S. R. Inherited human collagen lysyl hydroxylase deficiency: Ascorbic acid response. *J. Pediatr.* 92:378, 1978.

74. Epstein, E. H., Jr., Kraus, R. M., and Schackleton, C. H. L. X-linked ichthyosis: Increased blood cholesterol sulfate and electrophoretic mobility of low-density lipoprotein. *Science* 214:659, 1981.

75. Esterly, N. B. The ichthyosiform dermatoses. *Pediatrics* 42:990, 1968.

76. Falls, H. F., and Schull, W. J. Hallermann-Streiff syndrome. *Arch. Ophthalmol.* 63:409, 1960.

77. Felberg, N. T., and Michelson, J. B. The Immunologic Aspects of Pediatric Eye Disease. In R. D. Harley (Ed.), *Pediatric Ophthalmology* (2nd ed.), Vol. 2. Philadelphia: Saunders, 1983.

78. Feman, S., Apt, L. and Roth, A. M. The basal cell nevus syndrome. *Am. J. Ophthalmol.* 78:222, 1974.

79. Fischer, E., et al. Xeroderma pigmentosum patients in Germany: Clinical symptoms and DNA repair characteristics. *Arch. Dermatol. Res.* 274:229, 1982.

80. Fleishmajer, R., et al. Ultrastructure and composition of connective tissue in hyalinosis cutis et mucosae skin. *J. Invest. Dermatol.* 82:252, 1984.

81. Flynn, J. T. Neonatal Ophthalmology: Evaluation of Visual Function in the Neonate and Infant. In R. D. Harley (Ed.), *Pediatric Ophthalmology* (2nd ed.), Vol. 1. Philadelphia: Saunders, 1983.

82. Foroozonfar, N., et al. Bone-marrow transplant from an unrelated donor for chronic granulomatous disease. *Lancet* 1:210, 1977.

83. Franceschetti, A. The eye and inborn errors of metabolism. In D. Bergsma, A. J. Bron, and E. Cotlier (Eds.), *Birth Defects.* New York: Alan R. Liss., 1976.

84. François, J. Incontinentia pigmenti and retinal changes. *Br. J. Ophthalmol.* 68:19, 1984.

85. François, J. Ocular manifestations in aminoacidopathies. *Adv. Ophthalmol.* 25:28, 1972.

86. François, J. The Riley-Day syndrome. *Ophthalmologica* 174:20, 1977.

87. François, J., Hanssens, M., and Teuchy, H. Corneal ultrastructural changes in Fabry's disease. *Ophthalmologica* 176:313, 1978.

88. François, J., and Pierard, J. The François dyscephalic syndrome and skin manifestations. *Am. J. Ophthalmol.* 71:1241, 1971.

89. Fredrickson, D. S. Plasma Lipid Abnormalities and Cutaneous and Subcutaneous Xanthomas. In T. B. Fitzpatrick et al. (Eds.), *Dermatology in General Medicine* (2nd ed.). New York: McGraw-Hill, 1979.

90. Freedman, J. Corneal transplantation with associated histopathologic description in xeroderma pigmentosum occurring in a black family. *Ann. Ophthalmol.* 11:445, 1979.

91. From, L. Vascular Neoplasms, Pseudoneoplasms, and Hyperplasias. In T. B. Fitzpatrick et al. (Eds.), *Dermatology in General Medicine* (2nd ed.). New York: McGraw-Hill, 1979.

92. Fujiwara, Y., Goto, K., and Kano, Y. Ultraviolet hypersensitivity of Cockayne's syndrome fibroblasts. *Exp. Cell Res.* 139:207, 1982.

93. Fulk, C. S. Primary disorders of hyperpigmentation. *J. Am. Acad. Dermatol.* 10:1, 1984.

94. Furukawa, T., et al. Sturge-Weber and Klippel-Trenaunay syndrome with nevus of Ota and Ito. *Arch. Dermatol.* 102:640, 1970.

95. Gaasterland, D. E., Rodrigues, M. M., and Moshell, A. N. Ocular involvement in xeroderma pigmentosum. *Ophthalmology* (Rochester) 89:980, 1982.

96. Galijaard, H. *Genetic Metabolic Diseases, Early Diagnosis and Prenatal Analysis.* Amsterdam: Elsevier, 1980.

97. Gatti, R. A., et al. Ataxia-telangiectasia: A multiparameter analysis of eight families. *Clin. Immunol. Immunopathol.* 23:501, 1982.

98. Gedde-Dahl, T. Sixteen types of epidermolysis bullosa. *Acta Derm. Venereol. [Suppl.]* (Stockh.) 95:74, 1981.

99. Gedde-Dahl, T., and Anton-Lamprecht, I. Epidermolysis Bullosa. In A. E. H. Emery and D. L. Rimion (Eds.), *The Principles and Practice of Medical Genetics.* London: Churchill Livingstone, 1982.

100. German, J., Bloom, D., and Passarge, E. Bloom's syndrome: VII. Progress report for 1978. *Clin. Genet.* 15:361, 1979.

101. Goldberg, M. F. Waardenburg's syndrome with fundus and other anomalies. *Arch. Ophthalmol.* 76:797, 1966.

102. Goldberg, M. F., Payne, J. W., and Brunt, P. W. Ophthalmologic studies of familial dysautonomia. *Arch. Ophthalmol.* 8:732, 1969.

103. Goldberg, M. F., and Ryan, S. J. Intercalary staphyloma in Marfan's syndrome. *Am. J. Ophthalmol.* 67:329, 1969.

104. Goldberg, R. E., Pheasant, T. R., and Shields, J. A. Cavernous hemangioma of the retina: A four generation pedigree with neurocutaneous manifestations and an example of bilateral retinal involvement. *Arch. Ophthalmol.* 97:2321, 1979.

105. Goldsmith, L. A. Other Genetic Disorders of the Skin. In A. E. H. Emery and D. L. Rimion (Eds.), *The Principles and Practice of Medical Genetics.* London: Churchill Livingstone, 1982.

106. Goldsmith, L. A. Tyrosinemia II: Lessons in molecular pathophysiology. *Pediatr. Dermatol.* 1:25, 1983.

107. Goltz, R. W., et al. Focal dermal hypoplasia syndrome: A review of the literature and report of two cases. *Arch. Dermatol.* 101:1, 1970.

108. Gordon, H., Gordon, W., and Botha, V. Lipoid proteinosis in an inbred Namaqualand community. *Lancet* 1:1032, 1969.

109. Gorlin, R. J., Pindborg, J. J., and Cohen, M. M., Jr. *Syndromes of the Head and Neck* (2nd ed.). New York: McGraw-Hill, 1976.

110. Goudie, R. B., et al. Unstable mutations in vitiligo, organ-specific autoimmune diseases, and multiple adenoma peptic ulcer syndrome. *Lancet* 1:285, 1980.

111. Granek, H., and Baden, H. P. Corneal involvement in epidermolysis bullosa simplex. *Arch. Ophthalmol.* 98:469, 1980.

112. Griscelli, C., et al. A syndrome associating partial albinism and immunodeficiency. *Am. J. Med.* 65:691, 1978.

113. Hamada, T., et al. Incontinentia pigmenti (Ito). *Arch. Dermatol.* 96:673, 1967.

114. Hammerstein, W., Meiers, H. G., and Haensch, R. Die Hornhautveränderungen bei Ichthyosen. *Albrecht von Graefe's Arch. Klin. Ophthalmol.* 195:161, 1975.

115. Happle, R., and Hoehn, H. Cytogenetic studies on cultured fibroblast-like cells derived from basal cell carcinoma tissue. *Clin. Genet.* 4:17, 1973.

116. Happle, R., and Lenz, W. Striation of bones in focal dermal hypoplasia: Manifestation of functional mosaicism? *Br. J. Dermatol.* 96:133, 1977.

117. Hara, K., et al. Kinky hair disease: Biochemical, histochemical and ultrastructural studies. *Pediatr. Res.* 13:1222, 1979.

118. Havel, R. J. Approach to the patient with hyperlipidemia. *Med. Clin. North Am.* 66:319, 1982.

119. Hazen, P. G., et al. Premature cataracts in a family with hidrotic ectodermal dysplasia. *Arch. Dermatol.* 116:1385, 1980.

120. Hernandez, A., et al. A distinct variant of the Ehlers-Danlos syndrome. *Clin. Genet.* 16:335, 1979.

121. Hernell, O., et al. Suspected faulty essential fatty acid metabolism in Sjögren-Larsson syndrome. *Pediatr. Res.* 16:45, 1982.

122. Hidano, A., et al. Natural history of nevus of Ota. *Arch. Dermatol.* 95:187, 1967.

123. Hintner, H., and Wolff, K. Generalized atrophic benign epidermolysis bullosa. *Arch. Dermatol.* 118:375, 1982.

124. Ho, P. C., and Feman, S. S. Internuclear ophthalmoplegia in Fabry's disease. *Ann. Ophthalmol.* 13:949, 1981.

125. Hoar, D. I., and Waghorne, C. DNA repair in Cockayne syndrome. *Am. J. Hum. Genet.* 30:590, 1978.

126. Hoefnagel, D., and Benirschke, K. Dyscephalia mandibulo-oculo-facialis (Hallermann-Streiff syndrome). *Arch. Dis. Child.* 40:57, 1965.

127. Hollister, D. W. Clinical Features of Ehlers-Danlos Syndrome Types VIII and IX. In W. H. Akeson, P. Bornstein, and M. J. Glimcher (Eds.), *American Academy of Orthopaedic Surgeons Symposium on Heritable Disorders of Connective Tissue, San Diego, California, May, 1980.* St. Louis: Mosby, 1982.

128. Holubar, K., Matras, H., and Smalik, A. V. Multiple basal cell epitheliomas in basal cell nevus syndrome. *Arch. Dermatol.* 101:679, 1970.

129. Howard, R. O. Premature cataracts associated with generalized lentigo. *Trans. Am. Ophthalmol. Soc.* 77:121, 1979.

130. Hoyt, C. S., 3d. The ocular findings in infantile spasms. *Ophthalmology (Rochester)* 86:1794, 1979.

131. In, S., et al. Intraorbital optic nerve hemangioblastoma with von Hippel-Lindau disease. *J. Neurosurg.* 56:426, 1982.

132. Ishibashi, A. Histogenesis of hyalinosis cutis et mucosae. *J. Dermatol. (Tokyo)* 5:265, 1978.

133. Ishibashi, A., and Kurihara, Y. Goltz's syndrome: Focal dermal dysplasia syndrome. *Dermatologica* 144:156, 1972.

134. Jagell, S., Polland, W., and Sandgren, O. Specific changes in the fundus typical for the Sjögren-Larsson syndrome. *Acta Ophthalmol. (Copenh.)* 58:321, 1980.

135. Jaspers, N. G. J., and Bootsma, D. Genetic heterogeneity in ataxia-telangiectasia studied by cell fusion. *Proc. Natl. Acad. Sci. U.S.A.* 79:2641, 1982.

136. Jay, B., Blach, R. K., and Wells, R. S. Ocular manifestations of ichthyosis. *Br. J. Ophthalmol.* 52:217, 1968.

137. Jelinek, J. E., Bart, S. B., and Schiff, G. M. Hypomelanosis of Ito (incontinentia pigmenti achromians). *Arch. Dermatol.* 107:596, 1973.

138. Jerndal, T. Ectodermal dysplasia with infantile congenital glaucoma. *J. Pediatr. Ophthalmol.* 7:29, 1970.

139. Jorizzo, J. L., et al. Ichthyosis, brittle hair, impaired intelligence, decreased fertility, and short stature (BIDS syndrome). *Br. J. Dermatol.* 106:705, 1982.

140. Jorizzo, J. L., Crounse, R. G., and Wheeler, C. E., Jr. Lamellar ichthyosis, dwarfism, mental retardation, and hair shaft abnormalities. *J. Am. Acad. Dermatol.* 2:309, 1980.

141. Judisch, G. F., Waziri, M., and Krachmer, J. H. Ocular Ehlers-Danlos syndrome with normal lysyl hydroxylase activity. *Arch. Ophthalmol.* 94:1489, 1976.

142. Kampik, A., Sani, J. N., and Green, R. Ocular ochronosis: Clinicopathological, histochemical and ultrastructural studies. *Arch. Ophthalmol.* 98:1441, 1980.

143. Karpik, A. G., et al. Corneal transplantation in familial dysautonomia. *Am. J. Ophthalmol.* 88:993, 1979.

144. Keinke, T., Kaber, K., and Tosselson, A. Ota nevus, multiple hemangiomas, and Takayasu arteritis. *Arch. Dermatol.* 110:447, 1974.

145. Kirkham, T. H., and Werner, E. B. The ophthalmic manifestations of Rothmund's syndrome. *Can. J. Ophthalmol.* 10:1, 1975.

146. Kleinebrecht, J., et al. Sweat pore counts in ectodermal dysplasias. *Hum. Genet.* 57:437, 1981.

147. Kline, A. H., Sidbury, J. B., Jr., and Richter, C. P. The occurrence of ectodermal dysplasia and corneal dysplasia in one family: An inquiry into the mode of inheritance. *J. Pediatr.* 55:355, 1959.

148. Knox, D. L. Disorders of the Uveal Tract. In R. D. Harley (Ed.), *Pediatric Ophthalmology* (2nd ed.), Vol. 1. Philadelphia: Saunders, 1983.

149. Koppe, G., et al. X-linked ichthyosis. *Arch. Dis. Child.* 53:803, 1978.

150. Kroll, A. J., et al. Vitreous hemorrhage complicating retinal astrocytic hamartoma. *Surv. Ophthalmol.* 26:31, 1981.

151. Kurz, G. H., et al. The retina in type 5 hyperlipoproteinemia. *Am. J. Ophthalmol.* 82:32, 1976.

152. Laibson, P. R., and Waring, G. O. Diseases of the Cornea. In R. D. Harley (Ed.), *Pediatric Ophthalmology* (2nd ed.), Vol. 1. Philadelphia: Saunders, 1983.

153. Lazoff, S. G. Skeletal dysplasia, occipital horns, diarrhea, and obstructive uropathy: A new hereditary syndrome. *Birth Defects* 11(5):71, 1975.

154. Lerner, A. B. Vitiligo. *J. Invest. Dermatol.* 32:285, 1959.

155. Lerner, A. B., and Nordlund, J. J. Vitiligo: The loss of pigment in skin, hair and eyes. *J. Dermatol. (Tokyo)* 5:1, 1978.

156. Lerner, A. B., Nordlund, J. J., and Albert, D. M. Pigment cells of the eyes in people with vitiligo. *N. Engl. J. Med.* 296:232, 1977.

157. Lever, W. F., and Schaumburg-Lever, G. *Histopathology of the Skin* (6th ed.). Philadelphia: Lippincott, 1983.

158. Levin, P. S., et al. Histopathology of the eye in Cockayne's syndrome. *Arch. Ophthalmol.* 101:1093, 1983.

159. Lewis, R. A. Ocular albinism and deafness. *Am. J. Hum. Genet.* 30:57A, 1978.

160. Lewis, R. A., and Riccardi, V. M. von Recklinghausen neurofibromatosis: Incidence of iris hamartomata. *Ophthalmology (Rochester)* 88:348, 1981.

161. Loffredo, A., et al. Hereditary microphthalmos associated with ichthyosis. *Ophthalmologica* 184:78, 1982.

162. Lubin, J. R., Ni, C., and Albert, D. M. A clinicopathological study of the Vogt-Koyanagi-Harada syndrome. *Int. Ophthalmol. Clin.* 22:141, 1982.

163. Marchase, P., Holbrook, K., and Pinnell, S. R. A familial cutis laxa syndrome with ultrastructural abnormalities of collagen and elastin. *J. Invest. Dermatol.* 75:399, 1980.

164. Margolis, S., et al. Depigmentation of hair, skin and eyes associated with Apert Syndrome. *Birth Defects* 14:341, 1978.

165. Marshall, D. Ectodermal dysplasia. *Am. J. Ophthalmol.* 45:143, 1958.

166. Martyn, L. J., et al. Chorioretinal lesions in familial chronic granulomatous disease of childhood. *Am. J. Ophthalmol.* 73:403, 1972.

167. Maumenee, I. H. The eye in the Marfan syndrome. *Trans. Am. Ophthalmol. Soc.* 79:684, 1981.

168. Merenlender, J., and Rywlin, J. A. À propos de l'hérédité du vitiligo acquis (vitiligo dans 3 générations). *Acta Derm. Venereol. (Stockh.)* 21:583, 1949.

169. Milot, J., and Demay, F. Ocular anomalies in the de Lange syndrome. *Am. J. Ophthalmol.* 74:394, 1972.

170. Miranda, A., et al. Lipid storage myopathy, ichthyosis, and steatorrhea. *Muscle Nerve* 2:1, 1979.

171. Mishima, Y., and Mevorah, B. Nevus Ota and nevus Ito in American negroes. *J. Invest. Dermatol.* 36:133, 1961.

172. Misti, J., and Waldmann, T. A. A defect in antigen-specific antibody production due to a lack of T helper cells in a patient with ataxia-telangiectasia. *Trans. Assoc. Am. Physicians* 94:349, 1981.

173. Mohandes, T., et al. Regional assignment of the steroid sulfatase–X-linked ichthyosis locus: Implications for a non-inactivated region on the short arm of human X-chromosome. *Proc. Nat. Acad. Sci. U.S.A.* 76:5779, 1979.

174. Morris, T. J., Johnson, W. M. G., and Silvers, D. N. Giant pigment granules in biopsy specimens from café-au-lait spots in neurofibromatosis. *Arch. Dermatol.* 118:385, 1982.

175. Mosher, D. B., Fitzpatrick, T. B., and Ortonne, J. P. Abnormalities of Pigmentation. In T. B. Fitzpatrick et al. (Eds.), *Dermatology in General Medicine* (2nd ed.). New York: McGraw-Hill, 1979.

176. Muirhead, J. F., and Jackson, P. Lipoid proteinosis (of Urbach-Wiethe). *Arch. Ophthalmol.* 69:174, 1963.

177. Nelson, C. E., Dahl, M. V., and Goltz, R. W. Arcuate dermal erythema in a carrier of chronic granulomatous disease. *Arch. Dermatol.* 113:798, 1977.

178. Nelson, L. B. *Pediatric Ophthalmology.* Philadelphia: Saunders, 1984.

179. Nemet, P., et al. Ataxia telangiectasia. *Ophthalmologica* 181:330, 1980.

180. Nicholson, D. H., and Goldberg, M. F. Ocular abnormalities in the de Lange syndrome. *Arch. Ophthalmol.* 76:214, 1966.

181. Nordlund, J. J., et al. Halo nevi and the Vogt-Koyanagi-Harada syndrome: Manifestations of vitiligo. *Arch. Dermatol.* 116:690, 1980.

182. Nordlund, J. J., et al. The multiple lentigines syndrome. *Arch. Dermatol.* 107:259, 1973.

183. Noreiga-Sanchez, A., Markand, O. N., and Herndon, J. H. Oculocutaneous melanosis associated with the Sturge-Weber syndrome. *Neurology (Minneapolis)* 22:256, 1972.

184. Norwood, T. H., et al. Cellular aging in Werner's syndrome: A unique phenotype? *J. Invest. Dermatol.* 73:92, 1979.

185. Nyboer, J. H., Robertson, D. M., and Gomez, M. R.

Retinal lesions in tuberous sclerosis. *Arch. Ophthalmol.* 94:1277, 1976.

186. O'Donnell, F. E., Jr., et al. X-linked ocular albinism: An oculocutaneous macromelanosomal disorder. *Arch. Ophthalmol.* 94:1883, 1976.

187. Omenn, G. S., and McKusick, V. A. The association of Waardenburg syndrome and Hirschsprung megacolon. *Am. J. Med. Genet.* 3:217, 1979.

188. Orth, D. H., Fretzin, D. F., and Abramson, V. Collodion baby with transient bilateral upper lid ectropion. *Arch. Ophthalmol.* 91:206, 1974.

189. Ortonne, J. P., et al. Valeur diagnostique des taches café-au-lait. *Ann. Dermatol. Venereol.* 107:313, 1980.

190. Oxelius, V., Berkel, A. I., and Hanson, L. A. IgG2 deficiency in ataxia-telangiectasia. *N. Engl. J. Med.* 306:515, 1982.

191. Palestine, A. G., et al. Ocular findings in patients with neutrophil dysfunction. *Am. J. Ophthalmol.* 95:598, 1983.

192. Palmer, D. D., and Perry, H. O. Melanosis oculi, a variant of nevus of Ota. *Arch. Dermatol.* 85:740, 1962.

193. Partington, M. W. Waardenburg's syndrome and heterochromia iridum in a deaf school population. *Can. Med. Assoc. J.* 90:1008, 1964.

194. Paula-Barbosa, M. M., et al. Cerebellar cortex ultrastructure in ataxia-telangiectasia. *Ann. Neurol.* 13:297, 1983.

195. Pearce, W. G. Ocular and genetic features of Cockayne's syndrome. *Can. J. Ophthalmol.* 7:435, 1972.

196. Pearson, J. Familial dysautonomia (a brief review). *J. Auton. Nerv. Syst.* 1:119, 1979.

197. Pemberton, J. W., Freeman, H. M., and Schepens, C. L. Familial retinal detachment and the Ehler-Danlos syndrome. *Arch. Ophthalmol.* 76:817, 1966.

198. Petrohelos, M. A. Werner's syndrome: A survey of three cases, with review of the literature. *Am. J. Ophthalmol.* 56:941, 1963.

199. Pinnell, S. R., et al. A heritable disorder of connective tissue: Hydroxylysine-deficient collagen disease. *N. Engl. J. Med.* 286:1013, 1972.

200. Pipkin, A. C., and Pipkin, S. B. A pedigree of generalized lentigo. *J. Hered.* 41:79, 1950.

201. Pope, F. M. Historical evidence for the genetic heterogeneity of pseudoxanthoma elasticum. *Br. J. Dermatol.* 92:493, 1975.

202. Prentice, F. M., and Mackie, R. M. A case of focal dermal hypoplasia. *Clin. Exp. Dermatol.* 7:149, 1982.

203. Price, V. H., et al. Trichothiodystrophy: Sulfur-deficient brittle hair as a marker for a neuroectodermal symptom complex. *Arch. Dermatol.* 116:1375, 1980.

204. Pries, C., et al. The EEC syndrome. *Am. J. Dis. Child.* 127:840, 1974.

205. Privat, Y., et al. Nevus de Ota bilateral à localisation exclusivement oculaire et associé à un syndrome de dégénérescence spino-cérébelleuse. *Bull. Soc. Fr. Derm. Syph.* 75:213, 1968.

206. Proops, R., Taylor, A. M. R., and Insley, J. A clinical study of a family with Cockayne's syndrome. *J. Med. Genet.* 18:288, 1981.

207. Punnett, H. H., and Harley, R. D. Genetics in Pediatric Ophthalmology. In R. D. Harley (Ed.), *Pediatric Ophthalmology* (2nd ed.), Vol. 1. Philadelphia: Saunders, 1983.

208. Pyeritz, R. E., Bender, W. L., and Lipford, E. H., 3rd. Anderson-Fabry disease. *Johns Hopkins Med. J.* 150:181, 1982.

209. Rainbow, A. J., and Howes, M. A deficiency in the repair of UV and γ-ray damaged DNA in fibroblasts from Cockayne's syndrome. *Mutat. Res.* 93:235, 1982.

210. Rand, R. E., and Baden, H. P. The ichthyoses: A review. *J. Am. Acad. Dermatol.* 8:285, 1983.

211. Reed, W. B., Lopez, D. A., and Landing, B. Clinical spectrum of anhidrotic ectodermal dysplasia. *Arch. Dermatol.* 102:134, 1970.

212. Reed, W. B., et al. Pigmentary disorders in association with congenital deafness. *Arch. Dermatol.* 95:176, 1967.

213. Reed, W. B., and Sugarman, G. I. Unilateral nevus de Ota with sensorineural deafness. *Arch. Dermatol.* 109:881, 1974.

214. Reeve, E. B., et al. Development and calcification of skin lesions in thirty-nine patients with pseudoxanthoma elasticum. *Clin. Exp. Dermatol.* 4:291, 1979.

215. Reinke, R. T., Haber, K., and Josselson, A. Ota nevus, multiple hemangiomas and Takayasu arteritis. *Arch. Dermatol.* 110:447, 1974.

216. Riccardi, V. M. Neurofibromatosis heterogeneity. *J. Am. Acad. Dermatol.* 8:518, 1983.

217. Riccardi, V. M. The Phakomatoses. In A. E. H. Emery and D. L. Rimion (Eds.), *The Principles and Practice of Medical Genetics.* London: Churchill Livingstone, 1982.

218. Riccardi, V. M. von Recklinghausen neurofibromatosis. *N. Engl. J. Med.* 305:1617, 1981.

219. Riegel, E. M., et al. Ocular pathology of Fabry's disease in a hemizygous male following renal transplantation. *Surv. Ophthalmol.* 26:247, 1982.

220. Riley, H. D., Jr., and Smith, W. R. Macrocephaly, pseudopapilledema, and multiple hemangiomata: A previously undescribed heredofamilial syndrome. *Pediatrics* 26:293, 1960.

221. Rivat-Peran, L., et al. Immunoglobulins in ataxia-telangiectasia: Evidence for IgG4 and IgA2 subclass deficiencies. *Clin. Immunol. Immunopathol.* 20:99, 1981.

222. Robbins, J. H. Xeroderma Pigmentosum. In T. B. Fitzpatrick et al. (Eds.), *Dermatology in General Medicine* (2nd ed.). New York: McGraw-Hill, 1979.

223. Rogers, R. B., et al. Phenytoin therapy for junctional epidermolysis bullosa. *Arch. Dermatol.* 119:925, 1983.

224. Rosen, E. *Atopic Cataract.* Springfield, Ill.: Thomas, 1959.

225. Rosenthal, J. W., and Kloepfer, H. W. An acromegaloid, cutis verticis gyrata, corneal leukoma syndrome. *Arch. Ophthalmol.* 68:722, 1962.

226. Rostenburg, A., Jr., and Solomon. L. M. Atopic Dermatitis and Infantile Eczema. In M. Samter (Ed.), *Immunological Diseases* (2nd ed.), Vol. 2. Boston: Little, Brown and Co., 1971.

227. Salem, O. S., and Steck, W. D. Cowden's disease (multiple hamartoma and neoplasia syndrome): A case report and review of the English literature. *J. Am. Acad. Dermatol.* 8:686, 1983.

228. Schaumburg-Lever, G., and Lever, W. F. Electron microscopy of incontinentia pigmenti. *J. Invest. Dermatol.* 61:151, 1978.

229. Schmidt, A., von Samson, G., and Passarge, E. Hereditary Increase in Sister Chromatid Exchanges: The Bloom's Syndrome. In D. Müller et al. (Eds.), *Sister-Chromatid-Exchange Test.* Stuttgart: Thieme, 1982.

230. Schmoeckel, C., and Hohlfed, M. A specific ultrastructural marker for disseminated lipogranulomatosis (Farber). *Arch. Dermatol. Res.* 226:187, 1979.

231. Schwarts, M. F., Jr., et al. Hypomelanosis of Ito (incontinentia pigmenti achromians): A neurocutaneous syndrome. *J. Pediatr.* 90:236, 1977.

232. Scoggins, R. B., et al. Dyskeratosis congenita with Fanconi-type anemia: Investigations of immunologic and other defects (abstract). *Clin. Res.* 19:409, 1971.

233. Selmanowitz, V. J., and Porter, M. J. The Sjögren-Larsson syndrome. *Am. J. Med.* 42:412, 1967.

234. Shapiro, L. J. X-linked ichthyosis. *Int. J. Dermatol.* 20:26, 1981.

235. Shapiro, L. J., et al. Enzymatic basis of typical X-linked ichthyosis. *Lancet* 2:756, 1978.

236. Sher, N. A., Letson, R. D., and Desnick, R. J. The ocular manifestations in Fabry's disease. *Arch. Ophthalmol.* 97:671, 1979.

237. Sher, N. A., et al. Central retinal artery occlusion complicating Fabry's disease. *Arch. Ophthalmol.* 96:815, 1978.

238. Shindle, R. D., and Leone, C. R. Cicatricial ectropion associated with lamellar ichthyosis. *Arch. Ophthalmol.* 89:62, 1973.

239. Siccardi, A. G., et al. A new familial defect in neutrophil bactericidal activity. *Helv. Paediatr. Acta* 33:401, 1978.

240. Silver, H. K. Rothmund-Thomson syndrome: An oculocutaneous disorder. *Am. J. Dis. Child.* 111:182, 1966.

241. Simon, J. W., et al. Ophthalmic manifestations of the Hermansky-Pudlak syndrome (oculocutaneous albinism and hemorrhagic diathesis). *Am. J. Ophthalmol.* 93:71, 1982.

242. Simpson, J. L., et al. *Genetics in Obstetrics and Gynecology.* New York: Grune & Stratton, 1982.

243. Sirinavin, C., and Trowbridge, A. A. Dyskeratosis congenita: Clinical features and genetic aspects. Report of a family and review of the literature. *Med. Genet.* 12:339, 1975.

244. Skinner, B. A., Greist, M. C., and Norins, A. L. The keratitis, ichthyosis, and deafness (KID) syndrome. *Arch. Dermatol.* 117:285, 1981.

245. Smith, I., et al. Fetal damage despite low-phenylalanine diet after conception in a phenylketonuric woman. *Lancet* 1:17, 1979.

246. Soffer, D., et al. Cockayne syndrome: Unusual neuropathological findings and review of the literature. *Ann. Neurol.* 6:340, 1979.

247. Solomon, L. M., and Esterly, N. B. Epidermal and other congenital organoid nevi. *Curr. Probl. Pediatr.* 6:3, 1975.

248. Solomon, L. M., and Esterly, N. B. The Skin and the Eye. In M. F. Goldberg (Ed.), *Genetic and Metabolic Eye Disease* (1st ed.). Boston: Little, Brown and Co., 1974.

249. Solomon, L. M., and Keuer, E. J. The ectodermal dysplasias: Problems of classification and some newer syndromes. *Arch. Dermatol.* 116:1295, 1980.

250. Srsen, S. Alkaptonuria. *Johns Hopkins Med. J.* 145:217, 1979.

251. Srsen, S., and Varga, F. Newborn population screening for alkaptonuria in Slovakia. *Lancet* 2:576, 1978.

252. Steelenfreund, M. H., Gartner, S., and Vinger, P. F. The ocular pathology of Menkes' disease (kinky hair disease). *Arch. Ophthalmol.* 80:718, 1968.

253. Stenson, S. Ocular findings in xeroderma pigmentosum: Report of two cases. *Ann. Ophthalmol.* 14:580, 1982.

254. Stern, J., Jakobeic, F. A., and Horesepian, E. M. The architecture of optic nerve gliomas with and without neurofibromatosis. *Arch. Ophthalmol.* 98:505, 1980.

255. Strempel, I. Aggressives lidbasaliom bei erythrodermia ichthyosiformis congenita sicca. *Ophthalmologica* 176:53, 1978.

256. Taniguchi, N., et al. Impaired B-cell differentiation and T-cell regulatory function in four patients with Bloom's syndrome. *Clin. Immunol. Immunopathol.* 22:247, 1982.

257. Tasman, W. Diseases of the Retina and the Vitreous. In R. D. Harley (Ed.), *Pediatric Ophthalmology* (2nd ed.), Vol. 1. Philadelphia: Saunders, 1983.

258. Tasman, W. Retinal changes in congenital poikiloderma. *Am. J. Ophthalmol.* 72:979, 1971.

259. Thiele, U. Sjögren-Larsson syndrome. *Fortschr. Med.* 96:90, 1978.

260. Thiers, B. H. The mechanobullous diseases. *J. Am. Acad. Dermatol.* 5:745, 1981.

261. Thomas, J. V., et al. Ocular manifestations of focal dermal hypoplasia syndrome. *Arch. Ophthalmol.* 95:1997, 1977.

262. Tietz, W. A syndrome of deaf-mutism associated with albinism showing dominant autosomal inheritance. *Am. J. Hum. Genet.* 15:259, 1963.

263. Toumaala, P., and Haapanen, E. Three siblings with similar anomalies in the eyes, bones and skin. *Acta Ophthalmol. (Copenh.)* 46:385, 1968.

264. Tuppurainene, K., et al. Fabry's disease and cornea verticillata. *Acta Ophthalmol. (Copenh.)* 59:674, 1981.

265. Ufermann, K., Heege-Dohr, R., and Kosenow, W. Augenbeteiligung beim Cockayne-syndrome. *Klin. Monatsbl. Augenheilkd.* 162:655, 1973.

266. Utsunomiya, J., et al. Peutz-Jeghers syndrome: Its natural course and management. *Johns Hopkins Med. J.* 136:71, 1975.

267. Vermeer, B. J., et al. Xanthomatosis and other clinical findings in patients with elevated levels of very low density lipoproteins. *Br. J. Dermatol.* 100:657, 1979.

268. Vijayalaxmi, et al. Bloom's syndrome: Evidence for an increased mutation frequency in vivo. *Science* 221:851, 1983.

269. Waldmann, T. A., et al. Ataxia-telangiectasia: A multisystem hereditary disease with immunodeficiency, impaired organ maturation, X-ray hypersensitivity, and a high incidence of neoplasia. *Ann. Intern. Med.* 99:367, 1983.

270. Welch, R. B. von Hippel-Lindau disease: The recognition and treatment of early angiomatosis retinae and the use of cryosurgery as an adjunct to therapy. *Trans. Am. Ophthalmol. Soc.* 68:367, 1971.

271. Welshimer, K., and Swift, M. Congenital malformations and developmental disabilities in ataxia-telangiectasia, Fanconi anemia, and xeroderma pigmentosum families. *Am. J. Hum. Genet.* 34:781, 1982.

272. Weston, W. L. Disorders of phagocyte function. *Arch. Dermatol.* 112:1589, 1976.

273. Wheeler, J. M. Plexiform neurofibromatosis (von Recklinghausen's disease) involving the choroid, ciliary body, and other structures. *Am. J. Ophthalmol.* 20:368, 1937.

274. White, J. G., and Clawson, C. C. The Chédiak-Higashi syndrome: The nature of the giant neutrophil granules and their interactions with cytoplasm and foreign particulates. *Am. J. Pathol.* 98:151, 1980.

275. Whyte, M. P., and Dekaban, A. S. Familial cerebellar degeneration with slow eye movements, mental deterioration and incidental nevus of Ota. *Dev. Med. Child Neurol.* 18:373, 1976.

276. Wilund, D. A., and Weston, W. L. Incontinentia pigmenti. *Arch. Dermatol.* 116:701, 1980.

277. Williams, M. L. The ichthyoses: Pathogenesis and prenatal diagnosis. A review of recent advances. *Pediatr. Dermatol.* 1:1, 1983.

278. Williams, M. L., and Elias, P. M. Lamellar ichthyosis: Biochemical and clinical evidence of heterogeneity. *Clin. Res.* 31:152A, 1983.

279. Winder, A. F., Dodson, P. M., and Galton, D. J. Ophthalmological complications of the hypertriglyceridaemias. *Trans. Ophthalmol. Soc. U.K.* 100:119, 1980.

280. Witkop, C. J., Jr. Abnormalities of Pigmentation. In A. E. H. Emery and D. L. Rimion (Eds.), *The Principles and Practice of Medical Genetics.* London: Churchill Livingstone, 1982.

281. Witkop, C. J., Jr., Quevedo, W. C., Jr., and Fitzpatrick, T. B. Albinism, In J. B. Stanbury, J. B. Wyngaarden, and D. S. Fredrickson (Eds.), *The Metabolic Basis of Inherited Disease* (4th ed.). New York: McGraw-Hill, 1978.

282. Wolach, B., Baehner, R. L., and Boxer, L. A. Review: Clinical and laboratory approach to the management of neutrophil dysfunction. *Isr. J. Med. Sci.* 18:897, 1982.

283. Woo, S. L. C., et al. Prenatal diagnosis of classical phenylketonuria by gene mapping. *JAMA* 251:1998, 1984.

284. Woog, J. J., et al. Neurofibromatosis of the eyelid and orbit. *Int. Ophthalmol. Clin.* 22:157, 1982.

285. Yount, W. J. IgG2 deficiency and ataxia-telangiectasia. *N. Engl. J. Med.* 306:541, 1982.

286. Zelickson, A. S., et al. The Chédiak-Higashi syndrome: Formation of giant melanosomes and the basis of hypopigmentation. *J. Invest. Dermatol.* 49:575, 1967.

287. Ziprowski, L., et al. Partial albinism and deaf-mutism: Due to a recessive sex-linked gene. *Arch. Dermatol.* 86:530, 1962.

20

Therapy and Prevention of Various Genetic Eye Diseases

Edward Cotlier

In this review of therapy and prevention of genetic diseases affecting the eye, I shall discuss only therapies applied to humans, excluding therapeutic attempts in animal models, cells in culture, or model acellular systems. Ophthalmologists are involved in cataract surgery in galactosemic patients [25], surgery for dislocated lenses of homocystinuric patients [22], corneal transplantation in patients with mucopolysaccharidoses [15] or adult cystinosis, retinal detachment surgery and light coagulation therapy in patients with sickle cell anemia [10], strabismus surgery in children with glycogen storage disease (Pompe's) [21], and glaucoma surgery in children with Lowe's syndrome [1]. Furthermore, ophthalmolgists, with the cooperation of plastic surgeons, can reconstruct major abnormalities of the lids or lacrimal apparatus resulting from gene disorders [26]. This chapter will not discuss these treatments; rather I will concentrate on therapies for deficiencies of enzymes and accumulation of metabolites and therapy and prevention of inborn errors of metabolism.

DEFICIENCES OF ENZYMES AND ACCUMULATION OF METABOLITES

In the homozygous or hemizygous individual, the clinical and laboratory abnormalities of an inborn error of metabolism (IEM) often represent stored substrates resulting from partial or total enzyme deficiency (Fig. 20-1). Enzymes, like all other cellular proteins, are synthesized by exact amino acid alignment through RNA (ribonucleic acid) as specified by the genetic code (DNA, deoxyribonucleic acid). Thus enzyme deficiences indicate

alterations in the molecular composition of DNA or RNA or failure to transmit the proper information from DNA to RNA (transcription) or from RNA to protein (translation).

Interestingly enough, although in the homozygote an enzyme may be absent from all tissues and fluids of the body, clinical signs will appear only in selected tissues. For example, in Tay-Sachs disease, in which hexosaminidase A is absent in all tissues [3, 5], only the central nervous system and retina are clinically involved. It is obvious, then, that other tissues, such as the spleen, liver, cornea, or lens, do not require hexosaminidase A for their function, or that moderate accumulations of its substrate, ganglioside GM_2, do not show as clinical signs. Obligate heterozygotes for most inborn metabolic defects do not present clinical signs, even though enzymes may be reduced to levels of 50 percent or less. Corrective therapy in homozygotes, then, is geared to correct or prevent specific tissue damage.

THERAPY FOR INBORN ERRORS OF METABOLISM

Many theoretical possibilities for correcting defective genes are being considered. However, current therapy for IEM involves four main sites of attack: (1) dietary control, (2) chelation of excessive metabolites, (3) enzyme replacements, and (4) vitamin and cofactor therapy (Fig. 20-2).

Dietary Therapy

Inborn errors of metabolism that affect the eye and improve or reverse to normality after dietary

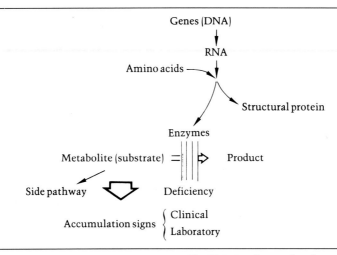

Fig. 20-1. *Biochemical pathway for transmission of genetic information and enzyme blockade resulting in inborn errors of metabolism.*

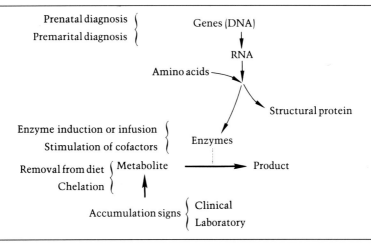

Fig. 20-2. *Sites where corrective measures result in prevention or treatment of inborn errors of metabolism.*

therapy are shown in Table 20-1. Galactosemia was selected from among these disorders for the more detailed discussion that follows.

GALACTOSEMIA

Immediately after a galactose-free diet is instituted, the main features of galactosemia, namely, hepatosplenomegaly, jaundice, and weight loss, begin to reverse. Cortical cataracts (vacuolation or cortical opacities) do not progress (and may even regress) after a galactose-free diet is begun, but mature cataracts do not regress and require surgical therapy. Donnell and colleagues recognize that "complete elimination of galactose has

been advocated, but absolute avoidance of this sugar in the diet is difficult if not impossible" [8]. Galactose-containing foods are generally replaced by casein hydrolysate (Nutramigen) or by a soybean formula (ProSoybee). The galactose content of these foods is neglible.

In galactosemia fetal brain damage or lens toxicity may begin in utero. Thus pregnant mothers known to be carriers of galactosemia must restrict their lactose intake.

Some practical and theoretical problems follow the administration of galactose-free diets: (1) It is very difficult for children to adhere strictly to such a diet, because cake, ice cream, and other lactose-containing foods are among children's favorites. Assay of galactose 1-phosphate in erythrocytes obtained at clinic visits is an excellent procedure for detection of dietary indiscretions. (2) Adherence to the galactose-free diet can be a source of psychological problems. (3) Galactose is required for the synthesis of complex brain and connective tissue glycolipids and glycoproteins, much needed at the time of brain maturation and body growth. Whether or not complete galactose deprivation may have an effect on the brain development of galactosemic patients has not been clearly established. As they grow up, galactosemic patients are able to metabolize galactose through alternate metabolic pathways [2].

Chelation or Removal of Stored Metabolites

Enzyme or transport protein deficiencies may result in the accumulation of a metabolite or metal with toxic effect to the tissues and clinical manifestations. For example, in Wilson's disease, decreased levels of serum ceruloplasmin, which is a glycoprotein attached to the α_2 globulin fraction, result in poor transport of free Cu^{2+} ions and storage of copper in tissues such as brain, liver, and cornea. The resultant clinical signs are basal ganglia degeneration, liver cirrhosis, and the Kayser-Fleischer ring. However, these clinical signs revert partially or totally after the administration of D-penicillamine, a chelator of Cu^{2+} ions at the tissue level [6]. Cupriuria follows penicillamine therapy. Other Cu^{2+} chelators, such as BAL (British anti-lewisite; dimercaprol), or copper-deficient diets, or both, can be given to reverse clinical signs of Wilson's disease (Table 20-2). The ophthalmologist can document the effect of therapy on the clearing of the Kayser-Fleischer ring by direct slit-lamp observation and gonioscopy.

Replacement of Deficient Enzymes (Plasma or Leukocyte Infusions)

In inborn errors of metabolism, most metabolites are stored within cells and sometimes only within cellular organelles such as lysosomes or endoplasmic reticulum. Thus any exogenous enzymes must be transported across capillaries and cell membranes and finally through specific cell organelle membranes before acting on the accumulated metabolite. The molecular weight of enzymes is large (e.g., glycosidases range between 50,000 and 200,000), and these enzymes may contain surface charges that oppose transport through the cell surface. Neufeld and Cantz, however, have found that thermolabile proteins (enzymes?) of 65,000 molecular weight secreted by normal cultured fibroblasts can penetrate into cultured cells from mucopolysaccharidosis patients (Hunter's or Hurler's syndromes) and can degrade stored mucopolysaccharides (MPS) [19]. In addition, these investigators have shown that normal urine contains similar "corrective factors" for fibroblasts from mucopolysaccharidosis patients.

Unfortunately, and contrary to the preliminary results [19], plasma and leukocyte transfusions in patients with Hunter's or Hurler's syndrome have not proven effective in reducing MPS storage in tissues or improving the clinical signs of these disorders (Table 20-3).

Plasma infusion in Fabry's disease has succeeded in decreasing, for a period of days, the plasma levels of ceramide trihexoside (the accumulated substrate), but clinical improvement was not detected [7]. Plasma infusion in patients with Tay-Sachs disease has not resulted in clinical or biochemical improvements [7]. Repeated transfusions of normal plasma in a patient with familial lecithin-cholesterol acyltransferase deficiency resulted in increase of plasma cholesteryl ester from 35 to 310 mg/100 ml, and the unesterified cholesterol decreased [9]. However, plasma triglycerides did not change significantly, and, although some lipoproteins of prebeta mobility appeared, de novo formation of α_1-lipoproteins was not found.

A persistently high level of replacement enzyme would be needed to treat diseases such as the mucopolysaccharidoses or sphingolipidoses on a "chronic" basis. As circulating enzymes are rapidly degraded or excreted by the kidney and may induce circulating antibodies, many failures of continuous serum enzyme infusions for IEM are anticipated. However, it is a promising avenue to pursue, since a slow-release depot preparation containing the deficient enzyme may be administered intramuscularly and may provide adequate therapy for days or weeks.

Vitamin Therapy

Two inborn errors of amino acid metabolism affecting the eye, namely, homocystinuria and gyrate atrophy of the retina, can be partially ameliorated by vitamin therapy (see Table 20-1). In homocystinuria, vitamin B_6 (pyridoxine) has been

Table 20-1. *Dietary Therapy*

Disease	Pathological findings		Therapy	Effect of therapy	
	Clinical	Laboratory		Clinical	Laboratory (serum)
Familial hyperlipoproteinemia Type I (hyperchylomicronemia)	Lipemia retinalis Eruptive xanthomas Abdominal pain Pancreatitis	Serum and lipoprotein electrophoresis: ↑ chylomicrons ↑ triglycerides ↓ postheparin lipolytic activity	Low-fat diet (40–60 g/day)	Reversal of lipemia retinalis	↓ Chylomicrons ↓ Triglycerides
Type II (hyperbetalipoproteinemia)	Xanthomas (palpebral, tendinous, tuberous) Corneal arcus Polyarthritis Vascular heart disease	Serum: ↑ Cholesterol ↑ β-lipoprotein (LDL) ↑ phospholipids	Type II diet: high in polyunsaturates, low in saturates, low in cholesterol Drugs: clofibrate, cholestyramine	↓ Heart disease Disappearance of xanthomas	↓ Cholesterol
Type III	Same as type II Also lipemia retinalis (rare)	↑ Cholesterol ↑ β-Lipoprotein ↑ Pre-β-lipoprotein	Type II diet	Same as type II	Same as type II
Type IV	Lipemia retinalis Eruptive xanthomas Angina pectoris (40%) Hepatosplenomegaly (rare)	↑ Triglycerides ↑ Pre-β-lipoprotiens (VLDL)	Reduce alcohol intake Low-fat diet Clofibrate: effective in 50% of cases	Reversal of lipemia retinalis	↓ Triglycerides
Type V	Same as type IV, plus abdominal pain, pancreatitis, hyperuricemia	↑ Triglycerides ↑ Cholesterol ↑ Chylomicrons ↑ Pre-β-lipoproteins (VLDL)	Low-fat and low-carbohydrate diet Nicotinic acid Norethindrone acetate	Same as type IV	↓ Triglycerides
Tyrosinosis	Corneal ulcers Cataracts Renal tubular acidosis	Serum: ↑ tyrosine Urine: ↓ tyrosine (↓ Million and phenolic substances)	Low-phenylalanine-tyrosine diet	Improvement of renal tubular acidosis Healing of corneal ulcers	Urine: ↓ tyrosine (↓ Million and phenolic substances)

Disease	Clinical manifestations	Laboratory findings	Treatment	Results	Screening
	Liver nodular cirrhosis Thrombocytopenia Skin pigmentation	Liver: ↓ soluble tyrosine amino transferase			
Galactosemia, "classic"	Cataracts Hepatosplenomegaly Mental retardation	Serum: galactosemia RBC, leukocytes: ↓ G1PUT ↑ G1P Aminoaciduria Galactosuria	Galactose-free diet: casein hydrolysate or soybean formula	Reversal of cataracts and hepatosplenomegaly Prevention of mental retardation	↓ Galactosemia and ↓ Galactosuria ↓ G1P in RBC
Galactokinase deficiency	Cataracts	Serum: galactosemia RBC: ↓ galactokinase ↑ galactitol Aminoaciduria Galactosuria	Galactose-free diet	Reversal or prevention of cataracts(?)	↓ Galactosuria
Refsum's disease	Retinitis pigmentosa Peripheral neuropathy Ataxia Skin and bone abnormalities	Serum, liver: ↑ phytanic acid	Low-phytanic-acid diet	Neurologic improvement	↑ Phytanic acid in serum
Homocystinuria	Ectopia lentis Thromboembolism Osteoporosis Mental retardation	Homocystinuria Serum: ↑ methionine ↑ homocystine Liver: ↓ cystathionine synthetase	Diets: 1. Low methionine 2. High cystine 3. Low methionine and cystine 4. Low methionine and cystine and methyl donor Pyridoxine (vitamin B$_6$) Vitamin B$_{12}$	None	↓ Homocystinuria Serum: ↓ methionine ↓ homocystine

↑ = elevated; ↓ = reduced; LDL = low-density lipoprotein; VLDL = very-low-density lipoprotein; RBC = red blood cells; G1PUT = galactose 1-phosphate uridyl transferase; G1P = galactose 1-phosphate.

Table 20-2. *Medical and Surgical Therapy*

Disease and therapeutic approach	Pathological findings		Therapy	Effect of therapy	
	Clinical	Laboratory		Clinical	Laboratory
Cystinosis; surgical and medical therapy	Corneal crystals Retinopathy Dwarfism Rickets Renal tubular acidosis Uremia	Aminoaciduria (generalized) Crystals in leukocytes and bone marrow cells	Renal transplantation Trial: dithiothreitol	Regression of corneal crystals (?) Improvement in uremia signs	—
Wilson's disease; chelation of metabolites	Kayser-Fleischer ring Liver cirrhosis Basal ganglia degeneration (tremor, etc.)	Serum: ↓ copper ↓ ceruloplasmin Aminoaciduria	D-Penicillamine BAL Avoid copper-high foods: liver, nuts, chocolate, mushrooms	Clearing of Kayser-Fleischer ring Improvement of tremor and CNS symptoms	Cupriuria
Abetalipoproteinemia; vitamin therapy	Retinitis pigmentosa ↓ Visual fields Abnormal dark adaptation Steatorrhea Ataxia	Serum: ↓ vitamin A ↓ carotene ↓ cholesterol ↓ triglycerides no betalipoprotein ↓ vitamin E	Vitamin A, 100,000–200,000 units	Improved dark adaptation No effect on retinitis pigmentosa	↓ Vitamin A in serum

↑ = elevated; ↓ = reduced; BAL = British anti-lewisite (dimercaprol); CNS = central nervous system.

Table 20-3. *Plasma or Leukocyte Infusion*

Disease	Pathological findings		Therapy	Effect of Therapy	
	Clinical	Laboratory		Clinical	Laboratory
Mucopolysaccharidosis I (Hurler)	Corneal opacities Gargoyle facies Dysostosis multiplex	Urine: ↑ dermatan sulfate ↑ heparan sulfate	Serum infusion	Skin changes	Urine: ↑ mucopolysaccharide (breakdown fractions)
Fabry's disease	Corneal verticillata Shooting pains of extremities Angiokeratoma Heart disease Nephropathy	Leukocyte: ↓ α-galactosidase Serum: ↑ ceramide trihexoside	Plasma infusion	None	Serum: ↓ ceramide trihexoside
Familial lecitin-cholesterol acyltransferase (LCAT) deficiency	Corneal infiltration and arcus Anemia	Serum: ↓ LCAT ↓ cholesterol esters ↑ free cholesterol RBC: target cells No pre-β-lipoprotein (VLDL) No α_1-lipoprotein (HDL)	Serum infusion, 8 times in 20 days	None	↑ Cholesterol esters ↓ Free cholesterol

↑ = elevated; ↓ = reduced; RBC = red blood cells;
VLDL = very-low-density lipoprotein; HDL = high-density lipoprotein.

tried, resulting in partial reversal of chemical signs: decreased homocystine accumulation in plasma and decreased homocystinuria [18]. The biochemical mechanism of vitamin B_6 action in homocystinuric patients has not been clarified, and only some homocystinuric patients respond to vitamin B_6 therapy.

PYRIDOXINE THERAPY FOR GYRATE ATROPHY
OF RETINA

Two therapeutic approaches have been attempted to stall the progressive retinal and choroidal atrophy in gyrate atrophy of retina (GA): pyridoxine administration and dietary therapy. Approximately 30 to 40 percent of GA patients with ornithine transaminase (OT) deficiency retain a pyridoxine-responsive mechanism that either via messenger RNA or direct enzyme protein stimulation induces OT in vivo or in vitro (fibroblast cultures). The result is a significant increase in ornithine excretion in urine and reduction of plasma ornithine levels. Therapy with 500 mg pyridoxine is required to improve GA patients biochemically, but whether diminished progression of retinal atrophy occurs is doubtful. The two significant series of patients are those of Weleber and associates [24] and Berson and co-workers [2]. Evaluation of other signs such as b wave amplitude on electroretinogram (ERG) indicates some temporary improvement after initiation of pyridoxine therapy. However, long-term results are not available.

For those patients unresponsive to pyridoxine, dietary attempts have been made to reduce ornithine plasma levels with low-arginine diets. Arginine is an ornithine precursor. Preliminary results appear hopeful, but here again whether retinal atrophy ceases to progress remains in doubt. Kaiser-Kupfer and co-workers treated 18 patients with low-arginine diets [16]. The diet is not very palatable, and thus compliance was poor. This therapeutic approach assumes ornithine is the pathogenic agent causing retinal and choroidal atrophy, which has not been demonstrated in experimental models. Furthermore, A. B. Rao, in our laboratories, has recently postulated that failure to metabolize keto acids may initiate or contribute to retinal destruction.

VITAMIN A THERAPY FOR RETINITIS PIGMENTOSA
IN ABETALIPOPROTEINEMIA

Two brothers with steatorrhea, acanthocytosis, abetalipoproteinemia, flat ERG, and decreased serum levels of vitamin A, carotene, Vitamin E, total lipids, total cholesterol, triglycerides, and phospholipid were treated with monthly injections of vitamin A (100,000 units/month for 2 months and 150,000 units the third month—see Table 20-2) [4]. ERGs recorded before vitamin A administration and 48 and 72 hours after each dose of vitamin A revealed no improvement in one sibling and formation of definite a and b waves in the other. In 2 other abetalipoproteinemia patients, Gouras and colleagues found improved dark adaptation threshold and increased ERG voltages when the serum levels of vitamin A were increased by oral supplement of vitamin A, 200,000 units two to four times monthly [13]. High levels of oral vitamin A given over a period of 3 years, however, failed to prevent the development of retinal degeneration in a 6-year-old patient [23].

**PREVENTION OF INBORN ERRORS
OF METABOLISM**

A family with one or more offspring with a serious or fatal IEM may suffer irreparable damage to finances and morale. In serious or fatal IEM, parents and affected children must endure tremendous emotional and physical ordeals, including frequent medical examinations and hospitalizations. These families fight the ever-present guilt of the two heterozygous carriers. The relatives and offspring must receive counseling on the genetic risks involved for future generations [7]. Medical care for a child affected by a serious or fatal IEM can drain the financial resources of a family and even mortgage their future. When medical care is fully provided at state institutions or state medical centers the cost to society of a child hospitalized with an IEM runs, after several years, into millions of dollars. Thus the efforts to prevent such births have been a target of genetic researchers, public health officials, and affected families for many years.

The prevention of IEM has become a reality through the techniques of aminocentesis, culture of amniotic fluid cells, and precise biochemical detection of disease in the homozygous fetus [3, 17]. Amniocentesis is applicable mainly in pregnancies of heterozygous parents (high-risk pregnancies). Basically, amniotic fluid containing amniotic cells is obtained by transabdominal amniocentesis between the fourteenth and twentieth week of pregnancy. Amniotic cells are separated from the fluid by centrifugation, and enzyme determinations are performed in the cells and the fluid. These assays in noncultured cells represent a rapid, economical, and simple screening technique. However, false-negative values are occasionally obtained, and tissue culture of the amniotic cells followed by enzyme determinations must back up studies in noncultured material. If an enzyme deficiency is found in the fetus, the parents must be properly advised, and if they desire, a therapeutic abortion can be performed.

The identification of affected homozygotes and separation from heterozygotes before birth appear to be marvelous technological advancements, and the benefits for the involved families are obvious. However, there are dangers for society at large. Before the application of amniocentesis diagnostic techniques, potential parents were willing to limit the size of their families to prevent birth of affected homozygotes. The result was a decreased number of heterozygous carriers as well. Now that amniocentesis diagnosis is available, a larger number of heterozygous carriers of autosomal recessive disorders are born and thus possibly increase the incidence of genetic disease in the population [12].

It is obvious that many obligate heterozygotes with one or more affected offspring willingly accept amniocentesis in all pregnancies. However, efforts are currently being made to identify heterozygous carriers before the first pregnancy. Thus certain requirements for heterozygote (carrier) identification and counseling have emerged:

1. Precise biochemical diagnostic tests are needed to separate accurately individuals with "low-normal" levels of an enzyme and individuals who are carriers for the gene and carry intermediate levels of the enzyme.
2. Genetic counseling by trained geneticists is required.
3. Planning and organization of genetic stations at the public health service level are also necessary.
4. Community education (of physicians, religious and civic leaders, and the public) must be expanded.
5. Ethical problems of genetic planning must be scrutinized with great care and insight.

GENETIC ENGINEERING

Genetic engineering techniques may be applicable to correct some IEM affecting the eye. Most such techniques involve the generation of enzymes by artificial bacterial systems or insertion of genetic material into cells in culture. Such proteins or cells could be transplanted to mammalian species or humans to correct localized tissue defects. Affected eye tissues in IEM could theoretically be treated, as they are accessible to external manipulations or depot preparations.

REFERENCES

1. Becker, B., and Shaffer, R. N. *Diagnosis and Therapy of the Glaucomas.* St. Louis: Mosby, 1961.
2. Berson, E. L., et al. A two-year trial of low protein, low arginine diets or vitamin B_6 for patients with gyrate atrophy. *Birth Defects* 18(6):209, 1982.
3. Brady, R. O., Johnson, W. G., and Uhlendori, B. W. Identification of heterozygous carriers of lipid storage disease: Current status and clinical applications. *Am. J. Med.* 51:423, 1971.
4. Carr, R. E. Abetalipoproteinemia and the eye. *Birth Defects* 12(3):385, 1976.
5. Cotlier, E. Tay-Sachs retina: Deficiency of acetyl hexosaminidase A. *Arch. Ophthalmol.* 86:352, 1971.
6. Danks, D. M. Hereditary Disorders of Copper Metabolism in Wilson's Disease and Menkes' Disease. In J. B. Stanbury et al. (Eds.), *The Metabolic Basis of Inherited Disease* (5th ed.). New York: McGraw-Hill, 1983.
7. Desnick, R. J., and Grabowski, G. A. Advances in the treatment of inherited metabolic disease. *Adv. Hum. Genet.* 11:281, 1981.
8. Donnell, G. N., Koeh, R., and Bergren, W. R. Observations on Results of Management of Galactosemic Patients. In D. Y.-Y. Hsia (Ed.), *Galactosemia.* Springfield, Ill.: Thomas, 1960.
9. Glomet, J. A., Norum, K. R. and Gjone, E. Familial Lecithin: Cholesterol Acyl Transferase Deficiency. In J. B. Stanbury et al. (Eds.), *The Metabolic Basis of Inherited Disease* (5th ed.) New York: McGraw-Hill, 1983.
10. Goldberg, M. F. The treatment of proliferative sickle retinopathy. *Trans. Am. Acad. Ophthalmol. Otolaryngol.* 75:532, 1971.
11. Gollance, R. B., and D'Amico, R. A. Atypical mucopolysaccharidosis and successful keratoplasty. *Am. J. Ophthalmol* 64:707, 1967.
12. Gordon, H. Genetic counseling: Considerations for talking to parents and prospective parents. *JAMA* 217:1215, 1971.
13. Gouras, P., Carr, R. E., and Gunkel, R. D. Retinitis pigmentosa in abetalipoproteinemia: Effects of vitamin A. *Invest. Ophthalmol.* 10:784, 1971.
14. Harris, M. (Ed.). *Early Diagnosis of Human Genetic Defects: Scientific and Ethical Considerations.* Fogarty International Center Proceedings No. 6., W.E.W. Publ. No. (NIH) 72-75. Washington: U.S. Government Printing Office, 1971.
15. Hughes, W. F. Corneal transplant for therapy of primary corneal dystrophies. *Birth Defects* 12(3):155, 1976.
16. Kaiser-Kupfer, M. I., et al. Visual results of a long-

term trial of a low-arginine diet in gyrate atrophy of choroid and retina. *Ophthalmology (Rochester)* 88:307, 1981.

17. Milunsky, A., et al. Prenatal genetic diagnosis. *N. Engl. J. Med.* 283:1370, 1970.

18. Mudd, H. S., and Levy, H. L. Disorders of Transulfuration. In J. B. Stanbury et al. (Eds.), *The Metabolic Basis of Inherited Disease* (5th ed.) New York: McGraw-Hill, 1983.

19. Neufeld, E. F., and Cantz, M. J. Corrective factors for inborn errors of mucopolysaccharide metabolism. *Ann. N.Y. Acad. Sci.* 179:580, 1971.

20. O'Brien, J. S. Ganglioside storage disease. *Annu. Rev. Hum. Genet.* 3:1972.

21. Smith, R. S., and Reinecke, R. D. Electron microscopy of ocular muscle in type II glycogenosis (Pompe's disease). *Am. J. Ophthalmol.* 73:965, 1972.

22. Spaeth, G. L., and Barber, G. W. Homocystinuria in a mentally retarded child and her normal cousin.

Trans. Am. Acad. Ophthalmol. Otolaryngol. 69:912, 1965.

23. Sperling, M. A., Hiles, D. A., and Kennerdell, J. S. Electroretinographic responses following vitamin A therapy in abetalipoproteinemia. *Am. J. Ophthalmol.* 73:342, 1972.

24. Weleber, R. G., Wirta, M. K., and Kennaway, N. G. Gyrate atrophy of the choroid and retina: Clinical and biochemical heterogeneity and responses to vitamin B_6. *Birth Defects* 18(6):219, 1982.

25. Wilson, W. A., Donnel, G. M., and Bergren: The dietary prophylaxis of cataracts in patients with galactosemia. *Birth Defects* 12(3):313, 1976.

26. Wood-Smith, D. Surgical Treatment of the Eyelid Defect in the Treacher Collins Syndrome: A Preliminary Report. In B. Smith and J. M. Converse (Eds.), *Proceedings of the 2nd International Symposium on Plastic and Reconstructive Surgery of the Eye and Adnexa.* St. Louis: Mosby, 1967.

Index

Index